TOXICO-TERRORISM
Emergency Response and Clinical Approach to Chemical, Biological, and Radiological Agents

NOTICE

TOXICO-TERRORISM
Emergency Response and Clinical Approach to Chemical, Biological, and Radiological Agents

Robin B. McFee, DO, MPH, FACPM

Assistant Professor, Department of Preventive Medicine
SUNY/Stony Brook
Assistant Professor, Department of Medicine
NYCOM, New York Institute of Technology
Toxicologist, Long Island Regional Poison Information Center
Winthrop University Hospital
Mineola, New York
Medical Director, Threat Science™

Jerrold B. Leikin, MD, FABMT, FACEP, FACMT, FAACT, FACOEM

Director of Medical Toxicology
Evanston Northwestern Healthcare—OMEGA
Glenbrook Hospital
Glenview, Illinois
Professor of Emergency Medicine
Feinberg School of Medicine
Northwestern University
Professor of Medicine, Pharmacology, and Health Systems Management
Rush Medical College
Chicago, Illinois

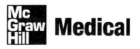

NEW YORK / CHICAGO / SAN FRANCISCO / LISBON / LONDON
MADRID / MEXICO CITY / MILAN / NEW DELHI / SAN JUAN
SEOUL / SINGAPORE / SYDNEY / TORONTO

Toxico-Terrorism: Emergency Response and Clinical Approach to Chemical, Biological, and Radiological Agents

ISBN: 978-0-07-147186-2
MHID: 0-07-147186-3

1 2 3 4 5 6 7 8 9 0   QPD/QPD   0 9 8 7

This book was set in Times Roman by International Typesetting and Composition Inc.
The editors were James Shanahan and Kim J. Davis.
The production supervisor was Catherine Saggese.
The index was prepared by Kathi Unger.
Quebecor Dubuque was printer and binder.

This book is printed on acid-free paper.

Library of Congress Cataloging-in-Publication Data

Toxico-terrorism : emergency response and clinical approach to
chemical, biological, and radiological agents / [edited by] Robin B.
McFee, Jerrold B. Leikin.
    p. ; cm.
Includes bibliographical references and index.
ISBN-13: 978-0-07-147186-2 (pbk. : alk. paper)
ISBN-10: 0-07-147186-3 (pbk. : alk. paper)
1. Bioterrorism—Prevention. 2. Emergency medical services. 3. Emergency management.
I. McFee, Robin B. II. Leikin, Jerrold B.
[DNLM: 1. Bioterrorism—prevention & control. 2. Disaster Planning.
3. Emergency Medical Services. WA 295 T755   2007]

RC88.9.T47T695   2007
363.325′3—dc22
                                        2007005124

With gratitude, love and in memory of Cinderella and Mac McFee—devoted, loving parents, insightful mentors, and my best friends.

Robin B. McFee

To Robin Ellen, Scott Michael, Eryn Nicole and D. J.
For their inspiration and support in the preparation of this book.

Jerrold B. Leikin

CONTENTS

CONTRIBUTORS

BRITNEY B. ANDERSON, MD
Chief Resident
Department of Emergency Medicine
Northwestern University
Division of Emergency Medicine
Northwestern Memorial Hospital
Chicago, Illinois

STEVEN E. AKS, DO, FACMT, FACEP
Associate Professor
Rush University
Director
The Toxikon Consortium
Section of Toxicology
Department of Emergency Medicine
Cook County (Stroger) Hospital
Chicago, Illinois

BRIAN L. BARDSLEY, JR, EMT-P, CCEMT-P
Police Officer
Chicago Police Department
Lieutenant, Stone Park Fire Department
Sergeant, Combat Medic, A Co 1-178th Infantry, ILANG
Chicago, Illinois

CHRISTINA HANTSCH BARDSLEY, MD, FACEP, FACMT
Associate Professor
Division of Emergency Medicine
Loyola University Chicago
Chicago, Illinois
Attending Physician, Emergency Medicine
  and Medical Toxicology
Loyola University Medical Center
Maywood, Illinois

SAPTARSHI BANDYOPADHYAY, MD
McGaw Medical Center
Northwestern University
Chicago, Illinois
Resident Physician
Department of Internal Medicine
Evanston Northwestern Healthcare
Evanston, Illinois

JONATHAN BANKOFF, MD
Emergency Department
Cook County Hospital
Chicago, Illinois

KIMBERLY A. BARKER, PharmD, DABAT
Clinical Operations Coordinator
Tennessee Poison Center
Vanderbilt University Medical Center
Nashville, Tennessee

EDWARD N. BARTHELL, MD, MS
Associate Clinical Professor
Medical College of Wisconsin
Milwaukee, Wisconsin
Executive Vice President
Infinity Healthcare
Mequon, Wisconsin
Chief Medical Officer
EMSystem
Milwaukee, Wisconsin

LAURA K. BECHTEL, PhD
Associate Researcher
Division of Medical Toxicology
Department of Emergency Medicine
University of Virginia
Charlottesville, Virginia

SHASHI KIRAN BELLAM, MD
Assistant Professor of Medicine
Feinberg School of Medicine
Northwestern University
Attending Physician
Evanston Northwestern Healthcare
Department of Medicine
Division of Pulmonary and Critical Care
Evanston, Illinois

DAVID M. BENEDEK, MD
Associate Professor
Assistant Chair
Center for the Study of Traumatic Stress
Department of Psychiatry
Uniformed Services University School of Medicine
Bethesda, Maryland

NICOLAS BERGERON, MD, FRCPC
Clinical Assistant Professor
Department of Psychiatry
Université de Montréal
Chief of Consultation-Liaison Psychiatry Service
Department of Psychiatry
Centre Hospitalier de l'Université de Montréal, Montréal,
  Québec, Canada

EDWARD M. BOTTEI, MD, FCCP
Clinical Assistant Professor in Clinical and Administrative
   Pharmacy Division, College of Pharmacy
Department of Occupational and Environmental Health,
   College of Public Health
Carver College of Medicine
Department of Internal Medicine
Carver College of Medicine
Department of Pediatrics
University of Iowa
Iowa City, Iowa
Department of Internal Medicine
St. Luke's Regional Medical Center
Sioux City, Iowa
Department of Internal Medicine
Mercy Medical Center
Sioux City, Iowa

RHONDA M. BRAND, PhD
Associate Professor
Department of Internal Medicine
Evanston Northwestern Healthcare and Feinberg School
   of Medicine at Northwestern University
Chicago, Illinois
Associate Professor
Division of Emergency Medicine and Department of Medicine
Evanston Northwestern Healthcare
Evanston, Illinois

SEAN M. BRYANT, MD
Assistant Professor of Emergency Medicine
Rush Medical College
Assistant Professor
Department of Emergency Medicine
Cook County-Stroger Hospital
Associate Medical Director
Illinois Poison Center
Chicago, Illinois

ANTHONY M. BURDA, BS PHARM
University of Illinois College of Pharmacy
Illinois Poison Center
Chicago, Illinois

RACHEL E. BURKE, MD
Attending Physician, Emergency Department
Rush University Medical Center
Chicago, Illinois

LARRY M. BUSH, MD
Clinical Associate Professor of Biomedical Science
Florida Atlantic University (FAU) Campus of the
   Miller School of Medicine-University of Miami
Boca Raton, Florida
Chief of the Division of Infectious Diseases
JFK Medical Center
Atlantis, Florida

ANDREA G. CARLSON, MD
Attending Physician in Emergency Medicine
Director of Medical Toxicology
Advocate Christ Medical Center
Oak Lawn, Illinois

CHRISTINA LYNNE CATLETT, MD, FACEP
Associate Director
The Johns Hopkins Office of Critical Event Preparedness
   and Response
Johns Hopkins University
Assistant Professor
Department of Emergency Medicine
The Johns Hopkins Hospital
Baltimore, Maryland

JOHN D. CHARETTE, MD
Department of Emergency Medicine
Madigan Army Medical Center
Tacoma, Washington

MANPREET S. CHHABRA, MD
Fellow
Department of Pediatric Ophthalmology
Cincinnati Children's Hospital Medical Center
Cincinnati, Ohio

DORAN M. CHRISTENSEN, DO
Volunteer Assistant Professor
College of Medicine
Department of Environmental Health
The University of Cincinnati
Cincinnati, Ohio
Associate Director and Staff Physician
Radiation Emergency Assistance Center/Training Site
   (REAC/TS)
Oak Ridge Institute for Science and Education (ORISE)—
   operated for the U.S. Department of Energy by Oak
   Ridge Associated Universities (ORAU)
Oak Ridge, Tennessee

ERIC COHEN, MD
Northwestern University
Chicago, Illinois
Evanston Northwestern Healthcare
Evanston, Illinois

KIRK L. CUMPSTON, DO, FACEP
Assistant Professor
Department of Emergency Medicine
Assistant Medical Director of the Virginia Poison Center
Medical College of Virginia Hospital
Virginia Commonwealth University Health Science Center
Richmond, Virginia

JORGE DEL CASTILLO, MD, MBA, FACEP
Associate Head
Division of Emergency Medicine
Evanston Northwestern Healthcare
Associate Professor Emergency Medicine
Northwestern University Medical School
Wilmette, Illinois

CAROL A. DESLAURIERS, PHARMD
Illinois Poison Center
Chicago, Illinois

KERSTIN DOSTAL, MD
Department of Emergency Medicine
Northwestern Memorial Hospital
Chicago, Illinois

AMY L. DRENDEL, DO, MS
Assistant Professor of Pediatrics
Pediatric Emergency Medicine
Children's Hospital of Wisconsin
Medical College of Wisconsin
Milwaukee, Wisconsin

ERIC ELTON, MD
Assistant Professor of Medicine
Northwestern University Feinberg School of Medicine
Chicago, Illinois
Director of Therapeutic Endoscopy
Evanston Northwestern Healthcare
Evanston, Illinois

TIMOTHY B. ERICKSON, MD, FACEP, FAACT, FACMT
Professor
Department of Emergency Medicine and Division of
    Clinical Toxicology
University of Illinois
Chicago, Illinois

CRAIG FEIED, MD
Director
National Institute for Medical Informatics
Washington, DC

A. SEATON GARRETT, MD, FACOEM
Radiation Emergency Assistance Center/Training Site (REAC/TS)
Oak Ridge Institute for Science & Education (ORISE)—
    operated for the U.S. Department of Energy by
    Oak Ridge Associated Universities (ORAU)
Former Medical Director
Oak Ridge National Laboratory (ORNL)
U.S. Department of Energy
Oak Ridge, Tennessee

MICHAEL GILLAM, MD
Research Director
National Institute for Medical Informatics
Washington, DC
Informatics Director
Division of Emergency Medicine
Evanston Northwestern Healthcare
Evanston, Illinois

MELISSA L. GIVENS MD, MPH
Staff Physician and Toxicologist
Madigan Army Medical Center
Tacoma, Washington

RACHEL GOLDSTEIN, DO, MSC
Department of Emergency Medicine
Holy Cross Hospital
Chicago, Illinois

DAVID D. GUMMIN, MD
Wisconsin Poison Center
Milwaukee, Wisconsin

PINCHAS (PINNY) HALPERN, MD
Senior Lecturer in Anesthesiology
Intensive Care and Emergency Medicine
Tel Aviv University
Sackler Faculty of Medicine
Chair
Department of Emergency Medicine
Tel Aviv Sourasky Medical Center
Tel Aviv, Israel

JONATHAN HANDLER, MD
Director of Development
National Institute for Medical Informatics
Washington, DC

DEBORAH A. HASSMAN, APN-CNP
Department of Emergency Medicine
Evanston Northwestern Healthcare
Evanston, Illinois

CHRISTIAN A. HERRERA, MD
Feinberg School of Medicine
Department of Emergency Medicine
Northwestern University
Chicago, Illinois

CHRISTOPHER P. HOLSTEGE, MD
Director
Division of Medical Toxicology
Associate Professor
Departments of Emergency Medicine and Pediatrics
University of Virginia
Medical Director
Blue Ridge Poison Center
University of Virginia Health System
Charlottesville, Virginia

STEPHEN HURWITZ, MD
Assistant Professor of Psychiatry
Northwestern University Feinberg School of Medicine
Chicago, Illinois
Director of Consultation-Liaison Psychiatry
Glenbrook and Highland Park Hospitals
Evanston Northwestern Healthcare
Evanston, Illinois

MAIRAJ JALEEL, MD
Evanston Northwestern Healthcare
Evanston, Illinois

OTIS W. JONES, MD, MPH
Radiation Emergency Assistance Center/Training Site (REAC/TS)
Oak Ridge, Tennessee

EJAAZ A. KALIMULLAH, MD
Chief Resident
Department of Emergency Medicine
Advocate Christ Medical Center
Oak Lawn, Illinois

RASHMI KAPUR, MD
Resident
Department of Ophthalmology
University of Illinois at Chicago
Chicago, Illinois

KENT KIRK, MD
Resurrection Hospital
Department of Surgery
Oak Park, Illinois

JERROLD B. LEIKIN, MD, FABMT, FACEP, FACMT, FAACT, FACOEM
Director of Medical Toxicology
Evanston Northwestern Healthcare—OMEGA
Glenbrook Hospital
Glenview, Illinois
Professor of Emergency Medicine
Feinberg School of Medicine
Northwestern University
Professor of Medicine, Pharmacology, and Health Systems
    Management
Rush Medical College
Chicago, Illinois

STEVEN D. LEVIN, MD
Assistant Professor of Orthopaedic Surgery
Feinberg School of Medicine
Northwestern University
Chicago, Illinois
Department of Orthopaedic Surgery
Evanston Northwestern Healthcare
Evanston, Illinois

SCOTT LILLIBRIDGE, MD
Professor of Epidemiology
Director
Center for Biosecurity and Public Health Preparedness
School of Public Health
University of Texas
Houston, Texas

J. MARC LIU, MD
Instructor
Department of Emergency Medicine
Medical College of Wisconsin
Assistant Director of Medical Services
Milwaukee County EMS
NAEMSP-Zoll EMS Resuscitation Fellow
Milwaukee, Wisconsin

JENNY J. LU, MD, MS
Clinical Instructor and Attending Physician
Department of Emergency Medicine
University of Illinois
Fellow
Medical Toxicology
Toxikon Consortium
Chicago, Illinois

NIRAJ MAHAJAN, MD
Fellow
Pulmonary and Critical Care
Department of Pulmonary and Critical Care
Rush University Medical Center
Chicago, Illinois

GERALD E. MALONEY, JR., DO
Senior Instructor in Emergency Medicine
Case Western Reserve University
Attending Physician
Emergency Medicine and Medical Toxicology
Department of Emergency Medicine
MetroHealth Medical Center
Cleveland, Ohio

KATHERINE A. MARTENS, MD
Loyola University Medical Center
Maywood, Illinois

ROBIN B. MCFEE, DO, MPH, FACPM
Assistant Professor
Department of Preventive Medicine
SUNY/Stony Brook
Assistant Professor
Department of Medicine
NYCOM, New York Institute of Technology
Consultant
Long Island Regional Poison Information Center
Winthrop University Hospital
Mineola, New York
Medical Director
Threat Science™

MARK B. MYCYK, MD
Assistant Professor
Department of Emergency Medicine
Northwestern University School of Medicine
Attending Physician
Department of Emergency Medicine
Northwestern Memorial Hospital
Attending Physician
Section of Toxicology
Cook County Hospital
Chicago, Illinois

RANDALL MYERS, MD
Division of Emergency Medicine
Northwestern Memorial Hospital
Chicago, Illinois

MARIA T. PEREZ, MD
Clinical Assistant Professor of Biomedical Science
Florida Atlantic University (FAU) Campus of the
    Miller School of Medicine-University of Miami
Boca Raton, Florida
Staff Pathologist
Division of Pathology and Laboratory Medicine
JFK Medical Center
Atlantis, Florida

SUSAN J. PIAZZA, MD
Evanston Northwestern Healthcare
Evanston, Illinois

MARY POWERS, RN, BSN, MS
Managing Director
Wisconsin Poison Center
Children's Hospital of Wisconsin
Milwaukee, Wisconsin

TRACEY H. REILLY, MD
Medical Toxicology Fellow
Department of Emergency Medicine
University of Virginia
Charlottesville, Virginia

MICHAEL REZAK, MD, PhD
Evanston Northwestern Healthcare
Evanston, Illinois

JAMES W. RHEE, MD
Assistant Professor of Medicine
Section of Emergency Medicine
University of Chicago
Attending Physician
Emergency Department
University of Chicago Medical Center
Chicago, Illinois

DANIEL R. RODGERS, MD
Assistant Professor of Emergency Medicine
Feinberg School of Medicine
Northwestern University
Northwestern Memorial Hospital
Department of Emergency Medicine
Chicago, Illinois

ROBERT ROSECRANS, PhD
Assistant Professor of Pathology
Feinberg School of Medicine
Northwestern University
Chicago, Illinois
Clinical Director of Laboratories
Glenbrook & Highland Park Hospitals
Evanston Northwestern Healthcare
Department of Pathology and Laboratory Medicine
Evanston, Illinois

BIJAN SAEEDI, MS
Manager, Lab Services
Head Chemist
SET Environmental, Inc.
Wheeling, Illinois

NIRAV A. SHAH, MD
Northwestern University
Chicago, Illinois

DANIEL H. SHEVRIN, MD
Associate Professor of Medicine
Feinberg School of Medicine
Northwestern University
Chicago, Illinois
Senior Attending Physician
Division of Hematology/Oncology
Evanston Northwestern Healthcare
Evanston, Illinois

TODD SIGG, PharmD
Illinois Poison Center
Chicago, Illinois

MARK SMITH, MD
Chair
Department of Emergency Medicine
MedStar Healthcare
Washington, DC

ERNEST STREMSKI MD, MBA
Associate Professor of Pediatrics
Medical College of Wisconsin
Milwaukee, Wisconsin

STEPHEN L. SUGARMAN, MS
Health Physics Project Manager
Radiation Emergency Assistance Center/Training Site (REAC/TS)
Oak Ridge Institute for Science and Education (ORISE)—
    operated for the U.S. Department of Energy by
    Oak Ridge Associated Universities (ORAU)
Oak Ridge, Tennessee

CHAD TAMELING, BS (ENVIRONMENTAL SCIENCE)
SET Environmental, Inc.
Wheeling, Illinois

BRIGHAM TEMPLE, MD
Instructor
Department of Emergency Medicine
Feinberg School of Medicine
Northwestern University
Chicago, Illinois
Chair of the Emergency Preparedness Committee
Division of Emergency Medicine
Evanston Northwestern Healthcare
Evanston, Illinois

RICHARD G. THOMAS, PharmD
Adjunct Clinical Instructor
Pharmacy Practice
Midwestern College of Pharmacy
Glendale, Arizona
Clinical Instructor
Pharmacy Practice
College of Pharmacy
University of Arizona
Tucson, Arizona
Phoenix Children's Hospital
Emergency Management Coordinator
Phoenix, Arizona

TREVONNE M. THOMPSON, MD
Assistant Professor of Medicine
Department of Emergency Medicine
University of Chicago
Attending Physician
Department of Emergency Medicine
University of Chicago Medical Center
Chicago, Illinois

RICHARD T. TOVAR, MD, FACEP
Medical College of Wisconsin
Delafield, Wisconsin

MICHAEL S. WAHL, MD
Managing Medical Director
Illinois Poison Center
Chicago, Illinois
Clinical Instructor
Department of Emergency Medicine
Feinberg School of Medicine
Northwestern University
Chicago, Illinois
Evanston Northwestern Healthcare
Division of Emergency Medicine
Evanston, Illinois

FRANK G. WALTER, MD, FACEP, FACMT, FAACT
Associate Professor of Emergency Medicine
Chief
Section of Medical Toxicology
Department of Emergency Medicine
University of Arizona College of Medicine
Director of Clinical Toxicology
University Medical Center
Tucson, Arizona

ERNEST E. WANG MD, FACEP
Assistant Professor
Division of Emergency Medicine
Feinberg School of Medicine
Northwestern University
Chicago, Illinois
Evanston Hospital
Evanston, Illinois

SUSAN SHOSHANA WEISBERG, MD, FAAP
Clinical Instructor
Department of Pediatrics
University of Illinois Medical Center
Chicago, Illinois
Attending Physician
Lutheran General Hospital
Park Ridge, Illinois

JACK WHITNEY, MD
Medical Director
Highland Park Hospital Emergency Medical Services System
Emergency Department
Highland Park Hospital
Highland Park, Illinois

ALBERT L. WILEY, JR., MD, PHD, FACR
Professor Emeritus
University of Wisconsin
Madison, Wisconsin
Director
Radiation Emergency Assistance Center/Training Site (REAC/TS)
Oak Ridge Institute for Science & Education (ORISE)—
    operated for the U.S. Department of Energy by
    Oak Ridge Associated Universities (ORAU)
Oak Ridge, Tennessee
Director
Radiation Medicine Collaborating Center
Radiation Emergency Medical Planning and Assistance
    Network (REMPAN)
World Health Organization (WHO)
Geneva, Switzerland

BRANDON K. WILLS, DO, MS
Clinical Assistant Professor
Division of Emergency Medicine
University of Washington
Staff Physician
Department of Emergency Medicine
Madigan Army Medical Center
Associate Medical Director
Washington Poison Center
Seattle, Washington

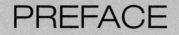

PREFACE

It was always difficult expressing the premise of the subject of this text to health professionals in a succinct manner. The terms "bioterrorism", "radiation incidents" and "chemical agent exposure" are frequently used and all imply a foreign substance invasion upon the human body from an environmental source (possibly intentional) that is limited to the properties of the specific substance. We thus came up with the term "Toxico-terrorism" to denote a comprehensive medical approach (from pre-hospital to public health organizations) of the intentional release, exposure, identification and management of chemical, biologic or radiological agents on a population. Realizing that the majority of terrorist events worldwide involve the use of explosives, we thought it was essential to provide an indepth discussion into preparing for and responding to this important threat. This text is divided into 8 sections ranging from organ system approach of the individual patient, to emergency medical system/emergency department preparation and public health considerations. Individual agents are discussed in detail in the appropriate section. Hopefully, this text will enable the reader to visualize a linear and comprehensive approach to this issue while keeping the focus on individual patient care. Since this field is always evolving, we welcome any feedback and look forward to continuing and expanding the discussion on the comprehensive approach to toxico-terrorism.

Robin B. McFee
Jerrold B. Leikin

ACKNOWLEDGMENTS

The creation of a textbook is a significant endeavor requiring the dedication and effort of so many people. The authors wish we could name everyone who made a contribution to *Toxico-terrorism*, but space restrictions preclude naming all the people to whom we are grateful. However, there are some individuals who warrant special mention: the team at McGraw-Hill, especially Jim Shanahan, Kim Davis, and Gita Raman for their insights and efforts. In the creation of this text, our goal has been to present the most practical, comprehensive and insightful book; toward that end we have selected as our contributors–the best of the best–with front line experience in WMD, HAZMAT and poison preparedness. We extend our gratitude to these wonderful professionals who generously shared their most precious resources–their talents and time.

Robin B. McFee
Jerrold B. Leikin

On a personal note, I want to convey deepest gratitude to my friend, colleague and co-author, Dr. Jerry Leikin with whom over the years I have enjoyed his friendship, professionalism, mentoring, and an exciting toxicological magical mystery tour in the land of WMD preparedness! Over the years I've been blessed with several amazing mentors in bioterrorism and toxicology–LtG (USA ret) Ron Blanck, DO, Dr. Howard Mofenson, Dr. Tom Caraccio, Dr. Ron Marino, and Dr. Jim Bernstein. Thank you to my "poison family" the Long Island Regional Poison Control Center team at Winthrop University Hospital of which I have been privileged to be part of for many years. My appreciation to Dr. Dorothy Lane of the Department of Preventive Medicine–SUNY/Stony Brook. Thank you to my friends, especially Judy Marcus Esq., Jeff Donaldson Esq., Sherry Reynolds RN, CSPI, Ken Korr MD, Dennis Maki MD, Dr. Tom McKibbens, Jay Connor, Beverly Travia, Archana Reddy, Bella Melikian, Betty Jane Martinelli, Sherry Aldi, Lynn Steeves, Dorothy Grosse and Janet Martin RN for their support and encouragement. Thank you to my colleagues at ASIS International, especially BG (USA ret) Jon Cofer, Dr. Kathleen Kiernan and fellow members of the Council on Global terrorism, Political Instability and International Crime. And last but not least, to the preparedness, security and intelligence professionals–government, military and private (some are friends) especially Howard Kaplan, Donald Sandel, Lt. Deena Disraelly, and David Quinn, whom I've worked with over the years and some who, in anonymity, work tirelessly on a daily basis putting their efforts *and* sometimes their lives on the line to protect our freedoms and our safety. We owe you much.

Robin B. McFee

This book would not be possible without the guidance and assistance from the clinical staff at Evanston Northwestern Healthcare. The dedicated clinicians from Evanston, Glenbrook, and Highland Park Hospitals were essential in contributing their expertise to this endeavor. Special thanks goes to the Emergency Department, Department of Medicine (especially Dr. Janardan Khandekar) and OMEGA Corporate Health at the above institutions. Lennie Espina and Julie Licata have been extremely helpful in manuscript preparation and coordination. I would also like to recognize the Illinois Poison Center, Wisconsin Poison Center and Toxicon Consortium for their invaluable assistance. Furthermore, it has been a true pleasure working with Dr. Robin McFee over the past three years on this and several other projects. She has been an inspiration to me because of her knowledge and enthusiasm on the subject of medical response to terrorism. Finally, I give my deepest appreciation to my family; my wife Robin, my children, Scott Michael and Eryn Nicole (and of course, D.J.) along with my parents, Evelyn and Mitchell and my father-in-law, Sam, for their tolerance and support of this seemingly never-ending project.

Jerrold B. Leikin

I

GENERAL PATIENT PRINCIPLES

INTRODUCTION

The approach to individuals exposed to an unknown agent varies whether a chemical, biological, radiological, or explosive substance is involved. Currently, evaluation of the medically ill individual is "hospitalcentric"—that is the entire evaluation process focused on one individual patient involves solely personal and equipment based at the hospital. With mass exposures, such "foreign" hospital procedures such as triage, field evaluation of nonbiological specimens, decontamination procedures all play a role in this process.

Individual patient care focuses on Toxidrome and Biodrome recognition as described in chapters 2 and 3. This section is then divided into an organ based systems approach to identifying and management of these issues. A focus on palliative care, special populations, and laboratory approach closes out this section.

1

TOXIDROME RECOGNITION

Ernest E. Wang and Timothy B. Erickson

S T A T   F A C T S

TOXIDROME RECOGNITION

- Many patients exposed to a biological, chemical, or radiological agent may display typical "toxidromes."
- Characteristic pattern of signs and symptoms relating to a toxin is known as a "toxidrome."
- Toxidrome recognition will aid the clinician in identifying a cohort of affected individuals.
- Most commonly described toxidromes include sympathomimetic, cholinergic (nerve agents), anticholinergic, and narcotic toxidromes.

INTRODUCTION

From a terrorist's standpoint, the ultimate success of an attack with a biological or chemical agent is the delayed or complete lack of recognition of the inciting agent and of the initially affected individuals. Ideal agents are colorless, odorless, tasteless, easily dispersed, and highly potent or contagious. The delay in recognition of the agent, particularly if it is a contagious agent, will allow for rapid transmission from person to person and prevent rapid quarantine of affected individuals. Moreover, a successful attack will instill fear in the general public and generate mass chaos.

Emergency health-care providers will most likely be the first to come into contact with these patients and have the greatest opportunity to alert the community and possibly prevent the spread of a potentially lethal agent. The Centers for Disease Control has a Web site entitled the *Emergency Preparedness and Response Web Site* that lists potential bioterrorism agents, their manifestations, and their management: *http://www.bt.cdc.gov/*

This chapter will focus on toxidrome recognition based on presenting symptoms and signs with an emphasis on the vital signs and physical examination.

TOXIDROMES

Certain classes of toxins will consistently present with a characteristic constellation of signs or symptoms (Table 1-1) called toxic syndromes, or toxidromes. Recognizing specific toxidromes will assist in detecting a cohort of affected individuals, as first responders often will not have the advantage of knowing the etiologic agent. A likely scenario would be a cohort of patients presenting with similar signs or symptoms that are out of character for the season or geographic location.

Classic Toxidromes

The most commonly described toxidromes include the sympathomimetic, cholinergic, anticholinergic, and narcotic toxidromes. Early recognition of these toxidromes may aid in the rapid diagnosis, management, and early quarantine of an outbreak.

Sympathomimetic Toxidrome

Sympathomimetic symptoms are usually caused by stimulants such as amphetamines, methylxanthines, cocaine, ephedrine, methylphenidate, nicotine, or phencyclidine. The toxidrome is characterized by a hyperadrenergic state and can include the following symptoms: tachycardia, hypertension, diaphoresis, restlessness, rapid or excessive speech, insomnia, hallucinations, tremor, excessive motor activity, euphoria, mydriasis, anorexia, paranoia, and seizures.

TABLE 1-1

TOXIC PHYSICAL FINDINGS

Miosis (COPS)			U	Uremia
C	Cholinergic agents, clonidine		D	DKA
O	Opiates, organophosphates		P	Paraldehyde, phenformin, phenol
P	Phenothiazines, pilocarpine		I	INH, iron, ibuprofen
S	Sedative hypnotics		L	Lactic acidosis
Mydriasis (SAW)			E	Ethylene glycol
S	Sympathomimetics (cocaine, amphetamines)		S	Salicylates, sepsis
A	Anticholinergics, atropine, antidepressants, amphetamines, antihistamines		**Elevated osmol gap (ME DIE)**	
			M	Methanol
W	Withdrawal (opiates, ETOH, benzodiazepines)		E	Ethylene glycol
Seizures (OTIS CAMPBELL)			D	Diuretics (mannitol), DKA (acetone)
O	Organophosphates		I	Isopropyl alcohol
T	Tricyclics, tetanus		E	Ethanol
I	INH, insulin		**Toxins requiring dialysis (STUMBLE)**	
S	Sympathomimetics, strychnine		S	Salicylates
C	Camphor, cocaine, cyanide, CO		T	Theophylline
A	Amphetamines		U	Uremia
M	Methylxanthines (theophylline, caffeine), monomethylhydrazine (gyromitrin mushrooms)		M	Methanol
			B	Barbiturates
P	PCP, phosgene		L	Lithium
B	β-Blockers, botanicals (water hemlock), bupropion (Wellbutrin), bioski (GHB)		E	Ethylene glycol
			Noncardiogenic pulmonary edema (MOPS)	
E	Ethanol withdrawal		M	Meprobamate, mustard agents
L	Lithium, lindane		O	Opioids, organophosphates
L	Lead, lidocaine		P	Phenobarbital, phosgene
Diaphoretic skin (SOAP)			S	Salicylates
S	Sympathomimetics		**Radiopaque toxins (CHIPS)**	
O	Organophosphates		C	Chloral hydrate, cocaine packets
A	ASA (salicylates)		H	Heavy metals (As, Hg, Pb)
P	PCP		I	Iron
Breath odors			P	Phenothiazines, packers
Bitter almonds	Cyanide		S	Sustained-release products (enteric coated)
Fruity	DKA, isopropanol		**Coma (LETHARGIC)**	
Oil of wintergreen	Methyl salicylates		L	Lead, lithium
			E	Ethanol, ethylene glycol
Rotten eggs	Sulfur dioxide, hydrogen sulfide		T	Trauma (drug-induced)
Pears	Chloral hydrate		H	Heroin (opioids), hypoglycemics, Haldol (neuroleptics), hypnotics (barbiturates, benzodiazepines)
Garlic	Arsenic, organophosphates, DMSO, nerve agents			
Mothballs	Camphor			
Freshly mowed hay	Phosgene		A	Alcohols, ASA, anticholinergics, arsenic
			R	Rodenticides
Metabolic acidosis with elevated anion gap (CATMUDPILES)			G	γ-Hydroxy Butyric Acid (GHB)
C	Carbon monoxide, cyanide		I	INH, insulin
A	Alcoholic ketoacidosis		C	CO, cyanide, cyclic antidepressants, cholinergic agents
T	Toluene, toxic seizures			
M	Methanol, metformin, massive amounts of any toxin			

Cholinergic Toxidrome

The cholinergic toxidrome is classically caused by nerve agents, organophosphates, and carbamate insecticides. It is characterized by salivation, lacrimation, urination, defecation, gastrointestinal (GI) distress, and emesis, which can be easily remembered with the mnemonic: SLUDGE. In addition, commonly noted signs include miotic pupils, diaphoresis, bronchorrhea, bradycardia, and bronchospasm (SLUDGEMDBBB). DUMBELS is another commonly used mnemonic to describe the symptoms: diarrhea, diaphoresis, urination, miosis/muscle fasciculations, bronchorrhea/brady-cardia/bronchospasm, emesis, lacrimation, and salivation.

Anticholinergic Toxidrome

This toxidrome can be recalled by the phrase, "Hot as a hare, red as a beet, dry as a bone, blind as a bat, and mad as a hatter." This mnemonic describes the manifestation of anticholinergic toxicity: hyperthermia, flushed skin, dry mouth, mydriasis, confusion, and delirium. The agents most commonly associated with this toxidrome include atropine, jimson weed, antihistamines, anti-Parkinson agents, and BZ.

The former military agent BZ (now used in pharmacology where it is known as QNB) is an anticholinergic compound that produces many effects similar to those of atropine such as mydriasis, drying of secretions, heart rate changes, and decreased intestinal motility. BZ, after an onset time of an hour or more, may produce confusion, disorientation, and disturbances in perception (delusions,

hallucinations) and expressive function (slurred speech). The antidote, physostigmine (Antilirium), reverses these effects for about an hour, and because the effects of BZ last for hours to days, repeated doses may be necessary.

Opioid Toxidrome

The opioid toxidrome is characterized by depressed mental status or coma, miosis, bradycardia, hypotension, and hypoventilation.

Infectious Toxidromes

Most of the biologic agents that have been used in the past present with a variety of symptoms. Patients will most likely present with delayed nonspecific flu-like symptoms. Depending on the organism, prominent symptoms include rash, cough, vomiting, diarrhea, and fever. Biologic agents that have been used in the past are listed alphabetically in Table 1-2.

TABLE 1-2

HISTORIC BIOLOGICAL AGENTS

A	P
• Anthrax (*Bacillus anthracis*)	• Plague (*Yersinia pestis*)
• Arenaviruses	• Psittacosis (*C. psittaci*)
B	**Q**
• *B. anthracis* (anthrax)	• Q fever (*C. burnetii*)
• Botulism (*Clostridium botulinum* toxin)	**R**
• *Brucella* species (brucellosis)	• Ricin toxin from *Ricinus communis* (castor beans)
• Brucellosis (*Brucella* species)	• *Rickettsia prowazekii* (typhus fever)
• *Burkholderia mallei* (glanders)	**S**
• *Burkholderia pseudomallei* (melioidosis)	• *Salmonella* species (salmonellosis)
C	• *Salmonella typhi* (typhoid fever)
• *Chlamydia psittaci* (psittacosis)	• Salmonellosis (*Salmonella* species)
• Cholera (*Vibrio cholerae*)	• *Shigella* (shigellosis)
• *C. botulinum* toxin (botulism)	• Shigellosis (*Shigella*)
• *Clostridium perfringens* (Epsilon toxin)	• Smallpox (variola major)
• *Coxiella burnetii* (Q fever)	• Staphylococcal enterotoxin B
E	**T**
• Ebola virus hemorrhagic fever	• Tularemia (*Francisella tularensis*)
• *Escherichia coli* O 157:H7 (*E. coli*)	• Typhoid fever (*Salmonella typhi*)
• Emerging infectious diseases such as Nipah virus and hantavirus	• Typhus fever (*R. prowazekii*)
• Epsilon toxin of *C. perfringens*	**V**
• *E. coli* O 157:H7 (*E. coli*)	• Variola major (smallpox)
F	• *V. cholerae* (cholera)
• Food safety threats (e.g., *Salmonella* species, *E. coli* O 157:H7, *Shigella*)	• Viral encephalitis (alphaviruses [e.g., Venezuelan equine encephalitis, eastern equine encephalitis, western equine encephalitis])
• *Francisella tularensis* (tularemia)	• Viral hemorrhagic fevers (filoviruses [e.g., Ebola, Marburg] and arenaviruses [e.g., Lassa, Machupo])
G	**W**
• Glanders (*B. mallei*)	• Water safety threats (e.g., *V. cholerae*, *Cryptosporidium parvum*)
L	**Y**
• Lassa fever	• *Y. pestis* (plague)
M	
• Marburg virus hemorrhagic fever	
• Melioidosis (*B. pseudomallei*)	

Source: http://www.bt.cdc.gov/agent/agentlist.asp

Chemical Toxidromes

Chemical agents that have known potential for use in a terrorist attack can be classified by their characteristic effects (Table 1-3). Biotoxins are primarily derived from plants or animals and include familiar agents such as ricin and strychnine. Blister agents (vesicants) and caustic agents are chemicals that primarily affect the eyes, mucous membranes of the respiratory tract, and skin. These agents include mustard gas in its various forms, phosgene, and hydrofluoric acid. Blood agents that primarily affect the body through absorption in the blood include cyanide in its various forms, sodium monofluoroacetate (compound 1080), and carbon monoxide. Nerve agents such as sarin and VX have received considerable attention in the press. Other classes include pulmonary agents, metals, and riot control agents/tear gas.

Other Toxidromes

Extrapyramidal
    Agents: Neuroleptics, haloperidol, phenothiazines
    Signs include choreoathetosis, trismus, opisthotonos, rigidity, tremor, and hyperreflexia
Hallucinogenic
    Agents: Cannabinoids, designer amphetamines, LSD (lysergic acid diethylamide), cocaine, phencyclidine, and indole alkaloids
    Signs include perceptual distortions, synesthesia, depersonalization, and derealization

PHYSICAL EXAMINATION

The physical examination should be performed with attention to the vital signs and characteristic physical findings correlative with a specific toxidrome. Many agents have characteristic effects on the temperature, pulse, respiratory rate, and blood pressure and can be recalled with the mnemonics listed in Table 1-4.

The practitioner should pay close attention to the mental status (depression/coma), pupillary size (miosis or mydriasis), skin examination (dry with anticholinergic poisoning or diaphoretic with organophosphate and sympathomimetic poisoning), and presence of seizure activity. The presence or absence of bowel sounds may also be useful in the setting of anticholinergic poisoning.

ACUTE RADIATION SYNDROME

Acute radiation syndrome (ARS) comprises several distinct toxidromes related to significant exposure to radiation. Each toxidrome has characteristic signs and symptoms that the clinician should be aware of when treating a patient who has been significantly exposed to radiation.

In order for exposed patients to become significantly exposed, five conditions must occur:

1. The radiation dose must be large (>0.7 Gy or 70 rads), although as little as 0.3 Gy or 30 rads can cause mild symptoms.
2. The source of the radiation must be externally applied (i.e., outside the patient's body).
3. The radiation dose must be high enough to penetrate the internal organs.
4. The entire body must be exposed.
5. The dose must be delivered in a short amount of time (within minutes).

The body's most sensitive cell lines—spermatocytes, lymphohematopoietic elements, and intestinal crypt cells—are the most affected by acute exposure to radiation. A predictable clinical course (Table 1-5) consisting of a *prodromal phase* (48 hours–6 days after exposure depending on severity), a *latent phase* (period of transient improvement for several days to a month), and finally the *manifest illness phase* (period of prolonged symptomatology from intense immunosuppression).

There are three well-described components of the *manifest illness* phase of ARS: bone marrow syndrome (or hematopoietic syndrome), gastrointestinal syndrome, cardiovascular (CV)/central nervous system (CNS) cerebrovascular syndrome, and cutaneous syndrome.

Symptoms are summarized in Table 1-6. The time course and severity of the development of these syndromes depends on the dose of radiation the victim is exposed to. (See Fig. 1-1.)

Bone marrow syndrome presents with anorexia, nausea, and vomiting beginning 1–2 hours after exposure. Subsequent to the exposure, patients will develop a hematologic crisis characterized by bone marrow aplasia resulting in pancytopenia. The patient is at significant risk for infection, bleeding, and poor wound healing, which ultimately may result in death. The highest predictor of mortality is the decline in absolute lymphocyte count. A 50% decline in absolute lymphocyte count within the first 24 hours of exposure, followed by a subsequent decline within the next 48 hours is potentially lethal.

Gastrointestinal syndrome is characterized by abdominal pain, nausea, vomiting, and watery diarrhea. Symptoms start within hours after high (>10 Gy) exposure, abate during the latent phases, which may last 5–7 days, then return again with the *manifest illness* phase. In addition to nausea, vomiting, and severe diarrhea, high fevers are common. Patients suffer and ultimately succumb to malnutrition and malabsorption, bowel obstruction from ileus, infection and sepsis, dehydration, cardiovascular collapse, electrolyte imbalance from fluid shifts, acute renal failure, anemia, and gastrointestinal hemorrhage. Survival is unlikely with this syndrome and death usually occurs within 2 weeks.

TABLE 1-3
POTENTIAL CHEMICAL AGENTS

Biotoxins

(Poisons that come from plants or animals)

- Abrin
- Brevetoxin (associated with red tides)
- Colchicine
- Digitalis
- Nicotine
- Ricin
- Saxitoxin
- Strychnine
- Tetrodotoxin
- Trichothecene

Blister agents/vesicants

(Chemicals that severely blister the eyes, respiratory tract, and skin on contact)

- Mustards
- Distilled mustard (HD)
- Mustard gas (H) (sulfur mustard)
- Mustard/lewisite (HL)
- Mustard/T
- Nitrogen mustard (HN-1, HN-2, HN-3)
- Sesqui mustard
- Sulfur mustard (H) (mustard gas)
- Lewisites/chloroarsine agents
- Lewisite (L, L-1, L-2, L-3)
- Mustard/lewisite (HL)
- Phosgene oxime (CX)

Blood agents

(Poisons that affect the body by being absorbed into the blood)

- Arsine gas (SA)
- Carbon monoxide
- Cyanide
- Cyanogen chloride (CK)
- Hydrogen cyanide (AC)
- Potassium cyanide (KCN)
- Sodium cyanide (NaCN)
- Sodium monofluoroacetate (compound 1080)

Caustics (acids)

(Chemicals that burn or corrode skin, eyes, and mucus membranes (lining of the nose, mouth, throat, and lungs) on contact)

- Hydrofluoric acid (hydrogen fluoride)

Choking/lung/pulmonary agents

[Chemicals that cause severe irritation or swelling of the respiratory tract (lining of the nose, throat, and lungs)]

- Ammonia
- Bromine (CA)
- Chlorine (CL)
- Hydrogen chloride
- Methyl bromide
- Methyl isocyanate
- Osmium tetroxide
- Phosgene
- Diphosgene (DP)
- Phosgene (CG)
- Phosphine
- Phosphorus, elemental, white or yellow
- Sulfuryl fluoride

Incapacitating agents

(Agents that cause confusion or cause an altered state of consciousness)

- BZ
- Fentanyls & other opioids

Long-acting anticoagulants

(Poisons that prevent blood from clotting properly, which can lead to uncontrolled bleeding)

- Super warfarin

Metals

(Agents that consist of metallic poisons)

- Arsenic
- Barium
- Mercury
- Thallium

Nerve agents

(Highly poisonous chemicals that work by preventing the nervous system from working properly)

- G agents
- Sarin (GB)
- Soman (GD)
- Tabun (GA)
- V agents
- VX

Organic solvents

(Agents that damage the tissues of living things by dissolving fats and oils)

- Benzene
- Toluene
- Xylene

Riot control agents/tear gas

[Highly irritating agents normally used by law enforcement for crowd control or by individuals for protection (for example, mace)]

- Bromobenzylcyanide (CA)
- Chloroacetophenone (CN)
- Chlorobenzylidenemalononitrile (CS)
- Chloropicrin (PS)
- Dibenzoxazepine (CR)

Toxic alcohols

(Poisonous alcohols that can damage the heart, kidneys, and nervous system)

- Ethylene glycol

Vomiting agents

(Chemicals that cause nausea and vomiting)

- Adamsite (DM)

TABLE 1-4
TOXIC VITAL SIGNS

Bradycardia (PACED)		Hypotension (CRASH)	
P	Propranolol (β-blockers), poppies (opioids)	C	Clonidine, carbon monoxide, cyanide, calcium channel blockers, cardioglycosides
A	Anticholinesterase drugs, organophosphates, nerve agents	R	Reserpine (antihypertensive agents), ricin
C	Clonidine, calcium channel blockers, cardioglycosides (Digitalis)	A	Antidepressants (tricyclic)
		S	Sedative hypnotics
E	Ethanol and alcohols	H	Heroin (opiates)
D	Digoxin, Darvon (opiates)	**Hypertension (CT SCAN)**	
Tachycardia (FAST)		C	Cocaine
F	Free base (cocaine), Freon (solvents)	T	Theophylline
A	Anticholinergics, antihistamines, amphetamines	S	Sympathomimetics
S	Sympathomimetics	C	Caffeine
T	Theophylline	A	Anticholinergics, amphetamines
Hypothermia (COOLS)		N	Nicotine
C	Carbon monoxide, cholinergics	**Tachypnea (PANTS)**	
O	Opiates	P	Phosgene, PCP
O	Oral hypoglycemics, insulin	A	Anticholinergics, asphyxiants
L	Liquor	N	Nerve agents
S	Sedative hypnotics	T	Toxin-induced acidosis
Hyperthermia (NASA)		S	Salicylates, solvents, sympathomimetics
N	Nicotine, neuroleptic malignant syndrome		
A	Antihistamines		
S	Salicylates, sympathomimetics		
A	Anticholinergics, antidepressants		

TABLE 1-5
PHASES OF RADIATION INJURY*

Dose Range, Gy	Prodrome	Manifestation of Illness	Prognosis (Without Therapy)
0.5–1	Mild	Slight decrease in blood cell counts	Almost certain survival
1–2	Mild to moderate	Early signs of bone marrow damage	Highly probable survival (>90% of victims)
2–3.5	Moderate	Moderate to severe bone marrow damage	Probable survival
3.5–5.5	Severe	Severe bone marrow damage; slight GI damage	Death within 3.5–6 weeks (50% of victims)
5.5–7.5	Severe	Pancytopenia and moderate GI damage	Death probable within 2–3 weeks
7.5–10	Severe	Marked GI and bone marrow damage, hypotension	Death probable within 1–2.5 weeks
10–20	Severe	Severe GI damage, pneumonitis, altered mental status, cognitive dysfunction	Death certain within 5–12 days
20–30	Severe	Cerebrovascular collapse, fever, shock	Death certain within 2–5 days

*Modified from Walker RI, Cerveny RJ, eds. (21). GI = gastrointestinal.

T A B L E 1 - 6
ACUTE RADIATION SYNDROMES

Syndrome	Dose*	Prodromal Stage	Latent Stage	Manifest Illness Stage	Recovery
Hematopoietic (Bone marrow)	>0.7 Gy (>70 rads) *(mild symptoms may occur as low as 0.3 Gy or 30 rads)*	• Symptoms are anorexia, nausea and vomiting. • Onset occurs 1 hour to 2 days after exposure. • Stage lasts for minutes to days.	• Stem cells in bone marrow are dying, although patient may appear and feel well. • Stage lasts 1–6 weeks.	• Symptoms are anorexia, fever, and malaise. • Drop in all blood cell counts occurs for several weeks. • Primary cause of death is infection and hemorrhage. • Survival decreases with increasing dose. • Most deaths occur within a few months after exposure.	• In most cases, bone marrow cells will begin to repopulate the marrow. • There should be full recovery for a large percentage of individuals from a few weeks up to two years after exposure. • Death may occur in some individuals at 1.2 Gy (120 rads). • The LD$_{50/60}$[†] is about 2.5–5 Gy (250–500 rads). • The LD$_{100}$[‡] is about 10 Gy (1000 rads).
Gastrointestinal (GI)	>10 Gy (>1000 rads) *(some symptoms may occur as low as 6 Gy or 600 rads)*	• Symptoms are anorexia, severe nausea, vomiting, cramps, and diarrhea. • Onset occurs within a few hours after exposure. • Stage lasts about 2 days.	• Stem cells in bone marrow and cells lining GI tract are dying, although patient may appear and feel well. • Stage lasts less than 1 week.	• Symptoms are malaise, anorexia, severe diarrhea, fever, dehydration, and electrolyte imbalance. • Death is due to infection, dehydration, and electrolyte imbalance. • Death occurs within 2 weeks of exposure.	
Cardiovascular (CV)/Central Nervous System (CNS)	>50 Gy (5000 rads) *(some symptoms may occur as low as 20 Gy or 2000 rads)*	• Symptoms are extreme nervousness and confusion; severe nausea, vomiting, and watery diarrhea; loss of consciousness; and burning sensations of the skin. • Onset occurs within minutes of exposure. • Stage lasts for minutes to hours.	• Patient may return to partial functionality. • Stage may last for hours but often is less.	• Symptoms are return of watery diarrhea, convulsions, and coma. • Onset occurs 5–6 hours after exposure. • Death occurs within 3 days of exposure.	• No recovery is expected.

* The absorbed doses quoted here are "gamma equivalent" values. Neutrons or protons generally produce the same effects as gamma, beta, or x-rays but at lower doses. If the patient has been exposed to neutrons or protons, consult radiation experts on how to interpret the dose.

† The LD$_{50/60}$ is the dose necessary to kill 50% of the exposed population in 60 days.

‡ The LD$_{100}$ is the dose necessary to kill 100% of the exposed population.

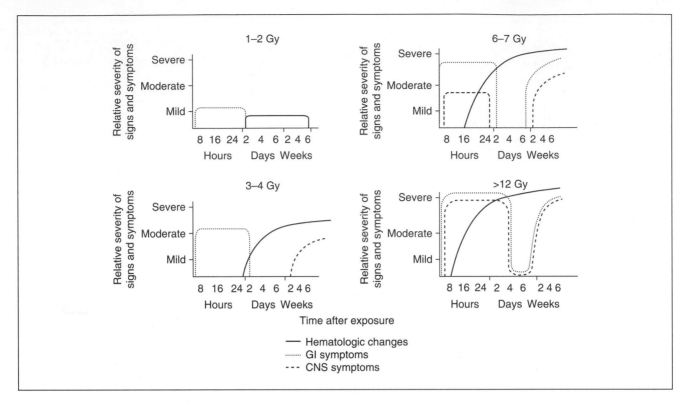

FIGURE 1-1

Approximate time course of clinical manifestations. Shown are approximate times for hematopoietic, gastrointestinal (GI), and central nervous system (CNS) symptoms at different ranges of whole-body radiation exposure. Hematopoietic changes include development of lymphopenia, granulocytopenia, or thrombocytopenia. GI symptoms include nausea, vomiting, or diarrhea. CNS symptoms include headache, impaired cognition, disorientation, ataxia, seizures, prostration, and hypotension. Note that the signs and symptoms of different organ systems significantly overlap at each radiation dose and that CNS symptoms do not appear until exposure to a high whole-body dose.
Source: From Waselenko JK, MacVittie TJ, Blakely WF, et al. Medical management of the acute radiation syndrome: recommendations of the Strategic National Stockpile Radiation Working Group. Ann Intern Med. 2004;140(12):1037–51.

Cerebrovascular syndrome is characterized by fever, hypotension, altered mental status and usually occurs with exposures between 20 and 50 Gy (2000–5000 rads). Onset of prodromal symptoms occurs within hours and is characterized by disorientation, confusion, prostration, loss of balance, and seizures. Physical examination is significant for papilledema, ataxia, absent or decreased tendon and corneal reflexes. The latent period lasts only for a few hours with rapid progression in 5–6 hours to manifest illness phase, which consists of sepsis-like symptoms: fever, watery diarrhea, respiratory distress, cardiovascular collapse, cerebral edema, and anoxia. Death occurs within 2–3 days secondary to circulatory collapse.

Cutaneous radiation injury (CRI) is another known manifestation of acute radiation exposure. Skin damage is manifested by transient itching, tingling, erythema, or edema. In severe exposures, penetration can be deep into the dermis and causes not only pain, but also tense edema,

blistering with hemorrhagic bullae, desquamation, and irreversible subcutaneous muscle ulceration and necrosis. Onset begins hours to days after exposure depending on the severity. This syndrome can occur independently of the other acute radiation syndromes.

CONCLUSION

Early recognition of a chemical or bioterrorism attack is essential for containment and treatment of affected individuals, before these contaminated individuals come in contact with the general public.

Working knowledge of the common toxidromes allows the practitioner to more readily recognize and classify presenting signs and symptoms into potential categories of toxic etiologic agents.

Suggested Reading

Acute Radiation Syndrome: A Fact Sheet for Physicians. 2005. (Accessed April 12, 2006, at *http://www.bt.cdc.gov/radiation/arsphysicianfactsheet.asp*)

Bioterrorism Agents/Diseases. 2006. (Accessed April 2006, at *http://www.bt.cdc.gov/agent/agentlist.asp*)

Chemical Agents. 2006. (Accessed April 2006, at *http://www.bt.cdc.gov/agent/agentlistchem.asp*)

Erickson TB, Thompson T.M., Lu, J.J.: The Approach to the Patient with an Unknown Overdose. *Emerg Med Clin N. Am* 2007:25:249–281.

Waselenko JK, MacVittie TJ, Blakely WF, et al. Medical management of the acute radiation syndrome: recommendations of the Strategic National Stockpile Radiation Working Group. *Ann Intern Med.* 2004;140(12):1037–51.

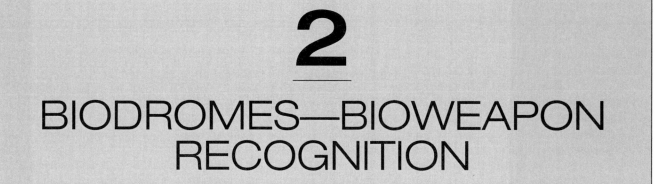

BIODROMES—BIOWEAPON RECOGNITION

Robin B. McFee

BIODROMES

Key to Biodromes

- Cascade of symptoms involving more than one organ system should alert the clinician to a potentially serious illness, especially with appropriate history.

Key Systems

Dermatological

Many bioweapons can have dermatologic manifestations. Examples from the CDC (Centers for Disease Control) Category A agents:

- *Plague*
  - Bubos (lymph nodes that become necrotic and quite visibly large). These enlarged lymph nodes are exquisitely painful.
  - Acral cyanosis—blackened, ischemic/necrotic appearance of digits/toes/nose and other areas
  - Pustular lesion(s)—at or distal to bite site if the result of flea exposure
- *Smallpox*—Rash is the hallmark diagnostic clue. Although there are generally four types of rash, the classic presentation is most common.
  - Common dermatologic presentation—lesions typically erupt on the face, hands, and feet and then work inward to the truck and appear on a given body region in the same development stage; as they progress, they will appear as pustules.
- *Tularemia*—Ulceroglandular lesion(s) is possible. Taken in context with vital signs and other clinical presentation, highly suggestive of illness. Nodules as well as lymphadenopathy possible.

- *Anthrax*—Classic black eschar associated with cutaneous anthrax. Usually accompanied by localized, often severe edema. Taken in context with history and clinical picture suggests diagnosis.
- *Viral hemorrhagic fevers (VHF)*—Hemorrhagic/capillary bed involvement suggested by ecchymosis, petechia (sometimes mildly firm to the touch) in skin, conjunctiva/eye lids, and easy bruisability. Rashes may accompany other skin manifestations and may be morbilliform in appearance.

Respiratory

- *Anthrax*
  - Inhalation anthrax causes severe pulmonary compromise including shortness of breath. (Table 2-1.)
  - Mediastinal widening on chest x-ray (CXR) is strongly suggestive.
- *Plague*
  - Pneumonic plague causes significant rapidly progressive respiratory symptoms. Multiple CXR findings possible.
- *Tularemia*
  - Symptoms are similar to severe pneumonia. CXR may show mediastinal lymphadenopathy or pneumonia. (See Table 2-2 also.)

Key Signs and Symptoms

- *Relative bradycardia or pulse-temperature dissociation— Fever is normally accompanied by an appropriate increase in heart rate. When the heart rate is unchanged or slows, that is, unexpectedly low in the presence of a fever, it is called relative bradycardia.* Few common illnesses present with fever that is unaccompanied by an increase in heart rate in the absence of cardiopulmonary illness or heart rate reducing medications. Fever, especially >102°F without tachycardia or elevated heart rate, is worrisome and warrants aggressive management. *Caveat:* The elderly may not be able to mount a febrile response to a virulent pathogen. The elderly may also have underlying cardiac disease or take heart rate suppression medication, which may confound the picture. *Consider severe respiratory illnesses/sepsis, especially in the context of relative bradycardia, rapidly progressive or fluctuating severe febrile illness, typhoid fever, tularemia, psittacosis, plague, viral hemorrhagic fevers, Q fever, malaria, Legionnaires' disease, rickettsia, Chlamydia pneumonia, intracellular gram-negative organisms.*

- *Rashes*—Infections preceded or accompanied by rashes warrant further investigation, especially involving high fevers >102°F. Rapidly progressive, synchronous rashes or pustules with a hemorrhagic appearance warrant investigation and possible respiratory precautions. Black, necrotic, or progressive lesions, especially accompanied by fever, warrant aggressive management and possible respiratory precautions. *Consider anthrax, plague, smallpox/poxviruses, rickettsia, psittacosis.*
- *Circumferential petechia*—After the blood pressure cuff is removed, often patients with hemorrhagic viral illnesses have petechia in the cuff location. The presence of bleeding stigmata in the presence of infection is worrisome. *Caveat:* The elderly often have easily bruised skin. Additionally many are on anticoagulants. Distinction— Such patients often have the petechia distal to the cuff compared to infectious etiologies. *Consider VHFs.*
- *Dyspnea—shortness of breath*—True shortness of breath rarely accompanies benign common respiratory illnesses. Any patient presenting with shortness of breath requires aggressive management. Respiratory precautions should be considered if underlying cardiac etiology without infection cannot be ruled out. *Consider inhalation anthrax, avian flu, pneumonic plague, tularemia, Legionella.*
- *Mental status changes*—Several bioweapons involve the central nervous system (CNS) and can cause behavioral changes, delirium or coma, including inhalation anthrax, brucellosis, and smallpox. *Caveat:* The elderly may be especially susceptible to the neuro effects of hypoxia associated with pneumonia or other infectious pulmonary illnesses, and may have altered mental status as a baseline. *Consider anthrax, brucellosis, smallpox.*

Preparedness

Train intake personnel/receptionists to identify worrisome symptoms and biodromes.

Waiting room prompts:

- Inquire about travel, key symptoms (high fever, cough, shortness of breath).
- Suggest respiratory hygiene and offer viral barrier tissues, wastebaskets, masks. (Should be available in waiting rooms and encourage use!)
- Tell the receptionist to alert you if
  - Patient has been in countries where illness of concern (today it's avian flu)
  - Patient and family members/colleagues/friends have similar illness

Important resources to be familiar with:

- Travel medicine expert
- Infectious disease expert
- Infection control team
- CDC—Office or Emergency Response
- State health department
- Laboratory response network (LRN) laboratory
- Local health department
  - Epidemiologist
  - Director

Equipment:

- Isolation
- Additional ventilators
- Negative pressure rooms—available: adaptable or permanent
- Personal protective equipment (PPE) including n95 masks *and* each team member is fit-tested and proficient in use
- PPE use protocols in place when to utilize
- Ability to isolate well from sick patients
- Respiratory hygiene products for waiting areas/patients
- CDC smallpox charts prominently displayed
- WHO avian flu charts prominently displayed

OVERVIEW

Bioweapon illness is not subtle! The pathogens are selected because they are highly virulent—causing death or significant morbidity. Do not try to make a serious illness look like a common one! If the patient comes in with a rapidly progressive febrile illness, especially with a rash, cardiac or pulmonary symptoms, consider this a significant illness. Obtain a careful history—circumstances of illness; timeline of symptoms; others with similar illness over a similar timeline; or sharing occupational, travel, or social activities.

Biodromes are like toxidromes. A toxidrome is a form of pattern recognition and represents symptoms that may appear to the uninitiated as unrelated but provides important clinical clues to either a class of specific toxin or toxicant when viewed collectively. An example of this is the toxidrome for anticholinergics. This class of medications can, in the toxic setting, result in multisystem

TABLE 2-1

INFLUENZA COMPARED TO SEASONAL FLUE AND INFLUENZA-LIKE ILLNESSES/UPPER RESPIRATORY INFECTIONS

Number of "+" Indicates Strength of Association	Inhalation Anthrax	Avian Flu (H5NI)	Seasonal Influenza (Flu)	Upper Respiratory Infection	Common Cold
Elevated temperature	+++	+++/++++	++	++	+/-
Fever/chills	++++	++++	++++	++++	
Cough	+++	+++	+++	+++	+++
Shortness of breath	++++	++++	+/-	+/-	-
Chest discomfort	+++	+++	++	++	+/-
Sore throat	+/-	+/-	+++	+++	++
Vomiting/nausea	+++	++	+	+	-
Diarrhea	++/+++	++	+(young children)	+/-	-
CNS/encephalopathy/seizures	++	++	-	-	-
Malaise/fatigue	+++	+++	+++	+	+/-
Runny nose/ watery eyes	+/-	+/-	+	++	+++
Headache/muscle ache	++	+++	+++	++	+/-
Young healthy at risk for serious illness	?	+++	+/-	+/-	-

*CNS = central nervous system

Source: From McFee RB, Bush L, Boehm K. Avian influenza: critical considerations for the primary care physician. JH Adv Studies Medicine. 2006;(6):10.

TABLE 2-2

CATEGORY "A" BIODROMES

Inhalation Anthrax
History of gastrointestinal symptoms 2–3 days precede respiratory worsening
Fever >101°F
Shortness of breath
Chest pain
Generalized malaise/fatigue
Laboratories—early relatively normal *but* may show hemoconcentration

Tularemia
Fever >101°F
Relative bradycardia
Ulceration, nodule, or other lesion possible
Respiratory complaints consistent with pneumonia

Plague
Fever
Constitutional symptoms (patients appear ill)
The 3 Hs: hematemesis, hemoptysis, hemorrhagic diarrhea
Pulmonary involvement
Early DIC

VHF
Fever >101°F

Evidence of capillary bed involvement including petechiae
Hypotension; may be severe and suggest hemorrhage/ circulatory collapse
Petechia at or distal to the cuff site possible, often circumferential
Relative bradycardia

Smallpox
Fever >101°F
Prostration
Rash dermal, firm with synchronous development starting on the head, hands, and feet then moving toward the trunk
Patients appear very ill
CNS involvement (delirium) possible

Botulinum
Bulbar nerve involvement bilateral
  Blurred vision
  Slurred speech
  Dysphagia
  Ptosis
Bilateral flaccid descending paralysis
Generalized weakness
Intact sensorium

CNS = central nervous system; DIC = disseminated intravascular coagulopathy; VHF = viral hemorrhagic fever involvement—each manifestation in isolation may not be specific but in the aggregate provides good support for the diagnosis. Often memorized with the mnemonic "red as a beet, mad as a hatter, hot as a hare, dry as a bone" simply suggests dermal, thermal, CNS, and fluid involvement. The same is true for the biodrome. An example of this would be the plague: high fever; the 3 Hs: hemoptysis, hematemesis, hemorrhagic diarrhea; and likely pulmonary involvement as well as signs of early disseminated intravascular coagulopathy (DIC).

Remember to take the entire clinical picture into consideration. For example, if the clinical presentation and suggested diagnosis seem unusual for the age of the patient or circumstances, this alone is rationale to further investigate. While most bioweapons or deadly emerging pathogens have a predilection for a specific organ system, such as the lungs for example, and that should be your first clue, nevertheless, these infectious agents often initiate more significant systemic or multiorgan illness than their natural counterparts—either by engineering or selection. An example of this is avian flu—the pulmonary involvement associated with H5N1 is dramatically more severe than seasonal influenza, and a cue to aggressive intervention!

Always obtain an *occupational* and *travel history* as well as inquire about similar illness among other members of family, circle of friends, coworkers, travelers encountered, workplaces, destinations, or countries visited.

BIODROMES—BIOWEAPON RECOGNITION

The emergency department (ED) is increasingly viewed as a frontline center for the early identification of potential outbreaks as well as resource for disease surveillance.

Given the close and often prolonged contact patients will have with ED staff, concerns arise that this setting is a potential source of infection propagation. Early diagnosis will be critical to containing emerging threats—intentionally released biological agents/bioweapons, as well as uncommon or relatively unknown pathogens.

Biological warfare—the use of microorganisms, pathogens for combat purposes—dates back to the Roman Empire and probably beforehand. Increasingly, terrorists have acquired several bioweapons such as *Bacillus anthracis* with intelligence sources indicating many other biologicals are of interest to and perhaps been purchased by a variety of terror organizations. The need therefore to detect biological agents that could be used in a bioterrorism attack is critical. Several are being developed to assist the clinician. Others are being developed for deployment in high-threat locations to protect strategically important facilities. In subsequent chapters, detection technology likely to aid the clinician will be discussed. Nevertheless, for the majority of clinical settings, the most likely early detection system we can at present rely upon is our clinical acumen and the ability to

diagnose the infected patient and identify the index patient early enough to initiate the response cascade. The importance of identifying the index patient cannot be understated. It is estimated that hundreds of lives were saved as a result of a community clinician rapidly recognizing the first intentional inhalation anthrax victim in 2001.

Diagnosing the cause of an illness, especially an infection or a poison, in an unconscious patient can be a daunting task. Identifying the poison involved from among a large array of potential toxicants can be a significant challenge to the clinician faced with an intoxicated patient. Without benefit of accurate information, basing the identification upon signs, symptoms, and tests can be difficult in isolation. The list of toxicants and pathophysiologic causes of hypotension alone is enormous! Narrowing the list of potential toxicants based upon isolated symptoms can take the clinician down many often contradictory paths. The concept of "toxidrome" thus emerged as a solution to this problem and became an invaluable tool to alert clinicians that the diagnosis of a poisoned patient and the identification of the offending agent often rests upon a cascade of clinical clues that when taken together suggests the toxicant. An example of this that virtually every medical student can recite even years after graduation is the toxidrome associated with anticholinergics: "red as a beet, hot/fast as a hare, mad as a hatter, dry as a bone." These represent the flush, fever, tachycardia, CNS, and fluid manifestations associated with this class of drug. From the toxicology literature, where Howard Mofenson first coined the term, which represented a refined form of symptom pattern recognition to the development of "syndromic surveillance," which has evolved from the concept of the "toxidrome," both remain useful clinical methods to identify offending agents. This same mindset applies to and is a rational, effective approach to the infected patient and thus the authors coined the term "the biodrome."

The same concept using the cascade of clinical findings as an approach to an infected patient offers similar value to that of the toxidrome. Global travel has set the stage for importing pathogens that were heretofore uncommon in the United States, but endemic in foreign lands—infectious diseases our health-care professionals have rarely seen or treated—and thus setting the stage for diagnostic challenges. Having a starting point in terms of identifying dangerous, rare, and emerging pathogens is critical. If a severe microbial illness exists anywhere in the world, the potential exists to weaponize it. Given the cornerstone to containing a biological threat—intentional biological weapon release or an emerging pathogen unintentionally spread by as a travel related illness—is rapid detection and diagnosis of the index patient, developing "biodromes" and disseminating information about hallmark clinical clues related to deadly or uncommon biologicals is essential. Since there is almost a parallel amount of pathogens to toxicants that can cause human illness, the use of "biodromes" is an important tool to diagnose illness resulting from biological weapons, as well as emerging pathogens and uncommon biological illnesses.

The cornerstone to diagnosing bioweapon illness is understanding that deadly pathogens often present with hallmark clues not likely to be present in more common, less virulent domestic infections. Bioweapon illness is rarely subtle; usually patients are far sicker than the common "look alike" illness one might be tempted to consider in the differential diagnosis. An example of this is inhalation anthrax compared to influenza illness (Table 2-1).

While it is tempting to think all respiratory illnesses present similarly, the fact is most patients do not present to their health-care provider the first day of the upper respiratory illnesses, including the flu (unfortunately given the optimal effectiveness from antiviral medications toward influenza occurs when administered within 48 hours), and thus by the time they present, the significant differences associated with each illness start to manifest—an advantage for the astute clinicians who carefully elicit a history and observe clinical findings. As Table 2-1 demonstrates, there are hallmark clues as well as a biodrome or cascade of symptoms that can aid the clinician in distinguishing between upper respiratory illness, avian flu, or inhalation anthrax. Note that as a hallmark clue, dyspnea or true shortness of breath is common among inhalation anthrax victims and avian flu but relatively uncommon among seasonal flu patients. This is a critical clinical distinction, as a solitary clinical finding it would suggest to the provider the patient has a serious illness and warrants further study even in the absence of bioweapon terrorism! The value of such distinguishing symptoms or biodromes to the patient is clear—even in the absence of concern about bioweapons, the finding of shortness of breath as Table 2-1 illustrates, especially in an otherwise healthy individual, is worrisome and should be investigated. In the end, a noninfectious cause may be found. Nevertheless, it is clear dyspnea should be a hallmark clue that triggers additional investigation. Applying the biodrome approach, if we take the history of most recent inhalation anthrax victims, there were several days of abdominal pains, diarrhea, and nausea—symptoms that rarely accompany adult seasonal flu patients. Add to this dyspnea, chest discomfort, and high fever, a biodrome emerges: several symptoms that in isolation may or may not yield the appropriate diagnosis but when taken together suggest both a serious illness and likely an emerging pathogen.

Therefore most common signs and symptoms associated with the pathogens—the biodrome—will be introduced in each chapter.

Important "look alike" illnesses that might create clinical confusion are introduced in the biological agent chapters along with key differences between the illnesses that the astute clinician will become alert to. An example of this is smallpox; often when clinicians are shown photographs of chickenpox or smallpox they cannot distinguish between the two. Not surprising given the number of clinicians who may have actually treated either! Both cause a pox-like exanthema even though chickenpox is not a true poxvirus! What are the major distinctions that a clinician can base the diagnosis upon? Chickenpox lesions are asynchronous—when you look at a patient with chickenpox you will notice the crop of lesions are in different stages of development: some are small and emerging while others are full and others are ready to crust over. Smallpox lesions are synchronous—the crop of lesions will appear at the same stage of development. Also, smallpox starts in the mouth, on the hands, head, and feet, working their way into the truncal region. Chickenpox rash usually starts on the trunk and works outwards toward the extremities. It is these types of key clinical distinctions that will be presented in the biological agent chapters that follow, which will enable you to rapidly make the diagnosis.

BIODROME: KEY ELEMENTS

In the chapters that follow, you will be introduced to the specific clinical findings associated with the biological agents discussed. Significant hallmark clues, such as relative bradycardia, patterns of petechia, rashes and black lesions, shortness of breath that should alert the clinician to a serious illness, and pertinent differential diagnostic features will be presented.

First and foremost, don't forget the basics! Vital signs—temperature, heart rate, respiratory rate, pain, and blood pressure—are critical and, taken together, often can strongly suggest or confirm the diagnosis.

Heart Rate

The usual heart rate response to fever is an increase in pulse rate. Pyrogens usually result in a 10–18-beats/min rise for every 1°C rise in febrile temperature, although individual variation occurs. The absence of an appropriate rise is referred to as relative bradycardia, or a pulse-temperature dissociation, and occurs with the following pathogens, some of which are bioweapons: VHFs, Q fever, tularemia. Plague, malaria, typhoid fever, leptospirosis, legionnaires' disease, and rickettsia may cause this as well. Patients taking medications, which can alter heart rate, may not manifest expected heart rate responses to fever. The elderly or individuals with underlying heart disease may not be able to develop an appropriate heart rate response.

Temperature/Fever

Most biological weapon illnesses are accompanied by fevers, often rapidly progressive and >102°F. Febrile illnesses that relapse may represent inadequately treated infections, especially if intermittent or low grade; these however are usually not typical of biological weapon-related infections such as malaria, although there are exceptions, including Q fever and certain tularemia infections. The elderly may not be able to generate the expected amplitude of febrile response owing to age-related physiological changes or may present with delayed fever and changes in mental status accompanied by low-grade fever.

Blood Pressure

Infections accompanied by hypotension generally are an ominous sign. VHFs, infections that may cause fluid shifts such as inhalation anthrax or avian influenza as well as septic shock and impending cardiovascular collapse are associated with hypotension. Petechia or ecchymosis at the cuff site supports vascular involvement although caution is essential in using this finding in the elderly who may be taking anticoagulants. Nevertheless, evidence of bleeding or capillary bed involvement in the setting of hypotension and infection suggests VHF.

Realizing infections target specific organ systems allows a ready diagnosis often by the predominant clinical features: dermatologic, pulmonary, or gastrointestinal are the leading entry points for most biologicals (contact, inhalation, ingestion), while inhalation is considered the most likely route for mass dissemination as well as contagion. Thus looking at route of possible infection, predominant symptoms as well as other signs and symptoms will facilitate identifying the appropriate biodrome.

Remember to take the patient in context of history bearing in mind travel, occupation, and social information along with identifying important signs and symptoms essential to diagnosis, especially a potential bioweapon illness or emerging pathogen.

Suggested Reading

Aronoff DM, Watt G. Prevalence of relative bradycardia in orientia tsutsugamushi infection. *Am J Trop Med Hyg.* 2003; 68(4):477–479.

Fever: Family Practice Notebook. *http://www.fpnotebook.com/ID44.htm* Last accessed April 3, 2006.

Henderson DA. Emerging Infectious Diseases—Special Issue—Smallpox: Clinical and Epidemiologic Features. *www.cdc.gov/ncidod/EID/vol5no4/henderson.htm*

Ippolito G, Nicastri E, Capobianchi M, et al. Hospital preparedness and maangement of patients affected by viral haemorrhagic fever or smallpox at the Lazzaro Spallanzani Institute, Italy. *Euro Surveill.* 2005;10;March 1–3:36–39.

Jones SW, Dobson ME, Francesconi SC, et al. DNA assays for detection, identification and individualization of select agent microorganisms: the armed forces institute of pathology, division of microbiology, Washington, DC. *Croat Med J.* 2005; 46(4):522–529.

McFee RB. Preparing for an era of weapons of mass destruction (WMD): are we there yet? Why we should all be concerned. Part 1. *Vet Human Toxicol.* 2002;44(4):193–199.

McFee RB. Bioterrorism and Weapons of Mass Destruction 2004: Physicians as first responders. The DO. 2004; Mar Suppl: 9–23.

McFee RB, Bush L, Boehm K. Avian influenza: critical considerations for the primary care physician. *JH Adv Studies Medicine.* 2006;(6):10.

O'Byrne WT, Terndrup TE, Kiefe CI, et al. A primer on biological weapons for the clinician, Part I. *Adv Stud Med.* 2003; 3(2):75–86.

Saini R, Pui JC, Burgin S. Rickettsialpox: report of three cases and a review. *J Am Acad Derm.* 2004;51:S137–S140.

Strambu I, Ciolan G, Anghel L, Mocanu A, et al. Bilateral lung consolidations related to accidental exposure to parrots. *Pneumologia,* 2006 July–September;55(3):123–127.

USAMRIID's Medical Management of Biological Casualties Handbook 4th Edition. 2001 U.S. Army Medical Research Institute of Infectious Diseases. Fort Detrick, Frederick, MD.

3

COUNTERMEASURES AND FACILITY PREPAREDNESS: AN OVERVIEW

Robin B. McFee

COUNTERMEASURES AND FACILITY PREPAREDNESS: AN OVERVIEW

Preparedness: Biologicals

Train intake personnel/receptionists to identify worrisome symptoms and biodromes.

Waiting room prompts:

- Inquire about travel, key symptoms (high fever, cough, shortness of breath)
- Suggest respiratory hygiene and offer viral barrier tissues, wastebaskets, masks (should be available in waiting rooms and encourage use!)
- Tell receptionist if
  - you have been in countries where illness of concern (today it's avian flu)
  - you and family members/colleagues/friends have similar illness

Important Resources:

- Post contact information in highly visible location about
- Develop working relationship with, and
- Integrate into preparedness planning/exercises
  - Travel medicine expert
  - Infectious disease expert
  - Infection control team
  - Centers for Disease Control (CDC)—Office or Emergency Response

- State health department
- Laboratory response network (LRN) laboratory
- Local health department
  - Epidemiologist
  - Director

Equipment:

- Isolation
- Additional ventilators and other means to aid the patient (Ambu-bags, etc)
- Negative pressure rooms—permanent or adaptable
- Personal protective equipment (PPE) including n95 masks *and* each team member is fit-tested and proficient in use
- PPE use protocols highly visible especially describing what to use and when to utilize
- Ability to isolate well from sick patients
- Respiratory hygiene products for waiting areas/patients
- CDC smallpox charts prominently displayed
- WHO avian flu charts prominently displayed

Medications:

- Antidotes, antimicrobials

INTRODUCTION

Preparedness suggests the ability to accomplish at a minimum three overarching, important functions: (1) respond to a wide variety of threats, (2) prevent unnecessary loss of life or injury, and (3) provide for the common good. It is a daunting task to protect a community and prepare for intentionally released toxicants or biologicals as well as emerging threats.

Preparedness against weapons of mass destruction largely depends upon trained responders, who are equipped with and knowledgeable about appropriate personal protective equipment (PPE) and other vital technology that includes communications, surveillance and monitoring, as well as having adequate clinical countermeasures such as medications, equipment that would include ventilators, decontamination apparatus, and other vital materials. Mandatory regular exercises and ongoing training are worthwhile activities if a successful response is expected. Hadassah University Hospital in Israel, arguably one of the most experienced health-care facilities (HCFs) in the world in responding to terrorism, takes part in ongoing training exercises with emergency services, and provides regular training to staff; senior medical students are required to attend a 2-week course on casualty management from terrorist attacks underscoring the importance and value of training health-care providers.

ANTIMICROBIALS AND ANTIDOTES

Bacillus anthracis (anthrax), Yersinia pestis (plague), and Francisella tularensis (tularemia) are all potential bioterrorism agents among a very lengthy list of available bacteria that are capable of causing significant death and disability. They are endemic in certain regions of the world, are highly virulent, and able to develop resistance to antibiotics making these particularly dangerous.

Countermeasures against biological weapons increasingly take into consideration the spectrum of physiologic damage that biological agents can inflict, and implement comprehensive strategies to improve the patients outcomes—such as enhancing the immune response with various colony stimulating factors, reducing pathogen load with antimicrobials—of which several subclasses exist, including antivirals, antibiotics antifungal, and complexing with or counteracting antitoxins, as well as other complementary symptomatic and supportive measures such as airway management, cardiovascular support, reverse isolation, and aggressive monitoring of multiple organ functions. These require adequate supplies of medications with training in the use and limitations of each therapeutic option.

Although certain toxins such as ricin and botulinum toxin are considered likely terrorist agents, most of the biological weapons of concern are bacterial or viral. While there are numerous antimicrobial agents available, fortunately from a logistics perspective, there are less than a dozen that the clinician should be completely familiar with as countermeasures against biological weapons. This section will concentrate on a general approach to antimicrobials and an overview of antibiotics and antivirals. Specific therapies will be discussed in each chapter.

It is important to recognize future biological weapons may be genetically engineered variations of the natural pathogens, in which case our current knowledge about treatments, including the utility of presently available countermeasures may not be valid, require additional treatment options or newer interventions.

Biological weapons agents, like pathogens in general, derive their pathogenicity, virulence, or ability to inflict harm to humans through a variety of mechanisms that may include all or some of the following: pathogen load, toxin production, impact on native immunity, and response to antimicrobial treatment. For example, β-lactam antibiotic-induced release of lipoteichoic acid or immunogenic cell fragments as occurs in gram-negative sepsis may have a direct impact upon patient recovery. Times have changed. "Name the bug, name the drug" is too simplistic an approach to biological weapons. Just selecting a drug that matches a bug is insufficient to conferring a survival advantage, as evidenced in the anthrax events of 2001. Anthrax was considered penicillin-sensitive, and thus was in some patients initially administered alone, subsequently or in combination to anthrax victims. Yet some died. Merely administering an antimicrobial for which the pathogen is sensitive fails to take into account the natural history and toxicity profile of the biological. Anthrax, as an example, not only can subject the victim to a large bacterial load, but produces lethal toxin and edema toxin—both of which initiate a serious cascade of physiologic derangements and contribute to the lethality of *Bacillus anthracis*. Penicillin is not an antitoxin. It is not believed to have the capability to interfere with protein synthesis associated with anthrax infection. Therefore, the astute clinician will be aware of the overall effects of the selected countermeasure that go beyond culture and sensitivity and attempt to counter the spectrum of deleterious and pathogenic capabilities of the bioweapon at hand, which will include the most appropriate antimicrobials.

Antibiotics

Antibiotics are medications that kill (bactericidal) or slow the growth (bacteriostatic) of bacteria. Antibiotics are not effective for other types of microbial pathogens such as viruses. Antibiotics are categorized based upon the structure, mechanism of action and also the spectrum of action that ranges from a general classification of targeting gram-positive or gram-negative bacteria, the organisms against which they are effective, the type of infections they treat (skin, respiratory) or more specific such as the ability to treat methicillin-resistant *Staphylococcus aureus* (MRSA) or vancomycin-resistant enterococcus (VRE). Individual antibiotics can vary widely in their effectiveness on various bacteria even within an overall class. For example, not all cephalosporins or penicillin class drugs attack similar bacteria, nor do they treat them equally.

Bactericidal antibiotics are regarded as superior to bacteriostatic agents for treatments of most infections; however, data remain lacking to support this position with the exception of a few severe infections such as endocarditis, meningitis, or bacteremia in a neutropenic patient.

Bacteriostatic or bactericidal activity (defined as a discrete end point as a 99.9% reduction in bacterial inoculum within a 24-hour period of exposure) is actually a continuum whereby a 99% reduction in the proper context could be considered bactericidal but at a slower rate. Bactericidal activity is not an invariable property of antibiotics. Depending upon the organism and growth conditions an antibiotic may be bacteriostatic or bactericidal. Chloramphenicol and erythromycin are protein synthesis inhibitors—classical bacteriostatic medications that target the ribosome. While *Staphylococcus aureus* is not killed by these antibiotics, *Streptococcus pneumoniae* is a susceptible organism and readily killed by these, as well as other antibiotics that would be considered bacteriostatic when administered to treat other bacterial species. Studies suggest clindamycin is bactericidal against *Bacillus anthracis,* yet bacteriostatic against other bacteria. Conversely, certain cell wall inhibitors such as penicillin and vancomycin, which are considered prototype bactericidal agents, do not produce a 99.9% kill of enterococci within 24 hours, and thus considered bacteriostatic against this organism. The same is true for fluoroquinolones, which typically kill *S. pneumoniae.*

Growth conditions affect the activity of bactericidal agents. For example, the β-lactam antibiotics, such as penicillin, require cells to be growing and dividing in order to achieve bactericidal action. Thus slow growth may impair the activity of the antibiotic. Conditions at the site of infection impacting the growth of bacteria may impact the effectiveness of the medication. Whether an antibiotic achieves bactericidal or bacteriostatic activity can vary by organism and conditions of growth.

Other factors to consider when selecting antibiotics to treat infections, especially rapidly progressive, multisystem, and potentially lethal ones are antimicrobial synergism and antimicrobial antagonism. In certain clinical cases, combining antimicrobials that individually have failed to realize their bactericidal activity allows them together to achieve a 99.9% kill rate. Such is the case of penicillin and vancomycin in the treatment of enterococcal endocarditis. Both agents fail to achieve 99.9% killing in 24 hours (thus considered bacteriostatic), yet when combined become bactericidal. On the other hand, there has been evidence that combining a cell wall inhibitory agent (penicillin), which depends upon bacterial growth to achieve bactericidal activity, with a reversible protein synthesis inhibitor (tetracycline), which interferes with cell growth, can actually decrease the overall effectiveness of treatment.

When treating rapidly progressive illnesses—whether aggressive pathogens or biological agents, selected to be used as terrorist weapons—it is essential for the astute physician to understand the pathogen, its impact on the host, and responses to various antimicrobial agents, including the potential value of antibiotic synergism such as with *Bacillus anthracis.* Bear in mind that certain antibiotic classes may exacerbate sepsis syndrome—not only gram-negative but gram-positive sepsis. While bactericidal agents should be considered preferred agents to treat serious, potentially life-threatening infections, selecting an antibiotic or combination of antibiotics should take into account not only bactericidal activity, but the impact on the cascade of effects caused by the pathogen and relies upon a keen understanding of the pathophysiology attendant to the microbe. An example of this is *Bacillus anthracis*—a gram-positive bacteria that produces toxins. These toxins lead to the cascade of serious clinical effects that ultimately can kill the patient. While still under study, it would appear there is a role for protein synthesis inhibitors, which may not only impact the bacteria, but may have some benefit on the dynamic interplay between host, bacterial death, and toxic proteins.

The effectiveness of antibiotics depends upon a variety of considerations. These include

1. The location of the infection.
   - Examples include the central nervous system, lower respiratory tract, bone, and skin.
2. The ability of the antibiotic to reach the site of infection.
   - Certain antibiotics may be able to target the specific bacteria, but may not be able to reach the site of infection. For example, certain antibiotics are unable to cross the blood-brain barrier—a significant limitation when treating a central nervous system infection.
3. The ability of the bacteria to resist or inactivate the antibiotic.
   - Bacteria are increasingly becoming resistant to β-lactams, even Ciprofloxacin resistance is emerging.
4. The cascade of factors contributing to the pathogenicity of the bacteria.
   - The ability of bacteria to cause illness is dependant upon multiple factors including toxin production, inactivation or derangement of host immune system, and modulators that include interferons, cytokines, and other immune response chemicals.
5. The toxicity/risk/adverse event profile of the antibiotic.
   - Adverse events ranging from mild gastrointestinal to anaphylaxis.
   - Certain antibiotics can be toxic, especially to specific organ systems. Vancomycin and aminoglycosides can be nephrotoxic.
   - Vancomycin and clindamycin along with other broad-spectrum antibiotics can kill native, benign intestinal flora allowing for pathogen overgrown, which can lead to clostridium difficile infection.
6. The underlying immune/health status of the patient.
7. The antibiotic capability of killing or slowing the bacteria from multiplying.

Also important to consider, what routes of administration is the antibiotic available? While parenteral may confer advantages, especially in a health-care setting, in a mass exposure event, the ability to treat as well as offer prophylaxis to large numbers of patients is better served by oral therapy.

The use of antibiotic combination therapy is being suggested in the treatment of bioweapon illness. Antibiotic combinations are considered to enhance antibacterial efficacy and to prevent the development of resistance. Numerous combinations are being evaluated. The reader is referred to the chapters discussing specific agents for more detail.

Given the highly lethal nature of biological weapons, new antibiotics are being developed and further research into the most effective treatments for emerging bioweapons and existing pathogens are ongoing. Physicians should remain vigilant for new treatments and become familiar with their routes of administration, side effects, and other critical nuances that underscore our ability to provide the best care to infected patients. Emergency physicians should ensure their department and health-care facility each have ample supplies and backup sources of essential antibiotics, a knowledge of second-line therapies if frontline agents become unavailable and provide appropriate training to staff, as well as ongoing input to facility preparedness protocols.

As of this writing, novel interventions not usually considered antimicrobials including Fe siderophores for Yersinia are being developed and may be approved after the publication of this text. The reader is alerted to emerging studies suggesting antibiotic cocktails may be more effective than monotherapy for such bioweapon illnesses as inhalation anthrax.

The goal of antimicrobial treatment is to achieve effective drug concentrations. Current antimicrobial dosing regimens are based upon research, some of which may be several years in the past, and utilized in the treatment of patients not critically ill. Bioweapon patients are likely to be critically ill. This has an impact upon the physiology of host immune defense, dynamic interplay of cytokines and other immunologic mediators, the pathogen and underlying health of the patient. Recent studies into antibiotic activity, for example, high peak/minimum inhibitory concentration (MIC) ratios for aminoglycosides, time above MIC for β-lactam antibiotics, pharmacokinetics such as volume of distribution and drug clearance, clearer insights into the mechanism of sepsis such as third space losses, altered renal clearance, inflammatory response to immunogenic products such as decreased serum albumin levels, all warrant reevaluation of antibiotic selection and dosing regimens for the bioweapon ill as well as critically ill septic patient. The effects of sepsis may lower antibiotic levels for optimal effectiveness. Of note, interventions to improve renal clearance or hepatic function may have an impact upon drug levels. Antibiotics that may contribute to the adverse effects of sepsis, such as have been well-described for β-lactams and gram-negative sepsis, require the physician to be knowledgeable about emerging trends in the management of acutely infected and critically ill patients, and the need to continuously evaluate the patient as well as the overall impact of multisystem interventions on the underlying cause of the illness and the countermeasures being utilized.

Antivirals

Currently there are few antivirals available for the treatment of viral biological weapons. These include Ribavirin, which may be useful for certain viral hemorrhagic fever (VHF) viruses such as Lassa, cidofovir, which, although still under investigation, may be helpful for smallpox victims, and acyclovir for varicella and zoster infections. Immune modulators such as interferon may play a role in the treatment of certain viral infections. Because there are also few viral illnesses that are treated by antivirals; symptomatic and supportive care in concert with preventing secondary bacterial infection remain a mainstay of treatment for certain bioweapon viruses. Emerging data suggest if survivors can be located that immune globulin may be an effective countermeasure for certain VHF viruses such as the Ebola virus, as well as other viral illnesses, especially in the absence of an approved antiviral medication. Oseltamivir and zanamivir may be used for avian influenza in addition to seasonal influenza, although resistance is emerging. An experienced virologist integrated with the ED (emergency department) preparedness team is a critical component to a viral pathogen response in addition to ample supplies of antiviral countermeasures and staff knowledgeable in the use of such interventions. The U.S. Army Military Research Institute for Infections Diseases (USAMRIID) in addition to the Centers for Disease Control and Prevention (CDC) are excellent resources both for the planning and response to viral bioweapons and highly pathogenic viral illnesses. USAMRIID is also conducting advance research into newer countermeasures against highly dangerous viruses.

Antidotes

Of note, there are numerous hazardous materials; radiation sources; and combinations of conventional, radioactive isotopes and chemical weapons that can be utilized to terrorize and harm a civilian population. Of the latter, it is possible that, like recent events in Tokyo, organophosphate toxicants, nerve agents, as well as cyanide may be used. Fortunately, there are antidotes available for these toxicants.

In the United States, the approved nerve agent antidotes include either a prepackaged set, the Mark I Nerve Agent Antidote Kit (NAAK), which contains atropine and pralidoxime (2-PAM) autoinjectors, although these are also available in stock bottles, as well as benzodiazepines, usually diazepam, and supportive care.

An in-depth discussion of antitoxins and other countermeasures will be specifically addressed in the appropriate agent chapters. Having adequate supplies, knowing where to obtain emergency quantities, as well as familiarity with front-line and second-line therapies is critical.

Recently a former Soviet agent was allegedly assassinated while in the United Kingdom with polonium 210. The omnipresence of radioactive materials, concerns over potentially unaccounted for weapons grade materials in the former Soviet Union (FSU) justify concern about and continued preparedness for radiation threats. While most medical specialties should be considered "nuanced" and requiring well-trained clinicians, radiation preparedness requires highly experienced professionals. In addition to having appropriate radiation antidotes, of which there is aggressive ongoing research and development of new interventions, as well as colony-stimulating factor medications, integral to effective preparedness is access to and familiarity working with a radiation health physicist and hematologists, given one of the critical effects of such poisoning includes suppression of white cells and increased risk of infection.

FACILITY PREPAREDNESS

Security

In the event of a terrorist or mass casualty event, the role of the hospital security department will be critical to protect the ED, control patient/victim flow, secure vital medications, integrating with law enforcement agencies, and ultimately ensuring that the disaster plans are successfully carried out.

The lack of surge capacity is no longer an unusual occurrence among U.S. HCFs. As such, hospitals are wrestling with the challenge caring for current levels of patient emergencies; nevertheless, hospitals/ED will be called upon to receive large numbers of patients and worried well. Orderly patient flow, the safety of staff, protection of materials, chain of custody for materials that may become evidence, crowd control, and open-entry corridors for essential transportation including supply shipments and ambulances will be the role of security. The ED physician should be aware of the vulnerabilities of the facility. International experience has demonstrated that most people exposed to a terrorist attack, whether chemical or explosive, will attempt to bypass crowd control measures to obtain immediate medical attention. Victims often arrive by means other than ambulances. Anxiety levels, escalating emotions, fear, and the potential for violence can occur. It is critical that the ED and hospital security, as well as local law enforcement agencies, collaborate in preparedness planning, drills, and coordinate efforts. Otherwise it is likely the facility will be overwhelmed, appropriate protocols not observed, such as decontamination procedures, further jeopardizing patients and providers as well.

Decontamination

Transference of toxicants from victims to rescuers, equipment, or facilities poses an exposure risk. The appropriate use of decontamination is critical to ensure safe transportation of patients with little risk of propagating toxicants and harming others. In the early days of the anthrax events of 2001, patients were inappropriately decontaminated with diluted bleach solutions and scrubbed with abrasive brushes. Soap and water are usually adequate for people, reserving chemical-based decontamination for surface cleaning. (See Table 3-1.)

It is important to understand the distinction between exposed and contaminated patients; the former do not require decontamination while the latter will need to have their clothes removed (often results in a decrease of 80% or more of the contaminant burden), and appropriately washed.

Whether using fixed decontamination structures or portable equipment, the key element is proper use of PPE, adequate cleaning of patients, and control of victim flow so that contaminated persons do not breach containment zones. Decontamination should occur away from the ED, regardless of the weather and number of patients. It should not occur in the ED as the risk attendant to contaminants could compromise the health of staff. Attention to wind direction to avoid downwind contamination, ample backup supply of water, contaminant runoff, patient flow, and providing towels and clean clothes for decontaminated patients is critical. Some jurisdictions require fire rescue to provide decontamination equipment

TABLE 3-1

DECONTAMINATION AND EMERGENCY DEPARTMENT EQUIPMENT—RADIATION

- Hospital greens and surgical gown (waterproof, with any openings in the gown taped shut)
- Surgical trousers taped to shoes
- Cap, face shield, booties (waterproof)
- Plastic apron
- Double gloves (inner layer taped to surgical gown)
- Pencil dosimeters
- Thermo luminescent dosimeters
- Survey meters
- Plastic (polyethylene) floor and wall coverings
- Ventilation filter paper
- Drapes
- Plastic bags
- Butcher paper
- Large garbage cans
- Radiation signs and tape
- Decontamination stretcher with drainage container tank
- Lead storage containers
- N95 masks
- Radiation detector (alpha, beta, gamma)
- Level A, B, C PPE (depending on response role)
- Neoprene industrial gloves

Source: From McFee RB, Leikin JB. Radiation terrorism: the unthinkable possibility, the ignored reality. JEMS. April 2005;78–93.

or services while others will rely on the HCF. Regardless of the approach, the ED team should practice regularly in interacting with decontamination teams. A more in-depth discussion of appropriate decontamination will be provided in the chemical chapters.

Personal Protective Equipment

- There are a variety of circumstances where PPE would be appropriate in the ED—from provider and patient worn respiratory protection to limit the spread of pathogens to gowns, gloves, goggles as standard precautions to Level C suits and positive air-powered respirators. The highest level of PPE most HCF have access to is Level C, yet this level is only protective under very specific circumstances that may not be readily known. The U.S. Occupational Health and Safety Authority (OSHA) states "The proper use of PPE requires considerable training by a competent person, and that wearing PPE without proper training can be extremely dangerous and potentially fatal." It appears incongruous that fire fighters and emergency personnel, especially hazardous material responders receive formal and frequent training in PPE, are required to wear Level A or B PPE when closely working with potentially contaminated patients, yet Level C is deemed reasonable protection for hospital staff. Of concern, sending hospital personnel into a contaminated area with very little experience or formal training in PPE beyond the one or two donning and doffing exercises is a potentially risky proposition. In addition to the danger of inappropriately using PPE, by virtue of inexperience, is the challenge of performing the range of medically important procedures wearing Level C equipment. Appropriate PPE will be discussed in respective chapters in the text. Practice prior to an actual event is essential to providing proper care with the least risk to the response team.

Suggested Reading

Aas P, Jacobsen D. Nerve gas: guidelines for care of victims of terrorism. *Tidsskr Nor Laegeforen.* March 17, 2005;125(6):731–735.

Athamna A, Athamna M, Nura A, et al. Is in vitro antibiotic combination more effective than single drug therapy against anthrax? *Antimicrob Agents Chemother.* April 2005;49(4):1323–1325.

Aurbek N, Thiermann H, Szinicz L, et al. Evaluation of HI 6 treatment after percutaneous VR exposure by use of a kinetic based dynamic computer model. *Toxicology.* April 20, 2007;233(1–3):173–9. Epub July 7, 2006.

Brouillard JE, Terriff CM, Tofan A, et al. Antibiotic selection and resistance issues with fluoroquinolones and doxycycline against bioterrorism agents. *Pharmacotherapy.* January 2006;26(1):3–14.

Bullard TB, Strack G, Scharoun K. Emergency department security: a call for reassessment. *Health Care Manag (Frederick).* September 2002;21(1):65–73.

Centers for Disease Control and Prevention. Rapid assessment of injuries among survivors of the terrorist attack on the World Trade Centre—New York City. September 11, 2001. *MMWR Morb Mortal Wkly Rep.* 2002;51:1–5.

Cethromycin: A-195773, A-1957730, ABT 773 Drugs RD 2007;8(2):95–102.

Chambers HF. *Bactericidal vs. Bacteriostatic Antibiotic Therapy: A Clinical Mini-Review.* NFID—Clinical Updates in Infectious Diseases 2003;VI(4):1–5.

Edwards NA, Caldicott DGE, Elisea T, et al. Truth hurts: hard lessons from Australia's largest mass casualty exercise with contaminated patients. *Emerg Med Australia.* 2006;18:185–195.

Ferreras JA, Ryu JS, Di Lello F, et al. Small-molecule inhibition of siderophore biosynthesis in Mycobacterium tuberculosis and Yersinia pestis. *Nat Chem Biol.* June 2005;1(1):29–32.

Garner A, Laurence H, Lee A. Practicality of performing medical procedures in chemical protective ensembles. *Emerg Med Austral.* 2004;16:108–113.

Gonzalez JC. Bio-terrorism, "dirty bombs," hospitals and security issues. *J Healthc Prot Manage.* Summer 2004;20(2):55–59.

Hick JL, Penn P, Hangling D, et al. Establishing and training health care facility decontamination teams. *Ann Emerg Med.* 2003;42:391–394.

Hogan DE, Waeckerle JF, Dire DJ, et al. Emergency department impact of the Oklahoma City terrorist bombing. *Ann Emerg Med.* 1999;34:160–167.

Kang SL, Rybak MJ, McGrath BJ, et al. Pharmacodynamics of levofloxacin, ofloxacin and ciprofloxacin alone and in combination with rifampin against methicillin-susceptible and resistant *Staphylococcus aureus* in and In Vitro Model. *Antimicrob Agents Chemother.* December 1994;38(12):2702–2709.

Lotz S, Starke A, Ziemann C, et al. *B*-lactam antibiotic-induced release of lipoteichoic acid from *Staphylococcus aureus* leads to activation of neutrophil granulocytes. *Annals Clin Microb Antimicrob.* June 2006;S15.

McFee RB, Bush L, Boehm K. Avian influenza: critical consideration for the primary care physician. *JH Adv Studies in Med.* 2006;6(10):431–440.

McFee RB, Leikin JB. Radiation terrorism: the unthinkable possibility, the ignored reality. *JEMS.* April 2005;30:78–93.

McFee RB. Bioterrorism and weapons of mass destruction 2004: physicians as first responders. The DO. March 2004;38 (suppl):9–23.

McFee RB, Leikin JB, Kiernan K. Preparing for an era of weapons of mass destruction are we there yet? Why we should all be concerned, Part II. *Vet Human Tox.* 2004;46(6): 347–351.

Moellering R. Treatment of enterococcal endocarditis. In: Sande M, Kaye D, Root R, eds. *Contemporary Issues in Infectious Diseases. Endocarditis.* Vol 2. New York. Churchill Livingstone, 1984:113–133.

Okumura T, Suzuki K, Fukuda A, et al. The Tokyo subway sarin attack: disaster management, part 1 : community emergency response. *Acad Emerg Med.* 1998, 2003;5:613–617.

Pinder M, Bellomo R, Lipman J. Pharmacological principles of antibiotic prescription in the critically ill. *Anaesth Intensive Care.* April 2002;30(2):134–144.

Rosenfeld JV, Fitzgerald M, Kossman T, et al. Is the Australian hospital system adequately prepared for terrorism? *Med J Aust.* 2005;183(11/12):567–570.

Ruiz ME, Gerrero IC, Tuazon CU. Endocarditis caused by methicillin-resistant *Staphylococcus aureus*: treatment failure with linezolid. *Clin Infect Dis.* 2002;35:1018–1020.

Shapira SC, Mor-Yosef S. Applying lessons from medical management of conventional terror to responding to weapons of mass destruction terror: the experience of a tertiary university hospital. *Stud Conflict Terrorism.* 2003;26:379–385.

Spreer A, Kerstan H, Bottcher T, et al. Reduced release of pneumolysis by *Streptococcus pneumoniae* in vitro and in vivo after treatment with nonbacteriolytic antibiotics in comparison to ceftriaxone. *Antimicrob Agents Chemother.* August 2003;2649–2654.

Szinicz L, Worek F, Thiermann H, et al. Development of antidotes: problems and strategies. *Toxicology.* July 14, 2006.

U.S. Department of Labor. Occupational Safety and Health Administration. OSHA guidelines. *http://www.osha.gov/ pls/oshaweb/owastand.display_standard_group?p_toc_level= 1&p_part_number = 1910*

4

SUPPORTIVE CARE

Edward M. Bottei and Jerrold B. Leikin

SUPPORTIVE CARE

- Good supportive care is the foundation of medical care for all patients.
- Acute hypoxemic respiratory failure (AHRF) is caused by intrapulmonary shunting and leads to hypoxemia. Therapy focuses on providing supplemental oxygen and decreasing oxygen demands.
- Hypercarbic respiratory failure (HRF) is caused by either a decreased drive to breathe or respiratory workload being greater than respiratory muscle strength. Therapy focuses on providing adequate alveolar ventilation while correcting the underlying cause.
- Shock leads to respiratory failure (RF) because of increased total body oxygen requirements in the face of decreased oxygen delivery to the respiratory muscles.
- Most shock states are initially treated with aggressive fluid resuscitation. The exception is cardiogenic shock in which gentle fluid resuscitation is used.
- Shock states not resolved by fluid challenges are treated with either a vasopressor (norepinephrine) or an inotrope (dobutamine).
- Patients in the ICU (intensive care unit) should have a list of housekeeping issues addressed daily so as to prevent complications of ICU care.

INTRODUCTION

In the world of medical toxicology and in medicine in general, the first and most important therapeutic intervention for all patients is good supportive care. While this textbook discusses many aspects of health-care preparedness for terrorism, only a few chapters will apply to any specific patient or group of patients. For example, decontamination is most useful within a few minutes of exposure, and antidotal therapy and enhancement of elimination techniques are used in less than 5% of poisoned cases. Supportive care applies to all patients and focuses on respiratory and circulatory considerations.

AIRWAY

Ensuring that the patient has a patent airway is the first step, since a patient with an obstructed airway will die within minutes. Common causes for loss of an airway include loss of protective reflexes (narcotic overdose), airway irritation or edema (ingestion of caustic agents or inhalation of airway irritants), and excessive secretions (nerve agent inhalation).

Restoration of airway patency is best achieved through orotracheal intubation. The oral route is preferred since larger diameter endotracheal tubes can be used and nasal-tracheal intubation is frequently complicated by sinusitis, otitis, and ventilator-associated pneumonia.

BREATHING

Classification of Respiratory Failure

Once the airway has been secured, the patient's oxygenation and ventilation needs to be assessed and supported if necessary. RF can be classified into one of four categories based on its pathophysiology and treatment: (I) AHRF, (II) HRF, (III) postoperative, and (IV) shock (Table 4-1).

Type I: Acute Hypoxemic Respiratory Failure

AHRF is caused by either flooding or collapsing of alveoli, resulting in an intrapulmonary shunt and systemic

TABLE 4-1

CLASSIFICATION OF RESPIRATORY FAILURE, CAUSES, AND TREATMENT

	Pathophysiology	Causes	Clinical Manifestations	Treatment
Type I AHRF	Alveolar flooding or collapse leading to intrapulmonary shunt	Pneumonia, pulmonary edema, atelectasis	Hypoxemia	• Increased Fio_2 • Judicious use of PEEP • Decreased oxygen requirements
Type II Hypercarbic Respiratory Failure	• Decreased respiratory drive *or* • Respiratory muscle load greater than respiratory muscle strength	• Decreased drive: narcotics. • Increased load: bronchospasm. • Decreased strength: botulism	Increased $Paco_2$	• Ventilatory support • Correcting the underlying cause
Type III Postoperative	Atelectasis and decreased respiratory drive	Pain, inhaled anesthetics, narcotics	Decreased Pao_2 and/or increased $Paco_2$	• Relief of pain • Wake patient up • Antiatelectasis maneuvers
Type IV Shock	Oxygen delivery insufficient for metabolic needs	Sepsis, hypovolemia, myocardial depression	Inappropriate end organ perfusion: mental status changes, decreased urine output, metabolic acidosis	Diagnose and treat underlying condition

AHRF, acute hypoxemic respiratory failure; PEEP, positive end-expiratory pressure.

Adapted from Hall JB, Schmidt GA, Wood LDH (eds). Principles of Critical Care Medicine. Third Edition. New York: McGraw-Hill, 2005, p. 420.

hypoxemia. There are many clinical states that can cause alveolar flooding: aspiration pneumonia, hydrocarbon aspiration, infectious pneumonias (community-acquired pneumonia, plague, tularemia, etc), high-pressure pulmonary edema (cardiogenic shock), low-pressure pulmonary edema (chemical pneumonitis from inhalation of phosgene, chlorine, or riot control agents), and increased secretions (inhalation of nerve and blister agents, etc). Atelectasis may be caused by hydrocarbon aspiration or pleural effusions from pulmonary anthrax. The clinical manifestations of AHRF are hypoxemia and the ensuing end organ dysfunction that results thereof. Treatment of AHRF includes increasing the percentage of inspired oxygen (Fio_2), judicious use of positive end-expiratory pressure (PEEP) if the patient is intubated, and decreasing oxygen requirements (treating fevers, decreasing work of breathing, etc).

Type II: Hypercarbic Respiratory Failure

HRF is also referred to as ventilatory failure and results from inadequate alveolar ventilation. There are three determinants of human ventilation: drive, strength, and load. There must be a central drive to breathe; this drive can be impaired by a stroke or a narcotic overdose. A classical example of central drive inhibition occurred in the Moscow theater hostage rescue in October 2002, when the Russian Spetsnaz rescue team pumped the narcotic carfentanil into

the theater to subdue the hostage takers. In the process, approximately 120 hostages also died from carfentanil overdose and the resultant central apnea. Respiratory load and muscle strength are inextricably linked together and must be in balance in order for a person to keep breathing. Strength can be decreased by such things as botulism, myopathies, or hypophosphatemia. Load can increase by bronchospasm caused by respiratory irritants, increased secretions caused by inhalation of nerve agents, or circumferential chest wall burns. When load is greater than strength, ventilatory failure will ensue. For those patients developing respiratory muscle weakness, a forced vital capacity less than 30% of the patients predicted is predictive for need for ventilatory support. Nerve agents are excellent at causing HRF because they cause both an increased work of breathing (from the muscarinic effects of bronchorrhea and bronchospasm) along with decreased respiratory muscle strength (from the nicotinic effects resulting in paralysis of the respiratory muscles). The clinical manifestations of HRF include a rising $Paco_2$ and CO_2 narcosis. Treatment of HRF includes intubation, bronchodilators, frequent suctioning, and sufficient ventilatory support to provide adequate minute volume and maintain appropriate alveolar ventilation.

Type III: Postoperative Respiratory Failure

Postoperative RF may be encountered in relation to terrorism when dealing with blast injuries and trauma. Type III

RF is caused by a combination of atelectasis and decreased respiratory drive. The atelectasis is a consequence of pain, either postoperatively or from broken bones, and the resultant shallow breathing. The use of inhaled anesthetics and narcotics can decrease respiratory drive. The combination of these two factors can produce either AHRF, HRF, or a combination of the two. Treatment of Type III RF includes control of pain, supplemental oxygen, waking the patient up without causing excessive discomfort, and anti-atelectasis maneuvers such as chest physical therapy and elevation of the head of the bed.

Type IV: Shock-Related Respiratory Failure

Shock occurs when the oxygen delivery to the body is inadequate in meeting the body's metabolic needs. RF occurs in the shock state because of a decreased oxygen delivery to the respiratory muscles combined with the increased metabolic needs of the body. Shock, and the ensuing RF, may be caused by many etiologies, including sepsis, hypovolemia, or myocardial depression. The signs and symptoms will depend upon the cause of the shock state. Likewise, treatment will focus on supporting oxygenation and ventilation while the underlying cause is treated. Shock is discussed further in the following section.

CIRCULATION

When assessing the adequacy of circulation, the focus needs to be on the adequacy of oxygen delivery to the tissues, not just on the vital signs. One study of trauma patients found that despite fluid resuscitation to normalize vital signs and urine output, 85% of the patients still had inadequate oxygen delivery to the tissues. Oxygen delivery is related to both the blood's ability to carry oxygen and the cardiac output.

Oxygen Carrying Capacity

Oxygen carrying capacity is the product of hemoglobin concentration and hemoglobin saturation. An absolute decrease in hemoglobin concentration may occur through either hemorrhage or red blood cell lysis, as can be seen in arsine exposures. A functional decrease in hemoglobin concentration occurs when hemoglobin is incapable of transporting oxygen. This can be seen in the conditions of carboxyhemoglobinemia, methemoglobinemia, and sulfhemoglobinemia. Decreases in hemoglobin saturation can result from conditions discussed in the section on AHRF.

Interruption of oxygen utilization on the cellular level can also lead to shock. Cyanide, sodium azide, hydrogen sulfide, and carbon monoxide all bind to mitochondrial cytochromes and stop production of adenosine triphosphate (ATP). In exposures to these cellular poisons, the cell will have to generate energy using anaerobic pathways, just the same as if there is no oxygen delivery to the tissues. If the exposure to these chemicals is severe enough, shock and death may ensue.

Cardiac Output

Cardiac output is the product of heart rate and stroke volume. Heart rate can affect cardiac output by being either too fast or too slow. When too fast, the left ventricle does not have time to fill properly. However, with bradycardia, the heart fills appropriately but contracts too infrequently to deliver an adequate amount of oxygen to the body. Stroke volume is determined by preload, contractility, and afterload. Preload can be decreased by hypovolemia or hemorrhage, and afterload may be decreased by excessive vasodilation. The causes of decreased myocardial contractility are many but include calcium channel blocker overdose, carbon monoxide, and heavy metal intoxication among others.

Diagnosis of Hypotension and Shock

As mentioned above, the goal of therapy is to restore oxygen delivery to normal, not just "fix the vital signs." A quick history and physical assessment should be performed in order to determine which of the three most common types of shock the patient has: hypovolemic, cardiogenic, or distributive (septic). The placement of a central venous or pulmonary artery catheter may be of benefit in determining which type of shock the patient is in, especially if the patient has a mixture of etiologies for their shock state. However, resuscitation efforts should never be delayed to gather this hemodynamic data. Gathering of data and treating the shock state should proceed together. In septic shock, the advent of early goal-directed therapy (EGDT) has established endpoints for central venous pressure (CVP), mean arterial pressure (MAP), urinary output, central venous oxygen saturation, arterial oxygen saturation, and hematocrit as keystones for targeting therapy.

Treatment of Hypotension and Shock

Fluid Resuscitation

The first intervention in the hypotensive patient is a fluid challenge. The choice of resuscitation fluid is based on the clinical scenario and the clinician's preference. Typically, 0.9% normal saline or lactated ringers are used. Transfusions of blood products to maintain a hematocrit near 30% has been shown to improve outcomes when part of EGDT in septic shock. The amount and rate at which to administer the fluid challenge is based on which type of shock the patient is in. Patients with hypovolemic or distributive shock usually need larger volumes infused quickly. Patients in cardiogenic shock, however, need smaller volumes infused more slowly so as not to develop pulmonary edema. The endpoint of fluid resuscitation is when there is either improvement of the patient's clinical condition (i.e., improvement of oxygen delivery) or a complication (pulmonary edema). In EGDT, endpoints for fluid resuscitation are CVP of 8–12 mm Hg and a MAP of 65–90 mm Hg.

Use of Vasopressors and Inotropic Agents

If fluid resuscitation has not achieved improvement in hemodynamic parameters and oxygen delivery, then the judicious use of either vasopressors and/or inotropic agents is appropriate (Table 4-2). In those patients who have a reasonable cardiac output but are vasodilated, norepinephrine is a reasonable vasopressor choice. If, however, the patient has a decreased cardiac output or decreased cardiac contractility, then inotropic support with dobutamine is a good choice. It is important to remember that dobutamine may cause hypotension from vasodilation if the patient has not been adequately fluid resuscitated before starting dobutamine. While phenylephrine, a pure α-agonist, may raise MAP, excessive use of phenylephrine may cause peripheral ischemia and decrease cardiac output by overly increasing cardiac afterload.

Treatment of Lactic Acidosis in Shock

For many years, physicians have treated lactic acidosis with sodium bicarbonate in the belief that normalizing the serum pH is beneficial to the patient. The pH of blood can be easily measured, but this measurement does not necessarily reflect the pH within tissues (heart, central nervous system [CNS], liver) or within cells or mitochondria. Therefore, normalizing serum pH does not necessarily normalize tissue or cellular pH. Also, while acidosis does have some harmful effects, it has also been shown that acidosis protects cells in a variety of organs from various insults, including hypoxia. The data supporting the belief that treating lactic acidosis with bicarbonate come from a few animal and in vitro studies and are marginal at best. There are equal amounts of data from animal and in vitro studies that show treating lactic acidosis with sodium bicarbonate is not efficacious and, in some studies, worsens the acidosis. There is also a lack of evidence supporting the use of bicarbonate in human lactic acidosis. There is an excellent review of this topic listed in the Suggested Readings. So, despite the physician's desire to want to "do something, anything" in the face of lactic acidosis and acidemia, we do not recommend the routine use of sodium bicarbonate. It is more important to identify and treat the underlying cause of the acidosis rather than push bicarbonate to "fix the pH."

TABLE 4-2

VASOPRESSORS USED TO TREAT SHOCK

Drug	Recommended Adult Dosing	Recommended Pediatric Dosing	Comments
Dobutamine	2.5–20 mcg/kg/min	2.5–15 mcg/kg/min	Maximum recommended dosing: 40 mcg/kg/min
Dopamine	1–20 mcg/kg/min	1–20 mcg/kg/min	The following ranges are approximate and may not hold for your particular patient: • Dopaminergic activity 1–5 mcg/kg/min • β-Adrenergic activity 5–10 mcg/kg/min • α-Adrenergic activity >10 mcg/kg/min Maximum recommended dosing: 30–50 mcg/kg/min
Epinephrine	1–10 mcg/min	0.1–1 mcg/ kg/min	Maximum recommended dosing: 1 mcg/kg/min
Norepinephrine	1–10 mcg/min	0.05–1 mcg/kg/min	Maximum recommended dosing: 2 mcg/kg/min in children and 30 mcg/min in adults
Isoproterenol	2–10 mcg/min	0.05–1 mcg/lkg/min	Maximum recommended dosing: 2 mcg/kg/min in children and 10 mcg/min in adults
Vasopressin	.01 to 0.04 U/min	Not studied	May be useful for septic shock and vasodilatory shock due to systemic inflammatory response

Note: All of these medications are given by a continuous intravenous infusion. Clinicians should start with low doses and titrate upward to clinical effect. If large doses of vasopressors are needed, invasive monitoring should be used to confirm the clinical diagnosis and to assess effects of therapy. Infiltration of these medications into the skin may cause skin necrosis and needs to be treated aggressively.

Notes on Resuscitation

Intraosseous infusions can be considered in children less than 6 years of age for the first 12 hours. Hypertonic solutions cannot be infused via the interosseous route due to possible occurrence of osteomyelitis. In order to avoid hypothermia in both children and adults, fluids may need to be warmed to 40°C to 42°C (104°F to 107.5°F).

HOUSEKEEPING ISSUES IN THE INTENSIVE CARE UNIT

When a patient is admitted to an ICU, there are certain ICU "housekeeping" issues that should be addressed every day. Addressing these issues helps decrease the complications and morbidity and mortality associated with ICU care.

1. If the patient is intubated or has a pulmonary artery catheter in place, then a daily chest x-ray should be performed to make sure the tube and line are in proper position and that no complications have developed (pneumothorax, movement of the tube or catheter).
2. Ensure that the patient has prophylaxis against the formation of deep venous thromboses with either an anticoagulant (heparin or enoxaparin) or sequential compression devices on the legs if the patient cannot be anticoagulated.
3. Ensure that the patient has stress ulcer prophylaxis with either an H_2-antagonist or a proton pump inhibitor.
4. If the patient is expected to be in the ICU for more than 24 hours, provide nutrition to the patient either via tube feedings into the stomach (preferred) or via total parenteral nutrition (TPN).
5. If the patient is pharmacologically sedated, wake the patient up daily to assess their mental status and their need for sedation. If the patient's clinical status is tenuous and waking the patient up will be detrimental to their condition, do not perform this maneuver until the patient is more stable.
6. Check all central venous and arterial lines to make sure they function properly and are not infected.
7. If the patient is intubated, make sure the head of the bed is elevated to at least a 30° angle to help prevent the development of ventilator-associated pneumonia.
8. Prevention and control of hyperglycemia has been shown to decrease mortality in ICU patients.

Suggested Reading

Bottei EB, Seger DL. Therapeutic Approach to the Critically Poisoned Patient. In: Brent J, Wallace K, Burkhart K, et al (eds). *Critical Care Toxicology: Diagnosis and Management of the Critically Poisoned Patient*. Mosby, Philadelphia, PA, 2005; Chapter 3.

Gehlbach BK, Schmidt GA. Bench-to-bedside review: treating acid-base abnormalities in the intensive care unit—the role of buffers. *Crit Care*. May 2004;8(4):259–265.

Holmes, C.L., Patel B.M., Russell J.A and Walley K.R.: Physiology of Vasopressin Relevant to Management of Septic Shock. *Chest* 2001;120:989–1002.

Mannucci, P.M., Levi., M.: Prevention and Treatment of Major Blood Loss *N. Engl. J. Med* 2007:356:2301–11.

Walley KR. Shock. In: Hall JB, Schmidt GA, Wood LDH (eds). *Principles of Critical Care*. McGraw-Hill, New York, NY, 2005; Chapter 21.

Wood LDH. The Pathophysiology and Differential Diagnosis of Acute Respiratory Failure. In: Hall JB, Schmidt GA, Wood LDH (eds). *Principles of Critical Care*. McGraw-Hill, New York, NY, 2005; Chapter 31.

5

DERMAL ISSUES

Rhonda Brand and Andrea Carlson

INTRODUCTION

The skin is a major target site for agents of terrorism due to both its large surface area and constant contact with the environment. Fortunately, intact skin acts as an effective barrier for the majority of natural and man-made toxins. However, penetration of chemicals possessing certain physical characteristics may occur even through healthy intact skin. Changes to the dermal barrier (e.g., burns and abrasions) can result in even greater absorption of toxins, further increasing the risk of injury and disease.

Why Is the Skin such an Effective Barrier?

The primary function of the skin is to maintain fluid homeostasis while preventing compounds from entering from the external environment. The skin is comprised of two layers: the epidermis and the dermis, with the epidermis being subdivided into the viable epidermis and the stratum corneum. The stratum corneum is the outermost layer and serves as the skin's principal barrier. It is approximately 15–20 μm thick in human skin and consists of terminally differentiated keratinocytes (corneocytes) that are embedded in a matrix of lipid bilayers similar to a "brick wall," with corneocytes serving as the bricks and lipids surrounding them as mortar. The viable epidermis is located just below the stratum corneum and is responsible for the production of the stratum corneum. The dermis is the innermost layer, comprised mainly of collagen fibers in an aqueous gel matrix. This configuration imparts elastic properties to the skin and provides the physiological support mechanism for the epidermis. The dermis also contains blood vessels, lymphatics, and nerve endings.

The lipids of the stratum corneum form a bilayer that becomes the major barrier to water and water-soluble chemicals. A chemical must therefore pass through the stratum corneum's "brick wall" to successfully penetrate through the skin. For a chemical to transverse this barrier, it must rely on partitioning into the lipid mortar surrounding the keratinocytes. It then remains in the lipids and diffuses around the keratinocytes until it has successfully passed through the entire stratum corneum. The chemical must then diffuse into the more hydrophilic viable epidermis before entering the blood vessels in the dermis. The need to partition into stratum corneum lipids and then into the hydrophilic bloodstream favors molecules that are moderately lipophilic.

Chemical absorption through the skin is therefore different from many other tissues because it relies on passive diffusion instead of active transport. Penetration demonstrates a linear relationship between exposure concentration and surface area. Dermal absorption can be modeled based on physical properties of the compound with the combination of molecular size and lipophilicity being the best predictor of dermal absorption. Smaller, uncharged chemicals penetrate better than larger, charged molecules. Hair follicles and sebaceous glands can also act as shunts for chemical absorption into the skin. The surface area of these appendages, however, is quite small when compared to the total surface area of skin and therefore they have a minor role in transdermal penetration.

PATHOPHYSIOLOGY

There are many types of chemical agents that are likely to be used in terrorist attacks. Some chemical agents of terrorism act as irritants or vesicants, and damage the skin directly. Nerve agents, in contrast, may be absorbed through the skin but cause little to no clinical effects until they are systemically distributed. Although these agents are structurally dissimilar and act by different mechanisms, they could be employed together for synergistic toxic effect. For example, vesicant application to the skin will result in local tissue damage and a decrease in skin integrity; this would enhance skin absorption of a subsequent nerve agent exposure.

Vesicant agents include nitrogen and sulfur mustards, and lewisite. There are three types of nitrogen mustards (HN-1, HN-2, HN-3) and all were developed as military agents beginning in the 1920s. To date, none have actually been used in warfare. HN-2 was transiently used in cancer therapy but has been replaced by less toxic alternatives. Sulfur mustard (bis-2-chloroethyl sulfide) is an oily, fat- soluble, light yellow-brown substance that smells like garlic. This agent has been employed many times in warfare. It is heavier than water and becomes liquid at room temperature. The liquid is rapidly absorbed through the skin due to its hydrophobic nature. A substantial reservoir of sulfur 14–36% has been measured in heat-separated epidermal membranes of the applied dose for up to 24 hours. Clinically, it is interesting to note that as little as 20 μg/cm^2 of liquid sulfur mustard and 4 μg/cm^2 of vapor sulfur mustard can cause injury to human skin. The difference is due to the fact that up to 80% of the liquid dose will evaporate before penetrating the epidermis. Interestingly, sulfur mustard is more toxic when administered through the percutaneous route compared to oral and subcutaneous routes, with an LD$_{50}$ of 5.7, 8.1, and 23 mg/kg respectively for each route.

Once absorbed into the skin, mustard induces a potent inflammatory response, with epidermal microblister formation; ulceration and necrosis; as well as dermal neutrophilic infiltration, hemorrhage, and necrosis. This intense response is due to activation of inflammatory cytokines and increased prostaglandin formation, which leads to extensive free radical formation. The end result is a disruption of the skin's cytoskeleton framework. The speed of onset of clinical effects correlates with the severity of exposure. This can range from 2 to 48 hours after exposure, but usually occurs within 4 to 8 hours. Erythema, with or without pruritis, is the most common initial skin finding and may progress to vesicles, blisters, and finally bullae. Partial to full thickness burns with skin loss may occur especially in the face,

armpits, groin, and neck. Dark coloration of the skin may also be seen at these sites as well as the flexor regions of the elbow and knee joints. Healing of lesions is very slow due to alkylation of cell types involved in the regeneration process.

Lewisite (2-chlorovinyl dichloroarsine) is an oily, clear liquid that smells like geraniums. Dermal absorption leads to degradation of laminin and Type IV collagen, causing dermo-epidermal detachment. It is absorbed more rapidly and is more potent than sulfur mustard, resulting in deeper lesions with a thicker roofed blister and more severe inflammatory reaction. Deep, aching pain may begin as early as 1 minute after exposure. After 5 minutes, the skin may develop the grey appearance of dead epithelium, and by 30 minutes, erythema and pruritis may ensue. Compared with sulfur mustard exposures, skin heals more rapidly following injury from lewisite. Lewisite absorption can also induce signs of systemic arsenic toxicity.

Nerve agents are absorbed through the skin with little to no local effect, and cause systemic disease. Nerve agents cause illness and death by preventing metabolism of muscarine and nicotine in the nerve synapse, leading to overstimulation of muscarinic and nicotinic receptors. Nerve agents are chemically similar to organophosphate pesticides; therefore, many conclusions drawn about pesticides can be extended to nerve agents. The greatest route of occupational exposure to pesticides is through the skin, with transdermal absorption rates during pesticide spraying being higher than from respiratory exposure. Furthermore, approximately 60–70% of all cases of unintentional acute pesticide poisoning are due to dermal occupational exposure. Depending on the specific agent, symptoms may be sudden, or delayed up to 18 hours after topical exposure.

When 50 μL soman (1,2,2-trimethylpropylmethylphosphonofluoridate) was applied over 3.1 cm^2 of the skin of animals, they died approximately 15 minutes later. This corresponded to a transdermal absorption rate of 0.27 μg/min/cm^2. As it is often impractical to work experimentally with chemical warfare agents, researchers often use substitute chemicals with similar molecular structures. Diethylmalonate acts as a simulant for soman because of its similar physical properties including volatility and solubility. It rapidly penetrates through human skin with maximum flux occurring at 5 hours after exposure. Approximately 16% of the dose penetrates in 24 hours, 45–50% turns to vapor, and the remainder persists in the lipophilic stratum corneum.

Exposing guinea pig skin to 25-μL sarin (isopropylmethylphosphofluoridate) over 3.1 cm^2 after pretreatment with ether or an anionic surfactant led to animal death in 7–19 minutes. The in vitro penetration of sarin (isopropylmethylphosphofluoridate) through human stratum corneum was found to range from 0.21 to 0.49 mg/cm^2/hr from a 7.8-mM donor solution, with absorption being dependent on the hydration state. Very few studies have been conducted examining the transdermal absorption of tabun (ethyl N,N-dimethylphosphoramideocyanidate). Tabun was applied to cat skin at a dose of 109 μL over 4.5 cm^2 and the animal died approximately 50 minutes later making it less toxic than soman. This corresponded to a transdermal delivery rate of 0.78 μg/min/cm^2.

Relative to the other nerve agents, the dermal absorption of VX is slow. Thus, VX is held foremost as a contact poison, rather than an inhalational hazard. The transdermal absorption of VX (o-ethyl-S-2[di-isopropylamino]ethyl) was found to be 0.6% ± 0.19% in human volunteers after a 6-hour exposure. This slow absorption of VX may increase the window of opportunity for decontamination efforts. VX is extremely potent, so absorption of even a minute's amount can result in life-threatening illness. A dose of 5.1, 11.2, 31.8, and 40 μg/kg placed on the cheek, forehead, abdomen, and forearm respectively produced a 70% depression in CHE levels. This inhibition occurred without any obvious effects on the skin.

Predictable, dose-dependent changes to the skin may also be seen after certain types of radiation exposure. Additionally, the skin may be the primary site of persistent contamination from larger α- and β-radioactive particles, necessitating clear and deliberate decontamination strategies. Further discussion of radiation injuries are discussed in Sec. 6.

Biological agents are rarely absorbed through intact skin, but may enter the systemic circulation through abraded skin or open wounds to cause disease. Some agents, such as anthrax spores, can cause disease limited to the skin. Additionally, skin-to-skin contact may transmit disease from one victim to another. A number of biological agents, including anthrax and the poxviruses, manifest classic skin lesions associated with systemic infection. Likewise, microvascular changes manifesting as petechiae or purpura can suggest infection with one of the hemorrhagic viruses. Specifics of disease from the above biological agents are covered in their respective chapters.

PROPERTIES OF EXPOSURE

Factors Influencing Transdermal Penetration

There are striking regional variations in the levels transdermal absorption for a given compound within different sites of the body. Variables influencing absorption include skin thickness, vascularity, moisture content, sweat gland activity, and surface temperature. For example, the percutaneous penetration of parathion across body site demonstrates that relative to the forearm (1.0), the palm of the hand (1.3), and ball of the foot (1.6) have slightly elevated absorption levels. The degree of penetration increases when the skin of the abdomen (2.1) or the back of the hand (2.4) is exposed. The enhancement is even greater in the head, where penetration is 3.7 times greater

for the scalp, 3.9 times greater for the jaw angle, 4.2 times greater for the forehead, and an amazing 7.4 times greater for the axilla. However, the region at the greatest risk for absorption is the thin skin of the scrotal area, which is 11.8 times more permeable than the forearm. Based on these findings, it is clear that exposure to some skin areas may result in greater toxicity than others. Therefore, anatomic location of the exposure should be a key component of the history obtained.

Penetration of toxins through the skin can be limited by the presence of clothing. In vitro studies using human skin and standard soldier clothing showed that the percentage of absorption of parathion was greatest on naked skin (1.78% ± 0.41%), and significantly reduced by both wet/sweated clothing (0.65% ± 0.16%, p = 0.000) and dry clothing (0.29 ± 0.17%, p = 0.000). Of note, even dry clothing permits some amount of absorption to occur, and in the event of a high-potency nerve agent, this exposure may still prove lethal. Chemically saturated clothing may cling to the skin, further increasing contact time with the toxin. For this reason, clothing should be removed as soon as possible after exposure.

Clothing can also serve as a major source of reexposure for bioterrorism agents, even after laundering. In a published case, three pesticide formulators from a manufacturing plant developed organophosphate poisoning due to residual parathion found in clothing that had been washed repeatedly. The first worker spilled a 76% parathion solution on his legs and his inguinal and scrotal areas. He immediately removed his clothes, showered, and changed coveralls. Two days later, he went to the emergency room with a plasma cholinesterase level of 340 U/L (normal range: 700–19,000 U/L). The patient was treated with atropine and pralidoxime, admitted for observation, and released the next morning. Eight days later, a second worker from the same plant was then sent to the emergency room and had a plasma cholinesterase level of 410 U/L. This formulator, however, had not been working with any organophosphates, so the method of his poisoning was unclear. A third worker at the plant became ill 3 days later while packing pesticides. His plasma cholinesterase level was 500 U/L and he also received antidotal therapy. The plant safety officer discovered that the coveralls from the original patient had not been bagged and burned after the initial spill, but instead were laundered for reuse. The worker wore them again and became ill. The same coveralls were laundered a second time and were subsequently worn by both of the other poisoning victims. This was confirmed by analyzing portions of the uniform where the spill had occurred for parathion using gas chromatography that demonstrated that 70,000 ppm (7%) of ethyl parathion remained in the coveralls. The clothes were then washed twice more, this time with soda ash, bleach, and detergent, and 2% of the organophosphate still remained. This case series illustrates the importance of proper disposal of contaminated clothing to prevent secondary exposure to organophosphate nerve agents.

Finally, environmental conditions (ambient temperature and humidity) can greatly influence the transdermal absorption of chemicals. For example, VX penetration ranged from 4% at 18°C to 32% at 46°C when applied to the cheek and from 0.4% at 18°C to 2.9% at 46°C when spread over the forearm. In vitro studies demonstrated that parathion absorption significantly increased when either the temperature was raised from 37°C to 42°C or when the humidity was raised from 20% to 90%. Temperature-dependent changes in the physical state of a toxin may reflect an increased ability to penetrate skin. Cutaneous vasodilation in response to heat permits a penetrating toxin greater access to the systemic circulation. Furthermore, the increase in heat and humidity will lead to more sweating. The transdermal absorption of parathion through a uniform saturated with sweat is significantly greater than absorption through a dry uniform (0.65% vs. 0.29%, p = 0.007). Finally, evaporation of sulfur mustard would be less in a humid environment, resulting in greater skin contact time.

DECONTAMINATION

The first principle of decontamination is to remove the source of contamination as soon as possible. Clothing should be removed immediately. This step can reduce contamination by an estimated 75–90% depending on the amount of clothing the victim was wearing at the time of the exposure. For most agents, the skin should be quickly washed with soap and warm water, or a 0.5% sodium hypochlorite solution (1 part standard household bleach to 5 parts water). Rapidly flushing the skin with water, for example, increased the lethal dose of sarin by 10.6 times. Furthermore, a 2-minute soap and water decontamination performed 15 minutes after application decreased the absorption of the pesticide azodrin from 14% to 2%. Decontamination guidelines demonstrating that flushing with water for 2–5 minutes should adequately remove most chemicals; however, that time should be increased to 5–6 minutes for patients who require critical care. The area should then be scrubbed again thoroughly with a single-use sponge, including nails, toenails, and hair, if appropriate. Vigorous scrubbing of the skin with stiff bristle brushes is discouraged, as the mechanical trauma may alter skin integrity and permit greater absorption. The area should then be washed again with soap and water and then rinsed with rubbing alcohol, followed by a final rinse of clear water. Clean clothing should then be put on and the contaminated clothing should be burned.

Fuller's earth was found to be effective as a skin decontaminant for sulfur mustard, reducing transdermal penetration by 91–95%. Aggressive strategies including dermabrasion and laser debridement have also been explored as methods to remove residual mustard. Cooling the skin after exposure has been experimentally demonstrated to slow absorption and ameliorate cellular injury from both mustard and lewisite.

A number of barrier creams have been evaluated for their protective effects against bioterrorism agents. Pretreatment of skin with these formulations may either increase or reduce lesions from sulfur mustard, depending on their composition. Perfluorinated barrier creams were effective at blocking sulfur mustard absorption under occluded conditions, but increased penetration when used under unoccluded conditions. Furthermore, some barrier creams reduced the effectiveness of fuller's earth as a decontaminant. It is hypothesized that the enhancement is due to prevention of sulfur mustard evaporation, which can account for up to 80% of the applied dose. Other barrier creams have been developed, which have been shown to effectively reduce the transdermal absorption of sulfur mustard, soman, and VX.

It is essential that the skin decontamination process does not itself enhance transdermal penetration. This can be tricky because both decontamination methods and barrier creams can actually increase the absorption of bioterrorism agents. For example, a number of different decontamination solutions were used to remove the soman agonist diethylmalonate. If they were not applied within the first 15 minutes after exposure, these solvents actually increased the penetration during the first 2 hours after decontamination. This can be explained by the fact that once a chemical has been absorbed into the stratum corneum, it cannot easily be removed by washing.

Chelating agents applied to the skin after chemical exposure may form complexes with the toxin and prevent its penetration into the skin. 2,3-Dimercaptopropanol (also known as British antilewisite or BAL) is recommended following exposure to lewisite. Recent research specific to the skin has centered on the development of postexposure therapy. Animal studies suggest an ointment containing zinc chloride and desferrioxamine may prevent nuclear damage and limit injury from nitrogen mustard. Povidone-iodine application may also reduce injury from sulfur mustard by reducing collagenolytic activity of the toxin.

CONCLUSION

This review has demonstrated that the skin is a major target for agents. Environmental factors, anatomical site, and skin integrity can significantly alter the quantity of chemicals that will be absorbed. Decontamination should be performed quickly after exposure, but care should be taken or penetration can actually increase after the decontamination procedure.

Suggested Reading

al-Saleh IA. Pesticides: a review article. *J Environ Pathol Toxicol Oncol.* 1994;13:151–61.

Chilcott RP, Brown RF, Rice P. Non-invasive quantification of skin injury resulting from exposure to sulphur mustard and Lewisite vapours. *Burns.* 2000;26:245–50.

Chilcott RP, Jenner J, Carrick W, et al. Human skin absorption of Bis-2-(chloroethyl)sulphide (sulphur mustard) in vitro. *J Appl Toxicol.* 2000;20:349–55.

Chilcott RP, Jenner J, Hotchkiss SA, et al. Evaluation of barrier creams against sulphur mustard. I. In vitro studies using human skin. *Skin Pharmacol Appl Skin Physiol.* 2002;15: 225–35.

Clifford NJ, Nies AS. Organophosphate poisoning from wearing a laundered uniform previously contaminated with parathion. *JAMA.* 1989;262:3035–6.

Craig FN, Cummings EG, Sim VM. Environmental temperature and the percutaneous absorption of a cholinesterase inhibitor, VX. *J Invest Dermatol.* 1977;68:357–61.

Cullander C, Guy RH. (D) Routes of delivery: case studies (6). Transdermal delivery of peptides and proteins. *Adv Drug Deliv Rev.* 1992;8:291–329.

Fredrikkson T. Influence of solvents and surface active agents on the barrier function of the skin towards sarin. *Acta Derm Venerol.* 1969;49:481–3.

Houston M, Hendrickson RG. Decontamination. *Crit Care Clin.* 2005;21(4):653–72.

Nelson P, Hancock JR, Sawyer TW. Therapeutic effects of hypothermia on Lewisite toxicity. *Toxicology.* 2006;222(1–2):8–16.

Rice P. Sulfur mustard injuries of the skin. Pathophysiology and management. *Toxicol Rev.* 2003;22(2):111–8.

Shelnutt S.R., Goad P., Belsito D.V., Dermatological Toxicity of Hexavalent Chromium. *Critical Reviews in Toxicology.* 2007:37:375–387.

Vijayaraghavan R, Kulkarni A, Pant SC, et al. Differential toxicity of sulfur mustard administered through percutaneous, subcutaneous, and oral routes. *Toxicol Appl Pharmacol.* 2005;202(2): 180–8.

Wester RM, Tanojo H, Maibach HI, et al. Predicted chemical warfare agent VX toxicity to uniformed soldier using in vitro human skin exposure and absorption. *Toxicol Appl Pharmacol.* 2000;168(2):149–52.

Wormser U, Brodsky B, Reich R. Topical treatment with povidone iodine reduces nitrogen mustard-induced skin collagenolytic activity. *Arch Toxicol.* 2002;76(2):119–21.

6

NEUROLOGIC ISSUES IN EMERGENCY BIOTERRORISM

Saptarshi Bandyopadhyay and Michael Rezak

NEUROLOGIC ISSUES IN EMERGENCY BIOTERRORISM

- Nausea and vomiting are sensitive indicators of contact with noxious stimuli.
- Terror attacks with toxins and chemicals will produce weakness, paralysis, seizures, and coma.
- Cerebral anthrax can cause headaches due to elevation of intracranial pressure.
- Mainstay therapy for seizure control is benzodiazepines.
- Central neurogenic hyperventilation may be present in individuals in a light coma.

INTRODUCTION

Though humans have arguably developed the most complicated nervous system of all living organisms, even primitive organisms (such as worms of the phylum *Mollusca*) display complicated behaviors in response to noxious stimuli. This behavior is mediated through connections between nociceptive receptors to the rest of the nervous system. Physicians interpret the manifestation of this behavior in humans as neurologic signs and symptoms. Living beings, no matter how primitive their nervous system, have a survival advantage if noxious stimuli can be detected at low levels and subsequently avoided. For this reason, neurologic signs and symptoms will often be the presenting feature of a toxidrome and, by extension, the first indication of a bioterror attack. Neurologic signs also appear without the normal intraspecies variability or gradation of symptoms seen

with other organ systems. Neurotoxicologists and emergency physicians are, therefore, fortunate that diseases and insults to the nervous system typically manifest promptly and obviously.

A recently published (and thorough) textbook of neurotoxicology reviewed more than 350 putative substances (natural compounds, synthetic chemicals, as well as biological toxins) known to cause damage to the nervous system of humans. To review all such compounds in the space allotted to this chapter would be an impossible task. Moreover, we attempt to present a symptom-oriented differential that would be diagnostically useful for what we believe will be the "likely" agents in a bioterror attack. However, there are a few principles which will help guide a clinician in understanding the neurological signs and symptoms of exposure to these agents.

The concept of "pathoclysis" is of major importance in determining why certain signs or symptoms predominate in the casualties of an attack with a specific bioterror agent. This hypothesis, as formulated and popularized by the neuroscientists Drs O. and C. Voight, states that each neuron is vulnerable to its own particular chemical or biological agent. While there is some theoretical disagreement regarding whether this vulnerability displays dose-response characteristics or an "all-or-none" phenomenon, this concept is useful in that it allows the physician to sometimes determine the nature of the agent of attack based on the presenting neurologic sign or symptom.

Another major idea useful in recognizing toxidromes is the concept of "fatiguability" as it relates to the nervous system. Comparing the early and late signs of a nicotinic agent attack illustrates the concept: initially, the toxidrome involves tachycardia due to the activity of the agent at nicotinic acetylcholine receptors in the sympathetic ganglia. However, after a few minutes (probably before the patient even presents for treatment), the opposite sign—bradycardia—will be present because of physiologic compensation towards muscarinic activity (relative to the nicotinic nerve endings) and because of the downregulation of nicotinic receptors and depletion of acetylcholine at the sites of nerve terminals within the sympathetic ganglia.

Ten common neurologic signs and symptoms that can be seen in a bioterror attack include nausea, dizziness and vertigo, headache, ocular and cranial nerve abnormalities, seizures, muscle fasciculations or weakness, paralysis, and coma. Biologic agents can cause almost any of these signs and symptoms and may herald the onset of nerve damage, whereas the presenting signs and symptoms in the case of a chemical attack mainly consist of weakness, paralysis, acute seizures, and coma. For the sake of continuity, only these 10 symptoms are discussed in this chapter. Other signs and symptoms, which may have a neurologic component, are discussed in more appropriate places: for instance, a discussion of delirium, hallucinations, and memory disturbance, inasmuch as it is related to bioterror, is deferred to in the Acute Psychiatric Issues section. Syndromes where neurologic manifestations are late and signs not prominent in making the diagnosis—for instance, vesicular smallpox—are also discussed separately.

The challenge in the case of a neurologic manifestation of a possible bioterror-related illness is to make a diagnosis as rapidly as possible—that is, to associate a particular neurologic symptom with one of the many syndromes to which it belongs. Not all neurologic signs will be related to a toxin-mediated syndrome (referred to as a "toxidrome"), and not all toxidromes are related to bioterror. The physician should be alert to the possibility that the neurologic sign or symptom may be a manifestation of an unrelated illness or cause. However, clinical suspicion of a bioterror event should be raised in "mass casualty" situations, when multiple patients present with similar signs and symptoms, and also when rare or unusual symptoms appear in a "high-profile" proband. Recognizing a bioterror toxidrome requires knowledge (or suspicion) of the route of dissemination, the careful evaluation of other organ systems in affected patients, judicious laboratory testing based on clinical suspicion and evidence, and possibly consultation with a neurologist or more experienced colleague.

A point of confusion (and contention!) may exist in determining when a specialist such as a neurologist is needed in the diagnosis and treatment of toxidromes. Some diseases and toxidromes are sufficiently distinct and rare to where a *single* incidence, especially of a "high-profile" nature, will be significant enough to warrant

consultation with a neurologist for accurate diagnosis and testing. Additionally, in case of a mass casualty with multiple neurologic complaints, the situation has the potential to quickly overwhelm the medical system. We feel in this case that it is appropriate to seek the assistance of a neurologist, especially when the agent of a possible bioterror attack is not known. Of course, it should go without saying that any physician who strongly suspects that his or her patient is the victim of a bioterror attack should notify local, state, and federal authorities.

Nausea and Vomiting

Neurologists recognize the chemotrigger zone (CTZ), located in the area postrema (dorsal portion) of the medulla near the caudal opening of the spinal canal, as the main mediator of the sense of "nausea" and the initiator of the involuntary reverse-peristaltic contractions that culminates in emesis. Ingested, inhaled, innoculated, or dermally absorbed toxins can stimulate the CTZ owing to the multiple ways in which chemical information reaches this sensitive zone: the CTZ collects nociceptive input from the stomach through the dorsal nucleus of the vagus, receives vestibular input through the cerebellar peduncles, and samples the chemical milieu of cerebrospinal fluid (CSF) via diffusion from the floor of the fourth ventricle. It is one of the "circumventricular organs" where the blood-brain barrier is porous or nonexistent. Ingested toxins stimulate nociceptive receptors in the stomach and activate the vagus nerve; inhaled toxins reach the CTZ through diffusion from the lungs to the bloodstream, or through the nerves in the cribriform plate into the olfactory bulb, then bypass the blood-brain barrier. Toxins innoculated or absorbed through the dermis may similarly bypass the blood-brain barrier or lead to metabolic derangements, which alter the chemical gradient of the blood-CSF barrier.

Nausea is, therefore, a sensitive symptom of contact with noxious stimuli. However, this symptom is also associated with many other signs and symptoms, some of which are discussed in this chapter. Vertigo and headache can directly produce nausea. Because there are multiple ways in which the CTZ can be stimulated, the phenomenon of nausea may *appear* to violate the principle of pathoclisis. However, there are billions of individual nerves, which can stimulate this important defense mechanism. For this reason, many state and local departments of health have suggested that "any unexplained gastrointestinal (GI) illness" is a potential indication of a bioterror event. Physicians should recognize nausea as a *nonspecific* symptom and a component of multiple toxidromes. See Table 6-1 for possible agents that induce nausea.

Ondansetron, a selective 5-HT$_3$ receptor antagonist, is very effective at controlling nausea. The adult dosing of

BIOTERROR AGENTS, WHICH INDUCE NAUSEA

Agent Class and Agent(s)	Toxidrome	Complications and Confirmatory Diagnostic Test	Specific Neurologic Therapy	Comments
Nicotinic agents Anatoxin-a Anatoxin-a(s) Epibatidine Nicotine (in DMSO)	Muscular twitching, weakness, and cramps; pallor with tachycardia and hypertension; seizures with loss of consciousness and apnea		Supportive therapy Mecamylamine (not readily available)	Avoid mouth-to-mouth ventilation
Muscarinic agents Muscarine Epibatidine Cyclopeptides: Amanita Mushroom	Increased secretions (saliva, tears, rhinorrhea, bronchorrhea, sweating);* bronchoconstriction with dyspnea; vomiting and diarrhea; bradycardia with hypotension; miosis; urinary incontinence		No antidote	See below
Organophosphates Diazinon Malathion Sevin Lannate Durisban Similar pesticides	Cholinergic crisis (nicotinic and/or muscarinic symptoms)	Multiple casualties in short period of time Diagnosed based on toxidrome Decreased RBC Acetylcholinesterase (AChE) activity is confirmatory Decreased RBC Butyrylcholinesterase (BChE) levels also present, but assay not commonly performed	Mark 1 Kit: Atropine 2 mg IM/IV Q5 minute titrate to effectiveness 2-PAM 600–1800 mg IM or 1 g IV over 30 minutes. Pyridostigmine 30–60 mg PO Q8H (adult dose) doesnot prevent seizures Diazepam or lorazepam 1 mg IV for seizures if >4 mg atropine given Ventilatory support Huperzine A, a plant-derived reversible and selective AChE inhibitor has been shown in European studies to prevent seizures, but may not be available in the United States	Differential includes occupational exposure to insecticides or pesticides, cyanide poisoning, myasthenia gravis
Nerve agents Tabun (GA) Sarin (GB) Soman (GD)	Muscarinic symptoms (See above)* Dim vision, miosis Eye and nose irritation Wheezing, rhonchi, respiratory arrest;			Erroneously called "nerve gas" in lay press

(Continued)

Agent Class and Agent(s)	Toxidrome	Complications and Confirmatory Diagnostic Test	Specific Neurologic Therapy	Comments
Cyclohexyl sarin (GF) VX	Heart block and other cardiac conduction abnormalities Decreased memory and concentration; (In high exposure: loss of consciousness, flaccid paralysis, and seizures) "Intermediate syndrome" (relapse) 5–18 days after therapy Late sequelae includes polyneuropathy Pyramidal signs and symptoms			Agents can be synthesized or obtained illegally in countries that formerly weaponized nerve agents
Chemical asphyxiants Hydrogen cyanide (AC) Cyanogen chloride (CK) Arsine (SA)	"Pink" skin and bright red venous blood Giddiness in seconds, to depressed consciousness Palpitations; dizziness, vomiting; headache, vertigo, delayed pupillary light reflex; eye irritation; tachycardia and hyperventilation; drowsiness; (In high exposure: immediate coma, seizures, convulsions, cardiorespiratory arrest, death within 1 to 15 minutes) Delayed toxic effects include parkinsonism, dysarthria, ocular abnormalities, and ataxia Cavitation of putamen and globus pallidus	Anion gap metabolic acidosis Increased serum lactate Venous O$_2$ saturation >85% Increased blood cyanide or thiocyanate levels Increased urine thiocyanate level	Decontamination 100% O$_2$ by face mask Intubation Cyanide antidote kit: Amyl nitrite amp Q5 min Sodium nitrite 300 mg IV over 10 minutes Sodium thiosulfate 12.5 g IV Hydroxocobalamin 2.5–5 grams is an alternative but somewhat impractical Adjust dosing based on weight and hematocrit	Only cyanogen chloride demonstrates bitter almond odor Differential includes industrial or occupational exposure to organic solvents, carbon monoxide poisoning, hypoglycemia, electrolyte disturbance, postictal state, hydrogen sulfide (H$_2$S) exposure, nerve agent poisoning
Vesicants/blister agents Sulfur mustard Lewisite Nitrogen mustard Mustard lewisite Phosgene-oxime Methyl bromide	Mucosal irritation and burning (eyes, mouth, nose) Skin erythema and blistering Swollen eyes Dyspnea Airway sloughing and pulmonary edema Tachycardia and hypotension Transient renal insufficiency Hepatic injury Sepsis Dizziness, headache, confusion, lethargy, seizures, coma	Metabolic abnormalities Neutropenia elevated urine thiodiglycol Pathologic findings on tissue biopsy	No antidote for mustards or methyl bromide Dimercaprol (BAL) 5 mg/kg; then, 2.5 mg/kg one or two per day for 10 days (if lewisite agent) Therapy in a burn unit Ventilatory support Ocular care Supportive care	Mustards demonstrate odor of garlic, horseradish, or mustard Differential includes industrial or accidental exposure to sodium hydroxide (NaOH), ammonia, or other caustic agents

Agent	Clinical features	Diagnosis	Treatment	Comments
Riot control agents Mace (CN) Malononitrile (CS) Bromobenzylcyanide (CA) Dibenz-oxazepine (CR) Pepper spray (OC) Adamsite (DM)	Mucosal irritation; burning, itching, red skin; dyspnea; diarrhea; abdominal cramping; headache; depression	Rarely, pulmonary edema on chest x-ray (most common cause of mortality)	No definitive treatment Skin decontamination Respiratory support Time for metabolism of agent	Considered a nonlethal agent, but can be lethal if exposure is massive as in, for example, an uncontrolled release
Anesthetic gases Chloroform (Freon) Phosgene Diphosgene Chloropicrin Halothane Cyclopropane Ethers Nitrous oxide (N_2O) Sulfur dioxide (SO_2)	Confusion; relaxation; dizziness and drowsiness; headache; dry mouth, oropharyngeal burning; choking and respiratory discomfort leading to pulmonary edema Pulmonary infiltrates, predisposing to lung abscess Hepatic and renal toxicity Cardiac arrest	Multiple casualties in short period of time Diagnosis made by toxidrome LFTs peak 3–4 days after exposure if hepatic toxicity present	Supportive, high-PEEP cardiorespiratory care N-Acetylcysteine for liver dysfunction shown efficacy in animals Steroids prevent pulmonary edema from nitrous oxide	Water solubility of the agent will determine amount of mucosal irritation and need for suctioning of secretions
Opiates and narcotics Aerosolized fentanyl 3-methyl fentanyl Carfentanil Trimethyl phentanylum Kokol-1 (Russian "knockout" gas)	Euphoria to drowsiness to depressed LOC to coma Respiratory depression (bradypnea, hypopnea) Miosis (pupillary dilation can be seen in hypoxic patients) Nystagmus Seizures Ventricular arrhythmias	Multiple casualties in short period of time Diagnosis made by toxidrome	Naloxone 0.4–2 mg SQ/IV Q2–3 minutes with response in 10 minutes	Differential also includes clonidine poisoning, cholinergic crisis, phenothiazine poisoning, PCP intoxication, pontine or subarachnoid hemorrhage
Phytotoxins Ricin (castor bean oil) Abrin (rosary pea toxin)	High fever	Initial leukocytosis ELISA for ricin or abrin toxin	No antidote Activated charcoal lavage	Small amounts (200 mcg of ricin, 1 mcg of abrin) are potentially lethal Differential includes tularemia, plague, Q fever, staphylococcal enterotoxin B, phosgene gas, and exposure to pyrolysis by-products of organofluorine polymers or other organo-halides, oxides of nitrogen
By ingestion	Abdominal pain Circulatory collapse and shock Necrosis of liver, spleen, and kidneys			

(Continued)

BIOTERROR AGENTS, WHICH INDUCE NAUSEA (CONTINUED)

Agent Class and Agent(s)	Toxidrome	Complications and Confirmatory Diagnostic Test	Specific Neurologic Therapy	Comments
By inhalation	Chest tightness, coughing, weakness Tracheobronchitis Pulmonary edema Necrotizing pneumonia			
By injection	Severe localized pain, muscle and regional lymph node necrosis Moderate hemorrhagic necrosis of visceral organs Lymphatic congestion Neuronal death in active cells (e.g., pacemaker neurons)			Has been used in the past by Romanian secret service in assassination attempts using inoculation device
Biologic toxins Botulinum toxin (inhaled) Saxitoxin	Ptosis and poorly reactive mitotic (dilated) pupils Disconjugate gaze, diplopia, facial diplegia Progressive, descending bulbar signs including dysphagia Muscular weakness, respiratory compromise	Normal NCV and SEPs Small motor unit potentials Incremental response to 50 Hz repetitive stimulation	Trivalent equine antitoxin (A, B, E) to botulinum toxin 10,000 IU slow IV infusion then 50,000 IU IM daily available from CDC Guanidine HCl 50 mg/kg has been tried Supportive therapy including mechanical ventilation for VC <15 cc/kg or NIF <20 cm H_2O	Differential includes Lambert-Eaton like myasthenia gravis, tick paralysis, pontine infarction, diphtheria, and Guillain-Barré (Miller-Fisher variant)
Staphylococcus enterotoxin B Shigatoxin (aerosolized)	Fever/chills Headache Myalgia Cough			
Trichothecene (T2) mycotoxins: Fusarium Myrothecium, Trichoderma, Verticinonosporium, Stachybotrys Ciguatera	Mucosal erythema and hemorrhage Red, blistering skin and mucosa (especially ocular) Increased salivation, coughing Dyspnea, pulmonary edema Hepatic and renal necrosis Hallucinations and dysesthesias (especially hot/cold reversal)	ELISHA for some agents available from commercial laboratories GC/MS of specific toxins in specialized laboratories	No antidote Supportive care Activated charcoal lavage Consider high-dose steroids	Differential includes exposure to choking agents including concentrated ozone, nitrous oxide, phosgene, ammonia though mycotoxins tend to produce more severe mucosal irritation

	Signs/Symptoms	Laboratory	Treatment	Comments
	Arthralgia, myalgia, polymyopathy Ataxia and lower extremity weakness Respiratory depression, paralysis, shock, seizures and coma in severe cases		Mannitol 1 g/kg IV for ciguatera toxin	
Scombrotoxin	Headache Pruritic erythema (from histadine) Vomiting, abdominal pain Dizziness Palpitations and tachycardia Breathlessness, wheezing Hypotension and shock in severe cases		Antihistamine such as Benadryl 1.25 mg/kg PO Q4-6H	
Inorganic toxins Mercury Arsenic Lead	Headache Intention tremor Confusion, ataxia, incoordination Dysarthria Change in behavior or mood ("mad hatter") Lethargy alternating with Irritability Abdominal pain, anorexia, weight loss (long-term) Renal Tubular Necrosis Stomatitis, metallic taste, hematemesis Encephalopathy	Microcytic anemia Heavy metal levels in urine	Gastric lavage (with proteinaceous fluid) Sodium formaldehyde sulfoxylate 250 mL in 5% solution to decrease absorption Dimercaprol (BAL) 4–5 mg/kg Q4H × 6 then Q6H × 8 then Q8H for 10 days, not to exceed 300 mg (adults) Mannitol 1g/kg IV as a temporizing measure until dialysis for renal failure	Mercury can be ingested (mercury salts), inhaled (mercury vapor), or dermally absorbed Symptoms may appear mildly and gradually months to years after exposure
Radiation 0.5–2 Gy	Anorexia and GI manifestations from mucosal sloughing Diarrhea Sepsis (from translocation of gut flora)	Leukopenia Toxidrome Mass casualty situation	Potassium iodide within 1 hour of exposure (competes with radioactive iodine)	Threshold for symptoms is 200 rads (about 2 Gy). Onset within 6 hours unless otherwise indicated Late sequelae include hypothyroidism and thyroid cancer due to absorption of radioactive iodine
2–10 Gy	Epilation, erythema, desquamation with necrosis Headache, vertigo, altered mental status, cerebral edema, seizures			
More than 10 Gy	Above symptoms, onset within 30 minutes			

* Often memorized using the mnemonic SLUDGE for Salivation, Lacrimation, Urination, Defecation, GI disturbances, and Emesis.

10 mg intravenously (IV), or the dosing based on the weight-based formula of 0.15 mg/kg body weight can be repeated every 4 hours. While ondansetron's mechanism of action has not been fully characterized, it is not a dopamine-receptor antagonist. Serotonin receptors of the 5-HT$_3$ type are present both peripherally on vagal nerve terminals and centrally in the chemoreceptor trigger zone of the area postrema. It is not certain whether ondansetron's antiemetic action in chemotherapy-induced nausea and vomiting is mediated centrally, peripherally, or in both sites; however, it is the most effective treatment for nausea. Alternatively, agents of the phenothiazine class such as prochlorperazine (Compazine) or promethazine (Phenergan) can be used to control nausea. Because of its antihistaminic properties, promethazine is considered a superior agent for treating vertigo and motion sickness than prochlorperazine. However, owing to the dopaminergic properties of the phenothiazines, both of these agents can theoretically cause dystonia, give rise to extrapyramidal symptoms, and worsen parkinsonism. Though promethazine is the less likely of the two agents to cause this side effect, all phenothiazines should be avoided in pediatric cases, cases involving 1-methyl-4-phenyl-1,2,3,6-tetrahydropyridine (MPTP) poisoning, and in the elderly with Parkinson's disease. Phenothiazines are dosed every 4 hours (like ondansetron) at a fixed dose as they are generally reserved for use in otherwise healthy adults.

Dizziness and Vertigo

Patients describe many sensory phenomena with the term "dizziness." This term can refer to

1. **True vertigo.** The illusion of "whirling," twisting, spinning, rotation, swaying, tilting, impulsion, movement of oneself or one's surroundings (oscillopsia), which may or may not be accompanied by autonomic symptoms of pallor, diaphoresis, nausea, or apprehension.
2. **Presyncope.** The sensation of an impending loss of consciousness or fainting (presyncope) possibly accompanied by the above autonomic symptoms.
3. **Disequilibrium.** A generalized feeling of leg weakness, muscular fatigue, imbalance, faintness, unsteadiness, or nonrotatory swaying.
4. **Pseudovertigo.** "Swimming sensation," "giddiness," "unreality," disassociation, double vision, or other unnatural experience.

Though there is a sizable overlap between these categories, and though patients may not be able to give information accurate enough to distinguish between these causes, it is crucial for the physician in a bioterror setting (just as it is crucial for a neurologist in a general setting) to *attempt* to distinguish what the patient means by the sensation of "dizziness," as the differential diagnosis can be greatly limited with this approach.

The causes of dizziness encompass neurolotoxic, ototoxic, cardiosuppressive, ophthalmoplegic, psychiatric, and other pathologic causes. In this sense, the number of potential causes is as varied as the causes of nausea. Table 6-2 lists the causes for each sensation and possible etiologies related to bioterror. A list encompassing etiologies of dizziness *not* caused by bioterror agents would be long and a full discussion is beyond the scope of this chapter; indeed, investigating the many causes of vertigo keeps many neurologists busy in their clinical practice. However, clusters of patients arriving in a short period of time through general patient intake (e.g., emergency room or urgent care clinic) should alert the physician to the possibility of exposure to a single common agent.

The main utility of recognizing dizziness and vertigo is another sensitive indicator of neurologic insult (Table 6-3). As such, the treatment of dizziness and vertigo in the mass casualty setting consists mainly of determining the underlying cause and treating appropriately. Clinical features that appear in the evaluation of vertigo include orthostasis, a useful indicator of vascular dysfunction, nystagmus, a useful indicator of vestibular malfunction, and a positive Nylen-Bárány maneuver, indicating a (benign) positional vertigo and for the most part ruling out a systemic cause.

The treatment of vertigo depends mainly on its cause—another reason for establishing the type of "dizziness" following a subjective complaint. Though disorienting and an uncomfortable sensation, to say the least, the symptoms of dizziness or vertigo by themselves are not life-threatening. However, when it prevents further evaluation or therapeutic measures, the following medications may be tried for symptomatic relief:*

- Diphenhydramine (Benadryl)
- Scopolamine (Transderm-Scop or Donnatal)
- Promethazine (Phenergan)
- Diazepam (Valium)
- Meclizine hydrochloride (Antivert)

---

* As there have been few uses of these agents in the setting of a bioterror attack, the indications and efficacy represent our best guess based on the mechanism of action of the medications and the known pathophysiology of the bioterror agents. Meclizine, in particular, is useful in Meniere's syndrome in which both the vestibular and auditory system is affected. Its effects as a treatment for bioterror agents is unknown, though it has central anticholinergic and antihistaminic action at the chemoreceptor trigger zone. It also decreases excitability of the middle ear labyrinth and blocks conduction in the middle ear vestibular-cerebellar pathways, and is thus one of the most powerful agents known for vertigo.

TABLE 6-2

DIFFERENTIAL CAUSES OF "DIZZINESS"

Type of Dizziness	Etiologic Factors	Key Findings	Possible Bioterror-Related Causes
Vertigo	Disturbance in peripheral or central nervous system pathways of vestibular system Direct neurotoxicity to vestibular nerve	Nystagmus Reduced response to caloric stimulation Abnormal auditory-evoked response	Posttraumatic vertigo Salicylate poisoning Anesthetic gas exposure Heavy metal exposure
Presyncope	Relative lack of cerebral perfusion, cardiac dysfunction, vascular stenosis Qualitative defect of blood, impaired oxygenation, decreased blood glucose	Orthostasis Low blood glucose or oxygenation Bradycardia or hypotension	Cyanide agents Carbon monoxide (from smoke inhalation or incendiary device)
Disequilibrium	Mismatch from vestibular, visual, and somatosensory (kinesthetic) systems Oculomotor disorders Ophthalmoplegia Diplopia	Oscillopsia	GABA-antagonists Heavy metal toxicity Antiepileptic medication (e.g., treatment of seizures on scene)
Pseudovertigo	Neuropsychiatric causes Hysteria Neurosis Depression Seizures Hyperventilation syndrome	Symptoms do not fit with recognized condition Symptoms not reproduced with physical maneuvers or testing	Posttraumatic stress syndrome Postepileptic fit

Headache

As a symptom of many afflictions of the nervous system and other parts of the body, the frequency of headache in the general population is so great—and its etiologies so diverse—that discussing the pathophysiology of this symptom would entail an entire book. The basic mechanisms of intracranial headache are

1. Traction on the great veins or venous sinuses of the brain.
2. Traction, distension, or dilation of the large arteries of the skull and brain, including the middle meningeal artery from hypertension, migraine headaches, a migraine variant, cluster headache, etc.
3. Infection or blockage of the frontal, maxillary, sphenoid, sinuses, or ethmoid air cells; or pain referred from ocular, oropharyngeal, aural, or nasal structures.
4. Inflammation or spasms near the pain-sensitive structures of the head and upper part of the spine (meninges, blood vessels, skin, periosteum, ligaments, muscles, cranial nerves V, VII, IX, X, the olfactory bulb, and the nerve roots of cranial nerves II and III).
5. Direct pressure on the same pain-sensitive structures.
6. Headaches of ocular origin, including those arising from eye strain, diplopia, raised intraocular pressure, uveitis, or iridocyclitis.
7. Miscellaneous causes such as exertion, psychogenic factors, or iatrogenic.

By history and context of presentation, the physician should be able to determine if the headache is of an acute nature or of a chronic, recurrent nature. Moreover, the quality, intensity, mode of onset, duration, location, precipitating or aggravating factors, time-intensity curve, and any family history of headaches should also be obtained through history, as this information could guide the physician to determine whether the headache is of a benign or organic cause (such is the case of the vast majority of headaches). Some common organic (noninfectious) causes of headache include migraine, cluster, or tension headaches, subarachnoid hemorrhage, intracranial mass lesions, temporal arteritis, and posttraumatic headaches. Vascular headaches are typically unilateral, periodic, *throbbing* (rarely, sharp) headaches that can be associated with nausea, phonophotophobia, and sensitivity to pressure. Migraine headaches and its variants are worse during times of hormonal flux (in women) and can be made worse by certain foods (caffeine, alcohol, salted meat, chocolate) and exposure to chemicals. The headaches of anoxia, carbon monoxide intoxication, circulatory insufficiency, foreign protein reactions, and hypercapnia are principally of vascular origin. Thus, a mass admission of patients with migraine- or cluster-type headaches should not prompt the physician to automatically eliminate a bioterror agent as a cause.

Headaches due to raised intracranial pressure can be seen in the toxidromes of meningoencephalitis and

TABLE 6-3

BIOTERROR AGENTS, WHICH INDUCE DIZZINESS OR VERTIGO

Agent Class and Agent(s)	Toxidrome	Complications and Confirmatory Diagnostic Test	Specific Neurologic Therapy	Comments
Antimuscarinic agents Jimson Weed "Agent Buzz" (QNB, BZ)	Anticholinergic syndrome* Mydriasis and loss of visual accommodation Dry mucous membranes Urinary retention Anhidrosis Hyperthermia Tachycardia Hypertension Confusion, delirium, memory loss Paresthesia, dysarthria, Hallucinations, folie-a-deux, mass hysteria Seizures Long-term sequelae may include phantom behaviors such as "wool-picking" or memory loss	No rapid tests enable a health-care provider to diagnose exposure to QNB Obtain extra blood and urine samples, as tests have been developed to confirm human exposure to QNB DIC is a potential complication Obtain CBC, clotting studies, LFTs and renal function tests	Physostigmine 1 mg IV/IM as a test dose Max dose 0.06 mg/kg IM in adults, 0.02 mg/kg IM in children	Stockpiled by armies for use as an incapacitating agent LD50 is 1000 times dose needed for incapacitation Avoid meclizine and scopolamine in this setting owing to their anticholinergic properties
Chemical asphyxiants Hydrogen cyanide (AC) Cyanogen chloride (CK) Arsine (SA)	Nausea and vomiting "Pink" skin and bright red venous blood Giddiness in seconds, to depressed consciousness Palpitations Headache Delayed pupillary light reflex Eye irritation Tachycardia and hyperventilation Drowsiness (In high exposure: immediate coma, seizures, convulsions, cardiorespiratory arrest, death within 1–15 minutes)	Anion gap metabolic acidosis Increased serum lactate Venous O_2 saturation >85% Increased blood cyanide or thiocyanate levels Increased urine thiocyanate level	Decontamination 100% O_2 by face mask intubation Cyanide antidote kit: Amyl nitrite amp Q5 min Sodium nitrite 300 mg IV over 10 minutes Sodium thiosulfate 12.5 g IV Hydroxocobalamin 2.5–5 g is an alternative but somewhat impractical Adjust dosing based on weight and hematocrit	Only cyanogen chloride demonstrates bitter almond odor Differential includes industrial or occupational exposure to organic solvents, carbon monoxide poisoning, hypoglycemia, electrolyte disturbance, postictal state, hydrogen sulfide (H_2S) exposure, nerve agent poisoning

Agent	Signs/Symptoms	Diagnosis	Treatment	Comments
Anesthetic gases Chloroform (Freon) Phosgene Diphosgene Chloropicrin Halothane Cyclopropane Ethers Nitrous oxide (N_2O) Sulfur dioxide (SO_2)	Delayed toxic effects include parkinsonism, dysarthria, ocular abnormalities, and ataxia Cavitation of putamen and globus pallidus Nausea Confusion Relaxation and drowsiness Headache Dry mouth, oropharyngeal burning Choking and respiratory discomfort leading to pulmonary edema Pulmonary infiltrates, predisposing to lung abscess Hepatic and renal toxicity Cardiac arrest	Multiple casualties in short period of time Diagnosis made by toxidrome. LFTs peak 3–4 days after exposure if hepatic toxicity present	Supportive, high-PEEP cardiorespiratory care N-Acetylcysteine for liver dysfunction shown efficacy in animals Steroids prevent pulmonary edema from nitrous oxide	Water solubility of the agent will determine amount of mucosal irritation and need for suctioning of secretions
Opiates and narcotics Aerosolized fentanyl 3-methyl fentanyl Carfentanil Trimethyl phentanylum Kokol-1 (Russian "knockout" gas)	Nausea Euphoria to drowsiness to depressed LOC to coma Respiratory depression (bradypnea, hypopnea) Miosis (Pupillary dilation can be seen in hypoxic patients) Nystagmus Seizures Ventricular arrhythmias	Multiple casualties in short period of time Diagnosis made by toxidrome	Naloxone 0.4–2 mg SQ/IV Q2–3 minutes with response in 10 minutes	Differential also includes clonidine poisoning, cholinergic crisis, phenothiazine poisoning, PCP intoxication, pontine or subarachnoid hemorrhage
Biologic toxins Botulinum toxin (inhaled)	Nausea Ptosis and poorly reactive miotic (dilated) pupils Disconjugate gaze, diplopia, facial diplegia Progressive, descending bulbar signs including dysphagia Muscular weakness, respiratory compromise	Normal NCV and SEPs Small motor unit potentials Incremental response to 50 Hz repetitive stimulation	Equine antitoxin to Botulinum toxin 550–850 IU slow IV infusion Supportive therapy including mechanical ventilation for VC <15 cc/kg or NIF <20 cm H_2O	Differential includes Lambert-Eaton—like myasthenia gravis, tick paralysis, pontine infarction, diphtheria, and Guillain-Barré (Miller-Fisher variant)

(Continued)

BIOTERROR AGENTS, WHICH INDUCE DIZZINESS OR VERTIGO (CONTINUED)

Agent Class and Agent(s)	Toxidrome	Complications and Confirmatory Diagnostic Test	Specific Neurologic Therapy	Comments
GABA antagonists Bicuculline Picrotoxin (cocculin) Tetramethylenedisulfo-tetramine (DSTA, TETS)	Epileptic symptoms including seizures, lethal convulsions,	Gas chromatography of serum sample for DSTA, if available	No proven antidote GABA-ergic agonist, e.g., benzodiazepines, and supportive care Pyridoxine 1 g PO QD and Baclofen PO 5–20 mg TID (max 80 mg/day) may be helpful	
Glycine receptor antagonist Strychnine	Painful muscular convulsions and spasms muscle fatigue Opisthotonus and "Sawhorse" stance Respiratory failure Mydriasis (late sign) and death	Toxidrome; characteristic whole-body muscle spasm	Diazepam 1 mg IV repeated with recurrence of symptoms activated charcoal	
Radiation 0.5–2 Gy	Nausea Anorexia and GI manifestations from mucosal sloughing Diarrhea Sepsis (from translocation of gut flora)	Leukopenia Toxidrome Mass casualty situation	Mechanical Ventilation Potassium iodide within 1 hour of exposure (competes with radioactive iodine)	If patient survives 24 hours, long-term prognosis is good Threshold for symptoms is 200 rads (about 2 Gy). Onset within 6 hours unless otherwise indicated
2–10 Gy	Epilation, erythema, desquamation with necrosis Headache, vertigo, altered mental status, cerebral edema, seizures			
More than 10 Gy	Above symptoms, onset within 30 minutes			Late sequelae include hypothyroidism and thyroid cancer due to absorption of radioactive iodine

* In addition to being the opposite of a cholinergic crisis, can be remembered with the pentad "blind as a bat, dry as a bone, hot as a hare, red as a beet, and mad as a hatter."

cerebral anthrax as well as in non-bioterror-related conditions such as pseudotumor cerebri. Despite the many confounders, the Illinois Department of Public Health considers any case of meningitis or encephalitis a "potential bioterror event." In these cases, papilledema is usually present and decreased visual acuity is a common finding, perhaps due to isolated sixth nerve palsies related to the pathogenesis of the condition. Regarding meningitis and encephalitis, sporadic cases are sufficiently common to warrant a lumbar puncture for common causes (see Table 6-4). A computerized tomography (CT) of the head should be performed to exclude intracranial mass lesions or hydrocephalus. When unavailable, technetium single photon emission computerized tomography (SPECT) (Tc-99 brain scans) or electroencephalograms (EEGs) are reasonable alternatives. In cases of intracranial mass lesions, CSF sampling is contraindicated for fear of brain herniation.

The headaches related to traumatic brain injury or the post-concussion syndrome (as would be seen, for example, after a violent explosion or physical trauma following the stampede after a bioterror attack) is characterized by vague descriptions, impaired concentration, dizziness, fatigue, photophobia, and nystagmus. Though this headache remits slowly, and though a small minority of patients will demonstrate structural abnormalities on CT scan of the head, this is largely considered to be "psychogenic" in origin.

In the mass casualty setting, a cluster of new-onset headaches in patients without a prior history of the above diseases should warrant suspicion that a bioterror agent is causing the symptom. Toxic headaches (called toxic-febrile headaches in the literature since they are characteristically more intense as body temperature rises) are encountered in a variety of biological attacks including typhoid fever, meningoencephalitis from any cause, and other agents listed in Table 6-4. Subarachnoid hemorrhage may also present with toxic headaches. The triad of fever, headache, and stiff neck should prompt an immediate infusion of antibiotics, a non-contrast CT of the brain, and a spinal puncture for a specimen of CSF, should contraindications not exist.

The treatment of headaches depends on the cause. In the setting of a bioterror event, some of the usual treatments available to a neurologist to treat headache are inappropriate or untested. For instance, the triptans and ergotamines, which have demonstrated their usefulness in migraine and migraine variants, have not been well-tested in episodes of chemical or biological weapons attack, and, moreover, these agents are theoretically dangerous because of their tendency to lower the seizure threshold. As seen in Table 6-4, headaches may herald an ominous prognosis. When specific antidotes are indicated, they should be administered; otherwise we favor supportive care with nonsteroidal anti-inflammatory drugs (NSAIDs) for headaches. Aspirin and acetaminophen in the customary doses provides relief for many patients with common headaches. Oxygen and dextrose should be administered to ensure adequate supply of these nutrients to the brain. In refractory cases (status migrainosus), glucocorticoids may be of benefit.

Movement Disorders

Terrorists utilize the fear of illness to achieve political aims. Perhaps no greater fear exists in the minds of the public than losing control over one's body—its muscle and purposeful movement—while still retaining consciousness and awareness of one's surroundings and circumstances. This idea, no doubt, has powerful attraction to the would-be terrorist: rendering their victim powerless yet cognizant, which is why in the setting of a bioterror attack, the physician should be acutely aware of neuromuscular complaints. The Illinois Department of Public Health, for this reason, advises any episode of flaccid muscle paralysis be considered a potential bioterror event.

The neuromuscular junction (NMJ) is one area where the blood-brain barrier (or, more accurately, the blood-neuron barrier) is porous. For this reason, muscle disorders (fasciculations, spasms, paresis, weakness, and paralysis) may be an early indication of a chemical or biological attack.

Biochemically, the physiologic contraction and relaxation of skeletal muscle occurs after a series of events:

1. Acetylcholine is preassembled from choline and acetyl-coenzyme A (a reaction catalyzed by the sulfhydryl-containing enzyme choline acetyl transferase [ChAT]) and stored in vesicles at the nerve terminal of a motor neuron.
2. Electrical impulses of membrane depolarization reach the axonal nerve terminal in sufficient quantities to cause the release of stored acetylcholine.
3. Acetylcholine is released into the NMJ in a controlled manner, and attaches to the acetylcholine receptor (AChR)/ion channel complex. This interaction with the acetylcholine receptor occurs in a rapid equilibrium, with a free- and bound-fraction of acetylcholine in the vicinity. (Note that the receptors are nicotinic receptors at the cellular level of muscle, but a similar interaction occurs with muscarinic receptors in the central nervous system [CNS].).
4. Acetylcholine binds to its receptor causing membrane depolarization and a subsequent intracellular flux of ions leading to the release of stores of calcium, which, in turn, activates the troponin-actin-myosin complex and propels the cross-bridging of light and heavy chains under the influence of ATP hydrolysis.
5. Free acetylcholine at the NMJ interacts with acetylcholinesterase, an enzyme in the NMJ, and is degraded into its inactive components, choline and acetate, ultimately removing its influence on the acetylcholine receptor and allowing restoration of the ionic gradients.

BIOTERROR AGENTS, WHICH INDUCE HEADACHE

Agent Class	Examples of Bioterror Agent(s) or Syndromes	Accompanying Symptoms and Signs	Diagnosis and Treatment
Meningoencephalitis	*Streptococcus* pneumonia	Headache, fever, neck stiffness	Lumbar puncture
	Hemophilus influenza	Kernig's and Brudzinski's sign	Dexamethasone 4 mg IV prior to
	Neisseria meningitides	Petechial rash (*Neisseria*)	antiobioticinfusion
		Seizure	Ceftriaxone 2 g IV daily (adult dose)
	Mycoplasma (Mycoplasma spp.)	Fever, sore throat, malaise	Cold agglutinins
		Persistent, dry, hacking cough	Complement fixation test
		Streaky infiltrate on chest x-ray	Sputum culture
		Incapacitating, but not life-threatening	PCR available in some centers
			Erythromycin 500 mg Q6H shortens duration
	Typhoid fever (*Salmonella typhi*)	Diffuse abdominal pain mimicking	Culture organism from blood, stool, or urine
		appendicitis	Ciprofloxacin 400 mg IV or Ceftriaxone 1 g
		Hepatosplenomegaly	IV daily (adult dose)
		Diarrhea	
		Rose spots on the abdomen	
		Sepsis	
		Osteomyelitis (especially in sickle-cell	
		patients)	
	Plague (*Yersinia pestis*)	Fevers, chills	Gram stain reveals gram-negative rods with
		Hemoptysis	bipolar staining at terminal ends
		Toxemia	Ciprofloxacin 400 mg IV or Doxycycline 200
		Regional lymphadenopathy and buboes	mg IV × 1 then 100 mg IV BID (adult dose)
		Conjunctivitis	until flea vectors eradicated
		Pneumonia (Pneumonic plague)	
		Sepsis	
		Respiratory failure, shock, DIC (late signs)	Those exposed to flea vectors should be
			offered prophylactic antibiotics
	Tularemia (*Francisella tularensis*)	Fevers, chills, malaise	Culture on cysteine-rich blood agar
		Ulceration at site of inoculation	Skin test or rise in IgG titer may be safer
		Regional lymphadenopathy (if inoculated)	than culture due to infectivity
		Pneumonia (if inhaled)	Gentamicin 3–5 mg/kg/day IV for 14 days or
		Abdominal pain (if ingested)	Cipro 400 mg IV BID until better, then 750 mg
			PO for 14 days

Category	Agent	Clinical features	Diagnosis/Treatment
Neurotropic viruses	Smallpox (Variola virus)	Fever, chills, malaise (prominent) Backache Bronchopneumonia (main cause of death) Thoracic lymphadenopathy Rigors Delirium Characteristic descending vesicular rash after 7–17 days	Cidofovir shows effectiveness in vitro Sandoglobulin or ribavirin may also be used Smallpox vaccine should be administered to those exposed to a patient with smallpox
Viral hemorrhagic fevers	Lassa virus and other arenaviridae Bunyaviridae Hantavirus Ebola and marburg viruses (Filoviridae) Yellow fever and dengue fever (Flaviviridae)	Malaise, fever, myalgia (initial symptoms) Vasculopathy, edema, coagulopathy Petechiae Internal and external hemorrhaging Hypotension, shock Renal and liver failure Endothelial dysfunction	Antigen-capture ELISA available for some viruses Patients should be kept in isolation due to high infectivity Treatment is mainly supportive with high morbidity regardless of efforts Ribavirin may be of benefit in Arenaviridae infections. Vaccines are under development
Viral encephalitis	Venezuelan equine encephalitis (VEE) Eastern equine encephalitis (EEE) Western equine encephalitis (WEE) (all viruses of genus *Alphaviridae*)	Chills, high fever, malaise Myalgia Vomiting Progresses to delirium, somnolence, coma. Neurologic residue in survivors includes epilepsy, paralysis, cranial nerve lesions	Leukopenia and elevated LFTs Lymphocytic leukorrhea in CSF ELISA test and viral isolation by culture are diagnostic Supportive therapy Vaccines are available, but poorly immunogenic
Bacterial infections	Anthrax (*Bacillus anthracis*) Cutaneous anthrax	Painless, pruritic papules evolving into vesicles rupturing and forming black eschar in 1 week (cutaneous anthrax)	ELISA for circulating anthrax toxin available Gram stain may help, but organism is difficult to culture
	Gastrointestinal anthrax	Pharyngeal ulcers and edema. Hemorrhagic mesenteric adenitis, ascites, hematemesis, hematochezia (gastrointestinal anthrax)	Ciprofloxacin 400 mg IV Q8H or Doxycycline 200 mg IV then 100 mg IV Q8H (adult dose) and Clindamycin 600–900 mg IV Q8H
	Inhalational anthrax	Malaise, fatigue, myalgia, nonproductive cough, fever Necrotizing hemorrhagic mediastinitis All forms can lead to confusion, blurred vision, visual distortion, syncope, and multiorgan failure Hemorrhagic meningitis with meningismus and coma is a major cause of death	Differential includes herpes encephalitis or rupture cerebral aneurysm

(*Continued*)

BIOTERROR AGENTS, WHICH INDUCE HEADACHE (CONTINUED)

Agent Class	Examples of Bioterror Agent(s) or Syndromes	Accompanying Symptoms and Signs	Diagnosis and Treatment
Biologic toxins	Staphylococcal enterotoxin B	Fever/chills	Usually self-limited illness
	Shigatoxin (aerosolized)	Nausea and vomiting	Supportive care
		Myalgia	
		Cough	
	Ciguatera toxin	Nausea, vomiting, diarrhea	Supportive therapy
		Paresthesias and dysesthesias (especially hot/cold reversal)	No antidote per se
		Lower extremity weakness	Mannitol 1 g/kg IV seems be useful adjunct in relieving symptoms
		Myalgia and pruritus	
		Arthralgia, malaise	
		Respiratory depression, paralysis, shock, convulsions (severe cases)	
	Scombrotoxin	Whole-body erythema	Elevated histidine in serum (not widely available)
		Nausea, vomiting, abdominal pain	
		Dizziness	Antihistamine such as Benadryl 1.25 mg/kg
		Palpitations and tachycardia	PO Q4–6H
		Breathlessness, wheezing	
		Hypotension and cardiovascular collapse	
Chemical asphyxiants	Hydrogen cyanide (AC)	"Pink" skin and bright red venous blood	100% oxygen by face mask
	Cyanogen chloride (CK)	Giddiness in seconds, to depressed consciousness	Two-stage detoxification by sodium nitrite 300 mg IV over 10 minutes
	Arsine (SA)	Palpitations	
		Dizziness, nausea, vomiting	Sodium thiosulfate 12.5 g IV
		Vertigo, delayed pupillary light reflex	
		Eye irritation	Hydroxocobalamin 2.5–5 g is an alternative but somewhat impractical
		Tachycardia and hyperventilation	
		Drowsiness	
		(In high exposure: immediate coma, seizures, convulsions, cardiorespiratory arrest, death within 1–15 minutes)	
		Delayed toxic effects include parkinsonism, dysarthria, ocular abnormalities, and ataxia	
		Cavitation of putamen and globus pallidus	

Category	Agents	Effects	Treatment/Notes
Vesicants/blister agents	Sulfur mustard Lewisite Nitrogen mustard Mustard lewisite Phosgene-oxime Methyl bromide	Nausea and vomiting Mucosal irritation and burning (eyes, mouth, nose) Skin erythema and blistering Swollen eyes Dyspnea Airway sloughing and pulmonary edema Tachycardia and hypotension Transient renal insufficiency Hepatic injury Sepsis Dizziness, confusion, lethargy, seizures, coma	No antidote for mustards or methyl bromide Dimercaprol (BAL) 5 mg/kg then 2.5 mg/kg one or two times per day for 10 days if lewisite agent
Riot control agents	Mace (CN) Malononitrile (CS) Bromobenzylcyanide (CA) Dibenz-oxazepine (CR) Pepper spray (OC) Adamsite (DM)	Nausea and vomiting Mucosal irritation Burning, itching, red skin Dyspnea Diarrhea Abdominal cramping Depression	No definitive treatment Skin decontamination Respiratory support
Anesthetic gases	Chloroform (Freon) Phosgene Diphosgene Chloropicrin Halothane Cyclopropane Ethers Nitrous oxide (N_2O) Sulfur dioxide (SO_2)	Confusion Relaxation Dizziness and drowsiness Nausea and vomiting Dry mouth, oropharyngeal burning Choking and respiratory discomfort leading to pulmonary edema Pulmonary infiltrates, predisposing to lung abscess Hepatic and renal toxicity Cardiac arrest	Supportive, high-PEEP cardiorespiratory care N-Acetylcysteine for liver dysfunction shown efficacy in animals Steroids prevent pulmonary edema from nitrous oxide
Hydrocarbons	Benzene Kerosene Toluene Hexane Xylenes	Dizziness, drowsiness Euphoria Difficulty with coordination Pulmonary edema Hepatotoxicity Convulsions and coma Cardiac arrhythmias (severe cases)	Gas chromatography/mass spectroscopy (GCMS) of liquid sample considered diagnostic Supportive care

(Continued)

TABLE 6-4

BIOTERROR AGENTS, WHICH INDUCE HEADACHE (CONTINUED)

Agent Class	Examples of Bioterror Agent(s) or Syndromes	Accompanying Symptoms and Signs	Diagnosis and Treatment
Inorganic heavy metal toxins	Mercury	Nausea and vomiting	Gastric lavage (with proteinaceous fluid)
	Arsenic	Intention tremor	Sodium formaldehyde sulfoxylate 250 mL in 5% solution to decrease absorption in acute setting
	Lead	Confusion, ataxia, incoordination	
		Dysarthria	
		Change in behavior or mood ("mad hatter")	Dimercaprol (BAL) 4–5 mg/kg Q4H = 6 then Q6H × 8 then Q8H for 10 days, not to exceed 300 mg (adults)
		Skin and nail changes	
		Lethargy alternating with irritability	
		Abdominal pain, anorexia, weight loss (long-term)	
		Renal tubular necrosis	Mannitol 1 g/kg IV as a temporizing measure until dialysis for renal failure
		Stomatitis, metallic taste, hematemesis	
		Encephalopathy	
	Tin (trimethyl tin chloride)	Dizziness	Characteristic changes on MRI
	Manganese vapor (arc welding)	Agitation and difficulty with concentration and visual focus	Supportive care
		Facial muscle twitching	
		Numbness	Patients may present with symptoms long after exposure
		GI symptoms and liver dysfunction	
		Immune dysfunction	
		Skin discoloration	
		Cough, respiratory discomfort	
Radiation			
0.5–2 Gy	"Dirty bomb"	Anorexia and GI manifestations from mucosal sloughing	Potassium iodide within 1 hour of exposure (competes with radioactive iodine)
		Nausea, vomiting, diarrhea	
		Sepsis (from translocation of gut flora)	
2–10 Gy	Strontium-90 radioactive generators (RTG from former USSR, NASA probes)	Epilation, erythema, desquamation with necrosis	Treatment of radiation poisoning is supportive
		Nausea, vertigo, altered mental status, cerebral edema, seizures	
More than 10 Gy	Nuclear Explosion	Above symptoms, onset within 30 minutes	

Some of the most potent chemical and biological agents of terrorism exert their effects on the peripheral nervous system (PNS) by inhibiting formation of acetylcholine, inhibiting or activating the release of acetylcholine, blocking or activating the acetylcholine receptor, or inhibiting the action of the acetylcholinesterase enzyme. For instance, organic mercury compounds have a high affinity for sulfhydryl groups, which contributes to its effect on enzyme dysfunction of choline acetyltransferase. This inhibition may lead to acetylcholine deficiency, and can have consequences on motor function. Botulinum toxin acts by suppressing the release of acetylcholine; whereas the venom from a black widow spider has the reverse effect (Table 6-5).

The standard approach by which a neurologist tests peripheral nerve function is through an electromyogram (EMG) and nerve conduction studies. However, newer tests such as current perception threshold (CPT) studies may constitute a more comprehensive approach to assessing neuromuscular function. While the literature on the use of CPT after neurotoxic exposure is still sparse, CPT is a well-established and sensitive test for peripheral sensory nerve function. Biopsy of the sural nerve may supply additional information if the gastrocnemius muscle function is compromised in a suspected bioterror attack. The biopsy is usually undertaken so that electron microscopy of the sample can differentiate between demyelinating diseases and axonal damage from a toxin. However, the majority of the time, the biopsy yields nonspecific information of limited value.

Of course, the ultimate control of skeletal muscle being voluntary, nerve impulses from the CNS are also involved in the proper control and coordination of muscle activity. Agents with sufficient penetration into the "higher centers" of motor control can similarly cause movement disorders and mimic well-known neurological diagnoses. For instance, certain heavy metals and the organic compound MPTP have an affinity for cells in the basal ganglia or substantia nigra and lead to parkinsonism, a condition characterized by "cogwheel" rigidity, flexed posture, bradykinesia, hypophonia, dysarthria, loss of postural reflexes, and "pill-rolling" tremor.

Diagnostic evaluation of CNS is performed by surface or invasive electrode placement. EEG, a far more complex procedure than EMG, is discussed in the next section. Physicians are fortunate, however, that the *clinical* evaluation of the CNS is less ambiguous. Changes in the CNS are usually manifested by the neurological signs and symptoms discussed so far, by alterations in cardiovascular function, changes in the pattern of respiration, and imaging of the brain through MRI (magnetic resonance imaging) and CT can also pinpoint different etiologic agents if these images are interpreted by a knowledgeable radiologist. Brain imaging is discussed later on under the section on "brain death."

Seizures

Physicians recognize seizures as potentially fatal, "aberrant, recurrent, and involuntary" electrical activity in the cerebral cortex. They manifest as subjective and objective phenomenon like elementary motor phenomenon to sensory disturbances, complex emotions, psychoillusory sensations, and hallucinations. For this reason, differentiating seizures from psychiatric disease, muscle weakness, and so forth is complicated. Seizures are potentially fatal due to the phenomenon of *excitotoxicity*: repeated excitation of a nerve leads to apoptosis. Numerous experiments have confirmed, for example, that repeated stimulation of a nerve with the neurotransmitter glutamate triggers the transcription of DNA segments associated with apoptosis. (That glutamate itself is used as a neurotransmitter is all the more surprising.) Moreover, unregulated activity in one part of the brain will quickly deplete the body's supply of glucose and essentially starve other parts of the brain. As neurons are postmitotic, recovery from the loss of a neuron requires the (slow) process of axonal branching of existing neurons; contrast this slow process from the rapidity with which apoptosis occurs.

Neurologists classify seizures according to whether the onset of seizures involves the entire cerebral cortex (generalized) or just a portion (partial). Generalized seizures are subsequently partitioned into absence seizures (no convulsions, preserved muscle tone), atonic (no convulsions, loss of muscle tone), tonic/clonic or grand mal seizures (convulsions with epileptiform EEG discharges), and myoclonic (convulsions without abnormal EEG discharges) types. Partial seizures are divided into *simple* partial seizures, which do not involve the loss of consciousness, and *complex* partial seizures, which do. However, physicians should be aware of the large amount of overlap of these conditions, making this distinction largely irrelevant in the acute care of affected individuals. Seizures are, by their nature, uncontrolled electrical discharges and need not follow rigid patterns or classifications. For example, partial seizures are sometimes said to undergo "secondary generalization," meaning that the aberrant electrical activity has spread to involve the entire cortex.

Space limits discussion of all of the precise pathophysiology, which produce seizures. The focus of this discussion will not be on the genetic, metabolic, nutritional, neoplastic, degenerative, or unknown causes. Rather, Table 6-6 focuses on the physical, circulatory, infectious, and toxic causes of seizures.

In the acute setting, there are two mainstays for controlling seizures: Lorazepam (Ativan) and Diazepam (Valium), which are administered IV and should control seizures within 10 minutes of administration. If the seizure recurs, these agents can be administered repeatedly for up to 30 minutes in an attempt to abort the attack.

AGENTS, WHICH ACT ON THE NEUROMUSCULAR UNIT

Agent	Site of Action	Mechanism of Action	Effects on Nerves/Muscle	Clinical Manifestations
Mercury	Choline acetyltransferase	Inhibits sulfhydryl-containing enzyme resulting in acetylcholine deficiency	Inhibitory; presynaptic neuron lacks neurotransmitter	Primary motor neuropathy Spontaneous arm/leg pain Dementia Stocking-glove neuropathy Acrodynia in pediatric patients
Arsenic	Unknown	Unknown	Inhibitory	Stocking-glove sensory neuropathy Painful, burning paresthesias Hyperhidrosis Distal motor neuropathy
Lead	Glutamate transmission (CNS)	Unclear; displaces other essential metals such as iron and calcium	Inhibitory; leading to weakness	Primary motor neuropathy Mononeuritis multiplex possible Arthralgia Cerebral edema (pediatric patients)
Thallium (nonradioactive)	Sodium and potassium channels	Replacement of cations and disruption of cellular processes		Stocking-glove sensory neuropathy ("hot coals" sensation) Distal neuropathy Alopecia Symptoms reverse with administration of Prussian blue (antidote)
Manganese	Globus pallidus, putamen, and caudate nucleus	Oxidative stress of neuromelanin-rich structures; neuronal degeneration	Dystonia	Manganism (Arc Welder's disease): behavioral changes parkinsonism Extrapyramidal symptoms Dystonia and ataxia
1-methyl-4-phenyl tetrahydropyridine (MPTP)	Subthalamic nuclei Substantia nigra	Necrosis	Repetitive movement	Parkinsonism

Botulinum toxin	Presynaptic vesicles	Inhibits release of acetylcholine	Inhibitory; nerve impulses not transmitted to muscle	Ptosis and poorly reactive mitotic (dilated) pupils Disconjugate gaze, diplopia, facial diplegia Progressive, descending bulbar signs including dysphagia Muscular weakness, respiratory compromise
Black widow spider venom		Stimulates over-release of acetylcholine	Excitatory; muscles stop in midcontraction and fail to relax	Latrodectism: muscle cramping, tremors, and painful muscle contractions Tetany Cholinergic crisis: headache, dizziness, diaphoresis and lacrimation nausea and vomiting anxiety, insomnia tachybradycardia, hypotension, tachypnea
Organophosphates Nerve agents Tetrodotoxin Saxitoxin Conotoxins	Acetylcholinesterase CNS/voltage-gated sodium ion channel	Inhibitory Blocking sodium channels and inhibiting neuronal depolarization	Paresis and paralysis Respiratory paralysis Irregular heartbeat	Perioral numbness or tingling (if ingested) Paresthesias of face and extremities Headache Epigastric pain, nausea, vomiting, diarrhea Respiratory distress, failure Convulsions and loss of consciousness Cardiac arrhythmias
Tetanospasmin (tetanus toxin)	Neuronal membrane via retrograde axonal transport	Inhibits neurotransmitters GABA and glycine by degrading the protein synaptobrevin	Overactivity in the muscles failure of inhibition of motor reflexes by sensory stimulation	Tetanic spasm Risus sardonicus Lockjaw (Masseter muscle first affected) Opisthotonus Fracture of long bones (severe cases)

(Continued)

T A B L E   6 - 5

AGENTS, WHICH ACT ON THE NEUROMUSCULAR UNIT (CONTINUED)

Agent	Site of Action	Mechanism of Action	Effects on Nerves/Muscle	Clinical Manifestations
β-oxalyl-L-α,β-diaminopropionic acid (ODAP, chicken vetch toxin, grass pea toxin)	CNS	Glutamate receptor agonist	Inhibitory	Neurolathyrism: Paralysis, characterized by lack of strength in or inability to move the lower limbs
Konzo (bitter cassava root toxin)	Unclear	Unclear. Cyanide-containing compound found in root	Spasms and cramping	Permanent spastic paraparesis of variable intensity. Arms and cranial nerves involved in severe cases
Mexican buckthorn fruit toxin				Motor polyneuropathy resembling Guillain-Barré syndrome
Ciguatera toxin (toxin of dinoflagellates found in tropical water fish and shellfish)	Unknown	Neurotoxin	Decrease contractile force	Muscle weakness and extreme fatigue Nausea/vomiting/diarrhea Paresthesia (hot/cold reversal) Memory loss Case reports of headache and coma
Nicotinic agents Anatoxin-a Anatoxin-a(s) Epibatidine Nicotine (in DMSO)	Acetylcholine receptor	AChR agonist	Excitatory (until fatigue)	Muscle twitching, weakness and cramping Pallor Tachycardia and hypertension Seizures Apnea Loss of consciousness
Phenothiazines Haldol Antihistamines (e.g., Benadryl) Tranquilizers Antipsychotics	Striatum	Histamine (H₁) receptor blocker; increases acetylcholine leading to relative lack of dopamine	Excitatory	Parkinsonism Dyskinesia and dystonia (mouth) Akathisia Neuroleptic malignant syndrome with hyperthermia

During these 30 minutes, the airway, breathing, circulation (ABCs), neurological examination, and vitals should be assessed; oxygen should be administered via intubation if necessary; blood should be drawn for chemistry, glucose, complete blood count (CBC), and other relevant tests; and an EEG should be ordered. If the seizures continue, the patient should be loaded with phenytoin or a phenytoin equivalent (PE), transferred to the intensive care unit (ICU), and monitored for changes in the electrocardiogram (ECG). The loading dose of phenytoin can be repeated once if the seizures are not controlled; however, if the seizures continue, at this point, the patient is considered to be in *status epilepticus*.

Status epilepticus is a true neurologic emergency requiring drastic action to break the cycle of seizure activity and to prevent mortality. Though convulsive status epilepticus is the most dramatic presentation, the physician should be alert to the possibility that nonconvulsive seizures also lead to status epilepticus. The patient should be transferred to the ICU immediately for institution of a barbiturate coma. The combination of barbiturates and anesthesia quiet all electrical activity in the brain, suppressing the seizure focus and epileptiform discharges on EEG. Once the seizures are suppressed, the brain is "reset" and the dosages lightened with the hope that seizures do not return as awareness and consciousness returns. The patient will require ventilator and vasopressor support during the coma due to the combined effects of barbiturates and anesthetics. By this time, the patient may also be suffering from hyperthermia due to the duration of uncontrolled seizure activity, and will require cooling blankets. Dosages listed below (Table 6-7) are for illustration only; the assistance and guidance of an epileptologist is crucial at this stage to adjust the dose of barbiturates and anesthesia according to brain activity.

Assuming that the seizure activity is broken, oral phenytoin or antiepileptic alternatives to phenytoin may be used prophylactically. The precise choice among these agents is most appropriately left to trained neurologists, as the agents have individual nuances, and may require close follow-up for side effects.

Confusion, Coma, and Brain Death

If the past history of terror attacks has any prognostic value, then, in future terror attacks, the physician can expect to have many casualties arrive with a loss of consciousness. When faced with this situation, it is imperative that the physician proceed in an ordered fashion to gather information, make a diagnosis, provide supportive care, and perform therapy that treats reversible causes of neurologic dysfunction while avoiding further neurological damage. This situation will test the clinical acumen and knowledge of a physician like no other (not to mention its emotional toll) as often the history will be unobtainable or vague, and the acuity of the situation demands prompt action. Physicians are therefore entrusted with the greatest responsibility while operating with minimal information, an unenviable situation.

Consciousness requires *awareness*, or the integration of sensory inputs at the cortical level, and *arousal*, which refers to the primitive responses encoded within the brain stem. Signs of awareness include responsiveness to tactile, visual, olfactory, or auditory stimuli. Signs of arousal include withdrawal to noxious stimuli, the corneal reflex, pupillary reactions, and the oculocephalic (Doll's eyes) and vestibulo-ocular (cold caloric) tests. A useful gauge of the depth of unconsciousness is the Glasgow Coma Scale (GCS), which, though initially developed for the assessment of trauma victims, is applicable to victims of terror attack as well. Patients without consciousness can be in various stages of unconsciousness from drowsiness to deep coma (Table 6-8). They are not *dead*, however, until cardiorespiratory functions cease or when it has been determined that the loss of *both* brain stem and cortical function is irreversible.

There are many bioterror-related causes and non-terror-related reasons that a patient may present in a coma. However, these causes can be classified into diseases which

- cause no focal neurological signs (opiates, hypoxia/anoxia, acidosis, shock, severe systemic infections, hyper/hypothermia, postictal states, concussions and traumatic brain injury, and acute hydrocephalus),
- cause meningeal irritation (any form of meningitis, any form of encephalitis, subarachnoid hemorrhage),
- cause focal brain stem or lateralizing signs (cerebral hemorrhage and infarction, brain stem or pontine stroke, brain abscess).

Arguably, no other medical issue carries as much legal, ethical, professional, and academic weight as the issue of death. In the spectrum from unconsciousness to persistent vegetative state to coma (Table 6-9), death occurs when a physician determines that either (1) all circulatory or respiratory function, or (2) the function of the entire brain and brain stem, has irreversibly ceased in accordance with accepted medical standards. It is this latter definition which constitutes the definition of "brain death" as accepted in the purview of the medical profession by law in more than 25 states in the United States, the World Medical Assembly, the Roman Catholic Church, the American Bar Association, the American Medical Association, the American Neurologic Association, and many other legal and medical bodies. Due to the many nuances of declaring brain death, it is helpful and appropriate for consultation with a neurologist before declaring someone dead as a consequence of a terror attack.

T A B L E 6 - 6

BIOTERROR AGENTS, WHICH INDUCE SEIZURES

Agent Class and Agent(s)	Toxidrome	Agent Class and Agent(s)	Toxidrome
Nicotinic agents Anatoxin-a Anatoxin-a(s) Epibatidine Nicotine (in DMSO)	Muscular twitching, weakness and cramps Pallor with tachycardia and hypertension Seizures with loss of consciousness and apnea	Vesicants/blister Agents sulfur mustard lewisite nitrogen mustard mustard lewisite phosgene-oxime methyl bromide	Mucosal irritation and burning (eyes, mouth, nose) Skin erythema and blistering Swollen eyes Dyspnea Airway sloughing and pulmonary edema; Tachycardia and hypotension Transient renal insufficiency Hepatic injury Sepsis Dizziness, headache, confusion, lethargy, seizures, coma
Ergot alkaloids Ergotamine Dihydroergotamine Rye fungus toxin	Ergotism Nausea, vomiting, and diarrhea Itching and desquamation Peripheral vasoconstriction and dry gangrene Paresthesias, burning sensation in fingers and toes Uterine contractions and placental abortion Hallucinations and insanity Convulsions, painful muscle spasms Unconsciousness	Opiates and narcotics Aerosolized fentanyl 3-methyl fentanyl Carfentanil Trimethyl Phentanylum Kokol-1 (Russian "knockout" gas)	Euphoria to drowsiness to depressed LOC to coma Respiratory depression (bradypnea, hypopnea) Miosis (Pupillary dilation can be seen in hypoxic patients) Nystagmus Seizures Ventricular arrhythmias
Chemical asphyxiants Hydrogen cyanide (AC) Cyanogen chloride (CK) Arsine (SA)	"Pink" skin and bright red venous blood Giddiness in seconds, to depressed consciousness Palpitations dizziness, vomiting Headache, vertigo, delayed pupillary light reflex Eye irritation	Tricoethecene (T2) mycotoxins: Fusarium Myrothecium Trichoderma Verticinonosporium Stachybotrys Ciguatera Scombrotoxin	Mucosal erythema and hemorrhage Red, blistering skin and mucosa (especially ocular) Increased salivation, coughing Dyspnea, pulmonary edema Hepatic and renal necrosis Hallucinations and dysesthesias (especially hot/cold reversal)

Agent / Dose	Manifestations
	Arthralgia, myalgia, polymyopathy
	Ataxia and lower extremity weakness
	Respiratory depression, paralysis, shock, seizures and coma in severe cases
	Headache
	Pruritic erythema (from histadine)
	Vomiting, abdominal pain
	Dizziness
	Palpitations and tachycardia
	Breathlessness, wheezing
	Hypotension and shock in severe cases
	Tachycardia and hyperventilation
	Drowsiness
	(In high exposure: immediate coma, seizures, convulsions, cardiorespiratory arrest, death within 1–15 minutes)
	Delayed toxic effects include parkinsonism, dysarthria, ocular abnormalities, and ataxia
	Cavitation of putamen and globus pallidus
Radiation	
0.5–2 Gy	Anorexia and GI manifestations from mucosal sloughing
	Diarrhea
	Sepsis (from translocation of gut flora)
2–10 Gy	Epilation, erythema, desquamation with necrosis
More than 10 Gy	Headache, vertigo, altered mental status, cerebral edema, seizures
	Above symptoms, onset within 30 minutes

TABLE 6-7

ANTIEPILEPTICS AND DOSAGE

Antiepileptic	Adult Dosing	Pediatric Dosing
Lorazepam (Ativan)	0.05–0.1 mg/kg IV over 2–5 minutes	Same
Diazepam (Valium)	5–10 mg IV Q 10–15 minutes × 3	0.2–0.5 mg/kg gel PR
Phenytoin (Dilantin)	20 mg/kg IV at 50 mg/min	Same
Fosphenytoin (Cerebyx)	20 mg/kg PE IV at 150 mg/min	Same
Phenobarbital (Luminal)	20 mg/kg IV at 50–75 mg/min	Consult epileptologist
Midazolam (Versed)	0.2 mg/kg IV then 75 mcg/kg/h	Consult epileptologist
Propofol (Diprivan)	1–3 mg/kg IV then 5–50 mcg/kg/min	Consult epileptologist

TABLE 6-8

CLASSIFICATION OF UNCONSCIOUSNESS

Level of Unconsciousness	Characteristics	Potential Causes
Confusion (GCS 12–14)	Inability to maintain coherent thought or action Awareness and arousal present, but response to stimuli is unusual or inappropriate	Toxic/metabolic encephalopathy Right parietal lobe lesion
Drowsiness (GCS 9–12)	Lacking awareness Arousal responses able to be evoked Able to respond verbally when aroused	Toxins including asphyxiants Hypoglycemia Sleep
Stupor (GCS 6–8)	Incomplete awareness of painful stimuli, but "fending-off" type motor response present Incoherent or absent verbal response when aroused Cheyne-Stokes breathing may be present	
Light coma (GCS 4–5)	Primitive and disorganized motor responses to noxious stimuli No response to attempts at arousal Central neurogenic hyperventilation or apneustic breathing may be present	Severe acidosis Toxins, poisoning Cerebral hemorrhage
Deep coma (GCS <4)	Loss of awareness and all arousal reflexes Ataxic and gasping (Biot's) respirations	Anesthetic gases

TABLE 6-9

CRITERIA FOR VEGETATIVE STATE AND BRAIN DEATH

Vegetative State	Brain Death
No awareness of surroundings	Coma without response to stimuli
No communication or emotional response	Apnea without ventilatory support
No comprehensible speech	No cephalic reflexes
Intact sleep-wake cycles	Body temperature > 34°C
Behavior, if present, is inconsistent with stimuli	Intact circulation
Variable brain stem and spinal reflexes	Negative toxicology screen
No voluntary movement*	Cessation of cardiorespiratory function for predetermined period of time
Intact cardiorespiratory function	Isoelectric EEG for 30 minutes at maximum gain
	No brain stem evoked response (BER)
	Absent cerebral circulation by scintigraphy, angiography, or Doppler ultrasound
	Absent brain function for duration determined by patient's age and underlying disease†

* May respond to noxious stimuli.

†Death from an irreversible metabolic or toxin-related condition usually has longer observation period than death from structural disease.

Source: Wijdiks EFM. Diagnosis of brain death. N Engl J Med. April 19, 2001;344(16):1215–1221.

Suggested Reading

Abrahams, B.C., Kaufman, D.M :Anticipating smallpox and monkeypox outbreaks: complications of the smallpox vaccine. *Neurologist* 2004:Sep;10(5):265–274.

PROJECT HEROES: Homeland Emergency Response Operational and Equipment Systems: a report to the National Personal Protective Technology Laboratory and the National Institute for Occupational Safety and Health by Occupational Health and Safety Division of the International Association of Fire Fighters (IAFF). Available at *http://www.cdc.gov/niosh/npptl/pdfs/ ProjectHEROES.pdf*

Baker PC, Bernat JL. The neuroanatomy of vomiting in man: association of projectile vomiting with a solitary metastasis in the lateral tegmentum of the pons and the middle cerebellar peduncle. *J Neurol Neurosurg Psychiatr.* 1985;48(11): 1165–1168.

Bleecker MI, Landgren KN, MJ Tiburzi. Curvilinear relationship between blood lead level and reaction time. *J Occup Env Med.* 1997;39:426–431.

Burt, AM. *Textbook of Neuroanatomy.* Philadelphia, PA: W.B. Saunders, 2003.

Center for Biological Defense, University of South Florida. *Recognition of and Response to Biological and Chemical Agents.* Available at *http://www.bt.usf.edu/*

Ciottone GR, ed. *Disaster Medicine.* 3rd ed. Chapters 91, 94–101, and 176. St. Louis, MO: Elsevier-Mosby, 2006.

Cleri DJ, Villota FJ, Prowancher RB. Smallpox, bioterrorism, and the neurologist. *Arch Neurol.* April 2003;60(4):489–494.

Cosgrove SE, Perl TM, et al. Ability of physicians to diagnose and manage illness due to category A bioterrorism agents. *Arch Intern Med.* September 26, 2005;165:2002–2006.

Grinker RR, Sahs AL. *Neurology.* 6th ed. Springfield, IL: Charles C. Thomas, 1966.

Harris JB, Blain PG. Neurotoxicology: what the neurologist needs to know. *J Neurol Neurosurg Psychiatr.* 2004;75 (Suppl. III): iii29–iii34.

Heuser G, Axelrod P, Heuser S. Defining chemical injury: a diagnostic protocol and profile of chemically injured civilians, industrial workers and Gulf War. Available at *http://www. iicph.org/docs/ipph_Defining_Chemical_Injury.htm and http://www.mcs-america.org/heuser.pdf*

Holstege CP, Bayulor M. CBRNE—Incapacitating Agents, 3-Quinuclidinyl Benzilate. E-Medicine review. Available at *http://www.emedicine.com/emerg/topic912.htm*

Illinois Department of Public Health. Bioterrorism Treatment Guidelines. Available at *http://www.idph.state.il.us/ Bioterrorism/pdf/BTFullGuidelines.pdf*

Jagminas L, Erdman DP. CBRNE—Evaluation of a Chemical Warfare Victim. E-Medicine. Available at *http://www.emedicine. com/emerg/topic892.htm*

Kandel ER, Schwartz JH, Jessell TM. *Principles of Neural Science.* 4th ed. New York, NY: Mcgraw-Hill, Health Professions Division, 2000.

Lucchini R, et al. Metals and neurodegeneration: research paper on heavy metals poisoning. Available at *http://www.bio. unipd.it/~zatta/metals/mangan.htm*

Martin CO, Adams HP, Jr. Neurological aspects of biological and chemical terrorism: a review for neurologists. *Arch Neurol.* January 2003;60:21–25.

Menkes JH, Sarnat HB, eds. *Child Neurology.* 6th ed. Lippincott Williams & Wilkins, Philadelphia, PA: 2000.

Meyer MA. Neurologic complications of anthrax: a review of the literature. *Arch Neurol.* April 2003;60:483–488.

Patocka J. Abrin and Ricin: two dangerous poisonous proteins. Available at *http://www.asanltr.com/newsletter/01-4/articles/ Abrin&RicinRev.htm*

Rotenberg JS, Newmark J. Nerve agent attacks on children: diagnosis and management. *Pediatrics.* September 2003;112(3): 648–658.

Rowland LP, ed. *Merritt's Textbook of Neurology.* 9th ed. Williams & Wilkins, Baltimore 1995.

Saary MJ, House RA. Preventable exposure to trimethyl tin chloride: a case report. *Occup Med.* 2002;52(4):227–230.

Samuels MA, ed. *Manual of Neurologic Therapeutics with Essentials of Diagnosis.* 3rd ed. Boston/Toronto: Little, Brown and Company, 1986.

Spencer PS, Schaumburg HH. *Experimental and Clinical Neurotoxicology.* 2nd ed. Oxford: Oxford University Press, 2000.

Victor M, Ropper AH. *Adams and Victor's Principles of Neurology.* 7th ed. McGraw-Hill, New York 2001.

White SM. Chemical and biological weapons: implications for anaesthesia and intensive care. *Br J Anaesth.* 2002;89(2):306.

Wijdiks, EFM. Diagnosis of brain death. *N Engl J Med.* April 19, 2001;344(16):1215–1221.

World Federation of Neurology. Terrorism and the neurologist. Available at *http://www.wfneurology.org/docs/pdf/WFN_ Neurotoxicology.pdf*

7

CARDIAC ISSUES

Jenny J. Lu and Sean M. Bryant

STAT FACTS

CARDIAC ISSUES

- The cardiovascular system is usually not the primary target for most weapons of mass destruction.
- Hypoxia/lactic acidosis should be investigated in patients with tachycardia.
- Muscarinic poisoning can result in pulmonary edema that can exacerbate tachycardia.
- Tachycardia is not a contraindication to atropine use in nerve gas exposure.

INTRODUCTION

Chemical, biological, and nuclear warfare agents will affect the cardiovascular system variably, depending on individual agent mechanisms of action and their routes and durations of exposures. Agents used for the purposes of mass destruction, for the most part, do not "directly" target the myocardium. However, heart rate and blood pressure are frequently affected and abnormalities should be both recognized and addressed. The goal of this chapter is to briefly review basic cardiovascular physiology and discuss how homeostasis is altered when either biological, chemical, or nuclear weapons are used in a mass casualty event.

CARDIOVASCULAR PHYSIOLOGY

Figure 7-1 illustrates the typical action potential of the myocardial cell (relating electrolyte flux across the cell membrane to the electrocardiogram [ECG]). Clinically relevant phases include phase 0, which represents depolarization of the membrane through rapid Na^+ channel activation, and phase 3 (final repolarization) indicating K^+ efflux from the cell. These two phases of the action potential reflect the QRS and QT interval lengths respectively.

Certain warfare agents are known to cause characteristic alterations in heart rate and blood pressure although the clinical picture will vary. One example includes nerve agents, which cause toxicity from acetylcholine accumulation through the inhibition of the enzyme acetylcholinesterase. Excessive levels of acetylcholine would be expected to produce increased vagal tone and thus bradycardia. However, tachycardia and hypertension are frequent findings secondary to nicotinic overdrive. Additionally, pulmonary edema from muscarinic poisoning producing hypoxemia may exacerbate the tachycardia.

Shock is classically defined as tissue hypoperfusion and can be divided into three broad categories (see Table 7-1). Hypovolemic shock from insufficient circulatory volume could potentially occur after exposure to any agent that causes significant vomiting and diarrhea (e.g., nerve agents and ricin) or bleeding. Cardiogenic shock, resulting from inadequate myocardial contractile function, can occur with cyanide poisoning. Cardiovascular shock is likely a result of systemic vascular damage from massive doses of radiation. Finally, biologic agents can cause a spectrum in severity from a systemic inflammatory response syndrome to frank sepsis and distributive shock.

APPROACH AND MANAGEMENT

The basic approach to the emergency patient always begins with the A, B, Cs (airway, breathing, and circulation). Appreciating vital sign abnormalities as well as performing a primary survey of the patient's condition helps to direct the appropriate care for the patient. Assuming airway and breathing are stable, the perfusion status of the patient should be assessed next. Simply obtaining a blood pressure and heart rate will give important clues to the

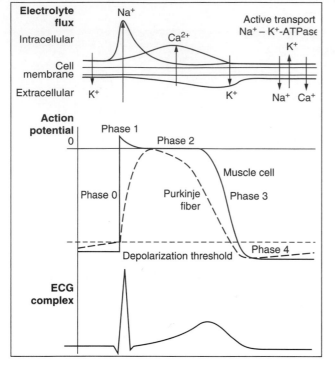

FIGURE 7-1

**RELATIONSHIP OF ELECTROLYTE MOVEMENT ACROSS
THE CELL MEMBRANE TO THE ACTION POTENTIAL AND
THE ELECTROCARDIOGRAM (ECG)**
*Source: From Hessler RA. Cardiovascular Principles. In:
Flomenbaum NE, Goldfrank LR, Hoffman RS, et al (eds).
Goldfrank's Toxicologic Emergencies. 8th Edition. New York, NY:
McGraw-Hill, 2002, p. 365.*

patient's condition. In addition, capillary refill, skin discoloration, strength/quality of pulses, and laboratory values (e.g., lactate levels, renal function indices like blood urea nitrogen [BUN] and creatinine, and myocardial markers of injury such as creatine kinase and troponin) suggesting end organ compromise secondary to poor perfusion must be taken into account. An electrolyte panel may be useful in situations where fluid abnormalities result from vomiting and diarrhea.

An ECG is essential in many patients presenting from exposure to a weapon of mass destruction, in conjunction with the exposure history, electrolyte levels (potassium and calcium), and vital signs to direct management. A widened QRS (>120 ms) can be treated with intravenous boluses of sodium bicarbonate (much like a tricyclic antidepressant overdose). Treatment of a prolonged QT (440 ms) is controversial. No study has indicated that magnesium is effective in "preventing" torsades de pointes; however, it is very effective in the treatment of this dysrhythmia.

Appropriate supportive care (fluid resuscitation, pressor supportives, antimicrobial treatments) is always the mainstay of care in any poisoned patient. Some agents may have specific antidotes (e.g., nerve agents and cyanide) to treat cardiovascular dysfunction. It should be noted that tachycardia is never a contraindication to atropine use in nerve agent poisoning, especially with the presence of a serious effect such as pulmonary edema. ACLS guidelines should be followed for the development of dysrhythmias or cardiac arrest. Please refer to Table 7-2 for an overview of

TABLE 7-1

CATEGORIES OF SHOCK

Categories of Shock	Main Mechanisms	Treatment
Hypovolemic	• Loss of circulating fluid volume	• Fluids and/or blood; treat cause
• Hemorrhagic	• Loss of whole blood	• Fluids
• Dehydration	• Depletion of tissue fluid	• Fluids, burn care
• Burn	• Loss of plasma proteins, altering colloid osmotic pressure	
Cardiogenic	• Impaired cardiac output, from excessive preload, reduced preload, excessive afterload	Small fluid boluses and/or pressors (dopamine, dobutamine, or norepinephrine)
Distributive	• Profound vasodilatation resulting in inappropriate	• Fluid, treat infection
• Septic	distribution of blood volume and inability to	• Fluid, epinephrine, diphenhydramine
• Anaphylactic	maintain adequate blood pressure	• Fluid, treat cause, consider traumatic
• Neurogenic	• Toxins from gram-positive or	cause (i.e., spinal cord injury)
	gram-negative organisms produce vasodilatation, with mediators of inflammation potentiating.	
	• Drastic, rapidly developing, IgE or non-IgE-mediated reactions	
	• Sympathetic nervous system (SNS) inhibition or parasympathetic nervous system (PSNS) stimulation causes vasodilatation and peripheral pooling. Spinal cord injuries block SNS.	

TABLE 7-2

CARDIOVASCULAR EFFECTS OF VARIOUS AGENTS

Agents	Cardiovascular Toxicity	Management/Approach
Nerve Agents		
Tabun	Bradycardia (muscarinic), tachycardia (nicotinic or resulting from pulmonary edema), hypertension, or hypotension with significant fluid loss	Atropine (repeat dosing until abatement of muscarinic signs, i.e., drying of pulmonary secretions)
Sarin	Bradycardia (muscarinic), tachycardia (nicotinic or resulting from pulmonary edema), hypertension, or hypotension with significant fluid loss	Atropine (repeat dosing until abatement of muscarinic signs, i.e., drying of pulmonary secretions)
Soman	Bradycardia (muscarinic), tachycardia (nicotinic or resulting from pulmonary edema), hypertension, or hypotension with significant fluid loss	Atropine (repeat dosing until abatement of muscarinic signs, i.e., drying of pulmonary secretions),
VX	Bradycardia (muscarinic), tachycardia (nicotinic or resulting from pulmonary edema), hypertension, or hypotension with significant fluid loss	Atropine (repeat dosing until abatement of muscarinic signs, i.e., drying of pulmonary secretions)
Vesicants		
Sulfur mustard	Hypertension, hypotension, tachycardia, weak cholinergic properties	Crystalloids
Lewisite	Hypertension, hypotension, tachycardia	Crystalloids
Phosgene	Hypertension, tachycardia	Supportive
Cyanide	Initial bradycardia and hypertension, followed by hypotension and reflex tachycardia, and terminal event being bradycardia and hypotension	Antidote kit: Includes sodium nitrite and sodium thiosulfate or hydroxocobalamin
Chlorine	Hypertension, dysrhythmias	Supportive
Riot Control Agents		
CN (chloroacetophenone)	Tachycardia, transient hypertension	Supportive
CS (o-chlorobenzilidene malononitrile)	Tachycardia, transient hypertension	Supportive
OC (oleoresin capsicum)	Tachycardia, transient hypertension	Supportive
Bacteria		
Anthrax	Hypertension followed by hypotension and tachycardia, septic shock	Supportive, antibiotics
Plague	Hypertension followed by hypotension and tachycardia, septic shock	Supportive, antibiotics
Tularemia	Hypertension followed by hypotension and tachycardia, septic shock	Supportive, antibiotics
Brucellosis	Hypertension followed by hypotension and tachycardia, endocarditis, myocarditis, pericarditis, aortic root abscess, pulmonary embolism, mycotic aneurysm	Supportive, antibiotics
Q fever	Hypertension followed by hypotension and tachycardia, pericarditis, myocarditis, endocarditis, septic shock	Supportive, antibiotics
Viruses		
Smallpox	Hypertension followed by hypotension and tachycardia, viremic shock	Supportive, experimental antivirals?
Viral hemorrhagic fevers	Hypertension followed by hypotension and tachycardia, viremic shock	Supportive, experimental antivirals?
Viral encephalitides	Hypertension followed by hypotension and tachycardia, viremic shock	Supportive, antivirals?

(Continued)

TABLE 7-2

CARDIOVASCULAR EFFECTS OF VARIOUS AGENTS (*CONTINUED*)

Agents	Cardiovascular Toxicity	Management/Approach
Toxins		
Botulinum	Hypotension and tachycardia, complications relating to respiratory failure	Supportive, antitoxin?
Ricin	Hypertension followed by hypotension and tachycardia, hypovolemic shock	Supportive
Staphylococcal enterotoxin B	Hypertension followed by hypotension and tachycardia	Supportive
Trichothecene mycotoxins	Hypertension followed by hypotension and tachycardia, hypovolemia and mycotoxic shock	Supportive
Nuclear	Hypotension and tachycardia, "vascular radiation syndrome," radiation-induced inflammatory changes to the heart	Supportive

the cardiovascular toxicity that results from the various agents found in later chapters of this book.

CONCLUSIONS

The cardiovascular system is not a primary target for most weapons of mass destruction. Injuries from explosions are not covered within this chapter but include penetrating or blunt cardiac trauma from shrapnel or blast force, which can lead to hemorrhage, pericardial tamponade, or myocardial infarction. Stress-related disorders may also contribute to cardiac sequelae. Supportive care is paramount in treating cardiovascular toxicity resulting from any warfare agent; rarely, specific antidotes can be used. Caveats include adequate decontamination to ensure the safety of the health-care team. Early consultation with a medical toxicologist would be prudent.

Suggested Reading

Finch SC. Acute radiation syndrome. *JAMA*. 1987;258:664–667.

Holstege CP, Kirk M, Sidell FR. Chemical warfare nerve agent poisoning. *Crit Care Clin*. 1997;13:923–942.

Keim M, Kaufmann AF. Principles for emergency response to bioterrorism. *Ann Emerg Med*. 1999;34:177–182.

Knudson GB. Operation Desert Shield: medical aspects of weapons of mass destruction. *Mil Med*. 1991;156:267–271.

Treatment of nerve gas poisoning. *Med Lett Drugs Ther*. 1995;37: 43–44.

Reeves GI: Radiation injuries. *Crit Care Clin*. 1999;2:457–473.

Richards CF, Burstein JL, Waeckerle JF, et al. Emergency physicians and biological terrorism. *Ann Emerg Med*. 1999;34:183–190.

Sidell FR, Borak J. Chemical warfare agents: II Nerve agents. *Ann Emerg Med*. 1992;21:865–871.

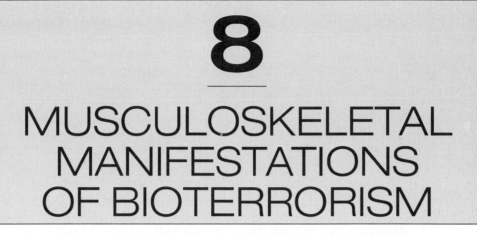

CHAPTER

8

MUSCULOSKELETAL MANIFESTATIONS OF BIOTERRORISM

Nirav A. Shah and Steven D. Levin

STAT FACTS

MUSCULOSKELETAL MANIFESTATIONS OF BIOTERRORISM

- Musculoskeletal injuries account for 60–70% of all war wounds.
- Broad-spectrum antibiotics should be initiated.
- Botulinum toxin does not penetrate intact skin.
- Skin necrosis with muscular dissemination is a late sign (black plague).

INTRODUCTION

The advances in orthopedic surgery over the second half of the twentieth century are largely attributed to our experiences in war. The majority of the advances in the orthopedic trauma world has come during wartime and helped to advance "damage control orthopedics." Secondary to recent events and the continued threat of terrorism, the musculoskeletal manifestations of biological and chemical warfare are on the forefront for the orthopedic surgeon.

Damage Control Orthopedics

Injuries of the musculoskeletal system have been the most common consequences of war in recent history and account for 60–70% of all wounds. Explosive devices are a preferred weapon of domestic and foreign terrorists secondary to the mutilation and explosive effects that wreak havoc in confined spaces such as modes of transportation and busy urban centers. The weapons cause primary blast injuries and secondary wounds from fragments of the weapons, which lead to a high incidence of infection and neurovascular injury. Damage control orthopedics emphasizes the immediate stabilization and control of the trauma with primary stabilization often with external fixation in the multiply injured patient. The goal in the multiply injured patient is to contain and stabilize orthopedic injuries so that all the other systems may begin their respective healing processes. Another important goal is to prevent a major second hit to the already damaged physiology by major orthopedic reconstructive surgery. Therefore, damage control orthopedics focuses on control of hemorrhage, management of soft tissue injury, and fracture stabilization without further systemic insults. Numerous studies have documented the large influx of a severe immunological reaction after the initial trauma-systemic inflammatory response syndrome (SIRS) that has dire consequences. The major obstacle now will be how civilian orthopedic surgeons will deal with these military weapons as they are used on domestic fronts by terrorists. The addition of biological agents to blast weapons will be the new challenge to juxtapose damage control orthopedics principles with the treatment, isolation, and control of the musculoskeletal response to chemical and biological warfare. Table 8-1 lists high priority chemical agents that the U.S. Food and Drug Administration (FDA) has listed as potential chemical agent threats. We have been unfortunately and unexpectedly ushered into an age of chemical and biological warfare but there have been some events historically that we have learned from in terms of specific diagnostics and treatments, and more importantly, we have seen the havoc these agents have created when used (Table 8-2).

The threat of biological and chemical warfare has been pushed upon us as a global and real threat. The

TABLE 8-1

PRIORITY CHEMICAL AGENTS POTENTIALLY USEFUL AS
WARFARE AND TERRORIST AGENTS, BY CATEGORY

Nerve Agents
Tabun
Sarin
Soman
Cyclosarin
VX

Blood Agents
Hydrogen cyanide
Cyanogen chloride

Blister Agents
Lewisite
Nitrogen and sulfur mustards
Phosgene oxime

Heavy Metals
Arsenic
Lead
Mercury

Volatile Toxins
Benzene
Chloroform
Trihalomethanes

Pulmonary Agents
Phosgene
Chlorine
Vinyl chloride

Incapacitating Agents
3-Quinuclidinyl benzilate

*Pesticides, Persistent and Nonpersistent Dioxins, Furans,
   and Polychlorinated Biphenyls, Explosive Nitro
   Compounds, and Oxidizers*
Ammonium nitrate combined with fuel oil

Flammable Industrial Gases and Liquids
Gasoline
Propane

Poisonous Industrial Gases, Liquids, and Solids
Cyanides
Nitriles

Corrosive Industrial Acids and Bases
Nitric acid
Sulfuric acid

*Source: Adapted from Greenfield RA, et al. Microbiological, biological,
and chemical weapons of warfare and terrorism. Am J Med. June 2002;323:
326–340.*

musculoskeletal and superficial skin manifestations may
at many times be the first indication for the clinician to
become suspicious of these agents and the disaster plan
may be evoked at that time. Treatment algorithms for the
patient have not yet been clearly identified secondary to a
paucity of experimental and clinical data. Global algorithms have been put into place with governing agencies,
primarily the Centers for Disease Control and Prevention
(CDC). The biological and chemical agents listed in this
chapter should be at the top of one's differential diagnosis
if any musculoskeletal manifestation is present. Clinicians
should have low thresholds to perform fasciotomies if the
agents have been injected under localized pressure; open
fracture treatment should be treated similarly based on the
grading of the injury, and diagnostic arthrocentesis and
subsequent incision and drainage (I&D) should be performed with a low threshold. (See Table 8-3.)

Current trauma protocol in civilian hospitals calls for
initiation of the adult trauma life supports (ATLS) algorithm. With the use of blast and chemical warfare, the addition of damage control orthopedic algorithms have been
put into place in various military hospitals (Fig. 8-1).

Evaluation for Biological Agents

When there is suspected bioterrorist activity with single or
multiple patients demonstrating multiple organ system
symptoms, initial workup should include a thorough physical examination, laboratory studies including complete
blood count (CBC) with differential, erythrocyte sedimentation rate (ESR), chemistry panel, urine analysis, chest
x-ray, and ECG. Blood cultures and skin biopsies should
also be considered if patients demonstrate a systemic
infection, or if localized skin lesions are noted. While the
patient is in isolation, no attempt should be made at surgical debridement of skin lesions as this has a high risk of
seeding possibly local cutaneous colonization to a systemic fatal distribution of the agent. Patients should be
monitored continuously and be well-oxygenated.

With weeping lesions that show musculoskeletal soft
tissue manifestations, broad span antibiotics should be initiated until the specific agent is notified.

In addition to treating the patient, some basic features
of the population being attacked can help rapidly differentiate between a chemical and biological attack. In a chemical attack, there are a large number of patients with very
similar symptoms seeking care simultaneously for multiple systems—especially respiratory, neurological, and
cutaneous chief complaints. Symptoms of chemical warfare include nausea, headache, eye pain, disorientation,
difficulty breathing, or convulsions. Biological organisms
present with an increased incidence in an otherwise
healthy population seeking care for generalized malaise
and symptoms involving the gastrointestinal and respiratory system in particular. While chemical and biological

TABLE 8-2

A BRIEF HISTORY OF CHEMICAL WARFARE AND TERRORISM IN THE 20th CENTURY

1917–1918	Germany employs chlorine, phosgene, and sulfur mustard in World War I
1930s	Botulinum toxin used by Japanese against Manchurian prisoners
1936	German chemist Gerhard Schrader synthesizes tabun
1937	Schrader and colleagues synthesize sarin (an acronym for group members' names)
1940–1945	Germany employs Zyklon B, a form of hydrogen cyanide, in their gas chambers
1942	Germany begins producing nerve agents at Dyhernfurth, these were never employed
1975–1981	Trichothecene (T-2) mycotoxins allegedly employed in "yellow rain" incidents in Laos, Cambodia, and Afghanistan
1978	Bulgarian exile Georgi Markov assassinated in London by ricin injection
1984	Iraq employs nerve agents against Iranian troops: 10,000 deaths
1988	Iraq employs various chemical agents against Kurdish rebels
1990s	Aum Shinrikyo attempts but fails at aerosol dissemination of botulinum toxin
1994	Aum Shinrikyo attacks apartment complex in Japan with sarin (GB): 300 injuries, 7 deaths
1995	Aum Shinrikyo launches multifocal Tokyo subway system attack with sarin: 1500 require medical treatment, 12 deaths

Source: Adapted from Greenfield RA, et al. Microbiological, Biological, and Chemical Weapons of Warfare and Terrorism. The American Journal of the Medical Sciences. June 2002;323:326–340. Source: Adapted from Greydanus DG, Homnick DN (eds). Disorders of the lung-pneumonia. In: Adolescent Medicine. Stamford, CT: Appleton & Lange, 1997.

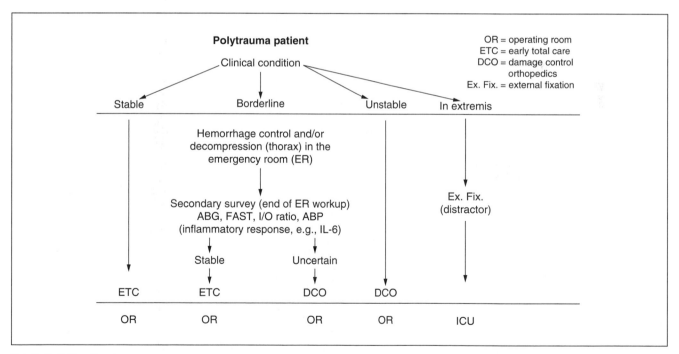

FIGURE 8-1

The current treatment algorithm from Hannover, Germany, for the use of damage control orthopedics is based on a prompt and accurate determination of whether the patient is stable, borderline, unstable, or in extremis. ER = emergency room, ABG = arterial blood gases, FAST = focused assessment sonography for trauma, I/O ratio = intake/output ratio, ABP = arterial blood pressure, IL-6 = interleukin-6, ETC = early total care, OR = operating room, DCO = damage control orthopedics, and ICU = intensive care unit.
Source: Adapted from Roberts CS. Damage control orthopedics: evolving concepts in the treatment of patients who have sustained orthopedic trauma. JBJS Am. 2005;87:434–449.

COMMON BIOLOGICAL AGENTS AND MUSCULOSKELETAL IMPLICATIONS

Agent	Musculoskeletal Manifestations	Organ System Findings	Diagnostics	Treatment
Anthrax	Cutaneous anthrax can develop into a necrotic eschar at times can lead to malignant edema and spreads to lymphatics and bloodstream that leads to papillary necrosis	Cutaneous anthrax—itching at inoculation site, followed by a popular lesion Inhalation anthrax—pulmonary edema followed by respiratory distress Intestinal anthrax—rapid ascites, cholera-like diarrhea and septicemia	Clinical evaluation	Supportive care, surgical treatment of necrotic lesions, and cutaneous edema is contraindicated secondary to risk of dissemination Ciprofloxacin or doxycycline. In bioterrorist activity, consider broad-spectrum treatment secondary to concerns of resistant strains being developed Universal precautions including burning or vaporizing clothing and materials possibly exposed to spores
Botulism	Intoxication with botulinum toxin is a neurological syndrome caused by presynaptic blockade of neuromuscular and autonomic cholinergic junctions Wound botulism also has been associated with the intramuscular or subcutaneous injection of black tar heroin. Intact skin is not penetrated by botulinum toxin, and person	The earliest clinical signs are usually blurred vision from dilated pupils, dry mouth, dysarthria, and dysphagia The speed and intensity of paralysis is dependent upon the amount of toxin absorbed	Definitive diagnosis requires identification of the toxin in serum, vomitus, gastric aspirate, or stool. More rapid antigen identification tests are in development	Supportive care and the administration of antitoxin Timely antitoxin administration will not reverse existent paralysis but will minimize progression The U.S.-licensed trivalent (A, B, E) equine antitoxin is available through state health authorities and the CDC. The dose per patient of licensed antitoxin is 10 mL (1 vial) diluted 10-fold in normal saline for slow intravenous (IV) administration once only Epinephrine and diphenhydramine should be on hand to treat adverse reactions Supportive therapy must include, as necessary, airway intubation and mechanical ventilation
	Botulism presents with acute, bilateral cranial nerve palsies that are followed by descending flaccid paralysis	Death due to botulism is attributable to aspiration-related events after loss of gag reflex or to ventilatory failure		

Hantavirus	As weakness descends, bulbar manifestations are followed by loss of head control, then more generalized deterioration in muscle tone. Deep tendon reflexes decline over days, and constipation and other autonomic dysfunctions may develop Mainly respiratory illness with migratory arthralgias and diffuse myalgias	Zoonotic virus with rodent hosts Mortality rate of 50 and secondary to ARDS or cardiac failure Clinical evaluation	Supportive care consisting of respiratory care to maintain oxygenation and adequate hemodynamic support and monitoring
Plague	Mostly diffuse myalgias after initial infection of the lymph nodes, there is painful lymphadenopathy followed by hemorrhagic dissemination that leads to systemic clinical findings—high-grade fever, headaches, chills, and abdominal distress. May also see draining sites of initial infection inoculation most commonly in groin, neck, and axilla. Skin necrosis leading to muscular dissemination is a late sequela, "black plague"	Bubonic—lymphatic system involvement Septicemic—blood infection Pneumonic Clinical evaluation	Antibiotics—streptomycin, gentamycin, tetracyclines, chloramphenicol Supportive care and isolation precautions
Smallpox	Characteristic epidermal lesions. The pustular fluid eventually dries up as the disease disappears and the lesions become filled with granular tissue, which forms scabs consisting of degenerated epithelial cells and leukocytes. Virus particles can be	Initial infection followed by prodrome of 2 weeks then fever then followed by onset of rash. Transmission from person to person through airborne respiratory particles.	The usual preliminary method of diagnosis of orthopoxvirus infections is by observing the characteristic brick-shaped virions in negatively stained pustular fluid or homogenates of scab material viewed by	There are no proven treatments for clinical smallpox; medical care is generally supportive Vaccination administered within 3–4 days postexposure can prevent disease or severe illness caused by variola virus. If a joint is

(Continued)

COMMON BIOLOGICAL AGENTS AND MUSCULOSKELETAL IMPLICATIONS (*CONTINUED*)

Agent	Musculoskeletal Manifestations	Organ System Findings	Diagnostics	Treatment
	present in large numbers in the scabs but are generally	Direct contact from rash can also transmit virus albeit less common then respiratory transmission	electron microscopy. See. Fig. 8-2.	infected by the virus it should be treated by urgent I&D and drain placement as described above
	Arthritis or "osteomyelitis variolosa": this complication occurred in approximately 1.7% in a case series review. It usually occurred after the fifteenth day and was accompanied by brief recurrence of fever during the scabbing stage. The elbow is the most commonly affected joint and symmetrical, bilateral involvement was frequently seen. This complication was most commonly caused by viral infection of the metaphyses of growing bones. Most cases resolved without permanent deformity.			
	Hemorrhagic smallpox: In patients with a highly compromised immune response, there is extensive multiplication of the virus in the spleen and bone marrow to produce a rare condition known as hemorrhagic smallpox associated with petechiae			
Ricin	Injection subcutaneously causes immediate muscle necrosis. After an 8-hour latent period, inhalational exposure produces necrosis of upper and lower respiratory epithelium causing tracheitis, bronchitis, bronchiolitis, and interstitial pneumonia with perivascular and alveolar edema	Protein cytotoxin derived from castor beans As an attack agent, it could be used to contaminate food or limited water supplies or aerosolized for inhalation	Specific antigen testing on serum and respiratory secretions and immuno-histochemical staining of tissues are useful if available, if not, seroconversion can be demonstrated	Treatment is supportive therapies only. The protective mask is effective in preventing aerosol exposure. Candidate vaccines are being developed

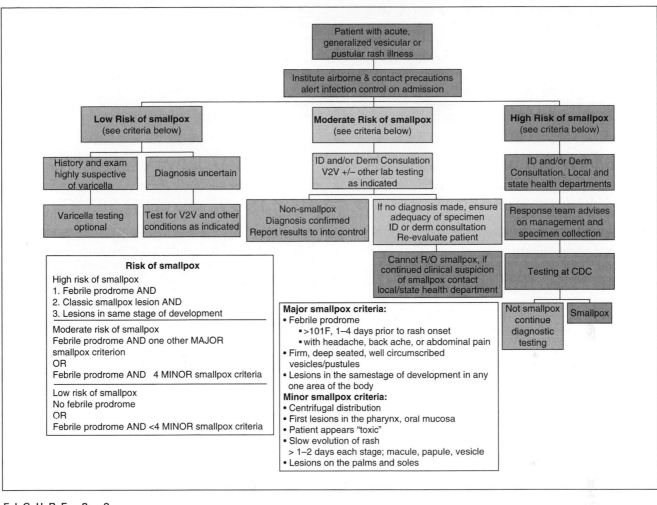

FIGURE 8-2

SMALLPOX EVALUATION AND TREATMENT ALGORITHM

agents will cause a large increase in sickness and death in the animal population, a sudden change in the insect population can help distinguish the category. Chemical agents will result in a lack of insects that are normally present, as opposed to biological agents that result in an unusual swarm of insects.

After the primary survey has been conducted and the patient has been stabilized, the secondary survey should include an evaluation of the back and the extremities with close inspection of the integument for lesions. When dealing with biologic agents or bacterial agents, it is pivotal to rule out a septic joint. If a septic joint is suspected and proven, it is mandatory to address it with urgent surgery, for any delay can cause irreparable articular cartilage damage.

Typically a patient with a septic joint demonstrates the following: severe pain on active or passive range of motion, erythema and/or calor of the affected joint, fever >101.5°F, malaise, and chills. One usually will see an elevated sed rate,

white blood cells (WBC), and C-reactive protein (CRP). If there is clinical suspicion of a septic joint, a sterile joint aspiration must be done and the specimen needs to be sent for stat gram stain, WBC count, and culture and sensitivity. A WBC count of >75,000 or a positive gram stain, or frank pus, are all indicative of a septic joint, and the patient must be taken to surgery for urgent irrigation and debridement and drain placement. Further cultures must be taken at the time of surgery. Many joints are amenable to arthroscopic surgery but some need to be addressed in an open fashion. The main principle, however, is that the joint be addressed to allow a path of egress of the affecting agent or bacteria.

After the initial I&D, intravenous (IV) antibiotics should be administered for a minimum of 48 hours and then a reassessment for repeat I&D based on clinical symptomology. The surgical drain is usually discontinued after 48 hours. It is also highly recommended to obtain an infectious disease consultation with any orthopedic infection.

Open fractures (fractures that communicate with the outside environment through a break in the skin) define another orthopedic emergency. There is a dearth of reported literature on the treatment of open fractures with exposure to biologic agents. Circumstances in which one encounters a patient with an open fracture exposed to biologic agents require the patient to be placed in isolation with an urgent initial evaluation that includes staging the open fracture based on the widely accepted Gustilo and Anderson open fracture classification. This helps delineate appropriate treatment and prognosis. Specific agent identification may require consideration of delaying irrigation and debridement secondary to concerns of seeding the agent systemically. Most open fractures are caused by significant energy to have concomitant soft tissue damage, which in turn causes these agents to seed deeper structures. At this juncture, damage control orthopedic protocols should be followed, especially if the patient begins to demonstrate systemic symptoms.

The initial steps of treatment of open fractures involves local sterile irrigation, coverage with Betadine-soaked sterile dressing and splinting. An IV cephalosporin (gram-positive coverage) should be administered (1 g). If there is a higher level of contamination, IV (gram-negative coverage) aminoglycoside is added (1 mg/kg). For gross contamination (barn yard and clostridium infections), high-dose IV penicillin is added (4 million U). IV therapy is additionally continued for at least 24 hours after the last I&D. A tetanus booster should be given for contaminated wounds. Formal radical debridement and irrigation should be accomplished within 6 hours. Debridement principles include wound extension in order to visualize the total wound environment, removal of all devitalized tissue, followed by copious sterile irrigation. Identification of the infecting agent although difficult in bioterrorist situations is always helpful. Skeletal stabilization should be accomplished after debridement providing a platform for soft tissue recovery. Highly contaminated wounds or severely damaged soft tissues should be returned to the operating room every 48 hours, until the wound is clean and only viable soft tissues remain. Exposed bone requires soft tissue coverage as soon as possible, (usually within 5 days). If bone grafting is required, a staged approach is employed usually within 6–8 weeks. (See Table 8-4.)

TABLE 8 - 4

OPEN FRACTURE CLASSIFICATION

Type	Definition
I	Open fracture with a clean wound <1 cm in length
II	Open fracture with a laceration of >1 cm long and without extensive soft-tissue damage, flaps, or avulsions
III	Either an open fracture with extensive soft-tissue laceration, damage, or loss; an open segmental fracture; or a traumatic amputation. Also: High-velocity gunshot injuries Open fractures caused by form injuries Open fractures requiring vascular repair Open fractures older than 8 hours
IIIa	Adequate periosteal cover of a fractures bone despite extensive soft-tissue laceration or damage High-energy trauma irrespective of size of wound
IIIb	Extensive soft-tissue loss with significant periosteal stripping and bone damage Usually associated with massive contamination
IIIc	Association with arterial injury requiring repair, irrespective of degree of soft-tissue injury

Source: From Gustilo RB, Mendoza RM, Williams DM. Problems in the management of type III (severe) open fractures. A new classification of type III open fractures. J Trauma 1984;24:742–746.

Suggested Reading

Born CT. Organizing the orthopaedic trauma association mass casualty response team. *Clin Orthop Relat Res.* 2004;422:114–116.

Department of Health and Human Services, Centers for Disease Control and Prevention. Emergency Preparedness and Response: Bioterrorism. February 15, 2007. Available at: *http://www.bt.cdc.gov/*

Greenfield RA, Brown BR, Hutchins JB, et al. Microbiological, biological, and chemical weapons of warfare and terrorism. *Am J Med.* June 2002;323:326–340.

Roberts CS. Damage control orthopaedics: evolving concepts in the treatment of patients who have sustained orthopaedic trauma. *JBJS Am.* 2005;87:434–449.

Roberts CS. Damage control orthopaedics: evolving concepts in the treatment of patients who have sustained orthopaedic trauma. *Instr Course Lect.* 2005;54:447–62.

9

OPHTHALMOLOGICAL ISSUES

Manpreet S. Chhabra, Rashmi Kapur, and Kent Kirk

STAT FACTS

OPHTHALMOLOGICAL ISSUES

- Ocular manifestations of exposure may occur via direct mucosal or systemic involvement.
- Reiter's syndrome can occur following shigella infection.
- Uveitis can be a complication of viral hemorrhagic fevers.

INTRODUCTION

Bioterrorism is the term applied to the unlawful use or threatened use of microorganisms or toxins derived from living organisms to produce death or disease in humans, animals, or plants. Some of these agents can cause ocular manifestations. It is important to identify them early so that the diseases can be recognized in time and appropriately treated.

Anthrax

Anthrax is an infection caused by the spore forming bacterium *Bacillus anthracis*. There are three routes of infection: inhalation leading to pulmonary disease, contact leading to cutaneous manifestations, or ingestion leading to gastrointestinal disease.

Pulmonary disease occurs when spores are inhaled and deposited in the alveolar spaces. There they germinate and cause infection, which leads to hemorrhage, pulmonary edema, and necrosis. This can be complicated by meningitis.

The cutaneous form occurs when the spores invade broken skin. The spores germinate and produce a toxin, which causes localized edema and a rash. Cutaneous anthrax can manifest itself on the eyelids leading to scarring cicatricial ectropion. The ectropion can lead to corneal scarring.

The gastrointestinal form occurs if spores are ingested and deposited in the gastrointestinal tract. Oral, esophageal, and intestinal ulcers can form leading to sepsis.

Anthrax is susceptible to ciprofloxacin, which must be administered before severe systemic disease occurs.

Botulism

Botulism is a skeletal muscle-paralyzing disease caused by a toxin made by the strictly anaerobic gram-positive *Bacillus* bacterium *Clostridium botulinum*. Human cases are usually caused by types A, B, or E. It is one of the most toxic substances known. Botulism is divided into five clinical types: classic or food-born botulism, infant botulism, wound botulism, hidden botulism, and inadvertent botulism.

- Food-born botulism is a public health emergency that is due to ingestion of food containing preformed neurotoxin, leading to illness within a few hours to days.
- Infant botulism occurs due to germination of spores of *C. botulinum* in their intestinal tract.
- Wound botulism occurs when wounds, especially injection drug sites, are infected with *C. botulinum* that secretes the toxin.
- Hidden botulism, also known as intestinal colonization botulism, refers to those cases of botulism in adults where there is no readily apparent source of botulinum toxin. It is also considered an adult form of infant botulism.
- Inadvertent botulism, the latest addition, refers to either an iatrogenic disease or an accidental occupational exposure occurring in laboratory workers.

Signs and symptoms of botulism poisoning occur within 12–36 hours after exposure. They usually begin in the cranial nerve territory with blurred vision, dysarthria, and dysphagia. The resulting paralysis descends from head to toe. This pattern distinguishes botulism from Guillain-Barré syndrome, which is characterized by ascending paralysis. Ocular effects of severe botulism almost always include marked extraocular muscle weakness, including ptosis. Weakness of the face, tongue, pharynx, and neck also occurs.

Weakness progresses for 4–5 days when it reaches a plateau. The weakness is usually bilateral although often asymmetric. The most fearful complication is respiratory collapse caused by paralysis of breathing muscles.

Ocular symptoms of botulism include marked extraocular muscle weakness leading to diplopia. Ptosis or drooping eyelids is the second most common symptom. Other symptoms may include abnormal pupillary reaction to light, impaired accommodation, nystagmus, and mydriasis.

Ophthalmological signs and symptoms are among the earliest disease manifestations in inhalational botulinum, and it has a dose-dependent onset. The public health department should be notified immediately if a case of botulism is suspected and the therapeutic antitoxin should be administered early to reduce the severity of symptoms.

It is important to keep the differential of botulism in mind if such patients present to the emergency room with initial ocular symptoms. Recovery is usually prolonged but nearly total. The major medical treatment is supportive.

Smallpox

Smallpox is a devastating disease caused by the variola virus, which was eradicated worldwide back in 1980. There are two World Health Organization approved repositories at the Centers for Disease Control in Atlanta and at the NPO (Scientific and Production Association) in the Novosibirsk region of the Soviet Union. The amount of clandestine stockpiles remains a matter of contention and concern. Smallpox presents as a potential threat to be used as a biological weapon. There has also been concern of the smallpox vaccine also being a tool for biological warfare. There are two clinical forms of smallpox with variola major being the most severe form. It is spread by aerosolized droplets, direct skin contact, and through fomites. There is an incubation period of 10–14 days before the advent of symptoms.

Ocular complications have been reported in 5–9% of cases of smallpox. These include generalized pustular rash on the eyelids, conjunctival pustules, and corneal involvement in the form of pustules. These pustules are painful and cause a tremendous inflammatory reaction and purulent discharge. They often extend to the cornea causing inflammation, scarring, and even perforation with loss of the eye. Disciform keratitis has also been reported, and corneal leukoma may occur after ulceration or disciform keratitis. Iritis, iridocyclitis, and secondary glaucoma may also occur. Other reported ocular symptoms include retinitis, chorioretinitis, and optic neuritis, paralysis of accommodation, paralysis of extraocular muscles, retrobulbar hemorrhage with proptosis, suppurative dacryocystitis, and ankyloblepharon.

Ocular vaccinia is the term referred to the accidental inoculation of vaccinia virus. It generally occurs when a patient accidentally rubs the eye after touching the smallpox vaccine site. It is also seen in individuals in close contact with the vaccine. Eyelid vaccinia has been reported to be the most common complication after smallpox vaccination and refers to raised, white, umbilicated pustules with a necrotic center surrounded by local erythema. Other complications include corneal perforation, disciform keratitis, interstitial keratitis, central retinal artery occlusion, pigmentary retinopathy, chorioretinitis, central serous retinopathy, exudative retinitis, optic neuritis, retrobulbar neuritis, transient strabismus, proptosis, limitation of ocular motility, and optic atrophy.

The long-term sequelae include entropion, symblepharon, eyelid margin defects, and loss of eyelashes. Treatment consists of topical antivirals such as idoxuridine, trifluridine, and vidarabine. Vaccinia immune globulin I used for ocular vaccinia in a dose of 0.3–0.5 mL/kg of body weight can be administered and needs to be repeated in 48 hours if there is no improvement. Topical steroids are given in combination with antivirals for disciform keratitis. Topical and/or oral antibiotics are used to prevent bacterial superinfection.

Shigellosis

Shigellosis refers to an infectious disease caused by *Shigella*. The symptoms of shigellosis include diarrhea, fever, and stomach cramps that develop 1–2 days after exposure of the patient to the pathogenic bacterium. Shigellosis usually causes bloody diarrhea and resolves in 5–7 days. The ocular significance of this disease can be seen in patients infected with *Shigella flexneri*. which leads to arthritis, irritation of the eyes, and painful urination, which is called Reiter's syndrome. It can last for months or years, and can lead to chronic arthritis, which is difficult to treat. This syndrome develops in genetically predisposed people and is caused by a reaction to *Shigella* infection. Treatment consists of antibiotics such as ampicillin, trimethoprim/sulfamethoxazole, nalidixic acid, or ciprofloxacin. Prevention is by frequent and careful hand washing with soap.

Escherichia Coli 0157:H7

Although most strains of *Escherichia coli* are harmless and live in the intestines of healthy humans and animals, 0157:H7 is a strain, which produces a powerful toxin and can cause severe illness. The ocular manifestations can be seen in *E. coli* infections complicated by hemolytic uremic syndrome, which leads to red blood cell destruction and kidney failure. The long-term complications include hypertension, seizures, blindness, and paralysis. Most patients recover without antibiotics in 5–10 days. Prevention is by cooking all ground beef thoroughly, drinking pasteurized milk, juice, or cider, washing fruits and vegetables thoroughly, and avoiding swallowing lake or pool water while swimming.

Ricin

Ricin, a poison made from the waste leftover from processing castor beans, acts by inhibition of protein synthesis by the cells of the body, leading to cellular destruction and eventually death. It can be in powder form, a mist, or a pellet, or it can be dissolved in water or weak acid. Effects of ricin poisoning depend on whether ricin was inhaled, ingested, or injected.

The eyes can be involved after exposure to the powder or mist form, which causes redness and pain. There is no antidote for ricin; so prevention of exposure is of prime importance. If exposure cannot be avoided, the most important factor is then washing the ricin off or out of the body as quickly as possible.

In the setting of ocular involvement, appropriate management consists of rinsing with plain water for 10–15 minutes. Contact lenses should be removed and discarded with the contaminated clothing. Eyeglasses should be washed with soap and water.

Viral Hemorrhagic Fevers

Viral hemorrhagic fevers (VHFs) refer to a severe multisystem syndrome caused by several distinct families of viruses. They are characterized by damage to the vascular system and impairment of the body to regulate itself. These symptoms are often accompanied by hemorrhage, which is rarely life-threatening. The Centers for Disease Control and Prevention (CDC) has developed a system for categorizing potential agents of bioterrorism into Categories A, B, and C. Ebola, Marburg, Lassa, Junin, Machup, Guanarito, and Sabie belong to Category A. VHFs are caused by viruses of four distinct families: arenaviruses, filoviruses, bunyaviruses, and flaviviruses. They are all RNA viruses and their survival is dependent on an animal or insect host, known as the natural reservoir. Humans are not the natural reservoir for any of these viruses. They spread to humans by accidental transmission. These viruses are extremely pathogenic, and have potential for transmission by fine particle aerosol. Hemorrhagic fever viruses have been used in biological weapon programs and are of interest to terrorist groups.

Specific signs and symptoms vary by the type of VHF, but initial signs and symptoms often include marked fever, fatigue, dizziness, muscle aches, loss of strength, and exhaustion. Symptoms of hemorrhagic fever include bleeding from the gums, nose, into the skin, red eyes, bloody stools, blood in vomitus, headache, vomiting, loss of appetite, diarrhea, weakness or severe fatigue, abdominal pain, generalized muscle or joint pain, difficulty swallowing, difficulty breathing, and hiccups. Severely ill patient cases may also show shock, nervous system malfunction, coma, delirium, and seizures. Some types of VHF are associated with renal failure. The ocular manifestations of Ebola hemorrhagic fever has been reported to include conjunctival injection, subconjunctival hemorrhage, ocular pain, photophobia, hyperlacrimation, and progressive visual loss and posterior uveitis. The pathogenesis of uveitis may be a delayed hypersensitivity reaction to viral antigens. Uveitis is also seen with Marburg virus. The clinical features of dengue hemorrhage fever include cells and flare in the anterior chamber and presence of vitreous cells. The main fundus findings have been reported to be macular and retinal hemorrhages, peripapillary hemorrhage, Roth's spot, diffuse retinal edema, blurring of the optic disc margin, serious retinal detachment, choroidal effusions, and nonspecific maculopathy. The mean interval between the onset of visual symptoms and the systemic manifestations of dengue fever is reported to be 7.26 days (range, 2–15 days, 62.5% between 5 and 8 days).

Local and state public health officials should be notified on suspecting any case of VHF. Patients with suspected or confirmed VHF infection should undergo specific infection-control recommendations, which include strict adherence to hand washing, double gloving and the use of impermeable gowns, N95 masks or powered air-purifying respirators, negative pressure isolation with 6–12 air exchanges per hour, leg and shoe coverings, and face shields or goggles. All contacts should be put under medical surveillance for signs of infection for 21 days.

Treatment is primarily supportive, as there is no treatment for established VHFs. Ribavirin, a nucleoside analog that reduces levels of guanosine monophosphate, guanosine diphosphate, and guanosine triphosphate, has been effective in treating some individuals with Lassa fever or hemorrhagic fever with renal syndrome, causing a significant reduction in mortality. An Ebola DNA plasmid vaccine that relies on a DNA "primer" from three strains of Ebola virus is in trial. There is availability of a live attenuated virus vaccine against Argentine hemorrhagic fever (Junin), which may also protect against Bolivian hemorrhagic fever (caused by Machupo virus). However, vaccination is of no use in the setting of a bioterrorist attack. Treatment with convalescent-phase plasma has been effective in a few patients with arenavirus infection. The prognosis is poor in patients with significant volume depletion and hemodynamic instability.

Avoidance of close physical contact with infected people and their body fluids is the most important way of controlling the spread of disease. Infection-control measures include isolating infected individuals; wearing protective clothing; and proper use, disinfection, and disposal of instruments and equipment used in treating or caring for patients with VHF.

Radiation Injury

Acute radiation syndrome (ARS) or radiation sickness is caused by irradiation of the whole body in a short span of time. The classic ARS syndromes are bone marrow syndrome, gastrointestinal syndrome, and cardiovascular/central nervous system syndrome. Cutaneous radiation syndrome is the term applied to complex pathological syndrome that results from acute exposure to the skin.

The effects of radiation injury to the eye include mild damage to radiation burns on the eyelid skin, injury to cornea causing immediate pain and vascularization, loss of transparency of the cornea, flare in the anterior chamber owing to leakage of proteins from the iris vessels, hyperemia and inflammation of the iris, pupillary miosis, cataract, retinal edema, burns and inflammation. All these effects may lead to decrease in vision. In the event of a radiation emergency, protection of eyes can be achieved by covering them to prevent effects of radiation.

Suggested Reading

Bioterrorism agents/diseases. November 19, 2004. Accessed February 11, 2006. Available at *http://www.bt.cdc.gov/agent/agentlist.asp*

Caya JG. Clostridium botulinum and the ophthalmologist: a review of botulism, including biological warfare ramifications of botulinum toxin. *Surv Ophthalmol.* July–August 2001;46(1):25–34.

Hom GG. Chemical, biological, and radiological weapons: implications for optometry and public health. *Optometry.* February 2003;74(2):81–98.

Kibadi K, Mupapa K, Kuvula K, et al. Late ophthalmologic manifestations in survivors of the 1995 Ebola virus epidemic in Kikwit, Democratic Republic of the Congo. *J Infect Dis.* February 1999;179 (Suppl 1):S13–4.

Lim WK, Mathur R, Koh A, et al. Ocular manifestations of dengue fever. *Ophthalmology.* November 2004;111(11):2057–64.

Maki DG. National preparedness for biological warfare and bioterrorism: smallpox and the ophthalmologist. *Arch Ophthalmol.* 2003;121:710–711.

Pigott DC. Hemorrhagic fever viruses. *Crit Care Clin.* October 2005;21(4):765–83.

Semba RD. The ocular complications of smallpox and smallpox immunization. *Arch Ophthalmol.* 2003;121:715–19.

World Health Organization. The Global Eradication of Smallpox: Final Repot of the Global Commission for the Certification of Smallpox Eradication, Geneva, Switzerland: World Health Organization; 1980.

10

RESPIRATORY AND CRITICAL CARE UNIT ISSUES

Niraj Mahajan, Mairaj Jaleel, and Shashi K. Bellam

STAT FACTS

RESPIRATORY AND CRITICAL CARE UNIT ISSUES

- Precautions for isolation of patients are crucial to prevent transmission of disease.
- Respiratory precautions for transmissible pathogens include the use of N95 masks or similar, gloves, eye protection, gowns, and if indicated, negative airflow ventilation.
- The SARS outbreak of 2002–2004 revealed that there can be a high rate of health-care worker infection during routine care of critically ill patients, but the use of appropriate precautions can greatly decrease the rate of transmission of illness.
- Full antichemical warfare protective equipment may decrease the ability to perform certain procedures as such, caregivers should be aware of potential limitations and consider appropriate alternatives, such as the use of laryngeal-mask-airways or noninvasive positive-pressure ventilation in lieu of endotracheal intubation.
- Ventilator circuits require additional use of expiratory-limb filters to prevent transmission of illness.
- Common respiratory symptoms include
  - Cough
  - Hemoptysis
  - Bronchospasm

THE ROLE OF PRECAUTIONS TO PREVENT TRANSMISSION OF ILLNESS

The use of standard precautions is recommended for the care of all patients in all health-care settings. Hands should be washed between patient contacts, after removing gloves, and after any potential contact with secretions, body fluids, or contaminated items. Gloves are recommended when touching mucous membranes, nonintact skin, and body fluids. The use of a protective gown is advised during procedures or patient-care activities when contact of clothing or exposed skin with blood, body fluids, or secretions is anticipated. A standard isolation gown should fully cover the front torso and arms, and should tie in the back. Gloves should cover the cuffs of the gown. The use of a mask, eye protection, or a face-shield is advised during any procedure or patient-care activity, which is likely to generate splashes or sprays of blood, secretions, or body fluids.

In many cases, the patient will require isolation to a single bedroom depending on the clinical scenario and if there is an increased risk of transmission. In addition to standard precautions, contact precautions should be implemented for specified patients known or suspected to be infected with microorganisms that can be transmitted by direct contact, that is, hand or skin-to-skin contact with the patient, or indirect contact including touching environmental surfaces or patient-care items in the patient's environment. The patient should be placed in a private room, if available. If a private room is not available, the patient should be placed in a room with a patient who has an active infection with the same microorganism, known as cohorting. In such situations, gloves should be worn when entering the room, removed when leaving the patient's room, and hands washed immediately. After glove removal and hand-washing, care should be taken to ensure that the hands do not touch any environmental surfaces or items in the patient's room.

Droplet precautions are designed to reduce droplet transmission of infectious agents. Droplet transmission involves contact of the mucous membranes of the nose or conjunctivae of a susceptible person with large-particle droplets containing microorganisms from a carrier. Droplets can be generated from the source person from sneezing, talking, coughing, or during procedures such as bronchoscopy. Transmission of large-particle droplets generally requires close contact between individuals as droplets generally do not remain suspended in air and tend to travel 3 feet or less. The patient should be placed in a private room if possible. If a private room is not obtainable, then the patient should be cohorted with an individual who is infected with the same microorganism and no other microorganism. If cohorting is not achievable, a spatial separation of at least 3 feet should be maintained between the infected patient and other patients in the room or visitors. In addition to standard precautions, a mask should be worn when working within 3 feet of the patient. Special air handling and ventilation are not required to prevent droplet transmission. The door of the patient room may remain open.

Airborne precautions are designed to reduce the risk of airborne transmission of infectious agents. Airborne transmission occurs by dissemination of airborne droplet nuclei of evaporated droplets that remain suspended in the air for long periods of time or dust particles, which contain the infectious agent. Microorganisms, which are carried in this manner, can be widely dispersed by air currents and inhaled or deposited on a susceptible host over longer distances from the source patient. Therefore, special air handling and ventilation are required to prevent airborne transmission. The patient should be placed in a private room that has (1) monitored negative air pressure in relation to surroundings, (2) 6–12 air exchanges per hour and, (3) appropriate discharge of air outdoors or monitored high-efficiency filtration of room air before the air is circulated to other areas of the hospital. The patient should be kept in the room, and the door should remain closed. The CDC advises the use of special respiratory protection, namely the N95 respirator for susceptible persons when entering the room of patients with known or suspected TB, rubeola, or varicella.

Antichemical warfare protective equipment includes the use of a full-body plastic suit, rubber gloves, and a gas mask with attached filter. As most physicians rarely or never have practiced medicine in full antichemical warfare protective equipment, the effects of such equipment on the ability to practice medicine (specifically, the ability to perform procedures) are generally unknown. Various studies have demonstrated decreased effectiveness in performing procedures with full antichemical protective equipment, including a significantly decreased success rate of procedures such as endotracheal intubation even in the hands of experienced physicians. In full antichemical warfare protective equipment, the use of laryngeal mask airways has been shown to be a more successful means of securing a temporary airway than attempting endotracheal intubation in simulated mass casualties. As such, clinicians should

have an appreciation that the use of protective equipment will change the ability and means to deliver health care, whether it be performing procedures, examining patients, or other aspects, in likely, some predictable and some unpredictable ways.

Mechanical Ventilation and Safety Issues Involving Ventilator Circuits

The SARS virus outbreak of 2002–2004 prompted much concern regarding safety issues related to the mechanical ventilation for patients in the setting of airborne infectious pathogens. Prior to this outbreak, guidelines for respiratory protection were generally unavailable or based on minimal data. The experiences in China, Hong Kong, and Canada provided not only an opportunity to create or update guidelines for respiratory precautions for dealing with a transmissible illness, but also provided a wealth of knowledge about the actual delivery of health care and subsequent outcomes. Patients who develop acute respiratory failure, or who have difficulty maintaining adequate oxygen levels, will likely require mechanical ventilation. However, the placement of an endotracheal tube provides a means for the virus or pathogen to be easily aerosolized, affecting caregivers, and ventilating such patients raising the concern that the virus or pathogen may exit the ventilator in droplet or aerosolized form along with the patient's exhaled air. The initial stage of the SARS virus outbreak was characterized by a high rate of health-care worker infection with the virus (51% of cases in the greater Toronto area from May to mid-April 2003). Among the cases of health-care workers who contracted SARS, there was a particularly high rate in physicians and nurses performing endotracheal intubation and mechanical ventilation, especially patients receiving noninvasive positive-pressure ventilation (NIV). Retrospective questionnaire surveys revealed ~9% (3 of 23) of physicians who intubated patients with SARS contracted the virus in the early period of the outbreak; in the later period of outbreak, the rate of health-care worker infection fell substantially (0 of 10). The later period of the outbreak was associated with a statistically increased use of personal protective devices, double gloves, N95 masks, or face shields. The official guidelines from the Health Canada Infection Control Guidelines Steering Committee include the use of an N95 mask of equivalent, gowns, and eye protection for health-care workers and the donning of a surgical mask by the patient with isolation from other patients.

Once intubated, the use of mechanical ventilators presents specific concerns with regard to prevention of transmission of illness, including but not limited to the use of filters on ventilators and ventilator tubing. To address this concern, the U.S. Centers for Disease Control and Prevention (CDC) has issued several statements regarding the use of filters on the exhalation limb of the ventilator in the setting of the SARS epidemic stating: "Submicron filters on exhalation valves of mechanical ventilators may prevent contaminated aerosols from entering the environment. Although the effectiveness of this measure in reducing the risk of SARS-CoV transmission is unknown, the use of such filters is prudent during high-frequency oscillatory ventilation of patients with SARS-CoV disease." The Emergency Care Research Institute has also advised the use of breathing circuit filters whenever SARS patients are mechanically ventilated. The use of breathing circuit filters would likely help reduce the risk of spreading airborne and aerosolized pathogens other than SARS. The proper use of breathing circuit filters also eliminates the need for cleaning and sterilizing any reusable components downstream of the filter. Some ventilators call for the use of a specific filter. If this filter does not offer adequate protection, then an additional filter should be placed upstream of the existing filter and exhaust valve. The CDC calls for the use of a HEPA (high-efficiency particulate air) filter in some of its recommendations including its guidelines for ventilator use and ground transport of SARS patients. Alternatively, breathing circuit filters, which have bacterial and viral filtration efficiencies of 99.97%, offer protection that is equal to or better than a standard HEPA filter. In general, the filter should be placed upstream of any reusable components. In an intensive care ventilator, the filter should usually be placed between the end of the exhalation limb tubing and the ventilator in order to prevent contamination of the exhalation valve. The installation of a filter or any new component in the breathing circuit can introduce risks. With filters, the most significant risk is that the filter can accumulate moisture, which would cause increased exhalation resistance or obstruction, which may lead to decreased effectiveness of ventilation or barotrauma. Manufacturer instructions should be followed in regard to the frequency of changing water traps so that the water trap does not overflow into the filter. The use of a heat-moisture exchanger can also be used where appropriate to minimize moisture in the breathing circuit and filter. During ventilation, one way to monitor for obstruction or increased resistance during exhalation is to monitor the expiratory flow, both for return of expiratory flow to baseline (zeroflow) before the next breath and for complete exhalation of the prescribed tidal volume.

NIV through the use of a face mask attached to a bilevel positive airway pressure system has been shown to be an effective means of mechanically ventilating patients in a variety of respiratory conditions. Due to fears of health-care worker contamination due to leakage from the mask-face interface, NIV was relatively infrequently used in the SARS epidemic. However, a retrospective review of the use of NIV in SARS patients in a hospital, which routinely used negative airflow rooms as well as personal protective equipment including N95 masks, protective eye wear, full-face shields, caps, gowns with full-sleeve coverage, and HEPA air purifying systems documented no cases of SARS in health-care workers. With the documented difficulties in performing intubation, while health-care workers are wearing full protective equipment, the well-proven track record of NIV for a variety of respiratory conditions, and the likelihood that in the event of a mass casualty, the number of traditional critical care ventilators will be limited, NIV may provide a means to safely and relatively easily provide mechanical ventilation in the event of respiratory failure. Pressure-cycled ventilators (such as those traditionally used for at-home therapy for obstructive sleep apnea) may be reasonable options for noninvasively ventilating patients after mass casualties when the supply of traditional ventilators is inadequate.

EVALUATION AND MANAGEMENT OF COMMON RESPIRATORY SYMPTOMS

Cough

Cough is defined as a deep inspiration followed by a strong expiration against a closed glottis, which then opens with an expulsive flow of air, followed by a restorative inspiration. It is a common symptom and is usually associated with infection. It can be divided into productive and nonproductive, as well as acute and chronic. Differentiation between acute and chronic cough is made by length of time; usually if cough persists more than 3 weeks, it is chronic. This discussion will be limited to acute cough. Common causes of acute cough are outlined in Table 10-1. Evaluation of cough including a detailed history (including details of frequency, timing, history of exposure to irritants, history of tobacco abuse, and whether cough is productive), and physical examination can reliably narrow the differential of possible diagnosis. Guided evaluation when indicated can include chest x-rays, spirometry or pulmonary function tests (particularly for the diagnosis of asthma or emphysema), 24-hour esophageal pH monitoring, CT (computerized tomography) of the chest, and bronchoscopy. The management of acute cough is generally limited to the treatment of any identifiable cause(s). Cough suppression may be indicated to limit discomfort or complications related to the cough itself. Codeine is the most common opiate antitussive. It acts centrally to inhibit cough and offers analgesia. Morphine may also be used for very severe intractable cough. Both drugs are narcotics and are not preferred because of the potential for abuse and side effect profile. Dextromethorphan is a commonly used over-the-counter medication. It is a d-isomer of codeine that does not have any addictive properties and as such has a better side effect profile and is a nonnarcotic antitussive. Dextromethorphan has been found in small studies to be equivalent to codeine in the prevention of acute and chronic cough. The use of mucolytics is not well proven,

TABLE 10-1

COMMON CAUSES OF ACUTE COUGH

Acute infections	Tracheobronchitis
	Bronchitis
	Pneumonia
	Chronic obstructive lung disease (COPD) exacerbations
	Pertussis
	Bronchiectasis exacerbations
Airway disorders	Asthma
	Chronic bronchitis
	Chronic postnasal drip
Lung parenchymal diseases	Interstitial lung diseases/fibrosis
	Emphysema
	Sarcoidosis
Tumors	Bronchogenic carcinoma
	Alveolar cell carcinoma
	Benign airway tumors
	Mediastinal tumors
Foreign bodies	Left ventricular failure
Middle ear pathology	Pulmonary infarction
Cardiovascular diseases	Thoracic aortic aneurysm
Others	Gastroesophageal reflux
	Recurrent aspiration
Drugs	Angiotensin-converting enzyme inhibitors

but may play a role in patients with excessive mucous production by decreasing sputum viscosity to increase clearance by expectoration.

Hemoptysis

Hemoptysis is defined as expectorated blood that originates in the lungs or bronchus. Massive hemoptysis is defined as the expectoration of blood more than 100–600 mL over 24 hours. Hemoptysis should be differentiated from bleeding from the upper gastrointestinal (GI) tract (hematemesis) or nasopharynx (pseudohemoptysis), as opposed to originating from the airway tract. Initial evaluation of hemoptysis should be directed to distinguishing from hematemesis or nasal blood loss, as frequently, hematemesis may be mistaken for expectorated blood. Symptoms such as nausea and vomiting would more likely indicate hematemesis. Cough would more commonly be experienced with hemoptysis. Evaluation includes visualization of the nasal passages for alternative sites of bleeding, CT scan of the chest to localize blood in the airways and for the presence of parenchymal lung lesions, and bronchoscopy to localize the site of bleeding. Chest CT and

bronchoscopy together likely have the highest diagnostic yield. Mild hemoptysis requires a detailed history, physical examination, imaging, and endoscopy as indicated, and then therapeutic interventions as indicated. Massive hemoptysis can be a life-threatening emergency. The primary therapy is airway protection and hemodynamic stabilization. Initial management includes intubation for poor gas exchange and protection of the airway to prevent aspiration with ongoing bleeding. An endotracheal tube at least size 8 or greater should be used to facilitate suctioning and diagnostic/therapeutic bronchoscopy. Coagulation studies should be obtained and coagulopathy corrected if present. In general, all patients with massive hemoptysis should be in the intensive care unit. At times the site of bleeding lung is known and the affected lung should be placed in a dependent position to protect the uninvolved lung from aspiration of blood. A double-lumen endotracheal tube should also be considered at this time to allow for continued aeration and minimized blood soiling of the unaffected lung. Localizing the site of bleeding is most effectively done in combination with a detailed history and physical (as the patient many times can be knowledgeable regarding what side the bleeding is originating) and a chest x-ray or chest CT scan to localize bleeding; however, there is no therapeutic benefit. Flexible bronchoscopy during active bleed will give a definitive source of bleeding. Angiography may also be done to localize the site of bleeding offering the therapeutic option of embolization. Rigid or flexible bronchoscopy may be considered both offering unique advantages. Rigid bronchoscopy offers better airway control, the ability to pass larger instruments during bronchoscopy, and better suctioning during the procedure but is less often used. Flexible bronchoscopy allows for better visualization. Most physicians prefer flexible bronchoscopy through an endotracheal tube when managing massive hemoptysis. There is no clear answer from the literature on which approach is most effective and choice is usually based on the individual caregiver experience and capability. Therapeutic intervention during bronchoscopy is preferred if an active site of bleeding is identified. Many methods of stopping bleeding have been studied. Lavage with ice water saline has been found very effective in control of bleeding. Topical agents such as epinephrine (1:20,000), as well as topical thrombin, fibrinogen, and vasopressin solutions have been used with variable observational results. No controlled trials have been done with these agents. Endobronchial tamponade involves inflating a balloon catheter in the affected segment allowing tamponade of bleeding as well as prevention of aspiration into the contralateral segments. In general, this method is more effective for larger bleeds. The balloon is usually left inflated for 24 hours. Compli-cations include mucosal injury and postobstructive pneumonia. Electrocautery and laser therapy should be considered if a clear lesion is visualized during bronchoscopy. These modalities are used more often in distal lesions. Angiography and embolization is another alternative. It is effective in many cases and may be used as a method to gain control of bleeding in the short term, but the rate of recurrent bleed is high and results are dependent on the experience of the angiographer. Potential complications of angiography include perforation of a blood vessel, emboli, and spinal artery infarction. Surgery is to be considered if source of bleeding is clearly identified and other measures to control bleeding have failed. Older studies clearly favor surgical over medical therapy; however, these were not randomized control studies and medical therapy was only tried in patients who were poor surgical candidates. In general, surgical resection may be preferred if bronchial embolization fails or bleeding is so brisk it cannot be controlled by embolization or other measures.

Bronchospasm

Bronchospasm is the temporary narrowing of the airways caused by contraction of the smooth muscles in the lung walls, edema of mucosa, or increased mucous production. Etiologies include irritant effects due to inhalation exposure to smoke, chemical irritants, cold air, or allergens; infection; exercise; food or medication allergy; and gastroesophageal reflux disease. The clinical presentation can include wheezing, cough (with or without production), dyspnea, pleuritic chest pain or tightness, and pulsus paradoxus. Management includes clinical assessment of severity (e.g., general appearance of the patient, is the patient speaking in full sentences, is there use of accessory muscles of respiration, is there cyanosis or hypotension or increase in pulsus paradoxus), spirometry to measure the forced expiratory value at 1 second (if less than 50% of predicted, then suggestive of severe bronchospasm), arterial blood gases (low arterial carbon dioxide partial pressure suggests hyperventilation, which can be seen in severe bronchospasm, a high arterial carbon dioxide partial pressure may suggest severe bronchospasm with inadequate alveolar ventilation—potentially an indication of impending respiratory failure). Medical therapy includes use of β_2-agonists via inhalation (metered-dose inhaler or nebulized). Use of a metered-dose inhaler with a spacer is therapeutically equivalent of the use of a continuous nebulizer. Anticholinergic inhalers have not been clearly shown to be beneficial in acute obstruction, but may have unproven benefit and are unlikely to have significant deleterious effects, so the use of inhaled ipratropium bromide is recommended. Intravenous magnesium has been used with anecdotal improvement with some trials demonstrating a significant effect, but an inconsistent one across the literature. Trials showing the greatest effect found benefit in patients with more severe obstruction—current recommendations suggest the use of magnesium should be reserved for patients that fail β_2-agonist therapy. Systemic

corticosteroids should be considered for patients with acute severe bronchospasm that have failed β_2-agonist therapy. Systemic corticosteroids have proven useful in control of airway inflammation, improvement in symptoms, and pulmonary function. Efficacy of oral corticosteroids has been almost equal to intravenous delivery, though the enteral rate of absorption is different for each individual. Most physicians prefer intravenous corticosteroids as it eliminates question of achieving maximum bioavailability. Heliox is a combination of helium and oxygen in the concentration of 70–80% helium with the remainder oxygen. It is an adjunctive therapy considered in patients with impending respiratory failure and can be used as a temporizing measure to reduce work of respiratory muscles giving more definitive therapies such as β_2-agonist and corticosteroids time to act. There are currently no guidelines for its use and requires more clinical trials. Limitations of heliox usage include physician inexperience and lack of ready availability in most hospitals.

The decision to intubate and mechanically ventilate a patient is a clinical one. Respiratory failure remains the only absolute indication. An individual assessment is to be made based on work of breathing, hemodynamic parameters, and presence of hypercapnia. Mechanical ventilation in a patient with bronchospasm is associated with complications related to elevated intrathoracic pressures such as pneumothorax, barotrauma, and decreased cardiac output. The mortality rates related to mechanical ventilation in patients with bronchospasm were significantly higher before the widespread use of the ventilator strategy of permissive hypercapnia. Permissive hypercapnia relies on the goal of adequate oxygenation while permitting an elevated arterial partial pressure of carbon dioxide. The risks of hypercapnia are lower than the risks of an elevated intrathoracic pressure. This strategy allows the patient more time for exhalation and avoids trapped gas within the thorax. A general strategy for permissive hypercapnia includes a minute ventilation of less than 115 mL/kg body weight, tidal volume of less than 8 mL/kg body weight, respiratory rate of 10–14 breaths/min, and an inspiratory flow rate of 80–100 L/min.

Suggested Reading

Booth CM, Matukas LM, Tomlinson GA, et al. Clinical features and short-term outcomes of 144 patients with SARS in the Greater Toronto area. *JAMA*. 2003;289:2801–9.

Caputa KM, Byrick R, Chapman MG, et al. Intubation of SARS patients: infection and perspectives of healthcare workers. *Can J Anesth*. 2006;53:122–129.

Cheung TM, Yam LY, So LK, et al. Effectiveness of noninvasive positive pressure ventilation in the treatment of acute respiratory failure in severe acute respiratory syndrome *Chest*. 2004;126:845–850.

Forler RA, Guest CB, Lapinsky SE, et al. Transmission of severe acute respiratory syndrome during intubation and mechanical ventilation. *Am J Resp Crit Care Med*. 2004;169:1198–1202.

Goldik Z, Bornstein J, Eden A, et al. Airway management by physicians wearing anti-chemical warfare gear: comparison between laryngeal mask airway and endotracheal intubation. *Eur J Anaesthesiol.* 2002;19:166–169.

Guideline for isolation precautions in hospitals. Accessed November 1, 2006. Available at *http://www.cdc.gov/ncidod/ dhqp/gl_isolation.html*

Infection control precautions for respiratory infections transmitted by large droplet and contact. Accessed November 1, 2006. Available at *http://www.phac-aspc.gc.ca/sars-sras/pdf/sars-icg-outbreakworld_e.pdf*

Nambiar M.P., Gordon, R.K., Rezk P.E., et al. Medical counter measure against respiratory toxicity and acute lung injury following inhalation exposure to chemical warfare nerve agent VX. *Toxicol Appl Pharmarocol.* 2007:219:142–150.

Newman, KB, Milne S, Hamilton C, et al. A comparison of albuterol administered by Metered-Dose inhaler and space with albuterol by nebulizer in adults presenting to an urban emergency department with acute asthma. *Chest.* 2002;121: 1036–1041.

Public Health Guidance for Community-Level Preparedness and Response to Severe Acute Respiratory Syndrome (SARS) Version 2, Supplement I: Infection Control in Healthcare, Home, and Community Settings. Accessed November 1, 2006. Available at *http://www.cdc.gov/ncidod/sars/guidance/ i/pdf/i.pdf*

Samet J.M., Geyh. A.S., Utell. M.J.: The legacy of World Trade Center Dust. *N. Engl J Med.* 2007: 356(23):2233–2236.

Smyrnios NA, Irwin RS, Curley FJ. Chronic cough with a history of excessive sputum production: the spectrum and frequency of causes, key components of the diagnostic evaluation, and outcome of specific therapy. *Chest.* 1995;108:991–997.

11

GASTROINTESTINAL AND HEPATIC ISSUES

Eric Cohen and Eric Elton

Eric Cohen and Eric Elton

STAT FACTS

GASTROINTESTINAL AND HEPATIC ISSUES

Phases of the acute radiation syndrome
- Prodromal phase
- Latent phase
- Manifest illness
- Recovery or death

Mean radiation dose to kill 50% of exposed victims at 60 days ($LD_{50/60}$): 3.25–4 Gy

Primary organ systems affected
- 0.7–4 Gy: hematological syndrome
- Above 8 Gy: gastrointestinal syndrome
- Above 20 Gy: cerebrovascular syndrome

Gastrointestinal manifestations
- Nausea and vomiting
- Diarrhea
- Gastrointestinal bleeding
- Ileus
- Malabsorption
- Electrolyte imbalances
- Bacterial translocation and sepsis

Interventions and therapy
- External decontamination
- Internal decontamination: gastric lavage, emetics, and purgatives
- Antiemetics
- Fluid and electrolyte replacement
- Acid suppression
- Blood product support
- Prophylactic antibiotics

INTRODUCTION

The purpose of this chapter is to provide medical professionals with a quickly accessible and accurate source of information about how clinical syndromes, as a result of terrorist activity, may present to an emergency department in the form of gastrointestinal illness. The chapter will be divided into three sections: radiation terrorism, bioterrorism, and chemical terrorism. The section on radiation will be presented in text format, and followed by tables. The bioterrorism and chemical terrorism sections are presented in Tables 11-1 and 11-2 with symptomatic cross-reference lists (Table 11-3) accompanying the former.

The myriad of agents described herein can cause insidious and fulminant symptoms. The list is by no means meant to be exhaustive and all-inclusive. There are hundreds of toxic chemicals in common use and many biological weapons that will cause some form of gastrointestinal illness. The agents listed here are a combination of the most likely, the most easily obtainable, and potentially the most dangerous weapons to which a terrorist organization might gain access.

In addition to recognition of the presenting symptoms, the emergency caregiver should be familiar with the acuity and progression of specific gastrointestinal illnesses; gastroenterology represents a field replete with diagnostic and therapeutic capabilities, both invasive and noninvasive. It should be remembered that the diagnostic and therapeutic recommendations listed in this chapter are based on the currently accepted standard. It is likely that the gold standard of recognition, diagnosis, and treatment would evolve along with the evolution of a real outbreak. Because there are so few recorded human cases in most instances, there is a dearth of literature regarding indications for endoscopic

BIOTERRORISM

Agent	Gastrointestinal Signs/Symptoms	Important Exam/ Labs/Imaging	Treatment Approach	Incubation
Anthrax (rare)	**Initial phase** Nausea, anorexia, vomiting, and fever progressing to severe abdominal pain, hematemesis, and diarrhea that is almost always bloody Acute abdomen picture with rebound tenderness may develop, can mimic appendicitis. Mesenteric adenopathy on computed tomography (CT) scan likely **Subsequent phase** 2–4 days after onset of symptoms, ascites develops as abdominal pain decreases. Shock, death within 2–5 days of onset. A form of GI anthrax involving the oropharynx has also been reported, where patients develop ulcers at the base of the tongue and/or the esophagus, along with dysphagia and regional lymphadenopathy. The mortality of GI anthrax is approximately 50%	Coordinate all aspects of testing, packaging, and transporting with public health laboratory/LRN Obtain specimens appropriate to system affected: blood (essential): will be positive within 12 hours ascitic fluid **Clues to diagnosis** • Gram-positive bacilli on unspun peripheral blood smear or ascitic fluid • Pharyngeal swab for pharyngeal form • Aerobic blood culture growth of large, gram-positive bacilli provides preliminary identification of Bacillus species • Upper endoscopy may reveal esophageal ulceration	Cipro 400 q 12 or Doxy 100 q 12, and 1 or 2 additional antimicrobials (may be resistant to Bactrim and extended spectrum Cephalosporins	Incubation 3–5 days for gas trointestinal anthrax
Brucellosis	GI symptoms may occur in up to 70% of patients. A significant percentage of patients may have GI complaints, primarily dyspepsia, although abdominal pain from hepatic abscesses and/or granulomas may occur (infiltrative hepatitis). Suspect hepatic abscesses in patients with signs of systemic toxicity and persistently elevated liver enzymes. The abscess can serve as a source of bacteremic seeding. There are also case reports of spontaneous bacterial peritonitis secondary to brucellosis infection. Other symptoms include anorexia, nausea, vomiting, diarrhea and/or constipation, ileitis and colitis	Blood and bone marrow cultures may be positive during the acute febrile phase. CT of the abdomen may reveal hepatic abscess	Doxycycline 200 mg qd plus Rifampin 600-900 mg qd for 6 weeks	Incubation 5–60 days
Cholera	The infection is often mild or without symptoms, but sometimes it can be severe. Approximately one in 20 infected persons has severe disease characterized by profuse watery diarrhea, vomiting, and leg cramps. Abrupt onset of vomiting and profuse, painless, watery-grayish diarrhea with flecks of mucus (rice water stool). Fluid losses can be significant (up to 20 L/day). Hypovolemic shock, hypokalemia, and metabolic acidosis can cause death within a few hours of onset, especially in children. Mortality, in untreated cases, is as high as 60%. Milder forms of the disease also occur, especially with the non-0-1 cholera. Fever is unusual	Darkfield microscopy showing large numbers of comma-shaped organisms with significant motility. However, this test is relatively insensitive and is nonspecific. Thiosulfate-citrate-bile salt-sucrose agar (TCBS) or alkaline peptone broth are used to facilitate growth and identification. Positive identification depends on serologic and biochemical testing	When fluid and electrolyte imbalances are corrected, cholera is a short, self-limiting disease lasting a few days. Doxycycline, tetracycline, co-trimoxazole, erythromycin, and furazolidone have all demonstrated effectiveness in decreasing the diarrhea and bacterial shedding in this disease	Incubation 2–5 days

T A B L E   1 1 - 1

BIOTERRORISM (*CONTINUED*)

Agent	Gastrointestinal Signs/Symptoms	Important Exam/ Labs/Imaging	Treatment Approach	Incubation
Clostridium botulinum	Ileus, gastric dilation, and constipation present, due to blockage of autonomic nerve impulse transmission. Nausea, vomiting, and abdominal pain are possible. GI symptoms are absent in wound botulism	Isolation of *C. botulinum* from stool or demonstration of the toxin by the mouse neutralization test establishes the diagnosis A low volume, normal saline, colonic irrigation may yield a useful specimen, since constipation predominates	Lavage (within 1 hour) with activated charcoal (sorbitol as a cathartic) may be useful to remove spores if there is a known ingestion; activated charcoal avidly binds to *C. botulinum*, type A neurotoxin. Avoid magnesium-based cathartics since magnesium may enhance neuro-toxicity	Incubation 12–36 hours
Glanders	Diarrhea and abnormal liver function tests can be seen.			
Yersinia pestis	Nausea (38%), vomiting +/- hematemesis (39%), diarrhea (28%), abdominal pain (17%); muco-purulent or watery sputum can become bloody. Intra-abdominal buboes may be accompanied by tenderness, guarding, and other peritoneal signs. Hepatomegaly can be present	Blood or sputum cultures	Doxycycline 100 bid, or Cipro 500 bid	Incubation of 2–8 days if flea-borne transmission
Francisella tularensis	Patients usually report a sore throat, abdominal pain (from mesenteric lymphadenopathy), nausea, vomiting, diarrhea, and, occasionally, frank gastrointestinal bleeding (from intestinal ulcerations). Necrotic, caseating granulomas can be found in liver	It can be grown from pharyngeal washings, sputum specimens, and even fasting gastric aspirates in a high proportion of patients with inhalational tularemia. It is only occasionally isolated from blood.	Streptomycin 1 g IM bid, or Doxycycline 100 mg IV bid	Incubation 3–14 days
Coxiella burnetii	Nausea, vomiting, diarrhea, abdominal pain, pancreatitis, mesenteric panniculitis. A majority of patients have abnormal liver function tests and some will develop hepatitis, which is associated with smooth-muscle and antiphospholipid or antinuclear antibodies. Hepatitis will present with hepatomegaly and jaundice	The indirect immunofluorescence assay (IFA) is the most dependable and widely used method. *It* may also be identified in infected tissues by using immunohistochemical staining and DNA detection methods.	Doxycycline 100 mg PO bid for 15-21 days. Quinolones are an alternative	Incubation 14–39 days
Smallpox	Severe disease can cause bleeding into the intestinal tract. Nausea and vomiting possible	PCR is helpful	No effective chemotherapy	Incubation 12–14 days
Venezuelan Equine Encephalitis	Nausea, vomiting, and diarrhea	VEE specific IgM in serum sample	Fluid and electrolyte balance, ventilation, and anticonvulsants if encephalitis develops	Incubation 1–5 days

TABLE 11-1

BIOTERRORISM (*CONTINUED*)

Agent	Gastrointestinal Signs/Symptoms	Important Exam/ Labs/Imaging	Treatment Approach	Incubation
Viral hemorrhagic fever (Filoviridae, Ebola, Marburg, Arenaviridae, Lassa, Argentine, Bolivian, Bunyaviridae, Hantaviurs, Congo-Crimean, Rift Valley fever, Yellow and Dengue fever	After 1–3 days, gastrointestinal symptoms develop, which may include nausea, vomiting, watery diarrhea, abdominal cramping and pain. Pancreatitis and jaundice may develop	Culture is positive during the acute stages, and laboratory confirmation via PCR and/or antigen detection may be used	Passive Ab for AHF, BHF, Lassa fever, CCHF. Ribavirin (CCHF, arenaviruses) 30 mg/kg IV initial dose, 15 mg/kg IV q 6 hours for 4 days	Incubation 4–21 days
Staphylococcal enterotoxin B	Acute salivation, nausea, vomiting progressing to abdominal cramps, and watery, nonbloody diarrhea	Aerobic blood culture; urine samples tested for SEB	Oxygenation, hydration; ventilatory support for inhalation exposure	Incubation 1–6 hours
Ricin	Resembles toxic mushroom ingestion and gastroenteritis if ingested. Nausea, vomiting, diarrhea (which may become bloody), and abdominal pain may occur within a few hours. Liver function tests may be abnormal, sometimes secondary to hepatic necrosis	Specific serum ELISA; nonspecific lab findings	Gastric decontamination with superactivated charcoal, followed by magnesium citrate after ingestion of more than 1 castor bean per 10 kg body weight	Incubation 18–24 hours
T-2 mycotoxin (Yellow Rain)	GI symptoms are similar to radiation syndrome. Vomiting is the most common symptom. The patient also may complain of significant crampy abdominal pain. Watery or bloody diarrhea typically is reported with ingestion of toxin. Anorexia also is a typical symptom of both ingested and absorbed intoxication	Gas-liquid chromatography, mass spectrometry: blood, tissue, environmental samples	No specific antidote; activated charcoal 2 g/kg PO for ingestions. Unproven treatments: metoclopramide, magnesium sulfate, sodium bicarbonate, and dexamethasone sodium phosphate	

Source: Data from Weinstein RS, Alibek K. Biological and Chemical Terrorism: A Guide for Healthcare Providers and First Responders. Thieme: New York, 2003; Keyes DC, Hail SL, Gracia R et al. Medical Response to Terrorism: Preparedness and Clinical Practice. Lippincott Williams & Wilkins: Philadelphia, 2005; PEPID database: Nuclear, Biological & Chemical Weapons. Can be accessed at www.pepid.com, Center for Disease Control: Biological and Chemical Weapons page. Can be Accessed at www.cdc.gov; LEXI Online. Lexicomp Corporation, Hudson, OH; Accessed at www.lexi.com on January 2006.

Agent	Gastrointestinal Signs/Symptoms	Important Exam/ Labs/Imaging	Treatment Approach
Ammonia	Swallowing ammonium hydroxide causes immediate burning in the mouth and throat. Concentrated solutions cause severe pain in the mouth, chest, and abdomen with swallowing difficulty, drooling, and persistent vomiting. Perforation of the esophagus or stomach may occur.	Upper endoscopy can help visualize an inflamed esophagus, although perforation of the esophagus is a concern.	Treatment consists of supportive measures. If ingested, give water or milk by mouth to dilute stomach contents. Do not induce emesis because the patient is at risk of abrupt seizures or coma. Do not administer activated charcoal. Gastric lavage with a small nasogastric tube is recommended to remove caustic material from the stomach and to prepare for endoscopic examination.
Chlora-mine	Burns of the esophagus and stomach; nausea and vomiting with the smell of chlorine in emesis; abdominal discomfort	Metabolic acidosis and hyper-chloremia	The pulmonary agents (3–10) have no specific treatment. Rest, airway and blood pressure management
Hydrochl-oric acid	Dysphagia, abdominal tenderness, guarding, crepitus, subcutaneous air (Hamman crunch)	Perform endoscopy for ingestions. Perform esophagoscopy and gastroscopy on all patients with symptomatic ingestions and on patients who are asymptomatic but have a history of a significant ingestion of a substance with the potential to cause major injury. Findings on esophagoscopy do not correlate well with physical signs and symptoms. Of patients with esophageal injuries, 2–15% have no oral burns. Burn findings are classified as superficial, transmucosal, or transmural. Esophagoscopy findings are used to guide further treatment. The presence of full-thickness or circumferential burns is associated with future stricture formation. The issue of whether to extend the endoscopic examination past the first site of injury is controversial.	
Sulfur dioxide	Nausea and vomiting are common within the first few hours after mustard exposure, beginning at approximately the same time the initial lesions become apparent. Early nausea and vomiting, which generally are transient and not severe, may be caused by the cholinergic activity of mustard, by a general reaction to injury, or by the unpleasant odor. Nausea and vomiting occurring days later probably are caused by the generalized cytotoxic activity of mustard and damage to the mucosa of the gastrointestinal tract.		

TABLE 11-2

CHEMICAL TERRORISM (*CONTINUED*)

Agent	Gastrointestinal Signs/Symptoms	Important Exam/ Labs/Imaging	Treatment Approach
Nitrous oxide	Nausea, abdominal pain, and hemoptysis		
Phosgene			
Perfluoroisobutylene			
Diphosgene			
Chloropicrin			
Cyanide	Nausea, vomiting. Bitter almond breath, burning taste	Look for high lactate and anion gap, cyanide in the blood, and unusually red venous blood	Amyl nitrite 1 amp crushed and inhaled over 30 seconds, q 3 minutes until sodium nitrite 300 mg is ready. Airway management
Sulfur mustard	The mucosal membrane of the GI tract can be damaged, resulting in nausea, vomiting, abdominal pain, bloody diarrhea, and dehydration		
Liquid mustard	Nausea, vomiting		There is no specific treatment. Treat symptoms
Lewisite	Nausea, vomiting, and diarrhea. A geranium odor		British Anti-Lewisite (BAL), given only if severe; or dimercaprol
(Nerve agents)	Nausea, vomiting, diarrhea, possibly fecal incontinence (GA-GD); seen with dermal or inhalational exposure	Erythrocyte cholinesterase activity levels < 10% of normal indicates severe exposure	Charcoal if ingested. Atropine 10-20 mg IV in 2–3 hours or Pralidoxime 1–2 g IV over 10 minutes
Tabun			
Sarin	In moderate dermal exposures, vomiting and/or diarrhea occur. Vomiting and/or diarrhea soon after exposure are ominous signs		
Soman	Fruity smell. In moderate dermal exposures, vomiting and/or diarrhea occur. Vomiting and/or diarrhea soon after exposure are ominous signs		
VX			
(Incapacitating agents)			
3-Quinuclidinyl benzilate	GI effects rare		
(Riot control agents)			
Pepper spray	GI effects rare		
Capsaicin			
(Arsine-based agents)	Nausea, vomiting, and crampy abdominal pain early; hepatomegaly and jaundice late	Look for signs of hemolysis	No specific treatment
Adarnsite			
Phenylchlorarsine			
Phenylcyanoarsine			
Phenylchloroarsine			

Source: Data from Weinstein RS, Alibek K. Biological and Chemical Terrorism: A Guide for Healthcare Providers and First Responders. Thieme: New York, 2003; Keyes DC, Hail SL, Gracia R et al. Medical Response to Terrorism: Preparedness ad Clinical Practice. Lippincott Williams & Wilkins: Philadelphia, 2005. PEPID database: Nuclear, Biological & Chemical Weapons. Can be accessed at www.pepid.com; Center for Disease Control: Biological and Chemical Weapons page. Can be accessed at www.cdc.gov; LEXI Online. Lexicomp Corporation, Hudson, OH; Accessed at www.lexi.com on January 2006.

TABLE 11-3

BIOTERRORISM: SYMPTOMATIC REFERENCE LIST

Vomiting	*Hematemesis*	*Diarrhea (nonbloody)*
Anthrax	Anthrax	Brucellosis
Brucellosis	*Y. pestis*	Cholera
Cholera	*F. tularensis* (possible)	Glanders
Clostridium botulinum	Smallpox (possible)	*Y. pestis*
Yersinia pestis		*F. tularensis*
Tularemia		*C. burnetti*
C. burnetti		Venezuelan equine
Smallpox		enciphalities
Venezuelan equine		Viral hemorrhagic fever
encephalitis		Staph enterotoxin B
Viral hemorrhagic fever		Ricin
Staph enterotoxin B		T2 mycotoxin
Ricin		
T2 mycotoxin		
Diarrhea (bloody)	*Hepatomegaly/Hepatitis*	*Granulomatis Disease*
Anthrax	Brucellosis	Brucellosis
F. tularensis	*Y. pestis*	
Smallpox (possible)	*C. burnetii*	
Ricin		
T2 mycotoxin		
Gastrointestinal Ulceration	*Abdominal/Mesenteric*	*Elevated Transminases*
Anthrax	*Adenopathy*	Brucellosis
F. tularensis	Anthrax	Cholera (if severe
Smallpox	*F. tularensis*	dehydration)
T2 mycotoxin		Glanders
		F. tularensis
		C. burnetii
		Venezuelan equine
		encephalitis
		Ricin

intervention. The recommendations herein have been formed with the consultation of practicing gastroenterologists and, therefore, are subjective by nature.

The following list of signs and symptoms will be useful to the emergency caregiver referencing this chapter of the book:

- Abdominal pain
- Acute abdomen
- Anorexia
- Ascites
- Constipation
- Diarrhea
- Hematemesis
- Hematochezia
- Hepatic necrosis
- Hepatitis
- Hepatomegaly
- Jaundice
- Liver failure

- Nausea
- Pharyngitis
- Tenesmus
- Urgency
- Vomiting

RADIATION TERRORISM

Because radiation effects are greatest in replicating cells, toxicity from high-level radiation exposure is most prominent in tissue with a rapid rate of turnover. The main organ systems affected by high exposure to radiation are, therefore, the gastrointestinal tract, the hematopoietic system, and the skin; the cerebrovascular system, while not characterized by rapid cell turnover, is also prominently affected at very high radiation doses. As the entire body would likely be exposed during a terrorist attack involving radiation, all of these effects would occur in concert, and it is somewhat artificial to separate out the effects on one system alone. Accordingly, while this section will focus on gastrointestinal issues, these will be discussed in the context of the effects of radiation on the body as a whole.

THE NATURE OF THE EXPOSURE

Types of Radiation

There are four basic types of ionizing radiation. In increasing order of potential for tissue damage, these are α-particles, β-particles, electromagnetic radiation (γ-rays and x-rays), and neutrons. α-Particles are large and therefore do not penetrate clothing or skin, although if internalized they can cause cellular damage within a short distance. β-Particles are lighter and are able to penetrate the skin to a depth of a few millimeters; this can lead to "beta burns," which are similar in appearance to thermal burns. γ-Rays are emitted during a nuclear detonation and fallout, as well as during exposure to certain radioisotopes. γ-Rays can easily penetrate tissue, and would be the most likely form of radiation leading to radiation sickness in a terrorist attack. The greatest potential for tissue damage comes from neutrons; these are released only with nuclear detonation or inside a nuclear reactor. Ionizing radiation damages cells either directly or through the formation of free radicals, resulting in the disruption of cell structures including deoxyribonucleic acid (DNA). This can lead to early cell death, or if the cell recovers, to an increased risk of eventual malignant transformation.

Types of Attacks

The primary experience with large-scale, high-level radiation exposure comes from the detonation of nuclear bombs over Hiroshima and Nagasaki, Japan, in 1945. While a terrorist attack involving a weapon of this scale is conceivable, other potential methods of attack, which are perhaps more likely include detonation of a smaller, improvised nuclear device; an attack on a nuclear power plant; an attack on another type of facility containing nuclear material, such as a radiotherapy clinic or radiopharmaceutical factory; and explosion of a radiation dispersal device—a so-called dirty bomb. Sources of radioactive material for a dirty bomb could include medical, research, and industrial facilities, as well as nuclear power plants and waste processing facilities or repositories. Exposure to radiation sources can be external or internal. External contamination occurs with the fallout of radioactive particles, which then adhere to the skin or clothing. Internal contamination follows the ingestion or inhalation of radioactive material; such material can also enter the body through open wounds or severely burned tissue. With respect to radionuclides entering the gastrointestinal tract, some of these will be absorbed into the systemic circulation, chiefly via the small intestine, while unabsorbable materials will pass through the length of the bowel and will eventually be excreted via the colon and rectum. Both local and systemic effects can occur during this process. The route of exposure should be kept in mind during initial decontamination, which is the first step in treating victims of radiation exposure.

Variables Affecting Toxicity

The main determinant of tissue effect is the total dose of radiation. Radiation dose is measured in grays (Gy), with 1 Gy defined as 1 J of ionizing radiation energy deposited in 1 kg of absorber. The mean dose required to kill 50% of exposed individuals at 60 days ($LD_{50/60}$) is estimated to be 3.25–4 Gy without medical care, and 6–7 Gy in patients receiving appropriate therapy. The effects of different levels of radiation exposure are shown in Table 11-4.

The rate of radiation delivery is also important in determining toxicity, as the same dose delivered over a shorter period leads to greater tissue damage. With slower exposures there is time for tissue repair, which limits overall injury. The same is true for radiation delivered in a fractionated manner, with intervening radiation-free intervals during which repair can occur. Other modifiers of radiation effect include the uniformity of exposure, age, sex, genetic susceptibility, concomitant injuries (chemical exposures, trauma, burns, and infection), and the type of medical care available.

THE ACUTE RADIATION SYNDROME

The acute radiation syndrome, also known as radiation sickness, occurs following exposures of at least 0.7 Gy. There are four phases: (1) a symptomatic prodromal phase, (2) a latent phase characterized by clinical improvement, (3) reappearance of symptoms—the so-called manifest illness, and (4) either recovery or death. The prodromal phase usually occurs within hours following exposure, although in some cases it can develop up to 6 days later. The predominant symptoms during this phase are nausea, vomiting, and fatigue. These resolve after 1–2 days, leading to a latent period lasting from several days to a month; the duration of the latent period is shorter for higher radiation doses. Following this, symptoms reappear and can last for weeks. It is the clinical course during this manifest illness phase, which determines outcome.

The organ systems most affected depend on the radiation dose. Between 0.7 and 4 Gy, the most prominent effects are hematological, with pancytopenia and resultant infection, bleeding, and anemia. With exposures above 8 Gy, gastrointestinal symptoms predominate; these are discussed in more detail below. At doses above 20–40 Gy, the cerebrovascular syndrome is most prominent, and is notable for an accelerated time course. During the prodromal phase, victims experience disorientation, confusion, loss of balance, and in some cases, seizures. Following a latent period, which lasts only hours, there is rapid development of hypotension, decreased consciousness, and fever. Death usually follows within 2 days.

TABLE 11-4

EFFECTS OF VARIOUS RADIATION DOSES

Dose (Gy)	Manifestations	Prognosis Without Therapy
0.0003 (e.g., chest x-ray)	No symptoms	No clinical effect
0.003 (e.g., dental x-ray)		No clinical effect
0.015–0.02 (e.g., total body CT scan)		0.08% risk of subsequent lethal cancer
0.1		0.5% risk of subsequent cancer
0.5–1.0 (e.g., Japanese A-bomb survivors)	Decreased cell counts	Almost certain survival; 5% risk of subsequent cancer
1–2 (e.g., average public exposure at Chernobyl)		>90% survival
2–3.5		Probable survival
3.5–5.5	GI damage	50% risk of death within 6 weeks
5.5–7.5		Probable death within 3 weeks
7.5–10 (e.g., maximum dose to Chernobyl fireman)		Probable death within 2.5 weeks
10–20	Pneumonitis, altered mental status	Certain death within 12 days
20–30	Cerebrovascular collapse, fever, shock	Certain death within 5 days

Sources: Data from Waselenko JK, MacVittie TJ, Blakely WF, et al. Medical management of the acute radiation syndrome: recommendations of the strategic national stockpile radiation working group. Ann Intern Med. 2004140:1037–51; Strom DJ. Health Impacts from Acute Radiation Exposure. Richland, WA: Northwest National Laboratory, 2003. Available at http://www.pnl.gov/bayesian/strom/pdfs/Strom2003G_PNNL-14424.pdf Accessed 14 November, 2005; Brenner DJ, Elliston CD. Estimated radiation risks potentially associated with full body CT screening. Radiology. 2004;232:735–8.

THE GASTROINTESTINAL SYNDROME

Gastrointestinal Kinetics

Because it is characterized by rapid cell turnover, the small intestine is the most prominent site of gastrointestinal toxicity from radiation. As they proliferate, mucosal cells move from the base of the intestinal crypts to the tips of the villi, from which they are eventually extruded. This process takes about 7–8 days. Crypt cells are particularly radiosensitive, and sustain damage characterized by mitotic inhibition or outright destruction within hours after exposure to high radiation doses. Because mature cells continue to migrate up the villi and are extruded, the lack of replenishment by new cells from the crypts leads to villous atrophy and denudation of the intestinal mucosa. At the same time, the effects of radiation on the microvasculature of the intestine lead to hemorrhage and fluid losses, which are most prominent 1–2 weeks after radiation exposure.

Clinical Manifestations

Clinically, the prodromal stage is characterized by crampy abdominal pain, watery diarrhea, nausea, and vomiting, which occur within hours of exposure. The interval between exposure and the onset of vomiting can be used to estimate the level of radiation exposure (biological dosimetry; see Table 11-5). A delay of >2 hours indicates a radiation dosage of <2 Gy; 1–2 hours a dosage of 2–4 Gy; 30–60 minutes a dosage of 4–6 Gy; 10–30 minutes a dosage of 6–8 Gy; and <10 minutes a dosage of >8 Gy. The acute onset of diarrhea generally corresponds to an exposure of >9 Gy. This initial estimate of dosage can be further refined in the ensuing 12 hours to 7 days using the absolute lymphocyte count and the rate of decline in lymphocyte number, which correlate well with cumulative dose.

TABLE 11-5

RELATIONSHIP BETWEEN THE TIMING OF ONSET OF VOMITING AND RADIATION DOSAGE

Onset of Vomiting after Exposure	Radiation Dosage	Expected Mortality
More than 2 hours	<2 Gy	<25% in 30–60 days
1–2 hours	2–4 Gy	25–50% in 30–60 days
<1 hour	4–6 Gy	50–75% in 20–35 days
10–30 minutes	6–8 Gy	75–99% in 20 days
<10 minutes	>8 Gy	>99% in days<

Source: Modified from Berger ME, Leonard RB, Ricks RC, et al. Hospital triage in the first 24 hours after a nuclear or radiological disaster. Oak Ridge, TN: Radiation Emergency Assistance Center/ Training Site, 2004. Accessed November 23 , 2005 Available at http://www.orau.gov/reacts/triage.pdf .

TABLE 11-6

MANIFESTATIONS AND MANAGEMENT OF THE THE GASTROINTESTINAL RADIATION SYNDROME

Mechanism	Manifestations	Appropriate Interventions
Mucosal sloughing	Diarrhea	Volume and electrolyte repletion
	Malabsorption	
	Hypovolemia	Antidiarrheals (e.g., loperamide)
	Electrolyte imbalances	
Mucosal ulceration	Gastrointestinal bleeding	Transfusion
		Acid suppression
Increased intestinal permeability	Bacterial translocation	Antibiotics
	Fever	
	Sepsis	
Altered intestinal motility	Ileus	Withhold oral intake
	Vomiting	Antiemetics (e.g., ondansetron or granisetron)

The prodromal stage is followed by a latent period of 5–7 days—relatively short owing to the high turnover rate of the small bowel mucosa. The manifest illness then follows, beginning with further vomiting and diarrhea. Clinical characteristics of the gastrointestinal radiation syndrome are shown in Table 11-6. Pathophysiologically, effects include mucosal sloughing and ulceration, impaired absorption and secretion, altered intestinal flora, increased intestinal permeability and a resultant decrease in resistance to bacterial translocation, destruction of gut lymphoid tissue, and altered intestinal motility. Additional clinical manifestations therefore include volume depletion (which can lead to acute renal failure or hypovolemic shock), malabsorption of nutrients, electrolyte imbalances, ileus, gastrointestinal hemorrhage, fever, and sepsis. Concomitant bone marrow suppression and leukopenia increase victims' susceptibility to infection. Death from the gastrointestinal syndrome generally occurs at 8–14 days following exposure.

A clinical grading system for the effects of radiation toxicity has been devised, rating symptoms on a 1–4 scale. For gastrointestinal manifestations, degree 1 is characterized by 2–3 bulky stools per day, occult bleeding, and minimal abdominal pain. At the high end of the scale, degree 4 is characterized by at least 10 watery stools per day, severe gastrointestinal bleeding, and excruciating abdominal pain. The use of this grading system may help guide the appropriate use of available resources.

Management

Most patients with the gastrointestinal syndrome die. If patients are known to have had very high (>10–12 Gy) exposures, interventions should be limited to comfort care and psychological support. With lesser or unknown exposures, initial management should assume that victims are salvageable. General aspects of care include stabilization of associated wounds and traumatic injuries, removal of contaminated clothing, and decontamination of skin and wounds. Removal of clothing and shoes will usually reduce a victim's contamination by 80–90%. Showering or washing the skin is the next step, the aggressiveness of which can be guided by the use of radiation detectors to assess residual contamination. Medical personnel should wear appropriate barrier clothing during the decontamination process, and they should themselves undergo decontamination following a patient's treatment.

If radionuclides have been ingested, gastric lavage and the administration of emetics and purgatives are indicated. Emetics include apomorphine and syrup of ipecac, while polyethylene glycol (PEG) solutions are useful as purgatives. For known internal contaminations with cesium 137, Prussian blue can be given. This works by trapping the cesium in the intestine, preventing the usual enterohepatic circulation (reabsorption from the gastrointestinal tract after excretion by the liver into the intestine). Aluminum antacids such as aluminum phosphate gel may decrease the absorption of strontium from the gut if given immediately after exposure.

More specific interventions for the gastrointestinal syndrome are shown in Table 11-6. Given the usefulness of the timing of onset of vomiting in assessing radiation dosage, prophylaxis against vomiting is undesirable. Measurement of serum amylase may be of some value as exposures of at least 0.5 Gy cause a significant increase in this enzyme, mainly of parotid gland origin. Once symptoms begin, antiemetics such as the serotonin receptor antagonists ondansetron and granisetron may be used. In patients with diarrhea and volume depletion, fluid and electrolyte replacement is of primary importance. Antidiarrheals such as loperamide may provide some symptomatic relief. Acid suppression to reduce the risk of gastroduodenal ulceration is reasonable, as is blood transfusion in the setting of significant gastrointestinal bleeding. If transfusion is required, blood products should be filtered and irradiated in order to reduce the number of leukocytes. This protects against transfusion-related graft versus host disease, to which victims are predisposed by concomitant immunosuppression.

Intravenous hyperalimentation is sometimes used, although nutritional status is unlikely to affect clinical outcome in the short-to-medium term. Prophylactic antimicrobials are appropriate in neutropenic patients (with an absolute neutrophil count of <500/mm^3); these often include a fluoroquinolone antibiotic as well as antiviral and antifungal agents. Gut prophylaxis has been shown to be disadvantageous in animal models of radiation toxicity, and is not recommended. Endoscopy should also generally be avoided, as the decreased mucosal integrity increases the risk of instrumentation, and as endoscopic findings are unlikely to alter management. Even in the setting of gastrointestinal bleeding, no discrete, endoscopically treatable lesion is likely to be found, given the diffuse nature of radiation-induced gastrointestinal injury.

For the hematopoietic syndrome, the administration of cytokines to stimulate the production of blood cells—particularly leukocytes—is generally accepted. A similar approach in the gastrointestinal syndrome has been contemplated, although there is little evidence to support it. In theory, cytokines or other growth factors could be used to increase the chance of stem cell survival and to hasten repopulation of the gut mucosa. However, while some growth factors have been shown under experimental conditions to reduce gastrointestinal injury from radiation when given prophylactically, they have not been shown to be useful when administered following radiation exposure.

CONCLUSION

Gastrointestinal symptoms are prominent in moderate-to-severe radiation exposures. The resultant fluid and electrolyte losses can lead to hypotension, hypovolemic shock, and renal failure, while the decrease in mucosal integrity can provide a portal for bacterial entry, leading to sepsis. These factors contribute significantly to the mortality of the acute radiation syndrome; in fact, most patients with the gastrointestinal syndrome die. Nonetheless, the provision of appropriate supportive care may allow some of these patients to survive.

Suggested Reading

Berger ME, Leonard RB, Ricks RC, et al. *Hospital Triage in the First 24 Hours After a Nuclear or Radiological Disaster.* Oak Ridge, TN: Radiation Emergency Assistance Center/ Training Site, 2004. Accessed November 23, 2005. Available at *http://www.orau.gov/reacts/triage.pdf*

Bertho JM, Griffiths NM, Gourmelon P. *The Medical Diagnosis and Treatment of Radiation Overexposed People.* Fontenay-aux-Roses, France: Institut de Radioprotection et de Sûreté Nucléaire. Accessed November 29, 2005. Available at *http://irpa11.irpa.net/pdfs/RC-7a.pdf*

Brenner DJ, Elliston CD. Estimated radiation risks potentially associated with full body CT screening. *Radiology.* 2004;232: 735–8.

Centers for Disease Control: *Biological* and *Chemical Weapons* page. Can be accessed at *http:/www.bt.cdc.gov/bioterrorism/* and *http:/www.bt.cdc.gov/chemical/*

Eng R, Jarrett D, Salter S, et al. *Medical Management of Radiological Casualties Handbook.* Bethesda, MD: Military Medical Operations, Armed Forces Radiobiology Research Institute, 2003. Accessed November 14, 2005. Available at *http://www.afrri.usuhs.mil/www/outreach/pdf/2edmmrchandbook.pdf*

Keyes DC, Hail SL, Gracia R, et al. *Medical Response to Terrorism: Preparedness and Clinical Practice.* Philadelphia, PA; Lippincott Williams & Wilkins: 2005.

LEXI Online... Lexicomp Corporation, Hudson, OH; Accessed at *www.lexi.com* on January 2006.

Strom DJ. *Health Impacts from Acute Radiation Exposure.* Richland, WA: Northwest National Laboratory, 2003. Accessed November 14, 2005. Available at *http://www.pnl.gov/bayesian/strom/pdfs/Strom2003G_PNNL-14424.pdf*

Walker RI, Cerveny TJ. Medical consequences of nuclear warfare. In: Zatchuk R, ed. *Textbook of Military Medicine.* Falls Church, VA: TMM Publications, Office of the Surgeon General, 1989. Accessed November 23, 2005. Available at *http://www.afrri.usuhs.mil/www/outreach/pdf/introduction.pdf*

Waselenko JK, MacVittie TJ, Blakely WF, et al. Medical management of the acute radiation syndrome: recommendations of the strategic national stockpile radiation working group. *Ann Intern Med.* 2004;140:1037–51.

Weinstein RS, Alibek K. *Biological and Chemical Terrorism: A Guide for Healthcare Providers and First Responders.* New York, NY; Thieme: 2003.

Yu CE. Medical response to radiation-related terrorism. *Pediatric Annals.* 2003;32(3):169–76.

12

ACUTE PSYCHIATRIC ISSUES

Stephen Hurwitz, Nicolas Bergeron, and David M. Benedek

STAT FACTS

ACUTE PSYCHIATRIC ISSUES

- An acute stress response comprising transient anxiety and hyperarousal will be the commonest presentation.
- An "outbreak of medically unexplained symptoms" (OMUS) involves the rapid spread of physical symptoms by psychological contagion followed by rapid remission.
- Delirium caused by direct exposure to chemical or infectious agents can exhibit high morbidity and mortality.
- Posttraumatic stress disorder (PTSD) can occur in up to 30% of exposed individuals.
- Recognized risk factors for the development of psychiatric disorders will assist in managing the anticipated demand surge in emergency settings.

INTRODUCTION

Events such as the 2001 anthrax attacks demonstrate that terrorists may achieve their primary goal of creating widespread fear and uncertainty without the production of mass casualties. While more effective dissemination of biological agents may certainly produce mass casualties and accompanying terror, additional factors such as the qualities of infectious agents rendering them difficult to detect (e.g., their odorless and colorless nature) are likely to intensify the psychological impact. So too are the realities that release may be accompanied by deliberate misinformation resulting in substantial confusion among community leaders and medical authorities, and that prior experience with such a large-scale event on a national level is lacking. These factors contribute to the argument that bioterrorism is "quintessentially psychological warfare." The preparedness of the community, its sociocultural characteristics, and the degree of competence with which a bioterrorist attack is managed will all play a role in the significance attributed to the event and the affected population's psychological response. Nevertheless, mistrust of the authorities, scapegoating, and discrimination of affected individuals are all expected to occur.

As there are no empirical data related to large-scale bioterrorism, reliance on data from other mass traumas, chemical accidents, and infectious disease outbreaks should be utilized in the planning of a response. The rates of psychiatric disorders following major terrorist attacks have been relatively high (as high as 4 to 20 psychological victims for every physical casualty), higher than those following natural or technological disasters. Anticipated emergency room (ER) psychiatric presentations following a bioterrorist attack, along with recommendations for their management, will be the focus of this chapter.

PSYCHIATRIC EFFECTS OF BIOTERRORISM

Overview

Psychiatric consequences will be most significant in the directly exposed victims of bioterrorism as well as those who erroneously believe that they were exposed. They will not, however, be confined to these groups. Other subgroups who may be indirectly involved include relatives, friends, and caretakers of the exposed (especially those observing the grotesqueries resulting from exposure or infection), persons experiencing the trauma vicariously through the news media, and first-line responders/direct health-care providers. Effects may be viewed from both a community and an individual patient perspective.

The well-described community response to traumatic stress provides a backdrop for the understanding of psychological responses to severe trauma (Table 12-1). The majority of the population will develop at least some of the described symptoms with a degree of individual variability regarding the phase-specific manifestations at given points in time. On average, symptoms peak in the days and weeks following the exposure, and then gradually decline over the period leading up to the 1-year mark. "Anniversary"-type exacerbations may be anticipated in a subsegment of the population.

TABLE 12-1
COMMUNITY RESPONSE TO TRAUMATIC EVENTS

Phases	Time Course	Responses
Immediate	During and immediately after acute traumatic event	• Strong emotions like shock, fear, and terror • Disbelief or denial • Numbness • Confusion • Anxiety and autonomic arousal • Heroic behaviors
Delayed	1 week to several months	• Persistance of autonomic arousal • Intrusive recollections • Combinations of anger, blame, guilt, sadness, grief, apathy, and social withdrawal • Somatic symptoms like fatigue, insomnia, headaches, dizziness, and nausea • Altruism and high social bonding
Chronic-recovery	2 months to 1–2 years	• Continued arousal and intrusive symptoms • Disappointment, resentment, and bitterness • Sadness for others • Weaker sense of community
Chronic-return to life	Up to several years	• Reestablishment of occupational and social identities • Rebuilding of lives • Refocusing on new challenges • Acknowledgment of some positive aspects of the experience

Source: Adapted from Benedek DM. Emergency mental health after a suicide bombing. In: Black SR, Levin D, Gibbs GS, Hauge L (eds). Terrorism and Disaster: What Clinicians Need to Know. Chicago, Illinois: Rush University Medical Center, 2005, pp. 1–10.

Group reactions of a pathological nature may also occur. An "outbreak of medically unexplained symptoms" (OMUS) involves the rapid spread of symptoms by psychological contagion, followed by a usually equally rapid remission. Typical presentations have included hyperventilation, dyspnea, dizziness, nausea, headache, syncope, abdominal distress, and agitation. In years past, unhelpful terms such as "mass hysteria" and "mass psychogenic illness" were used to describe these presentations. "Mass panic" is a collective phenomenon involving disorganized flight in a desire to escape, or alternatively behavioral "freezing." It is a rarely described; rather, adaptive and helpful community behavior is the norm.

While the predictable community responses help to explain the overall surge in demand for medical services, individual patient responses will be the focus in clinical settings such as the ER, clinics, and primary care offices. Distress responses and somatic manifestations of anxiety (Table 12-2) not meeting criteria for psychiatric disorder will account for much of the initial burden. Due to both the incubation periods of infectious agents and the possible delay in the development of trauma-induced psychiatric disorders, presentations of more clearly defined psychiatric

illnesses may be removed in time and space from a "release" event, with the overall psychiatric burden not becoming clear for 3–6 months.

While posttraumatic stress disorder (PTSD), has been "traditionally" identified as *the* psychiatric consequence of severe trauma (and does occur in up to 30% of those

TABLE 12-2
PHYSICAL SYMPTOMS OF ANXIETY AND AUTONOMIC AROUSAL

• Chest pain/tightness	• Dizziness	• Anorexia
• Palpitations	• Light-headedness	• Dry mouth
• Tachycardia		• Nausea
• Dyspnea	• Faintness	• Vomiting
• Hyperventilation	• Diaphoresis	• Diarrhea
• Paresthesias	• Flushing	• Urinary frequency
• Muscle tension/aches	• Pallor	
	• Headaches	• Tremors

Source: Adapted from Lacy TJ, Benedek D. Terrorism and weapons of mass destruction: managing the behavioral reaction in primary care. South Med J. 2003;96:394–399.

directly exposed), the scope of potential mental health consequences is far greater than this. Other psychiatric and neuropsychiatric disorders such as adjustment disorder, acute stress disorder (ASD), major depression, panic disorder, and delirium will occur, as will subsyndromal states such as those involving disturbances of sleep or mood or the regression of children to earlier developmental stages. "Downstream" consequences of a psychological or social nature will include negative effects on work performance and attendance, family dysfunction (related to separation, relocation, violence, or substance abuse), reluctance to travel, and economic adversity. Psychiatric casualties may be reluctant to seek assistance related to real or perceived stigma.

The medical management responses to bioterrorism, including restrictive measures (such as protective gear and quarantine), decontamination, mass immunization, and mandated medical treatments, may be just as psychologically traumatic as the experience of bioterrorism itself. For example, patients in quarantine may have guilt about having exposed others or about the inability to fulfill a typical caretaker role such as that of parents or health-care providers. Also, ASD and depressive symptoms have been described in health-care personnel quarantined during the SARS epidemic. Agents such as mustard gas and smallpox cause disfiguring cutaneous lesions that may worsen the traumatic effect of the exposure for both directly affected persons as well as caretakers and loved ones.

Emergency Room Presentations

Acute Stress Response and Distress-Related Behaviors

An acute stress response as described in the immediate and delayed phases of the community traumatic stress response is the most common psychological and behavioral presentation following severe trauma (Table 12-1). Symptoms of anxiety and hyperarousal will be especially frequent. While the response contains elements of ASD/PTSD symptomatology, this normal, potentially adaptive response to highly stressful situations does not meet criteria for these or any other psychiatric disorders and typically resolves spontaneously without sequelae. The physiologic basis of these symptoms includes activation of the sympathetic autonomic nervous system ("fight-or-flight" response) and a triggering of the hypothalamic-pituitary-adrenal axis with the dynamic release of glucocorticosteroids and peripheral catecholamines. Distress-related behaviors include reduced work productivity (due to distractibility) and work absenteeism, health-risk behaviors such as increased tobacco or alcohol use, and lack of adherence to public health interventions (e.g., vaccination plans, shelter-in-place recommendations, or guidance on self-monitoring for symptoms of infection). Management of the acute stress response as described below may serve to reduce these behaviors.

Medically Unexplained Symptoms of a Physical Nature

Medically unexplained symptoms of a physical nature and misattributed by the patient as resulting from exposure to chemical or infectious agent(s) will occur. These symptoms may range from those with acute onset and rapid resolution to those of chronic duration, and may involve isolated cases or group presentations. Most frequently, these physical symptoms represent elements of the normal acute stress response that are misattributed in etiology (Table 12-2). Such misattribution may lead to further physiologic signs of anxiety. Unlike the majority of individuals experiencing autonomic arousal, these patients are not easily reassured regarding the normal and "explainable" nature of their symptoms, which may also mimic the reported effect of a chemical or biological agent. Presentations may occur in both exposed and unexposed individuals creating a challenge for triage. Chronic cases of medically unexplained physical symptoms (MUPS) have included arthralgias, rashes, and dysesthesias.

The term "worried well" has been applied to these patients but is best avoided, as their symptomatology is real (despite a misattribution of etiology). Moreover, any insinuation that they *are* "well" will only serve to heighten their mistrust and strengthen their belief that they have serious medical pathology that is being glossed over. The categorization of these disorders as "somatoform" in type may similarly polarize patients and physicians. Thus, a somatoform diagnosis is usually best reserved for clear-cut cases of pseudoneurologic symptomatology (conversion disorder) or chronic cases of MUPS where such categorization facilitates more effective management.

Psychiatric Disorders

The diagnostic criteria for *psychiatric disorders*, as distinguished from *psychological/behavioral* symptoms not amounting to disorders, include the requirement for either clinically significant distress or impairment of functioning (Table 12-3). Subgroups at the greatest risk for their development will include those in Table 12-4.

Exposure to a life-threatening traumatic event along with the symptomatic domains outlined in Table 12-5 form the cornerstones of diagnosing ASD and PTSD. Individuals who meet syndromal criteria, and whose symptoms have been present for at least 2 days but no longer than the 4-week period following the event itself, will be diagnosed as having ASD. Those meeting syndromal criteria whose symptoms are present for more than 1 month will be diagnosed as having PTSD, which represents a failure of the natural recovery process following an acute trauma. For the majority of individuals with PTSD, the disorder resolves, with symptoms declining most rapidly over the first 12 months; however about one-third develop chronic non-remitting symptomatology.

TABLE 12-3

PSYCHIATRIC DISORDERS SEEN IN THE AFTERMATH OF A BIOTERRORIST ATTACK

Diagnosis	Description/Symptoms	Time Course	Functional Impact
Adjustment disorder	Development of emotional or behavioral symptoms in response to an identifiable stressor in excess of what would be expected (for example with depressed or traumatic stress disorder-type symptoms)	Occurring within 3 months of stressor	Disturbance causes
Panic disorder	• Recurrent unexpected panic attacks • Persistent worry or significant change in behavior related to the panic attacks	>1 month	clinically significant
Acute stress disorder	• Exposure to a traumatic event in which the person experienced or witnessed a life-threatening event that was associated with intense emotions • Dissociation • Reexperiencing of event • Avoidance • Hyperarousal	>2 days and <4 weeks	distress or impairment
Posttraumatic stress disorder	• Exposure to a traumatic event in which the person experienced or witnessed a life threatening event that was associated with intense emotions • Reexperiencing of event • Avoidance and numbing • Hyperarousal	>1 month	in social,
Phobic disorder	• Marked and persistent fear that is excessive or unreasonable, cued by the presence or anticipation of a specific object or situation • Avoidance of phobic situation	>6 months	occupational,
Major depression	Depressed mood or anhedonia associated with weight loss or gain, insomnia or hypersomnia, retardation or agitation, fatigue or energy loss, worthlessness or inappropriate guilt, poor concentration, and thoughts of death/suicide	>2 weeks	or other
Traumatic grief	• Has experienced the death of a significant other • Intrusive thoughts about the deceased • Sadness and yearning for the deceased • Feelings of bitterness, futility, emptiness, or numbness • Shattered worldview	At least 2 months after the loss	important areas of
Somatoform disorder	Physical complaints or symptoms that cannot be fully explained by a general medical condition or effects of a substance	Usually >6 months	
Substance abuse	Maladaptive pattern of substance use	Occurring within a 12-month period	functioning
Delirium	• Disturbance of consciousness with attentional deficits • Change in cognition or perceptual disturbance • Caused by a medical condition or a substance	Subacute onset and fluctuating presentation	

Source: Adapted from American Psychiatric Association. Diagnostic and Statistical Manual of Mental Disorders, 4th Edition, Text Revision, Washington, DC: American Psychiatric Association, 2000.

TABLE 12-4

AT-RISK GROUPS FOR MENTAL HEALTH PROBLEMS IN THE AFTERMATH OF A BIOTERRORIST ATTACK

Trauma Experience	Vulnerability	Support
• Intensely exposed to traumatic event • Injured • Bereaved survivors • Having severe symptoms as a result of the trauma	• Children • Elderly • Women with children at home • Having a preexisting psychiatric disorder	• Having a poor social network • Belonging to a community with depleted resources

Sources: Norris FH, Friedman MJ, Watson PJ, et al. 60,000 disaster victims speak, Part I: An empirical review of the empirical literature: 1981–2001. Psychiatry. 2002;65:207.
Hall RCW, Ng AT, Norwood AE. Disaster Psychiatry Handbook. American Psychiatric Association, 2004.

Other psychiatric disorders will be relatively frequent as well. Major depression will be a significant diagnosis several weeks into the disaster, and about 50% of PTSD patients will have this disorder as a comorbid illness. Those with ASD/PTSD "type" symptoms, who don't meet syndromal criteria for these disorders, may meet criteria for an adjustment disorder. Other diagnoses will include traumatic grief, substance abuse, and anxiety disorders (such as panic disorder and specific phobias). Brief psychotic disorder and malingering will be encountered, but only rarely.

Finally, patients with preexisting psychiatric disorders such as schizophrenia, bipolar disorder, and panic disorder may suffer a relapse or exacerbation as a result of an attack. For the chronically mentally ill, the disruption of access to their medications and other routine aspects of their care as well as the previously described stressors associated with fear of exposure may precipitate emergency department presentation.

TABLE 12-5

EXAMPLES WITHIN SYMPTOM DOMAINS OF TRAUMATIC STRESS DISORDERS

Reexperience of traumatic event	Hyperarousal
• Recurrent thoughts • Flashback • Nightmares	• Insomnia • Poor concentration • Hypervigilence • Exaggerated startle response
Avoidance of stimuli that arouse recollections of the trauma	**Dissociation/Numbing** • Reduction in awareness of surroundings • Sense of numbing, detachment, or absence of emotional responsiveness

Source: Adapted from American Psychiatric Association. Diagnostic and Statistical Manual of Mental Disorders. 4th Edition, Text Revision. Washington, DC: American Psychiatric Association, 2000.

Neuropsychiatric Effects Induced by the Agents of Bioterrorism

Neuropsychiatric syndromes in the form of direct central nervous system effects of chemical or infectious agents are well-described. Examples include frank presentations such as cognitive disturbance; hallucinations or delusions; or more subtle manifestations such as anxiety, lethargy, or depression. Within this category, delirium is an especially important disorder with a high morbidity and mortality.

MANAGEMENT OF PSYCHIATRIC PRESENTATIONS FOLLOWING BIOTERRORISM

General Principles

Primary prevention and mitigation of the psychiatric sequelae of bioterrorism involves medical and societal preparation prior to the event's occurrence. Components include educating the general public, first responders, and medical personnel to provide a realistic appreciation of the threat of bioterrorism, planning the locations of psychiatric "holding areas," setting up referral networks for ongoing psychiatric treatment, providing linkages with community agencies, establishing mechanisms to identify and monitor at-risk populations, and having methods in place to help connect survivors with loved ones. Periodic reevaluation of such predisaster planning is essential, along with regular practice drills.

Secondary prevention involves psychiatric assessment and treatment in the immediate aftermath of the event. The rapid identification and effective treatment of exposed and infected individuals is an important aspect of promoting safety and calmness. Following medical evaluation and stabilization, the administration of "psychological first aid" to exposed individuals will be a basic but key component. Objectives of this intervention include (1) promoting safety, for example, by helping people to obtain food, shelter, and emergency medical attention, (2) promoting calmness, for example, by compassionate listening and the provision of accurate information, (3) promoting connectedness, for example, by bringing together dispersed family members, (4) promoting self-efficacy, for example, by giving people practical suggestions on how to help themselves, and (5) promoting hope, for example, by directing people to available community services and alerting them to others that will be forthcoming. Because of the likely scope of an attack, it is anticipated that not only psychiatrists but also first responders, other mental health workers, ER physicians, primary care physicians, hospital chaplains, and trained lay people will all play a role in providing these services. Implementation of a previously established mechanism for identification of vulnerable subsections of the population (e.g., children, the homeless, and the chronically mentally ill) and initiation of health surveillance for purposes of early recognition of distress or emergent psychiatric disorder are also an important part of preventive efforts. Appropriate use of the mass media by the authorities is an essential component of disaster management. The propagation of clear and redundant information to the population at large regarding the medical realities and recommended courses of action should reduce the likelihood of maladaptive collective and individual responses, and supplement the beneficial effects of psychological first aid.

The ER will be the primary area of general medical and psychiatric triage and treatment. Ideally, patients who are medically cleared but require additional observation and/or treatment should be moved to a separate psychiatric holding area preferably close to the main medical triage and treatment area. Such a setting facilitates continuity, while providing a less stimulating environment to help reduce hyperarousal. It also allows for patients to be transferred back to the main ER if necessary. Psychosocial interventions will incorporate and extend elements of psychological first aid including (1) the provision of psychoeducational materials regarding anticipated psychological responses, (2) a written handout detailing resources for outpatient psychiatric follow-up or social assistance, and (3) the collection of victims contact information and permission to visit them in the community.

Psychopharmacologic intervention is a valuable and at times essential treatment modality. The primary medication categories for administration in the ER itself will be the benzodiazepine anxiolytics, the atypical antipsychotics, and the conventional antipsychotic haloperidol, the latter where parenteral medication is required. In addition, nonbenzodiazepine hypnotics, antidepressants, and other psychotropic categories may be prescribed for outpatient usage.

Not least, the psychological needs of medical and rescue personnel need to be attended to in order to avoid burnout and attrition. Appropriate work/rest scheduling is essential. Regular group debriefings of the staff in the emergency department, involving frank and open discussion (e.g., "lessons learned"), generally foster cohesion and help morale.

Tertiary prevention involves the provision of psychiatric treatment (psychosocial and psychopharmacologic) to persistently symptomatic patients and the utilization of community resources beyond the emergency department. Outreach for the screening and tracking of known casualties and at-risk populations (Table 12-4) and the continued constructive use of the media to provide factual information and dispel rumors are key components. In this setting, mental health providers should facilitate coping and resilience in survivors and rescue workers. Treatment plans need to be sensitive to the cultural characteristics of the population(s) in question.

Management of Psychiatric Presentations in the Emergency Department

Acute Stress Response and Distress-Related Behaviors

Patients with an acute stress response may experience their most significant symptoms very transiently, and thus be suitable for a prompt discharge, or benefit from additional observation and management in a psychiatric holding area. Psychoeducation in the form of supportive reassurance and the provision of clear, simple guidance on signs or symptoms that should prompt reevaluation may minimize distress and distress-behavior in such cases. Deciding who to rapidly discharge (with its own potential advantage of promoting "normalcy" and self-efficacy) and who to observe will be based on symptom severity, available supports, and psychiatric risk factors.

Patients should be reassured that their reactions are not pathologic but rather "a normal and common reaction to a highly stressful situation." Most people cope well in their own way, benefiting from small quotients of support and information. For those managed in the psychiatric holding area, principles of "psychological first aid for disaster management" such as the provision of rest, support, and the distribution of psychosocial fact sheets (housed in a holding area supply box) will typically facilitate their discharge within hours. It is usually best to encourage patients to return to work and other regular activities, as for them not to do so will tend to reinforce guilt and social withdrawal. Critical incident stress debriefing (CISD), conducted as a form of group therapy requiring people to describe their experiences in detail with associated emotional catharsis, has not been consistently demonstrated to prevent PTSD. Moreover, CISD may even exacerbate psychiatric symptoms in some situations and thus is not recommended.

A minority of acutely distressed patients will require psychotropic medications; most typically sedative-hypnotics (benzodiazepines such as lorazepam 0.5–2 mg bid to tid or nonbenzodiazepine hypnotics such as zolpidem 5–10 mg qhs) to treat anxiety or insomnia. For those requiring take-home prescription medications, quantities should be limited but sufficient to cover the time interval leading up to an anticipated outpatient appointment.

Medically Unexplained Physical Symptoms

Patients with MUPS should not have their problems discounted or dismissed, as doing so will likely prolong their symptomatology and incapacity. Rather, their concerns should be validated and they should be provided with support in a calm, assertive, but nonconfrontational fashion. Care should be taken not to become locked in a debate over "contested causation." In cases of OMUS, individuals should be physically separated to minimize the role of suggestibility, while in chronic cases patients should be shown support and concern while avoiding the performance of unnecessary medical tests.

Psychiatric Disorders

Patients with psychiatric disorders, either new onset or preexisting, may also require a brief period of management in a psychiatric holding area. Thereafter, follow-up evaluation and treatment will be required. Outpatient referral will be the norm, with inpatient psychiatric hospitalization generally reserved for those with psychiatric disorders who are acutely suicidal, homicidal, or frankly psychotic and agitated.

Psychosocial management in the ER typically encompasses supportive and educative measures as described previously. Cognitive behavioral therapy (CBT) is a form of psychotherapy incorporating reexposure to the traumatic event (either in imagination or in real-life simulation) coupled with anxiety management training such as relaxation, breathing techniques, and cognitive restructuring. Although CBT has been established to be effective in the treatment of PTSD and may also have a role in its prevention, it may be impractical to provide in an ER setting.

Regardless of etiology, persistent anxiety, or insomnia may be both very distressing and disabling for patients. For depressed or anxious patients who require rapid relief of these symptoms, sedative-hypnotics (including a limited prescription quantity for use postrelease) are once again a sound choice. Patients should be especially alerted to the potential side effect of sedation, which may affect driving or the operation of heavy machinery. They should also be advised to review the ongoing need for these medications with their outpatient clinicians; for example, the benzodiazepines do not treat the core symptoms of ASD and PTSD and may possibly even worsen the course of these disorders. Selective serotonin reuptake inhibitor antidepressants (SSRIs) such as paroxetine and sertraline have an established role in the treatment of major depressive disorders and anxiety disorders such as panic disorder and PTSD. Though less well-supported by clinical research to date,

they may also be reasonable options for treating ASD. They are, however, usually best initiated by the outpatient clinician who can manage potential treatment-emergent side effects, rarely dangerous, but with the potential to alienate patients from taking medications in the future. The antidepressants, fluoxetine, mirtazapine, and venlafaxine, may also be effective options for the treatment of PTSD, although they are not specifically U.S. Food and Drug Administration (FDA) approved for this indication. Pharmacologic intervention designed to prevent the occurrence of PTSD is an area of active investigation. While various medications including the β-blocker propranolol have demonstrated promise, no pharmacotherapy (including the sedative-hypnotics or SSRIs) is currently recommended for this purpose specifically. Acutely psychotic patients who are cooperative enough to take medications orally should be administered for an atypical antipsychotic agent such as risperidone 0.25–2 mg or olanzapine 2.5–10 mg, approximately every 2 hours as needed.

Delirium and Other Behavioral Emergencies

Patients who are severely agitated, assaultive, or grossly uncooperative with medical treatment (e.g., attempting to remove intravenous lines) will require the provision of general safety measures such as constant observation, emergency medication, or physical restraint, as well as diagnosis-specific general medical and psychiatric management.

In the case of delirium, the management includes not only the imperative elements of attending to the safety of patients and staff and treating the underlying medical cause(s), but usually also the administration of antipsychotic agents to target agitation and the other core symptoms of the disorder. For relatively cooperative patients, oral administration of an atypical antipsychotic agent is appropriate, while for those who require rapid sedation and/or are unable to take medication by mouth, intravenous haloperidol (although not FDA approved by this route) is recommended. Bolus dosages of 2–5 mg every 20 minutes as needed are a typical initial strategy; however, other dosages in the range of 0.5–20 mg may be required. In severe refractory cases, haloperidol may also be administered as a continuous intravenous infusion of 5–25 mg/h. Unless access is not available, the intravenous route of administration is preferred over the intramuscular; greater efficacy, ease of administration, and lower (indeed rare) occurrence of extrapyramidal symptoms (even at higher dosages) being some of the advantages. The ECG should be monitored, and a QTc interval longer than 450 millisecond or more than 25% over baseline may warrant cardiology consultation, dose reduction, or discontinuation. Benzodiazepines are generally not recommended for the management of delirium (other than that due to alcohol or sedative-hypnotic withdrawal); however, intravenous lorazepam may be given, either in combination with haloperidol, if additional sedation is required, or as monotherapy in patients intolerant of haloperidol. Lorazepam 0.5–2 mg intravenously every 20 minutes as needed is then an appropriate initial strategy. The administration of physostigmine should be considered for the management of delirium secondary to anticholinergic agents.

For severe agitation or noncompliance with medical treatment, secondary to acute psychosis or mania, and where the patient does not have intravenous access, intramuscular haloperidol 2–5 mg every 30 minutes as needed, along with intramuscular lorazepam 1–2 mg every 30 minutes as needed, is generally indicated. Patients should be monitored for the potential development of extrapyramidal symptoms such as acute dystonia and akathisia or rarely the potentially fatal neuroleptic malignant syndrome.

CONCLUSION

Following a bioterrorist attack, there will be a demand surge in ERs related to an influx of the truly exposed and those misattributing the physical symptoms of the acute stress response to the biological agent or agents. Mental health presentations are expected to be relatively common and quite broad in type. These presentations will frequently fall into one or combinations of three domains: (1) emotional distress such as anxiety or fear; a normal response not meeting criteria for a psychiatric disorder and responding to basic reassurance, (2) maladaptive symptoms or behaviors such as insomnia, work absenteeism, or excessive alcohol use; also not meeting syndromal criteria but often benefiting from short-term psychosocial or medication intervention, (3) new-onset psychiatric/neuropsychiatric disorders such as major depression, PTSD and delirium or exacerbations of preexisting psychiatric disorders such as schizophrenia, requiring acute clinical intervention, followed generally by longer-term psychiatric treatment. ER physicians and staff, by identifying and treating exposed individuals, providing psychoeducational and supportive measures during the triage process, and treating emergent psychiatric disorders with psychosocial and psychopharmacologic interventions, will help reduce the overall psychologic sequela of a large-scale event.

SUGGESTED READING

Allen MH, Currier GW, Carpenter D, et al. Treatment of behavioral emergencies 2005. *J Psychiatr Pract*. 2005;11:5–108.

American Psychiatric Association. Practice guideline for the treatment of patients with delirium. *Am J Psychiatr*. 1999;156 (Suppl 5):1–20.

Benedek DM. Emergency mental health after a suicide bombing. In: Black SR, Levin D, Gibbs GS, Hauge L (eds). *Terrorism and Disaster: What Clinicians Need to Know*. Chicago, Illinois: Rush University Medical Center, 2005, pp. 1–10.

Benedek DM, Holloway HC, Becker SM. Emergency mental health management in bioterrorism events. *Emerg Med Clin North Am*. 2002;20:393–407.

Clauw DJ, Engel CC Jr, Aronowitz R, et al. Unexplained symptoms after terrorism and war: an expert consensus statement. *J Occup Environ Med*. 2003;45:1040–1048.

Foa EB, Cahill SP, Boscarino JA, et al. Social, psychological, and psychiatric interventions following terrorist attacks: recommendations for practice and research. *Neuropsychopharmacology*. 2005;30:1806–1817.

Hall RCW, Ng AT, Norwood AE. *Disaster Psychiatry Handbook* American Psychiatric Association, 2004.

Lacy TJ, Benedek D. Terrorism and weapons of mass destruction: managing the behavioral reaction in primary care. *South Med J*. 2003;96:394–399.

Norris FH, Friedman MJ, Watson PJ, et al. 60,000 disaster victims speak, Part I: an empirical review of the empirical literature: 1981–2001. *Psychiatry*. 2002;65:207.

Ritchie EC, Friedman M, Watson P, et al. Mass violence and early mental health intervention: a proposed application of best practice guidelines to chemical, biological, and radiological attacks. *Mil Med*. 2004;169:575–579.

Ursano R, Norwood AE. *Trauma & Disaster: Responses & Management*. Washington, DC: American Psychiatric Publishing, 2003.

Ursano RJ, Fullerton CS, et al. Trauma and disaster. In: Ursano RJ, McCaughey BG, Fullerton CS, (eds). *Individuals and Community Responses to Trauma and Disaster: The Structure of Human Chaos*. Cambridge, MA: Cambridge University Press, 1994, pp. 3–27.

Weiner, D: Emergency Preparedness in Handbook of Bioterrorism and Disaster Medicine, (eds). Antosia, R.E., Cahill, J.D. Springer, New York, New York, 2006, pp. 411–416.

13

PALLIATIVE AND EXPECTANT (BLACK TAG) CARE

Daniel H. Shevrin

STAT FACTS

PALLIATIVE AND EXPECTANT (BLACK TAG) CARE

- Nociceptive pain is generally responsive to opiate agents.
- It is important to assess pain intensity by numerical pain scales.
- Nonopioid pain medication includes ketorolac, ketamine, corticosteroids, and lidocaine.
- Treatment of nausea/vomiting includes dopamine antagonists, histamine antagonists, serotonin antagonists, cerebral cortical agents, or prokinetic agents.
- Short-acting benzodiazepines are the agents of choice to treat anxiety.

INTRODUCTION

Given the focus of this book on the care of patients in the emergency department (ED) following an act of bioterrorism, the classic definition of palliative care should probably be slightly amended. The classic definition of palliative care is the comprehensive management of physical, social, spiritual needs of patients whose diseases are not responsive to curative treatment, the goal being to achieve the best possible quality of life through relief of suffering and control of symptoms. Since the focus of this chapter is on patients who have suffered a bioterrorist attack of some type, and who are unlikely to survive, that is, given the "black tag" designation, it would seem that the goals of treatment should be more narrowly defined to emphasize symptom management and relief of suffering in a very short time frame to individuals who are likely to die from their injuries within hours to days.

In some respects, palliative care management of patients involved in a bioterrorist attack shares features with the management of military personnel who suffer injuries during battle. This is particularly relevant now since weapons are more likely to include biologic and chemical agents. Also relevant is the recent experience in New Orleans, LA, when many people suffering injuries, trauma, and exacerbation of underlying illnesses in the aftermath of Katrina were managed with palliative intent in makeshift EDs.

Particularly since September 11, we acknowledge that a terrorist attack resulting in mass injuries, suffering, and death could certainly occur again. As outlined in this book, there are a wide range of potential "weapons," including biologic (infectious) agents, various toxins/toxicants, radiation, and explosives. It is not the purpose of this chapter to review the specific injuries each of these agents could cause; those details are adequately outlined elsewhere in the book. Moreover, this chapter will address the specific symptoms resulting from these injuries. To the extent that many of these agents result in common symptoms, that is, pain, this chapter will be structured to address management of the most common major symptom groups. These will include pain and symptoms related to the gastrointestinal (GI), pulmonary, and neurological systems. In addition, the issues of family support, spiritual guidance, and ethical considerations will be discussed.

SYMPTOM MANAGEMENT IN THE EMERGENCY DEPARTMENT

Assessment of Prognosis

The emergency physician (EP) must be able to assess prognosis based on the patient's general condition and realistic treatment possibilities and goals and be able to communicate them to the patient or their surrogate to determine whether these treatments are desirable. For the patient who presents with death imminent, the EP must be able to discuss this with the patient or family and help determine an appropriate code status. Most patients will not have an advanced directive and the physician will need to use their judgment to help advise/advocate whether to recommend resuscitation or to die by "natural" causes. If extending time or restoring function is not feasible and/or desirable, then the EP must be capable of providing comfort and relief of suffering.

Doctrine of Double Effect

Double effect is the delivery of adequate medication by a physician that *unintentionally* hastens death but is provided with the *intent* to relieve suffering. This is different from physician-assisted suicide in which treatment is *intended* to cause a patient's death. The U.S. Supreme Court sanctions double effect whereas physician-assisted suicide is illegal in all states but Oregon. This doctrine is described in more detail later in this chapter.

PAIN MANAGEMENT

Pain Classification

Proper management and relief of pain remains the mainstay of palliative care. Patients arriving at the ED following a bioterrorist attack have suffered various forms of tissue injury, which lead to pain. An excellent review of pain management in the ED can be found in the book by Mace et al. Physical pain is classified as nociceptive (somatic or visceral) and neuropathic.

- *Nociceptive* pain is produced by damaged tissue or organs.
- *Somatic nociceptive* pain is produced if the body part is musculoskeletal or cutaneous.
- *Visceral nociceptive* pain is produced if the body part is an internal organ, such as the liver, pancreas, or stomach.
- *Neuropathic* pain is produced if the sensory afferent nerve itself is damaged or destroyed.

In general, nociceptive pain is responsive to opiates and neuropathic pain has a variable response to opiates. In many cases, particularly when a patient has suffered major trauma, burns, chemical exposure, or exposure to a biologic agent, the pain is a combination of both types.

Pain Assessment

The characteristics of pain combined with associated symptoms constitute the pain pattern. Relevant features of a pain pattern include site of pain, radiation, quality/character, severity, duration, aggravating and relieving factors, response to previous and current analgesic therapies, and associated signs and symptoms. Responses to these questions can help differentiate nociceptive from neuropathic pain. Most patients with neuropathic pain have more than one pain quality, such as burning, jabbing, knife-like, shooting, and/or skin sensitivity. There may be radiation of the pain that follows the dermatome distribution of cranial and peripheral nerves. Although patients often have mixed syndromes of nociceptive and neuropathic pain, the knowledge that neuropathic pain is present is important, as effective management includes nonopioid medications. Knowledge of previous opioid treatment and the patient's response to this treatment is also helpful in determining pain management. Patients receiving opioids for chronic pain conditions will require higher doses of pain medication than opioid-naive patients. The degree of response to a dose of opioid by a paramedic on the way to the ED can help determine subsequent doses of narcotics. Excellent general reviews of pain management can be found in the books by Benzon et al. and Macintyre and Ready.

Pain Scales

It is critical to assess the patient's pain intensity, initially to help determine the appropriate dose of pain medication, and, subsequently, to determine the response to the treatment. The most commonly used pain scale is the Numerical Rating Scale, which typically consists of a series of numbers and is administered verbally. Patients rate their pain from 0 to 10, whereby 0 represents "no pain" and 10 represents "the most intense pain imaginable." It is easy to administer and easily understood. The level of pain intensity measured by this scale is divided into three levels:

- Pain 1–3: Mild
- Pain 4–6: Moderate
- Pain 7–10: Severe pain—Pain emergency

Individuals suffering a bioterrorist attack that results in pain will most likely experience severe pain, that is, pain rated $\geq$7. The following discussion will focus on the management of severe pain, which always includes the use of opioids that are typically administered parenterally.

Pharmacology of Opioids

Opioids act primarily at μ-receptor sites. They are all capable of producing the same degree of pain relief and can be made equianalgesic if adjustments are made for dose and route of administration. Table 13-1 outlines commonly used opioids along with their equianalgesic doses and half-lives. Examples of conversions from one opioid to another will be given later in the chapter.

TABLE 13-1

EQUIANALGESIC DOSING OF COMMONLY USED OPIOIDS

Analgesic	Parenteral Dose (mg)	Oral Dose (mg)
Morphine	10	30
Hydromorphone	1.5	7.5
Fentanyl	0.1	—
Oxycodone	—	20–30
Hydrocodone	—	30
Codeine	—	200

- Morphine

  Morphine is the protypical μ-opioid receptor agonist against which all other opioids are compared for equianalgesic potency. It can be administered parenterally (IV, IM, SC), orally, or via epidural or intrathecal routes. When given parenterally, onset of analgesia occurs within 5 minutes and peak analgesic effect occurs within 10–20 minutes. Morphine has a relatively longer analgesic effect (4–5 hours) compared to its plasma half-life (2–3.5 hours), thereby minimizing its accumulation and contributing to its safety. Morphine's elimination is dependent on hepatic mechanisms and should be used with caution in patients with hepatic insufficiency. Its metabolites are excreted through the kidneys and the dose should be adjusted in those with significant renal impairment. Morphine can cause histamine release resulting in opioid-induced hypotension, skin rash, and flushing. Morphine is also available for oral administration (immediate or sustained release), but its relatively low bioavailability and slow onset of action (30–60 minutes) make this route less desirable in the setting of acute pain in an ED.

- Hydromorphone

  Hydromorphone (Dilaudid) is an analogue of morphine with strong μ-opioid receptor agonist activity and a similar duration of analgesic effect (3–4 hours). Hydromorphone's milligram-to-milligram potency is five to seven times that of morphine. Its onset of action when given parenterally is within 5 minutes and peak analgesic effect occurs within 8–20 minutes. Side effects of pruritus, sedation, and nausea/vomiting occur less frequently with hydromorphone than morphine.

- Fentanyl

  Fentanyl (Sublimaze) is a synthetic opioid analgesic with agonist effects at μ-opioid receptors. It is highly lipophilic, which allows for transdermal and transmucosal administration for the management of chronic and breakthrough pain, respectively. Given parenterally, it has a faster onset of action than morphine but also a shorter duration of action. It causes no significant histamine release and may be preferred for use in patients with reactive airway disease. Additionally, since histamine-mediated vasodilatation does not occur, it may be a safer choice in patients with hemodynamic instability.

- Meperidine

  Also a synthetic analgesic with similar effects at μ-opioid receptors as morphine, meperidine (Demerol) causes central nervous system (CNS) excitability, including altered mental status, myoclonus, and seizures. This is due to active metabolites, which can have a very long half-life. Given the availability of other opioids with less toxicity and equal to superior analgesia, use of meperidine is not recommended.

- Oxycodone

  Oxycodone is a semisynthetic congener of morphine that is only available in oral form. It is available in both a short-acting and long-acting formulation.

- Methadone

  This low-cost opioid has very unpredictable pharmacokinetics, which makes it undesirable for use in the acute setting. It is mainly used in its oral formulation in the setting of chronic pain.

Other Pain Medications

There are several nonopioids that may be useful for management of acute pain in the ED in the setting of a bioterrorist attack.

- Ketorolac

  Ketorolac (Toradol) is currently the only parenteral nonsteroidal anti-inflammatory drug (NSAID) for clinical analgesic use in the United States. It is given parenterally at a dose of 60 mg, which is followed by 30 mg q 6 hours. It has analgesic efficacy similar to morphine for moderate pain. In contrast to opioids, it does not cause sedation, respiratory depression, or nausea, which makes it useful in situations in which these side effects must be avoided.

- Ketamine

  Ketamine is a dissociative anesthetic that has sedative effects with amnestic and analgesic properties. When used for acute pain management, its major advantages are that it causes minimal respiratory depression, has bronchodilating effects (making it useful in asthmatics or those suffering respiratory symptoms from inhalation of noxious agents), and increases systolic blood pressure (making it useful in patients with hypotension). Ketamine may result in various degrees of agitation known as an emergence reaction. This can be treated with benzodiazepines, such as midazolam. A typical dose is 150 mcg/kg given IV or IM.

- Corticosteroids

  This class of drugs is thought to relieve pain by anti-inflammatory effects. These drugs may also reduce neuropathic pain by a reduction in ectopic pulse generation via their sodium channel-blocking activity. Parenteral steroids have a relatively rapid onset of action and include dexamethasone (Decadron) and methylprednisolone (Solumedrol). A typical dose of dexamethasone is 10 mg IVP and of methylprednisolone is 100 mg IVP.

- Lidocaine infusion

  Systemic infusion of lidocaine has been shown to produce significant pain relief in patients with severe neuropathic pain. Pain relief typically occurs with blood levels well below the antiarrhythmic range. The typical dose is 2–5 mg/kg infused over 30 minutes.

PAIN MANAGEMENT: STEP-BY-STEP PLAN

Step 1—Determine Goals of Treatment

Since the majority of victims of a bioterrorist attack brought to the ED are unlikely to survive, the immediate and most important goal is relief of suffering from pain. The EP must explain the concept of double effect to the patient and family that aggressive treatment of pain may unintentionally hasten death, but that the goal of treatment is to relieve the patient's pain and suffering. If the patient's condition prevents comprehension of this concept and/or family is not present, it is the obligation of the EP to provide adequate treatment to relieve pain. At this time, the EP should consider initiating a discussion concerning the patient's wishes regarding resuscitation and intubation, that is, do not resuscitate (DNR) status.

Step 2—Determine Route of Drug Administration

The IV route is recommended, as it is the most convenient and effective route of drug administration. Since immediate IV access may not be available, the subcutaneous (SC) route is an effective alternative. Intramuscular injections are not recommended since SC injections are less painful and equally efficacious.

Step 3—Determine Equianalgesic Dosing

Most patients suffering a bioterrorist attack seen in the ED are not currently receiving chronic opioids (opioid naive). In those who are already taking opioids, it is necessary to convert opiates to morphine equivalents in order to determine the appropriate initial dose and to avoid underdosing. Morphine equivalents are the total milligrams of all opiates used in 24 hours converted to morphine (IV or oral).

The conversion equation is

$$\frac{\text{Pain dose desired}}{\text{Dose equivalent}} = \frac{\text{Actual pain dose}}{\text{Dose equivalent}}$$

(Desired pain medicine) (Actual pain medicine)

For example, a cancer patient is taking MS Contin (sustained release morphine) 120 mg q 12 hours and hydromorphone 4 mg PO four times daily. In order to convert to morphine equivalents (IV), *first convert total oral morphine to IV morphine*

$$\frac{X \text{ mg IV morphine}}{10 \text{ mg}} = \frac{240 \text{ mg oral morphine}}{30 \text{ mg}}$$

(dose equivalent) (dose equivalent)

30X = 2400

X = 80 mg IV morphine over 24 hours

Then convert total oral hydromorphone to IV morphine:

$$\frac{X \text{ mg IV morphine}}{10 \text{ mg}} = \frac{16 \text{ mg oral hydromorphone}}{7.5 \text{ mg}}$$

(dose equivalent) (dose equivalent)

7.5X = 160

X = 21.3 mg IV morphine over 24 hours

***Total dose IV morphine* = 80 + 21 ~ 100 mg**

The recommended bolus dose is 10–20% of the total 24-hour dose. Since the patient is probably in severe pain, the patient should receive 20 mg IVP morphine as an initial dose (see Step 4 for other guidelines for initial dose determination).

Step 4—Initiate Rapid Titration of Parenteral Opioids

Rapid titration involves an initial parenteral opioid infusion (preferably IV) that is followed by repeated opioid infusions until pain is relieved. Suggestions for the initial dose ranges were obtained from opioid-naive patients using morphine by patient-controlled analgesia (PCA) after major surgery and are age related. A general guideline is to approximate the 24-hour morphine requirement for patients over 20 years old (100 − age in years) and divide by 8.

For example, for a 75-year-old opioid-naive patient

$$\frac{100 - 75}{8} = \frac{25}{8} = 3 \text{ mg}$$

The range would be 2–5 mg IVP morphine.

For a 25-year-old opioid-naive patient

$$\frac{100 - 25}{8} = \frac{75}{8} = 9 \text{ mg}$$

The range would be 7–12 mg IVP morphine.

This calculation provides a "ballpark" morphine dose to begin the titration process. Hydromorphone, which is ~ six to seven times more potent than morphine, can be substituted and would be 0.5–1 mg IVP for the 75-year-old and 1–2 mg IVP for the 25-year-old. Fentanyl, which is

100 times more potent than morphine, can also be substituted and would be 0.03–0.05 mg IVP for the 75-year-old and 0.05–0.1 mg for the 25-year-old. After the initial opioid dose is given, the patient is closely monitored for pain response. The pain response should be assessed at 15 minutes. If there is minimal to no relief 15 minutes after the initial dose, then the patient should receive a dose double the size of the initial dose. If there is partial relief at 15 minutes, then the patient should receive a dose that is 25–50% greater than the initial dose. If there is complete relief, then hold further opioids. The 15-minute assessment interval applies for morphine and hydromorphone. If fentanyl is given, then pain assessment should be at 5 minutes. Providing an adequate initial dose of opioid followed by repeat dosing at a rapid interval based on pain response will allow the EP to rapidly relieve pain in most patients. This rapid titration scheme is shown in Fig. 13-1.

Step 5—Initiate Use of Adjuvant Medication

If pain is not responding adequately to opioids, then there could be a neuropathic component to the pain. This may be particularly relevant in burns or nerve damage from trauma or chemical agents. Administration of parenteral steroids should be strongly considered. There is also evidence to support the use of a lidocaine infusion in severe neuropathic pain.

Step 6—Address and Treat Side Effects of Opioids

Respiratory depression and death as a result of opioid administration is feared by most physicians. In practice,

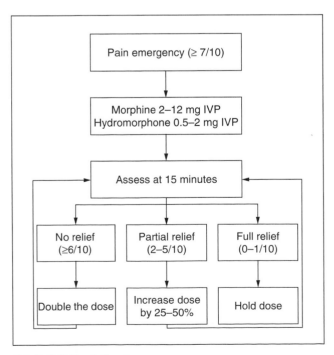

FIGURE 13-1

RAPID TITRATION SCHEME FOR PAIN MANAGEMENT

this is a very uncommon event. In a patient whose death is imminent due to major trauma or massive exposure to a biologic agent, this may be an acceptable mode of death (see concept of double effect). If the patient is expected to survive and aggressive interventions are anticipated, then significant respiratory depression (respiratory rate <6/min usually accompanied by oxygen saturation <90%) should be treated with naloxone:

- Dilute 0.4 mg of naloxone in 10 mL sterile water (0.04 mg/mL) and give 0.1–0.2 mg IV q 1–2 minutes until patient is alert.
- Reversal of respiratory depression with naloxone will likely result in rapid recurrence of pain. Repeat opioid doses should be 25–50% less than previous doses.

Urticaria and pruritus should be treated with antihistamines. Nausea should be treated with parenteral prochlorperazine (10 mg), metoclopramide (10 mg), or Phenergan (25 mg).

GASTROINTESTINAL SYMPTOMS

General Concepts

GI symptoms that would likely result from a bioterrorist attack mainly include nausea/vomiting and diarrhea. Although a search for the mechanism of these symptoms is generally recommended to guide therapy, the EP will probably not have the luxury of time to make this determination. In addition, it is unlikely that the cause of these symptoms, that is, infectious agent, chemical exposure, radiation, or other toxin can be reversed or adequately treated. Treatment is, therefore, empiric and focused on relieving the symptom.

Nausea/Vomiting

There are multiple potential causes of nausea and vomiting; probably the most important distinction the EP must make to direct therapy is the presence of bowel obstruction. If present, then antiemetic agents are unlikely to relieve symptoms; placement of a nasogastric tube is the treatment of choice. Otherwise, treatment is empiric and there are a number of agents that are available, which have efficacy.

Medications for Treatment of Nausea/Vomiting

- Dopamine antagonists: haloperidol (Haldol), droperidol (Inapsine), prochlorperazine (Compazine), metoclopramide (Reglan), promethazine (Phenergan)
- Histamine antagonists: diphenhydramine (Benadryl), hydroxyzine (Atarax)
- Serotonin antagonists: ondansetron (Zofran), granisetron (Kytril)
- Cerebral cortical agents: dexamethasone (Decadron), lorazepam (Ativan)
- Prokinetic agent: metoclopramide (Reglan)

Treatment of mild to moderate nausea

- Compazine 10 mg IVP
- Phenergan 25 mg IVP
- Ativan 0.5–1 mg IVP (helpful in anxiety, agitation)

Treatment of severe nausea or vomiting

- Haldol 1–2 mg IVP + Benadryl 50 mg IVP or Phenergan 50 mg IVP
- Haldol 1–2 mg IVP + Ativan 1 mg IVP (helpful in anxiety, agitation)
- Add Decadron 10 mg IVP to above if ineffective
- Zofran 16 mg IVP + Decadron 10 mg IVP (probably no more effective than above choices and very expensive; high efficacy for radiation-induced nausea/vomiting)
- Consider adding PPI (proton pump inhibitor) if vomiting to reduce gastric irritation: Pantoprazole (Protonix) 40 mg IVP

Diarrhea

There are multiple causes of diarrhea that could result from a bioterrorist attack, particularly due to infectious agents and radiation, but treatment should be empiric.

- Loperamide (Imodium): 4 mg PO initial dose, then 2 mg after each loose stool
- Diphenoxylate (Lomotil): 5 mg PO initial dose, then 2.5–5 mg q 4–6 hours
- Codeine: 10–60 mg PO q 4 hours
- Octreotide (Sandostatin): 50–100 mcg SC q 8–12 hours (if unable to take PO)

PULMONARY SYMPTOMS

General Concepts

The most common pulmonary symptom faced by the EP in the aftermath of a bioterrorist attack is dyspnea. This symptom can be caused by a wide range of infectious agents and by chemical inhalation. Other pulmonary symptoms are hemoptysis, cough, and excessive secretions. The approach should be empiric with the goal being relief of the symptom(s), even if the intervention may hasten death (see concept of double effect).

Dyspnea

This is an extremely unpleasant symptom, often described as air hunger, which requires immediate and effective treatment. The mainstay of treatment is opioid therapy. Opioids decrease the perception of breathlessness, the ventilatory drive, and oxygen consumption. Mild dyspnea can be treated with oral morphine, such as Roxanol, but parenteral morphine is the most efficacious.

Morphine for treatment of dyspnea

- Morphine 1–2 mg IVP every 5–10 minutes until dyspnea is relieved
- Morphine as continuous infusion
  - Calculate the total dose necessary to control the dyspnea, and half of that dose is administered per hour as continuous infusion.
  - In opioid-naive patients, typically 1–2 mg/h continuous infusion is effective.
  - If dyspnea persists while on continuous infusion, give a bolus equal to 150% of the hourly dose and increase the hourly dose by 50%.
- Nebulized morphine: This route is helpful if no IV access or if IV morphine is ineffective.
  - 5 mg morphine in 2 mL sterile water and administer via nebulizer.

Other treatments of dyspnea

- Ativan can be very effective for anxiety that accompanies dyspnea.
  - Ativan 1–2 mg IVP q 1–2 hours as needed
  - May give as continuous infusion at 1–5 mg/h
  - Diazepam (Valium) 2–5 mg IVP q 4–6 hours (longer half-life)
- Corticosteroids: Glucocorticoids are recommended in patients who have bronchospasm, edema, or bronchial obstruction.
  - Decadron: 10–20 mg IVP
- Anticholinergic agents: These agents are used for excessive secretions.
  - Atropine 0.4–1 mg IVP
  - Hyoscyamine (Levsin) 0.125 mg PO or SL q 6
  - Scopolamine transdermal patch 1.5 mg
- Midazolam (Versed): Use in dyspnea refractory to above agents.
  - Versed 2–4 mg IVP followed by continuous infusion at 2–5 mg/h

NEUROLOGIC SYMPTOMS

General Concepts

Individuals involved in a bioterrorist attack are likely to experience neurologic symptoms, ranging from mild anxiety to preterminal delirium. These symptoms may be a direct result of a specific offending agent or a nonspecific reaction to their condition and the overall horror of the situation. The concept of double effect is relevant, particularly in the patient with preterminal delirium, as effective treatment for this condition will almost certainly hasten death.

Anxiety

Short-acting benzodiazepines are considered to be the agents of choice for anxiety in patients who are critically ill. Alprazolam (Xanax) and lorazepam (Ativan) are the best studied.

- Ativan: 0.5–1 mg IVP *or* 1–2 mg PO q 3–6 hours prn
- Xanax: 0.25–2 mg PO q 6 hours prn

When anxiety is severe or occurs with paranoia, hallucinations, or agitation, the use of a major tranquilizer is required. A short-acting benzodiazepine such as Ativan should not be given due to the likelihood that the patient will experience a paradoxical reaction, in which the patient "fights" the sedating effect of the drug and becomes even more agitated. It can be used *after* administration of a major tranquilizer if further sedation is desired.

- Haloperidol (Haldol) is the drug of choice: 1–5 mg IVP q 4 hours prn, but can be repeated in 1 hour if necessary.

Palliative Sedation in the Dying Patient

Under the circumstances of a bioterrorist attack, the EP will be confronted with patients who are experiencing severe agitation/delirium as a consequence of the offending agent and/or as a condition occurring immediately prior to death. The EP must then seriously consider administration of palliative sedation. When a patient has suffered an insult (such as that experienced during a bioterrorist attack) that is certain to result in their death within a relatively short period of time and they are suffering from intolerable symptoms that cannot be relieved even by expert palliative care, administering sedatives to induce unconsciousness is an acceptable treatment to relieve suffering. The term palliative sedation is used to avoid any implication that the intention of the treatment is to cause the patient's death. Is this a form of euthanasia? The answer is "no" as outlined below in a description of the doctrine of double effect.

Doctrine of Double Effect

This doctrine draws a moral distinction between what a person intends and what is accepted as a foreseen but unintended consequence. According to this doctrine, intentionally causing death is wrong. However, the physician must administer sufficiently high dose of sedatives and opioids to achieve the goal of relief of suffering. The doctrine of double effect also requires that (1) the giving of sedatives and opioids must not be morally wrong, (2) the secondary untoward effect (respiratory depression or death) must not be the means to accomplish the primary beneficial effect (relief of suffering), (3) there must be proportionality between the intended primary effects, and the unintended but foreseen secondary effects, and (4) there must be no less harmful option for achieving the goal of relief of suffering.

When the EP determines that palliative sedation is required, then it is imperative that a frank discussion occur with the patient, family, and medical team. When available, an expert in palliative medicine should be consulted. The EP must be explicit about the goals of treatment and the anticipated outcome. Questions about the dying process and requests to hasten it must be addressed. Efforts to provide comfort and closure for the patient and family are necessary. The hospital chaplain and/or other religious personnel should be involved to provide spiritual guidance and closure. Social workers and other mental health workers should be included to provide support and counseling to the families of the victims.

Pharmacologic Intervention in Palliative Sedation

- Midazolam
  Midazolam (Versed) is the most commonly used drug for palliative sedation, with a rapid onset of action and short half-life.
  - 2–5 mg (0.04–0.08 mg/kg) IVP for immediate sedation but a continuous infusion is required.
  - Start infusion at 0.5–1 mg/h and titrate upward; expectation is that the final dose will likely range from 4 to 10 mg/h.
  - In some patients, midazolam produces a paradoxical agitation; other agents will then be required.
- Phenobarbital
  Give 200 mg IVP, then continuous infusion at 25–60 mg/h.
- Propofol
  Propofol is an anesthetic agent that can be used for palliative sedation. Give 10 mg/h infusion titrated up by 10 mg/h every 15–20 minutes.
- Adjunctive medications
  - Parenteral opioid infusion if pain is an issue
  - Haloperidol 1–5 mg IVP for agitated delirium
  - Dantrolene for myoclonus (may occur as toxicity from opioid infusion)

CONCLUSION

This chapter has hopefully provided some useful guidelines for the successful palliative management of victims of a bioterrorist attack seen in the ED. Since most patients are not expected to survive such a horrific event, then every effort must be made to relieve suffering. We now have effective drugs to relieve pain, dyspnea, nausea/vomiting, and agitation, and the EP should have the expertise to administer adequate doses of these drugs. Finally, the EP must be prepared to provide palliative sedation under circumstances when symptoms cannot be relieved. The doctrine of double effect provides a sound ethical, legal, and medical justification for this treatment.

Suggested Reading

Beauchamp TL, Childress JF. *Principles of Biomedical Ethics,* 5th ed. New York, Oxford University Press, 2001; p. 128.

Benzon HT, Raja SN, Molloy RE. *Essentials of Pain Medicine and Regional Anesthesia,* 2nd ed. Philadelphia, Elsevier Churchill Livingston, 2005.

Boyle J. Medical ethics and double effect: the case of terminal sedation. *Theor Med Bioeth.* 2004;25:61.

Jackson KC, Lipman AG. Delirium in palliative care patients. In: Lipman AG, Jackson KC, Tyler LS (eds.). *Evidence Based Symptom Control in Palliative Care.* Binghamton, New York, Haworth Press, 2000; p. 59.

Johnston K. Staff at New Orleans hospital debated euthanizing patients. CNN, Oct 13th, 2005.

Krauss B. Management of acute pain and anxiety in children undergoing procedures in the emergency department. *Pediatr Emer Care.* 2001;17:115.

Lo B, Rubenfeld G. Palliative sedation in dying patients. *JAMA.* 2005;294:1810.

Mace SE, Ducharme J, Murphy MF. *Pain Management and Sedation: Emergency Department Management.* New York, McGraw-Hill, 2006.

Macintyre PE, Ready LB. *Acute Pain Management: A Practical Guide.* London, W.B. Saunders, 2001.

Schrebner S, Yoeli N, Paz G. Hospital preparedness for possible nonconventional casualities: the Israeli experience. *Gen Hosp Psych.* 2004;26:59.

Storey P, Knight CF, Schonwetter RS. *Pocket Guide to Hospice/Palliative Medicine.* Glenview, Illinois American Academy of Hospice and Palliative Medicine, 2003.

Tyler LS. Dyspnea in palliative care patients. In: Lipman AG, Jackson KC, Tyler LS (eds.): *Evidence Based Symptom Control in Palliative Care.* Binghamton, New York, Haworth Press, 2000; p. 109.

Tyler LS. Nausea and vomiting in palliative care. In: Lipman AG, Jackson KC, Tyler LS (eds.). *Evidence Based Symptom Control in Palliative Care.* Binghamton, New York, Haworth Press, 2000; p. 163.

14

SPECIAL POPULATIONS: PEDIATRICS

Amy L. Drendel and David D. Gummin

STAT FACTS

SPECIAL POPULATIONS: PEDIATRICS

- Children present a unique challenge to health-care providers preparing for and responding to terrorism threats; they are *not* just small adults.
- Though children may be sentinel cases in terrorism events, the early signs and symptoms associated with biological weapons are difficult to differentiate from common childhood illnesses.
- The provider must appreciate differences in resuscitating children, compared to adults.
- Triage protocols appropriate to the pediatric patient ensure that the greatest good is done for the greatest number of children. Application of adult protocols to children is inappropriate.
- Differences in pediatric physiology emphasize the vulnerability of this population to bioterrorism.
- Attention to psychological needs is essential to the assessment and treatment of children in a bioterrorism event.
- The provider must be familiar with unique pediatric treatment regimens, as many of these differ from adult protocols.

INTRODUCTION

The assessment and treatment of children is a unique challenge to health-care providers preparing for and responding to terrorism threats. Anecdotal and uncontrolled studies suggest that children have physical, psychological, and social needs that differ from adults. Compared to adults, children are more likely to first manifest symptoms, to present in proportionately larger numbers for care, to have more severe symptoms, to be more difficult to identify and to care for, and require greater resource utilization. Simply modifying current practices for adults is insufficient; a specific approach for the pediatric patient is best. The provider who anticipates specific pediatric needs, and who demonstrates expertise in the assessment and treatment of children, will assure the success of a pediatric bioterrorism disaster plan.

RECOGNITION CHALLENGE

The early signs and symptoms incited by biological weapons may be difficult to discern from common childhood viral illnesses. Initial presenting symptoms associated with many biological agents include fever and respiratory complaints—two very common complaints for pediatric patients in the emergency and clinical setting. Furthermore, many children will not be able to communicate the details of their symptoms effectively. This complicates the initial assessment of the pediatric terror victim. Clustering of severe symptoms and rapid progression of symptoms should raise suspicion. Inhaled anthrax, plague, and tularemia typically progress from fever with respiratory complaints to fulminant pneumonia. Specific rashes are associated with the febrile illnesses of anthrax and smallpox. Mild exposure to nerve agents can produce nausea, vomiting, and weakness, which are difficult to differentiate from viral gastroenteritis. Acuity of onset (seconds to minutes) and clustering of patients should alert the clinician to the possibility of a terrorist threat.

Children may be sentinel cases in terrorist events since some agents demonstrate shorter incubation periods in children. Relatively greater exposure occurs in children, with higher dose for weight, because of their smaller mass. Clinicians caring for children may be the first to recognize bioterrorist activity for all of these reasons, but a high index of suspicion is required. Syndromic surveillance, a technique for monitoring presenting health complaints for unusual illness clusters, is currently being utilized to improve detection. Early detection is problematic, but is the critical first step for medical and public health responders to deliver appropriate and timely treatment and containment.

RESUSCITATION DIFFERENCES IN CHILDREN

It is essential for the bioterrorism responder to appreciate the ways in which pediatric resuscitation differs from adult resuscitation. Importantly, cardiopulmonary arrest in children typically results from the progression of respiratory distress to respiratory failure. It is rarely a primary cardiac event. Attention to the child with respiratory insufficiency can prevent progression and facilitate recovery from impending cardiopulmonary arrest.

Airway

Pediatric airways are much smaller in diameter and length. This poses a challenge to those managing the airway, but also makes children more susceptible to airway compromise. Excessive secretions and bronchospasm are seen with some bioterrorism agents. The child's relative large tongue can obstruct the airway unless properly positioned. Obstruction of the nares can cause significant respiratory compromise, since young children are relative nose breathers. Many pediatric airways can be maintained simply with a head tilt–chin lift (sniffing position) or a jaw thrust in those who require cervical spine precautions. A towel roll under the shoulders can reduce airway obstruction from neck flexion (because of the prominent occiput) that invariably occurs in supine young children. The use of airway adjuncts and interventions requires smaller airway equipment (airways, masks, nasal cannulae, laryngoscopes, endotracheal tubes, suction catheters, and tracheostomy tubes) and an appreciation for anatomical differences in the pediatric patient.

Breathing

Acute respiratory failure can develop in children more rapidly than in an adult. It is critical to recognize the initial signs and symptoms of respiratory insufficiency. The child's high metabolic rate leads to a high oxygen demand per kilogram of weight. Oxygen consumption in an infant is 6–8 mL/kg/min compared to 3–4 mL/kg/min in adults. Inadequate ventilation and hypoxemia can develop more rapidly. Children also have limited endurance of their accessory muscles of breathing. Slowed or irregular respiratory rate is an indication of deterioration. Altered mental state, retracting, grunting, and diminished air entry may be the only signs of respiratory compromise. Bag-mask ventilation of children requires pediatric self-inflating bags or anesthesia bags that deliver smaller volumes. The rate of ventilation must be increased for children.

Circulation

Children will maintain a normal blood pressure in the face of significant hypovolemia. Careful attention to heart rate and perfusion is necessary. Assessment of pulses is easiest at the femoral or brachial sites, particularly in younger children. Evidence of poor perfusion can be identified by cyanosis, mottling, poor capillary refill, and altered mental status.

Children have smaller fluid reserves and circulating blood volume. They are more likely to require volume resuscitation, though vascular access can be particularly difficult to obtain. Small intravenous needles can improve success. Intraosseous lines can be placed in the proximal medial tibia for rapid access to treat shock. Initial fluid administration should be with isotonic normal saline or lactated Ringer's solution in 20 mL/kg boluses, but might require 80 mL/kg of crystalloid or more.

Disability

Limited cognitive and developmental capabilities of children make them especially vulnerable, as they may be unable to escape attack or to make decisions to evacuate. Their limitations also can present a challenge to the rescuer. Inability to communicate symptoms limits the assessment and makes interventions difficult. A simple objective assessment of level of consciousness that can be useful, is the mnemonic AVPU (alert, responds to voice, responds to pain, or is unresponsive).

Exposure

Exposure of children for assessment of injury as well as for decontamination puts them at risk of hypothermia. Their large body surface-to-mass ratio facilitates rapid loss of heat. Children are notoriously difficult to care for in personal protective equipment. Bulky protective clothing may impair the caregiver's ability to resuscitate children.

TRIAGE PROTOCOLS

Objective triage guidelines for patients of all ages can help ensure that the greatest good is done for the greatest number of casualties. Triage protocols specific to pediatric patients are best. Adult protocols should not be applied to the pediatric patient, as these tend to provide insufficient emphasis on acute, correctable, ventilatory pathology. Adult protocols inadequately address the nonambulatory pediatric patient. Triage intervention may be complicated by unavailability of age-specific equipment in the field. The JumpSTART triage protocol (Fig. 14-1) is an adaptation of the most common mass-casualty triage system used in the United States and many other countries. Distinctions include modification of decision points to match the range of pediatric norms, recognition that the primary pathway to death is respiratory failure/arrest, and recognition that not all children will be ambulatory.

Succession of normal vital signs with age makes triage assessment difficult, increasing the risk of errors, and adding delay. Experience has shown that pediatric-specific zones offer many advantages to both providers and children. Designated personnel and devices like the Broselow tape are important tools that providers can use for weight- and size-based norms. Rescuers skilled at engaging the cooperation of children (or at observing those children who cannot communicate) can play an important role in the triage of children in a bioterror event.

PHYSIOLOGIC DIFFERENCES IN CHILDREN

Physiologic differences in children make them more vulnerable than adults to bioterror attacks. The most apparent difference between children and adults is their relative size. The smaller mass of a child allows relatively lower doses of toxic or infectious agents to produce more severe effects or even death. Chemical, radiation, and biological agents cause dose-dependent effects, so that children will generally present earlier and with greater severity than will adult counterparts.

Children, it's often said, are not simply small adults. Toxicokinetic differences increase their risk in bioterrorism events. They are likely to absorb larger doses for a number of reasons: Younger children have shorter stature and are closer to the ground. This increases their potential exposure to radioactive materials from nuclear fallout. High-density, aerosolized chemical and biological agents also tend to concentrate near the ground. *Sarin*, the nerve agent made infamous by its use in two civilian terrorist acts, has a high vapor density. Similarly, chlorine gas concentrates near the ground and increases the child's potential exposure.

Young children exhibit frequent hand-to-mouth activity that increases their risk of exposure by ingestion. Children have higher ventilation rates and increased alveolar uptake. This increases risk of exposure by inhalation. Transdermal absorption (e.g., nerve agents) is increased by the relatively large surface-mass ratio and the higher permeability of their poorly keratinized skin. These differences lead to more severe injury due to corrosives and vesicants. A case series of children in Iran showed faster onset and more severe dermal lesions after mustard exposure in children. Decontamination of these patients risks hypothermia because of increased heat loss resulting from the increased surface-mass ratio.

Children have a relatively immature ability to metabolize drugs and also to detoxify many chemical agents, prolonging effective exposure to agents such as organophosphates.

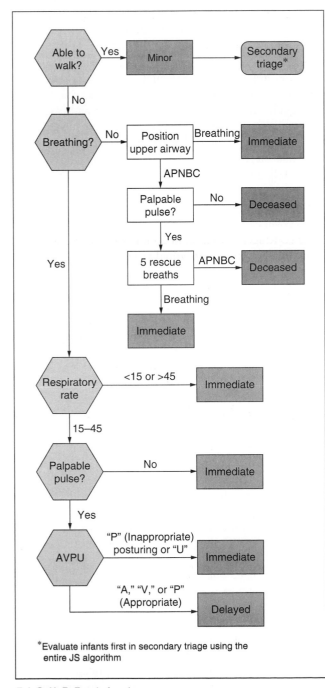

FIGURE 14-1

UMPSTART PEDIATRIC MCI TRIAGE
Source: Reproduced with the permission of Lou Romig MD, FACEP.

Paraoxonase detoxifies organophosphate pesticides, but levels at birth are half of those found in adults.

In some instances, children simply respond differently than adults to exposures. Children exposed to anticholinesterase pesticides have disproportionately more depressed sensorium and muscle weakness, without peripheral muscarinic effects seen in adults. Children in cholinergic crisis may not manifest miosis. Infants and children exposed to nerve agents are more prone to seizures than adult counterparts. Some of these differences may be attributed to an immature blood-brain barrier or to increased sensitivity of receptors.

Radiation-induced cancers occur more often in children than in adults exposed to the same dose. Young children have little or no naturally acquired immunity, which places them at particular risk of severe disease with biological agents. More than 80% of the adult population is no longer immune to smallpox because of its worldwide eradication, while 100% of children are susceptible. In some cases, children appear to be more susceptible to biologic agents. Most adults who contract Venezuelan equine encephalitis fully recover. Children, however, develop severe and often fatal encephalitis in 4% of cases.

PSYCHOSOCIAL NEEDS

The psychological effects of disasters on children are neither uniform nor universal. Outcome depends upon the nature of the disaster, the level of exposure, and individual characteristics of the children. Important characteristics include the child's age and developmental stage. The different needs and vulnerabilities of preschoolers, children, and adolescents demand an appreciation for the range of mental health issues that may ensue. Infants and toddlers may not comprehend the implications, but they are affected by the loss of routine and of loved ones. This can lead to regression and detachment. Younger children are generally unable to understand the intentions and rationale of terrorism, but may focus on specific details of the event and on their own personal safety. This age-group does not understand the permanence of death. They are likely to experience sleep disruption and behavioral regression, with increased temper tantrums. School-age children are more likely to be cognitive of the intent and implications of an event. They tend to display more empathy for families affected by the crisis, and to become focused on the safety of society as a whole. These children can have sleep disorders and may react with anxiety and depression or with aggression and behavioral problems. Adolescent responses most closely resemble adult reactions. They are at risk of depression and anxiety. Teens who are still developing coping skills and establishing their own identity are more susceptible to major psychiatric disorders. This age-group can isolate themselves or react with defiance and risk-taking behaviors. Because of psychological immaturity, children have less coping skills and require special attention to their psychological needs.

Some subsets of children may be at increased risk for adverse psychological reactions. Children with poor social support, a history of psychopathology, or a shy or fearful nature are at increased risk. Those who have a high level of exposure or who have experienced previous losses have higher risk for an adverse reaction to terrorism. Because children are intimately dependent on their parents, a child's anxiety can be compounded by parents' fears and distress. Parents should be advised to present information to children simply, honestly, and at the level of the child's developmental and cognitive abilities.

Early intervention is essential to promote postdisaster resilience in children and families. Postdisaster psychological and emotional functioning of parents and caretakers positively impacts outcomes in children. This underscores the importance of postdisaster family interventions. It is important to recognize the stages of a child's response to disaster. In the first few days, children will generally experience fright, disbelief, denial, grief, and relief. This is followed over the next few weeks by regression and emotional distress: anxiety, fear, sadness, depression, anger, hostility, apathy, sleep disturbance, and somatization. Children with adverse stress reaction and behavioral symptoms for longer than 1 month are at risk for developing posttraumatic stress disorder or violent, delinquent behaviors later in life.

UNIQUE PEDIATRIC TREATMENT REGIMENS

Antibiotics, vaccines, and antidotes have a fundamental role in treatment and prophylaxis after bioterrorism events. Proper doses have been recommended for many agents, but some doses have not been established for children.

Antibiotics of choice for bioterrorism are not those typically used in the treatment of childhood infections. Lack of experience with their use in this population implies that few pharmacies and clinics stock these medications in liquid form. Further, pediatricians are not typically familiar with many of these drugs, since many are relatively contraindicated for use in childhood. Tetracycline antibiotics may discolor teeth in children younger than 8 years of age, and rarely, skeletal growth may be retarded. There is concern that fluoroquinolones may cause arthropathy. Generally spoken, the risk of morbidity and mortality from a biological agent-induced illness far outweighs the minor risk that may be associated with short-term use of these antibiotics. For this reason, the Food and Drug Administration has specifically approved their use for children in this setting. Chloramphenicol, however, is not considered safe in children younger than 2 years of age because of the risk of "gray baby syndrome."

Many vaccines have been approved for use in those over age 18, but efficacy in children is not documented. The smallpox vaccine has been well-studied in children, but pediatric patients more commonly experience severe complications including encephalitis, particularly under 1 year of age. Yellow fever vaccine is inappropriate for use in infants because of the risk of developing encephalitis. Only infant botulism and smallpox vaccine are approved for children older than 1 year of age. Vaccines are available or being developed for anthrax, plague, tularemia, Q fever, and Venezuelan equine encephalitis.

Prepackaged drugs (auto injectors for atropine and pralidoxime) and kits (cyanide antidote), stockpiled for terrorist attacks, are not appropriate for use in children. In dire emergencies, these auto injectors, with 0.8-inch needle insertion length and 2 mg atropine or 600 mg pralidoxime, might be useful in children older than 2 years (and at least 13 kg). Consult appropriate resources for recommendation on their use.

Recommendations for the treatment of children with radiation exposure are well-defined. Potassium iodide (KI) is specifically indicated for children for the prevention of thyroid cancer. It works by saturating the thyroid and blocking uptake of radioiodine. Exposed children should receive KI, ideally within 2 hours of exposure. Of note, a single serum TSH level 2–4 weeks after dosage of KI should be sufficient to identify any transient decreases in thyroxine. This is most commonly seen in newborns treated with KI.

Suggested Reading

American Academy of Pediatrics. Chemical and biological terrorism and its impact on children: a subject review. *Pediatrics.* 2000;105:662–670.

American Academy of Pediatrics. Psychosocial implications of disaster or terrorism on children: a guide for the pediatrician. *Pediatrics.* 2005;116(3):787–795.

American Academy of Pediatrics. Radiation disasters and children. *Pediatrics.* 2003;111(6):1455–1466.

American Academy of Pediatrics. The pediatrician and disaster preparedness. *Pediatrics.* 2006;117(2):560–565.

Cieslak TJ, Henretig FM. Ring-a-ring-a roses: bioterrorism and its peculiar relevance to pediatrics. *Curr Opin Pediatr.* 2003;15:107–111.

Henretig FM, Cieslak TJ, Eitzen EM. Biologic and chemical terrorism. *J Pediatr.* 2002;141(3):311–326.

Karr CJ, Solomon GM, Brock-Utne AC Health effects of common home, lawn and garden pesticides. *Ped. Ar Clin North Am.* 2007;54:63–80.

Quail MT, Shannon MW. Pralidoxime safety and toxicity in children *Prehosp Emerg Care* 2007;11:36–41.

More information about JumpSTART: *http://jumpstarttriage.com* Accessed March 29, 2006.

More information about pediatric disaster preparedness: *http://www.chawisconsin.org/traumapreparedness_flash.htm* Accessed March 29, 2006.

Patt HA, Feigin RD. Diagnosis and management of suspected cases of bioterrorism: a pediatric perspective. *Pediatrics.* 2002;109(4):685–692.

Rotenberg JS, Newmark J. Nerve agents attacks on children: diagnosis and management. *Pediatrics.* 2003;112(3):648–658.

Stocker JT Clinical and Pathologic Differential diagnosis of selected potential bioterrorism agents of interest to pediatric health care providers *Clin Lab Med* 2006 Jun;26(2):329–44,VIII.

White SR, Henretig FM, Dukes RG. Medical management of vulnerable populations and comorbid conditions of victims of bioterrorism. *Emerg Med Clin North Am.* 2002;20:365–392.

15

GERIATRICS: BIOTERRORISM, EMERGING THREATS, AND EMERGENCY PREPAREDNESS: SPECIAL CONSIDERATIONS FOR GERIATRIC PATIENTS

Robin B. McFee and Scott Lillibridge

STAT FACTS

GERIATRICS: BIOTERRORISM, EMERGING THREATS, AND EMERGENCY PREPAREDNESS: SPECIAL CONSIDERATIONS FOR GERIATRIC PATIENTS

- The elderly are not merely older versions of adults. The anatomic and physiologic changes associated with aging, as well as ethnic, social, and economic influences impact diagnosis, management, and follow-up.
- Infectious diseases may progress more rapidly among older adults, especially the frail elderly.
- Coexisting illnesses or medications may confound the diagnosis.
- Countermeasures may be especially problematic. For example, the syringe size and force associated with the nerve agent autoinjectors found in the Mark I Nerve Agent Antidote Kits (NAAK)—designed as intramuscular injections for strong war fighters—may ostensibly become interosseous by virtue of the loss of muscle mass of older individuals.
- It is important to understand the impact of aging upon the response to illness and the risks in addition to the benefits of countermeasures as they pertain to older persons.

Preparedness for Elders "DISASTER"

D Diagnose early
I Impaired communication by elders
S Supplies—especially elder appropriate

A Animal treatment
S Scripts (prescriptions)
T Transportation needs
E Emotional response/needs
R Rapid diagnosis and response is critical

Potential unusual pathogen or bioterrorism especially if increased numbers of similarly presenting patients beyond normal seasonal epidemiology

Overall

- Change in behavior
- Unusual clinical symptoms or signs
- Rapidly progressive symptoms
- History suggestive of unusual exposure

Important Clinical Symptoms

- Relative bradycardia
- An important and reliable clue to an uncommon pathogen or biological weapon; may also indicate a serious decline in health among patients with infectious disease

- Elderly patients may not manifest this important clue either owing to the fact that older patients may not mount an appropriate pyrexic response until late in the illness, or are likely to be taking medications that can suppress heart rate.

Other Important Clues:

- Change in mental status
- Pulmonary complaints with GI complaints
- Dyspnea accompanying influenza-like illness (ILI)
- Petechia or vascular dermatologic signs
- "BP cuff sign" (petechia at the site of where the blood pressure cuff was applied)
- CXR unexpected for pt/present/age/sit
- Sleep disruption
- Rapidly elevating temperature—any high fever in the elderly is worrisome

Pre-Event Preparedness Considerations— The Elderly

Communications

Make certain your facility and response teams address communication with individuals who

- Do not speak English
- Are visually impaired
- Are hearing impaired
- Cannot verbally communicate
- Are cognitively impaired

Access

Consider the impact of communications, physical and cognitive impairments on patient access and delivery of care.

Training

In-service training concerning the significant differences in clinical presentations and treatment of geriatric patients compared to nonelder adults or children.

Equipment

- Countermeasures (antidotes/medications) that may impose additional risk to elderly patients or require special adjustments for aging patients should be identified, as should safer alternative interventions.
- Nerve Agent Antidote Kits (Mark I Kits) contain 2 mg atropine and 600 mg pralidoxime autoinjectors.
  - The needle size of the autoinjectors was developed to penetrate military garb worn by physically fit male warfighters, not frail, thin elderly.
  - Dosing considerations based upon mg/kg and comorbidities.
- Where feasible, personal protective equipment (PPE) should be available

- Personnel should be fit tested for and trained in the appropriate selection and use of equipment prior to an event.
- Consideration should also be given to shelter in place strategies and the equipment needs or actions associated with that preparedness modality.

Key Diagnostic Considerations

Biodromes (cluster of symptoms when together strongly suggest the diagnosis) associated with various bioweapon illnesses may present similar to or different from the classical presentations of the agents when elderly patients are affected.

- **Fever**
  - Most bioweapon illnesses present with fever.
  - The elderly may not mount an early febrile response compared to nonelder adults.
  - High fever in the elderly is worrisome and requires aggressive attention.
- **Cardiovascular**
  - Fever usually is accompanied by an elevated heart rate.
  - Biological agents as well as unusual pathogen can cause a decline in heart rate in the presence of high fever (pulse-temperature dissociation or relative bradycardia).

The following may affect heart rate response to fever in the elderly:

- Rate-reduction medications: Ex/β-adrenergic antagonists
- Implantable cardiac devices
- Underlying cardiac disease

Bioweapon illnesses may present with fever *and* heart rate reduction often referred to as "pulse-temperature dissociation" or "relative bradycardia." Delayed temperature elevation and/or inability to increase heart rate may confound the finding of relative bradycardia—a hallmark clue that may be found in tularemia, viral hemorrhagic fevers, and other bioweapon illnesses.

- **Neurologic**
  - Unexpected changes in behavior, memory, or consciousness warrant aggressive clinical care and are rarely benign; while such events can occur in the elderly, in the acute setting these may reflect stroke, trauma, or infection. Several bioweapon agents are associated with CNS involvement including anthrax, brucellosis, and smallpox. Other severe infections like avian flu, toxins, toxicants, or disease processes can also cause altered mental status.
- **Dermal**

Petechia, ecchymosis may indicate viral hemorrhagic fevers, septicemic plague, or other bioweapon illnesses that may reflect hematological involvement.

- Anticoagulant use is widespread among the elderly; this predisposes the patient to various dermal manifestations of bleeding.
- Elder skin is often fragile and may be readily bruised, simulating the effects of bleeding diathesis.

INTRODUCTION

The events of the last few years—bioterrorism, suicide bombings, and another Persian Gulf War, tsunamis and deadly earthquakes, SARS, emerging infectious diseases such as Marburg and more deadly strains of influenza—all demonstrate the fact that we are part of a global world. Threats such as terrorism as well as emerging infectious diseases once thought remote and unlikely to cross our shores have been shown with avian flu, 9-11, even anthrax, and monkeypox to pose a clear risk to our communities. While local and often predictable natural disasters such as hurricanes, floods, mudslides, blizzards, and fires should remain paramount in our preparedness efforts, protecting our communities is not a zero-sum game; an all hazards approach that encompasses a wide range of threats, especially as pertain to the aging community, is critical. Preparedness for an unknown terrorist event with an undisclosed target or timetable is a daunting task. Significant progress has been made to remedy local, regional, and national vulnerabilities. Nevertheless, certain populations remain especially vulnerable, including older people, children, women who are pregnant, persons with disabilities, and certain minorities with linguistic differences. While there are commonalities to preparedness shared across populations, the differences unique to special populations must be addressed to minimize the effects of emergencies on diagnostic considerations, including identifying patients, patients' ability to participate in their own rescue or treatment, and the availability of long-term follow-up.

Bioterrorism and emergency preparedness for any population is a daunting task when one considers the training, resources, logistics, political and practical issues involved that are necessary to identify and remedy a myriad of local, regional, and national vulnerabilities and to protect a broad range of people and subpopulations. This is especially challenging for the aging population. Unlike the younger populations, the elderly, even the robust elderly, are undergoing declines in physiologic function, mobility, sensory interpretation such as hearing or vision, and often are marginalized within the broader population due to a variety of factors including lower socioeconomic status, ageism, institutionalization, disability, or isolation.

Emergency physicians and other health-care providers need to prepare for as well as provide an appropriate response to biological weapons, especially in the protection of vulnerable subpopulations, especially an aging community and elderly patients. Preparedness considerations to care for the elderly incorporate traditional planning plus incorporate issues that are unique to aging patients. These include potential physical and cognitive limitations, atypical presentations of bioweapon illness, and limited ability to convey important details about the history of present illness. Often the elderly live alone and may have limited access to care or reside in group housing. The elderly may also have service or companion animals. The ability to provide care, decontamination, or other veterinary services is important to address before an emergency given there are numerous examples of patients presenting with their animal companions or service animals.

There is a wide range of potential terrorist events that could occur in the community—chemical, biological, or radiological; this chapter will emphasize the potential differences in clinical presentation elders may demonstrate compared to adults. It is important when preparing for any of the chemical, biological, radiological, nuclear, or explosive (CBRNE) threats that the clinician recognizes potential age-related changes that may influence the identification or treatment of CBRNE among the elderly.

The impact of infectious diseases disproportionately affects older persons, accounting for 40% of deaths among the elderly. This is largely due to the effects associated with aging, including biological, institutional, and cultural influences. Decreased physical reserves, a compromised immune system, greater susceptibility to stress all contribute to their vulnerability to infections. Underlying comorbidities not only enhance the risks associated with infection but may influence the body's ability to manifest symptoms or provide confounding clinical clues. For example, temperature is an important screening tool to identify infection; older persons may not manifest fever early in the course of illness. Thus this early marker for viral or bacterial infection may be lost and may delay diagnosis unless the astute clinician takes into account the entire spectrum of illness—the biodrome.

PHYSIOLOGIC CHANGES OF AGING

Unlike nonelderly adults, the aging patient often has multiple preexisting illnesses with symptoms that may mimic those associated with a bioweapon illness. Even the presentation of common illness in the elderly such as community-acquired pneumonia is often atypical. For example, fever, typically considered a hallmark of infection in the nonelderly population, may not occur in an older patient. As we age, virtually every major organ system may demonstrate age-related changes that confound diagnosis, predispose to greater risk of adverse outcome, hamper rescue or enhance vulnerability. The age- and nutrition-related decline in immune system function overall can predispose the elderly to a more severe response to a bioweapon. In addition to these immunophysiological differences between elderly and nonelderly, there are others including but not limited to hematological (anticoagulant therapy, fragile skin, declines in platelet count/bone marrow dysfunction), cognitive (cerebral vascular disease, medication, dementia, depression, Alzheimer's), and cardiovascular (heart disease, medications, pacemakers). Higher respiratory rates may predispose to inhaling larger doses of biological pathogens while decrease in pulmonary health may hasten deadly outcomes (Tables 15-1 and 15-2).

TABLE 15-1

SYSTEMS APPROACH: COMORBID CONDITIONS/ SYMPTOM ALTERATION

Cardiovascular

- Underlying health as starting point
- Heart rate response
  - Response to pathogen/toxicant
  - Response to intervention
- Comorbidity
- Medications

Dermal

- Delicate skin
- Chronic breakdown
- Chronic lesions
- Ecchymosis

Central Nervous System

- Mentation
- Cerebral flow
- Lipid solubility ~ drug metabolism
- Sleep
- D/dx
  - Organic brain syndrome
  - Depression
  - Alertness and Orientation

Ocular

- Medications
- Cataracts
- Underlying eye disease

Auditory

Hearing loss
- Medications
- Underlying hearing loss
- Tumors

Tinnitus

- Medications
- Explosive event
- Cardiovascular disease

Pulmonary

- COPD/chronic bronchitis
- Underlying cardiac disease
- Asthma

Musculoskeletal

- Degenerative diseases
- Benign tremors
- Endocrine
- Neurological

TABLE 15-2

BIOTERRORISM PEARLS: THESE FINDINGS ARE IMPORTANT CLUES TO BIOWEAPON ILLNESS. AGE-RELATED INFLUENCES THAT MIGHT MIMIC OR ALTER THESE CLUES

- Relative bradycardia
  - Comorbid cardiac disease
  - Heart rate reducing medications
  - Attenuated febrile response
- Change in mental status
  - Organic brain disorders
  - Medication effects
  - Psychiatric disorders
- Pulmonary complaints with GI complaints
  - Underlying pulmonary and GI diseases
- Dyspnea accompanying ILI
  - Underlying cardiovascular disease
  - Underlying pulmonary disease
- Petechial or vascular dermatologic signs
  - Anticoagulant therapy
  - Underlying dermatologic disorder
  - Abuse
- BP cuff sign
  - Anticoagulant therapy
- CXR unexpected for pt/present/age/sit
- Sleep disruption
  - Medications
  - Underlying psychiatric illness
  - Chronic illness

While bioweapon illnesses initially may present with seemingly nonspecific signs and symptoms in the early stages, as the illness progresses, often there are hallmark clues that suggest the diagnosis. These include uncommon clinical findings such as petechial rashes or other dermal manifestations, relative bradycardia, painless solitary or myriad synchronous lesions, and rapid onset with early multisystem involvement. Several biological weapons including tularemia and certain viral hemorrhagic fevers (VHF) can cause high fevers (a strong clinical clue, especially among the young) without an appropriate elevation in heart rate that typically accompanies fevers; a pulse-temperature dissociation, which also is referred to as relative bradycardia. Relative bradycardia—whereupon the heart rate fails to increase appropriately with the increase in fever—is highly uncommon except in unusual illness or fulminant decompensation from highly aggressive infection. In addition to a general inability to mount a febrile response, which would all but guarantee losing this important clinical finding, many elders are taking medications that may control heart rate, such as β-adrenergic blockers, or have implanted pacemakers, as well as a limited capacity to demonstrate fever, thus leading to total loss of the relative bradycardia clue among elderly patients.

Some biological agents that might be used in biological terrorism, including brucellosis, may contain neurotoxins that directly or indirectly affect neurological function and alter behavior. Other bioweapons may present with or have deleterious affects on mental status, neurological function, or level of cognitive function, negatively impacting the ability to obtain an accurate history as well as mimicking delirium, dementia, or other age-related cognitive deficits or behaviors including "sundown psychosis." Nerve agent victims, even when treated rapidly and appropriately, may exhibit long-term sequelae that include nightmares and personality changes. Because elderly patients may have coexisting neurobehavioral illness, distinguishing the effects of weapons of mass destruction (WMD) or crisis from underlying symptoms may be challenging.

HISTORY AND CONTEXT OF ILLNESS

All patients should be asked about recent travel, and any alterations in their routine activities, including dining, work, caregivers, or friends. Caregivers and family/friends should also be included in obtaining the history if available and as necessary, especially if the patient suffers from memory deficits. In addition, a careful timeline about the clinical presentation, any and all changes in health, symptoms, and complaints should be elicited, even those seemingly insignificant. It bears repeating that while taken separately, many of the signs and symptoms associated with biological weapons may seem to be exacerbations of the underlying comorbidities of the patient, taken together and in the appropriate context may represent the constellation of findings associated with the bioweapon. Inquiring if the presentation is similar or different from prior experiences and distinguishing between a rapid onset versus a slowly evolving presentation will also assist in the diagnosis. A thorough examination—follicles to feet—should be conducted if there is any suspicion of unusual illness, keeping in mind the normal and expected hallmark clues associated with bioweapons and the expected alterations that may result from normal physiologic changes associated with aging.

This chapter will discuss the special considerations attendant to the elderly as pertaining especially to bioterrorism threats. The reader is referred to the chapters addressing the specific CBRNE agents for a more in-depth discussion.

CDC Category A Agents: Diagnostic Considerations in the Elderly

(See Chap. 39 for more in-depth discussions of the following agents).

Bioweapons are usually derived from highly pathogenic and uncommon microbes.

Bacillus Anthracis/Inhalation Anthrax

Inhalation anthrax may appear with initial symptoms similar to influenza-like illness. Patients with chronic obstructive pulmonary disease (COPD) may experience exacerbation of illness, which may be inaccurately attributed to preexisting pulmonary disease, bronchitis, or new-onset viral respiratory infection. If several patients present with similar illness especially developing over a relatively short period of time or unexpectedly severe, this warrants concern. Inhalation anthrax causes a rapidly progressive illness. In addition, an unexpected constellation of symptoms involving nonpulmonary systems suggests a diagnosis other than influenza. The flu rarely causes true dyspnea, chest pain, nausea, and vomiting, unlike inhalation anthrax in which these are common. However these symptoms can also be attributed to acute coronary events. Since cardiac disease is prevalent in the elderly, a thorough investigation is imperative. Gastrointestinal disturbances are not uncommon among the elderly; looking at the appropriate timeline of illness is critical to the diagnosis. Patients complaining about significant shortness of breath in an appropriate context, with rapidity of clinical onset and severity ought to alert the clinician to a serious illness warranting aggressive investigation including laboratory analysis and management. Inhalation anthrax is a febrile illness; a high temperature in the elderly is worrisome, especially given the fact physiologic changes of aging often result in a blunted febrile response early in the illness. The elderly may also take medications, which have antipyretic effects. One of the keys to early diagnosis in the anthrax cases of 2001 was chest x-ray (CXR) and a thorough history. *The time from exposure to illness* was very short. It is also likely you will see increasing numbers of *severely ill* patients.

Variola/Smallpox

In smallpox, the elderly, especially immunosuppressed and nutritionally deficient, may be at increased risk. While the clinical presentation of the most common form of smallpox and the cascade of associated findings would seem to be unmistakable, the early presentation may be mistaken for chickenpox or shingles (herpes zoster), drug eruptions or disseminated herpes simplex. Studies suggest clinicians have a difficult time distinguishing images of smallpox from chickenpox. Since smallpox erupts as a synchronous rash in a centrifugal pattern, unlike the dermatomal distribution of shingles or the asynchronous rash of chickenpox, the diagnosis should not be missed, especially in the appropriate context of headache, high fever, altered mental status. Unfortunately as discussed earlier, the high fever normally associated with smallpox may not be evident in the elderly, who may only present therefore with delirium, which may be confused by other underlying conditions including dementia. Careful history, attention to syndromic symptoms, and awareness of other similar patients are critical to recognizing smallpox exposure and bioweapon attack. However, without some history of smallpox within the community it may be difficult to rapidly identify an index case.

Botulinum Toxin/Botulism

Unlike the other Category A bioweapons, which cause elevated temperature, and can cause alteration in mental status, *botulinum toxin would cause a flaccid descending paralysis starting with the bulbar musculature, without fever or alteration in mental status.* Another disease, which has been labeled a mimic of botulism, is the Miller-Fisher variant of the Guillain-Barré syndrome (GB). This disease also has been known to present with diplopia, ophthalmoplegia, ptosis, and facial and extremity weakness. However with this condition usually comes a history of antecedent infection, ascending paralysis, paresthesias, and early areflexia. On cerebrospinal fluid (CSF) examination, an increase in protein content of the fluid exists, which is characteristic of GB. Often confused with other acute neurologic events, the fact that botulinum presents with intact sensorium, bilateral neuromuscular involvement starting with the cranial nerves then proceeding distally are strongly suggestive of the diagnosis.

Typically patients initially present with dysphonia, dysarthria, diplopia, and dysphagia. These signs also manifest in CNS (central nervous system) diseases not infrequently affecting the elderly and may lead to misdiagnosis of stroke, malignancy, underlying neurological disease, or CNS infection. The common tremors of aging should not be confused with botulinum. However, it is important to realize elderly patients with underlying tremors may also have been exposed to botulinum toxin. Careful examination, thorough history, and presence of several patients with similar symptoms would alert the clinician to a botulinum attack. As botulinum toxicity progresses, respiratory function becomes impaired; a life-threatening exigency mandating early recognition and intervention. Long-term ventilatory support may be necessary. Antitoxin only scavenges "free" toxin and does not reverse the effects of neurotoxicity. Use caution with antitoxins owing to the risk of severe reactions since most are equine derived.

Yersinia Pestis/Plague

Like inhalation anthrax, the very early symptoms of pneumonic plague may be flu-like, and thus the elderly patient might be misdiagnosed with influenza, bacterial pneumonia, or influenza-like illness. It is important to recognize the rapidly progressive nature of the illness. Plague has been associated with hemoptysis, which can occur within 24 hours and hematemesis. Other infections or diseases can cause blood-tinged sputum, which may be mistaken for the true hemoptysis of plague, including COPD. Those patients, unlike true plague victims, will not have high fevers or a rapidly fulminant clinical course. Again bear in mind, elderly patients may not present with high fevers. However the cascade of rapid deterioration, pulmonary complaints, hemoptysis, progressive altered mental status (which might be misdiagnosed as meningitis) suggests plague especially in the presence of other patients with similar symptoms. Enzyme-linked immunosorbent assay (ELISA) and dipstick (immunochromatographic) tests to detect F1 antigen are highly sensitive and specific. The F1 antigen monoclonal antibody dipstick assay is a rapid and valuable test especially given reliable results may be obtained in 15 minutes. Since 1999, the World Health Organization (WHO) considers the detection of the F1 antigen in appropriate samples, in addition to symptoms and history consistent with *Yersinia pestis* to be a presumptive criterion for diagnosing plague.

Tularemia

While there are several forms of tularemia, the pneumonic form is most likely to be utilized as a biological weapon. Constitutional symptoms include severe systemic illness with rapid onset, relative bradycardia, substernal chest pain, and cough. Relative bradycardia is an important clue. This important, uncommon clinical finding should alert the clinician to significant illness resulting from bioweapon, sepsis or dangerous, emerging pathogens. The elderly may not manifest fever early in the illness owing to general physiologic changes of aging. Additionally, medications used in the treatment of comorbid conditions may blunt the heart rate response falsely appearing as relative bradycardia. Nevertheless, a high (>101°F) or rapidly rising fever is usually worrisome in the elderly. Respiratory symptoms consistent with pneumonia are possible. Pharyngitis may also be present. Some of these symptoms are associated with patients having underlying coronary artery or pulmonary disease. However sudden fever, constitutional symptoms especially rapid in onset may suggest other than coronary artery disease (CAD) especially if other similarly appearing patients are observed.

Viral Hemorrhagic Fevers

VHFs refer to a wide variety of worldwide RNA (ribonucleic acid) viruses, of which Ebola virus is one of the most feared and widely recognized as a deadly pathogen (hence likely to cause psychological morbidity). The former Soviet Union (FSU) worked extensively with Ebola and other VHF. Several VHFs are associated with high-case fatality rates with few therapeutic options unlike the bacterial bioweapons. The VHFs are a diverse group of viruses. As such each may have specific clues not common to other members of the category, and beyond this introduction. Nevertheless, VHFs as a group cause a variety of bleeding dyscrasias ranging from petechia, which may evolve to profound ecchymosis, epistaxis, hematuria, or severe hemorrhage leading to cardiovascular collapse. Patients undergoing anticoagulant treatment—especially chronic warfarin use, not uncommon among the elderly—may exhibit bleeding diathesis not dissimilar to those caused by VHF. Using a sphygmomanometer, inflating the cuff to over 200 mm Hg may cause circumferential petechia if the patient is infected with a VHF; however, this finding may occur among elderly patients taking antiplatelet or anticoagulant therapy. However, this latter group may demonstrate petechia distal to the cuff and consistent with other ecchymoses located on multiple places on the patient. Owing to capillary bed involvement and bleeding, resulting in VHF victims may be hypotensive; again this may not be uncommon among elderly patients with CAD or are dehydrated. Pulse temperature dissociation or relative bradycardia is possible. High fevers usually accompany the VHF, but may be blunted in the elderly, which may confound this important clue. VHF risk factors should be sought. These include recent travel to regions with endemic illness (Africa, Asia, Peru). The constellation of multiorgan symptoms—bleeding, fever, hypotension, thrombocytopenia, headache, GI complaints in the appropriate context—should alert the clinician of a possible emerging infectious disease or bioweapon illness. The context of illness is critical to early diagnosis, and while time consuming and possibly challenging in the emergency department setting, nevertheless, an index of suspicion for highly pathologic infections is essential if such illnesses are going to be quickly identified and contained.

EXPLOSIVES AND OTHER MASS CASUALTY EVENTS

Explosives and other mass casualty events may create significantly noisy disturbances. The blast injury associated with explosives may cause hearing impairments limiting communications and further confounding diagnosis. However it should be remembered that the elderly may have preexisting hearing impairment; hearing assistive devices may be lost in the confusion, also potentially confounding the clinical evaluation. The elderly may have preexisting pulmonary illness; the astute clinician should nevertheless consider the potential for lung injury associated with the blast.

NERVE AGENTS (ORGANOPHOSPHATES)

Nerve agents may cause ocular changes such as early mydriasis followed by sustained miosis. The elderly may have underlying eye disease or take medications that alter the pupillary response typical of organophosphate toxicity.

Fasciculations and other manifestations of nerve agents may also be mimicked by neuromuscular illnesses or medications. Though more common among children, when occurring at all, nightmares and sleep disturbances, the latter not being uncommon among the elderly, are associated with NA, even after appropriately treated. Gastrointestinal symptoms are also associated with NA exposures; again these must be distinguished from normal patient history. Respiratory and cardiovascular symptoms should be readily distinguished from preexisting changes related to aging. Most telling is the intensity, frequency, and severity of symptoms; NA can cause severe diarrhea as well as lacrimation, salivation, bronchorrhea. NA patients are "wet"!

While the toxidrome associated with nerve agent, including a likely identifiable exposure, should become obvious as increased numbers of victims appear; nevertheless, the challenge arises in the proper identification, decontamination, and treatment of the index case. It is important to recognize that certain insecticides are chemically similar to nerve agents and when used improperly can cause the expected toxidrome associated with organophosphates. Context will be critical to determine an accidental exposure from a planned event. Regardless of the exposure, decontamination and precautions to protect the health-care facility are essential in the management of the patient.

The usual treatment for OP toxicity includes atropine and pralidoxime, usually found in the Mark I Nerve Agent Antidote Kits (NAAK). Of concern, the syringe size and force associated with the nerve agent autoinjectors found in the Mark I NAAK—designed as intramuscular injections for strong war-fighters—may ostensibly become interosseous by virtue of the loss of muscle mass of older individuals.

RADIATION

The symptoms of radiation toxicity in the early stages such as weakness, gastrointestinal complaints can appear similar to constitutional ailments of aging. Acute radiation syndrome (ARS) is a well-defined pattern of illness. The progression of symptoms and involvement of systems characterized as having rapidly reproducing cells—hematologic, gastrointestinal, as well as dermal systems and hair—should alert the clinician of potential exposure. The reader is referred to the section on radiation. Clinicians should be alert to the fact that the hematological changes associated with radiation toxicity may also initially appear similar to cytopenias of aging or chronic illness.

CONCLUSION

The elderly community is not a homogeneous population. On the contrary, it is comprised of the frailest of frail on one extreme and robust, healthy, and active persons who regularly engage in travel, exploration, and a variety of activities at the other extreme. The latter individuals may become exposed overseas or during international travel to bioweapons or uncommon illness, and in spite of overt good health, are still undergoing age-related biopsychosocial changes that may manifest when illness is contracted. The frail may become exposed from intentional release or from visitation with infected individuals. This is often the case during influenza season. The number of Americans over 65 continues to increase dramatically. And while infectious disease is generally not one of the leading causes of death among the young, it accounts for 40% of deaths among the elderly.

A critical consideration to diagnosing exposure to biological agents in the elderly is to understand the clinical pattern of these weapons and illnesses in the nonelderly and how the changes associated with aging can affect the hallmark clues, often making them more subtle or nonexistent. In addition, while potentially dangerous illnesses may be mandatory reportable diseases this system of surveillance relies upon active participation from providers to public health. Therefore, by the time a pattern of apparently similar illnesses is recognized, the outbreak may be well underway before emergency physicians and other clinicians are alerted. Adding to the challenge of early identification among elderly patients, it is likely that victims may present symptoms the patients have had in the past, and thus the decision "had it before, must be the same today" has led to a pattern of medical decision-making with the elderly that can compromise accurate diagnosis from infectious diseases, including biological warfare agents. Compounding this some bioweapon illness may present to the uninitiated with seemingly nonspecific complaints not unlike normal complaints common to older persons, which include generalized aches, pulmonary or "flu-like" upper respiratory symptoms. Therefore, a more effective method reverts to time-honored basics—a good physical examination focusing on combinations of symptoms (biodromes) in addition to obtaining a thorough history from patient, caregiver and/or friends/family. Having an index of suspicion and focusing beyond merely one organ system (biodrome) will facilitate identifying sentinel cases, since many bioweapons involve multiple organs. For example, while the early anthrax victims in 2001 presented with severe pulmonary complaints, most had gastrointestinal symptoms early in the illness. The sentinel case was admitted with significant CNS involvement and had severe gastrointestinal complaints prior to pulmonary symptoms—all uncommon in influenza.

It is important to recognize elders may be dependent upon service animals or animal companions—while important to their activities of daily living, provisions in preparedness planning do not always ascribe the same importance, and thus resources for these animals remains limited. Stories of elders refusing to evacuate their homes without their animal companions underscore the importance

TABLE 15-3

SGEC ETHNOGERIATRIC TIPS FOR BTEPEE (BIOTERRORISM AND EMERGENCY PREPAREDNESS FOR ETHNIC ELDERS)

Evaluate risk to ethnic elder

Translate technical information to simple, indigenous terms

Help the senior communicate her/his special needs

Negotiate/navigate pathways to trust-relationship

Intervene with culturally appropriate plans

Collaborate with family, community, and ethnic media

Explain how to access local/neighborhood resources

Label survival kits with English and other languages

Differentiate between stress-induced anxiety and language difficulties

Educate senior, family, and community leaders

Respect traditional healing practices and rituals

Support with nonverbal behaviors

of addressing this issue as part of overall preparedness planning. Access to veterinary medicine expertise and the ability to provide for the needs of service animals during the care of the elderly patient is important.

In the event of an intentional release of a biological weapon or other terrorist action, treating large numbers of victims may strain an already overburdened health-care facility (Table 15-3). Recognizing the impact of CBRNE agents upon special populations before an event may enhance the likelihood of successfully identifying the index case as well as improved medical care.

Suggested Reading

Al-Sous MW, Bohlega S, Al-Kawi MZ, et al. Neurobrucellosis: clinical and neuroimaging correlation. *AJNR Am J Neuroradiol.* March 2004;25(3):395–401.

Borio L, Inglesby T, Peters CJ, et al. Hemorrhagic fever viruses as biological weapons: medical and public health management. *JAMA.* May 8, 2002:287(18):2391–2405.

CDC Plague Homepage. *http://www.cdc.gov/ncidod/dvbid/plague/index.htm*

Dennis D, Chu M. A major new test for plague. *Lancet.* 2003;353: 361:191–192.

Johnson A, Howe JL, McBride MR, et al. Bioterrorism and Emergency Preparedness in Aging (BTEPA): HRSA-Funded GEC Collaboration for Curricula and Training. *Gerontology & Geriatrics Ed.* 2006;26(4):63–86.

Leikin JB, McFee RB, Walter F, et al. A primer for nuclear terrorism. *Dis Mon.* August 2003;49(8):485–516.

Leikin JB, McFee RB, Walter FG, et al. *Chemical and nuclear agents of terrorism.* In: Stephen Hessl, ed. Clinics in Occupational & Environmental Medicine, Law Enforcement. August 2003;3(3).

Lillibridge S. New developments in health and medical preparedness related to the threat of terrorism. *Prehosp Emerg Care.* January–March 2003;7(1):56–58.

McFee RB. Bioterrorism and Weapons of Mass Destruction 2004: Physicians as first responders. Special Supplement Edition of *The DO* 2004; March: 9–23.

McFee RB. Preparing for an era of weapons of mass destruction (WMD) – are we there yet? Why we should be concerned. *Vet Hum Toxicol.* 2002;44 (4):193–199.

McFee RB, Leikin JB, Kiernan K. Preparing for an era of weapons of mass destruction (WMD)—are we there yet? Why we should be concerned. Part II. *Vet Hum Toxicol.* 2004;46:347–351.

McGough M, Frank LL, Tipton S, et al. Communicating the risks of bioterrorism and other emergencies in a diverse society: a case study of special populations in North Dakota. *Biosecur Bioterror.* 2005;3(3):235–245.

Miller AK, Daniels WJ. Biologic agents of terrorism *in* clinics in occupational and environmental medicine. *Law Enforcement Worker Health.* August 2003;3:457–476.

Norkina OV, Kulichenko AN, Gintsburg Al, et al. Development of a diagnostic test for Yersinia pestis by the polymerase chain reaction. *J Appl Bacteriol.* 1994;76(3):240–245.

Plague. In: WHO report on global surveillance of epidemic prone infectious disease, 2000. *http://www.wo.int/emc-documents/ surveillances/docs/whocdcsrisr2001.html/plague/plague.html #history*

Stephenson J. Plague rapid diagnostic test. *JAMA.* 2003;289(6): 691.

Tumosa N (ed.). Position Statement of the NAGEC Bioterrorism Preparedness Committee. *Aging Successfully,* 2003; XIII (1):21.

Tumosa N (ed.). Position Statement of the NAGEC Bioterrorism Preparedness Committee. *Aging Successfully,* 2004; XIV(3): 1–24.

World Health Organization (WHO). 1999 Plague Manual: epidemiology distribution, surveillance and control (WHO/CDS/ CSR/EDC/99.2), 9–4.

16

SPECIAL POPULATIONS: WOMEN WHO ARE PREGNANT

Kirk L. Cumpston

STAT FACTS

SPECIAL POPULATIONS: WOMEN WHO ARE PREGNANT

- Use the same decontamination, diagnostics, and treatment for the pregnant woman as is indicated for the nonpregnant patient.
- Use the same dosing regimen of pharmaceuticals in the pregnant patient as is routinely done in the nonpregnant patient.
- Intra-amniotic methylene blue, penicillamine, ribavirin, and amyl nitrite should be avoided in the pregnant patient.
- Common pharmaceuticals, which are usually contraindicated in pregnancy like tetracyclines and fluoroquinolones are routinely used in the pregnant woman to treat and prophylax against biological weapon exposure.
- Smallpox vaccine is indicated in the pregnant woman exposed to smallpox despite known complications to the mother and fetus.
- The physiological changes in pregnancy can make the pregnant more susceptible or more resistant to weapons of mass destruction.
- The hypotensive pregnant woman should be first resuscitated with intravenous fluids and positioned in the left lateral decubitus position to decrease pressure on the inferior vena cava.

INTRODUCTION

In the unfortunate circumstance of a mass casualty chemical/biological/radiological/explosive event, certain groups in our population are viewed as being especially vulnerable. Included in this category are children, elderly, the immuno-compromised, the disabled, and the pregnant woman. The inherent physiological change in the pregnant woman, and the potential effects on two patients, complicates diagnostic testing and therapeutic endeavors. The simplistic approach to this interlaced problem is the common interjection of "Treat the mother and you treat the baby!" In a general sense, this underlying principle still holds true, but nevertheless there exists salient wisdom on how to optimize care of both the mother and her fetus. This chapter will focus on the effects of the aforementioned mass casualty events on the gestational woman and her unborn fetus, and will not undertake a discussion about the general clinical presentations, laboratory studies, and pathophysiology because this will be conveyed in the specific chapters for each agent.

PERSONAL PROTECTIVE EQUIPMENT/DECONTAMINATION

Depending on which trimester of gestation the woman is in, her body habitus may inhibit proper fitting of personal protective equipment. If the pregnant woman can physically bestow a Level A suit, preexisting increased body temperature, decreased functional residual capacity, decreased peripheral vascular resistance, peripheral edema, and nausea may lead to a still greater increase in body temperature, expanded work of breathing, orthostatic syncope, improper application of gloves, and emesis, respectively. There may be many practical restrictions for the pregnant woman successfully using the highest level of protection or even the less cumbersome options.

The same principles of dermal decontamination that are applied to the nonpregnant patient should be applied to the pregnant patient as well, with some notable differences. The pregnant woman has a greater body surface area, which makes her more vulnerable to dermal toxicity and absorption. Aggressive and thorough irrigation with special attention to evacuation of contaminants in body folds is of utmost importance. Water and a mild detergent would not be expected to harm the fetus. Dermal decontamination should always include ocular decontamination with copious amounts of normal saline until physical evidence of the removal of the contaminant and resolution of symptoms.

RESOURCES

The pregnant woman will require considerably more resources for a single person than the nonpregnant patient. Depending on the time of gestation, she may need fetal monitoring; ultrasound; neonatal monitoring and critical care; warmers; facilities for emergent cesarean delivery and vaginal delivery; adult intensive care unit; obstetricians, neonatologists, perinatologists, and genetic councilors. In addition to antidotes, adequate stocking of the standard medications used to treat complications of pregnancy.

SPECIFIC AGENTS

Chemical Agents

Nerve Agents

The nerve agents tabun, sarin, soman, and VX have important unique chemical characteristics but in general have the same mechanism of toxicity by inhibiting acetylcholinesterase. The pregnant patient may be more susceptible to the toxic effects of dermal and respiratory exposure due to an increased body surface area, increased respiratory rate and tidal volume, and reduction in the amount of plasma cholinesterase concentration decreases during pregnancy. Because of the lipophilicity of the nerve agents, it is expected to pass through the placenta and cause death or congenital abnormality. Adverse fetal effects have been reported from gestational exposure to organophosphates and likewise in the offspring of survivors from Iraqi chemical attacks during the Iran/Iraq war. The most common chemicals used were mustard gas, nerve gas, cyanide, damper gas, and mixtures of nauseating and immobilizing agents and some of the victims (13.8%) did not know which gas they were exposed to. They excluded fetal

demise and only looked at gross congenital anomalies. The incidence of congenital malformations was 258/1000 in the gas exposed and 33/1000 in the nonexposed cohort.

Five pregnant women were exposed to sarin gas during the Tokyo subway attack. One elected for a therapeutic abortion and postabortion examination is unknown. Two more women, who were 16 and 36 weeks pregnant, received atropine, pralidoxime, and oxygen and delivered normal term infants. The final two women received atropine only and recovered. In response to questionnaires, no fetal malformations were reported at 1 month and 1 year. More data are known about maternal-fetal effects after exposure to organophosphate insecticides, which can be applied to all the organophosphate nerve agents.

Both atropine and pralidoxime are U.S. Food and Drug Administration (FDA) Pregnancy Class C antidotes. The risk of morbidity or mortality after withholding these critical antidotes far outweighs the risk of administering these without knowing the effect on the fetus. Restoring the mothers to a homeostatic state will benefit the fetus as well. Atropine and pralidoxime are expected to pass through the placenta and could potentially affect the fetus in a positive or negative way.

Blister Agents

The blister agents include mustard gas, lewisite, and phosgene oxime. The pregnant woman may be more susceptible to the toxic effects of dermal and inhalational mustard gas exposure because of a larger body surface area and skin that is stretched thin during late pregnancy, increased peripheral circulation, and increased respiratory rate and tidal volume. As the name implies, the vesicants will cause dermal injury and absorption of the vesicant toxicants with the exception of phosgene oxime. The mustard agents in particular require extra vigilance when implementing dermal decontamination because of the oily nature of these agents. Otherwise the clinical effects and treatment of the pregnant woman should be identical to the nonpregnant patient. Like the mustard gases, lewisite can also be systemically absorbed through skin, gastrointestinal, and respiratory routes and is expected to cross the placenta and affect the fetus. However, lewisite has not been found to cause teratogenesis. The fact that immediate symptoms are seen after lewisite exposure may protect the pregnant women because it can serve as a deterrent. Comprehensive supportive care and antidotal treatment of the mother is the foundation of the treatment to the fetus after the aforementioned vesicant exposures. Because phosgene oxime is generally not systemically absorbed and has mucous membrane irritating effects, supportive treatment of the irritation to the maternal respiratory tract to ensure adequate ventilation and oxygenation will effectively care for the fetus.

The mechanism of toxicity of the mustard agents involves alkylation of DNA, RNA, and proteins and they are known mutagenic and carcinogenic toxicants in humans. One would intuitively expect teratogenic effects in the fetus during organogenesis or fetal demise at anytime during the pregnancy after exposure to these highly lipophilic agents, which can penetrate the placenta. The limited number of studies about the toxicity of mustard gases and lewisite include experimental animal studies and the effects on workers in factories that produced the vesicant agents. These found no negative effects, even on the offspring of pregnant workers. One must consider that these are chronic exposures. The extent of presenting and delayed effects on the fetus after a large chemical release is unknown.

The antidote Dimercaprol or British Anti-Lewisite (BAL) can be used to treat a lewisite exposure (Table 16-1). The FDA Pregnancy Category is C. This antidote has been used to chelate pregnant women with lead poisoning, without any ill effects on the fetus related to Dimercaprol.

Chemical Asphyxiants (Cyanide)

Cyanide causes cellular asphyxia by inhibition of cytochrome oxidase in the cells of every organ system, including the placenta and fetus. The primary routes of exposure are inhalational or possibly orally from contamination of the water supply. The toxicity results in a severe lactic acidosis, hypotension, dysrhythmias, and seizures. If the exposure is to just cyanide gas, dry dermal decontamination can be performed. If the exposure is aqueous in nature, standard dry and wet decontamination should be executed. When the skin is intact, there is no concern about systemic absorption from only a dermal exposure. Numerous antidotes are available for treatment of cyanide toxicity around the world. In the United States, amyl nitrite, sodium nitrite, and sodium thiosulfate are the only approved antidotes. Hydroxycobalamin is attainable in Europe and may become approved for use in the United States.

Amyl nitrite is used in the prehospital setting and considered FDA Pregnancy Category X by one reference. The FDA Pregnancy Category for sodium nitrite is often unlabeled, and is Category C for sodium thiosulfate. Prophylactic sodium thiosulfate along with a sodium nitroprusside infusion in gravid ewes has been shown to prevent cyanide toxicity. The sodium thiosulfate did not cross the placenta but was hypothesized to bind the cyanide as it crossed the placenta from the fetus to the maternal circulation down the concentration gradient. Hydroxycobalamin is an FDA Pregnancy Category C rated drug. The benefit of reversing severe life-threatening cyanide toxicity in the pregnant woman outweighs the known risks. In a mass casualty setting resulting from cyanide, the antidote reserves will quickly be utilized and many of the patients will have to be managed with ventilatory, metabolic, and hemodynamic support.

TABLE 16-1

FDA PREGNANCY CATEGORY OF ANTIDOTES AND ANTIBIOTICS

Pharmaceutical	FDA Pregnancy Class
Aluminum hydroxide	C
Amoxicillin	B
Amyl nitrite	C*, X[†], unknown[‡]
Anthrax vaccine	C
Atropine	C
Botulinum antitoxin	Unknown
Chloramphenicol	C
Ciprofloxacin	C
Diethylene triamine penta-acetic (DMPA)	
Zn-DMPA	C
Ca-DMPA	D
Dimercaprol	C
Doxycycline	D
Edetate calcium disodium, Ca	B
Erythromycin	B
Filgrastim (Colony stimulating factor)	C
Gentamicin sulfate	D
Hydroxycobalamin	Unknown
Iodide, potassium	D
Levofloxacin	C
Lorazepam	D
Magnesium sulfate	B
Methylene blue, intra-amnionic	X
Ofloxacin	C
Penicillin G	B
Penicillamine	D
Phosphate	C
Polyethylene glycol	C
Pralidoxime chloride	C
Prussian blue	Unknown
Pyridostigmine bromide	C
Ribavirin	X
Rifampin	C
Sargramostim (GM-CSF)	C
Smallpox vaccine	C
Sodium bicarbonate	C
Sodium nitrite	Unknown
Sodium phosphate (enema)	Unknown
Sodium thiosulfate	C
Streptomycin sulfate	D
Succimer (DMSA)	C
Sulfamethoxazole/Trimethoprim	C
Tetracycline	D

*Sifton DW. PDR Guide to Biological and Chemical Warfare Response. Montvale, NJ: Thomson/Physicians' Desk Reference, 2002.
[†] Leikin JB, Paloucek FP: Leikin & Paloucek's Poisoning Toxicology Handbook. 3rd ed. Hudson, OH: Lexi-Comp, 2002.
[‡] Olson KR. Poisoning & Drug Overdose. 4th ed. New York: McGraw-Hill, 2004.

Flammable Industrial Gases/Liquids

The primary concern for the pregnant women after exposure to flammable gases or liquids is trauma secondary to an explosion and burn management. If ignition has not occurred, standard practice of dermal decontamination should be completed. Whenever ingestion of a hydrocarbon has occurred, the potential for aspiration must be considered.

Chloroform is a hydrocarbon that may be embryotoxic. It can be absorbed through inhalation, oral, and dermal exposure and diffuses across the placenta. No increased frequency of congenital malformations has been noted after maternal exposure during the first trimester, but there is strong evidence that chloroform is mutagenic and carcinogenic.

The fetal effects of maternal trihalomethane exposure in drinking water have undergone extensive epidemiological study. There appears to be an increased chance of intrauterine growth retardation, which is influenced by a genetic predisposition. However in one study, the normal range of trihalomethane concentrations in drinking water were not associated with an increased pregnancy loss. A different study found small excess risk in stillbirth and intrauterine growth retardation when exposed in the second and third trimesters associated with high trihalomethane water concentrations. It is reasonable to assume that if a population of pregnant women were exposed to high levels of trihalomethane in the water used as a chemical weapon, there could be increased intrauterine growth retardation and possibly stillbirth. If the pregnant woman suffered an inhalational exposure, it is difficult to predict what fetal effects would occur imminently or subsequently. If any acute effects occur supportive care of the mother and fetus is the only option without an antidote.

Corrosive Industrial Agent

The same principles used in diagnosing and treating the corrosive exposure in the nonpregnant patient should be applied to the pregnant patient. If the exposure is dermal, proper decontamination is indicated along with local burn care. If the exposure is inhalational or oral, monitoring (endoscopy) and treating the complications is still indicated in the pregnant patient. There are the usual concerns for systemic absorption of fluoride-containing acids and chelation of calcium and magnesium. Calcium supplementation occurs during pregnancy and no adverse effects have been reported. There are two cases of calcium used to treat poisoning in overdose during pregnancy and no adverse fetal effect was noted.

Heavy Metals

Arsenic: After acute arsenic exposure, the fate of the fetus will depend on the clinical manifestations in the mother and her subsequent treatment. One epidemiological study in Texas found no increased incidence of neural tube defects in the offspring of women chronically exposed to environmental arsenic and mercury. In the Bangladesh population, the incidence of stillbirth was increased six times in mothers who were exposed to high levels of arsenic. It is justifiable to expect a similar or greater risk if pregnant women were exposed to high levels of arsenic in the drinking water after a chemical attack. Respiratory exposure to arsenical gases can present with hemolysis of both maternal and fetal red blood cells and methemoglobinemia. Intra-amniotic injection of methylene blue is considered teratogenic because of cases of jejunal atresia and fetal death. The implication of these findings to intravenous methylene blue remains unknown. Decontamination and antidotal treatment with dimercaprol or succimer should not be withheld in the pregnant woman. Their FDA Pregnancy Categories are both C. Penicillamine should not be used to treat arsenic, lead, or mercury poisoning in pregnancy because it is considered a teratogen and there are more effective alternative chelators (Table 16-1).

Lead: Lead poisoning in pregnancy is generally related to chronic exposures. This could occur after a chemical or explosive attack, which also contained lead contaminants. The pregnant woman may have increased lead toxicity because bone resorption during pregnancy leads to greater lead mobilization. Lead can cross the placenta and effects are seen in the fetus and mother such as maternal hypertension, spontaneous abortion, and developmental impairment. If lead is seen on an abdominal radiography, gastric decontamination can be performed with whole-bowel irrigation. Dimercaprol and succimer are used to chelate the lead in the red blood cells and attempt to lower the body burden. Edetate calcium disodium is another chelating agent, which can be used to treat high blood lead levels and lead encephalopathy. Its FDA Pregnancy Category is B (Table 16-1). As stated previously, penicillamine should be avoided in the pregnant patient.

Mercury: Chronic elemental mercury exposure could lead to toxic effects from mercury in the mother and the fetus. Volatilized elemental mercury results in pulmonary toxicity and delayed neurological effects. Treatment is a combination of chelation and supportive care. Inorganic mercury exposure can lead to gastrointestinal corrosive effects, renal failure, and neurological effects. Treatment is supportive and possibly chelation therapy. Because of tragic environmental methylmercury exposures in Japan and Iraq, and epidemiological studies of human populations with large fish consumption, it is clear that methylmercury can be toxic to the mother and fetus. The maternal effects are discussed elsewhere. The list of toxic fetal effects includes chorea, ataxia, tremors, seizures, cerebral palsy, microcephaly, psychomotor retardation, dysarthria, deafness, and death. If the ground and water became contaminated with methylmercury after a chemical attack, these effects would likely be seen. Dermal decontamination should not differ from standard methods.

Gastric decontamination is ineffective due to rapid absorption. Chelation for organic mercury exposure is controversial and potentially harmful, depending on the agent used. If chelation is desired, the safest choice is succimer with the same regimen as the treatment of lead poisoning. Chelation of organic mercury is often futile because damage to the central nervous system has already occurred.

Pulmonary Agents: The important similarities and differences of the clinical manifestations and treatments of chlorine and phosgene gas toxicity are discussed in another chapter. The pregnant woman's treatment should be identical. The fetal effects will be primarily related to oxygenation and ventilation of the gravid mother. If these life-threatening consequences to the mother are addressed appropriately the fetus should do well. External decontamination should follow the general principles applied to these exposures. There are no effective antidotes. Symptomatic treatment and 24-hour observation for delayed pulmonary edema after a phosgene exposure should be adequate.

Vinyl chloride gas exposure can cause frostbite injury to the skin and a narcotic-like sedation similar to other hydrocarbons. Dermal decontamination is dually important because of its caustic nature and potential absorption. Supplemental oxygen and symptomatic treatment are the extent of treatment. Vinyl chloride is a known human carcinogen, which causes angiosarcoma of the liver. There are reports of central nervous system defects, genital defects, gastrointestinal defects, and clubfoot in children exposed to vinyl chloride during pregnancy.

Pesticides: There are many different groups of pesticides, each with its unique toxicity and possible toxicity and teratogenicity to the fetus, nevertheless organophosphate pesticides will only be discussed here because it is the most likely agent to be used, and most severe acute threat. Organophosphate poisoning results in muscarinic and nicotinic clinical manifestations identical to the nerve agents discussed above. Decontamination and antidotal treatment should replicate what has already been discussed. The fetus also has been found to have a diminished level of red blood cell cholinesterase, which may make it more susceptible if this truly correlates with the level of neuronal cholinesterase. Organophosphate poisoning in pregnancy has been associated with fetal demise, vertebral deformities, limb defects, polydactyly, intestinal hernia, cleft palate, and hydroureter. There is one case in which an abortion was performed in the third trimester of pregnancy, and two cases in which the fetus was delivered successfully after acute organophosphate poisoning in the second and third trimesters, and the two patients suffered from intermediate syndrome.

Riot Control Agents: The riot control agents are o-chlorobenzlidine malononitrile (CS), 1-chloroacetophenone (CN, tear gas, or mace) and dibenzoxazepine (CR), and oleoresin capsicum (OC, pepper spray). All of these agents cause irritation to the mucous membranes of the eyes, nose, and respiratory tract of the pregnant woman. In a closed space, serious pulmonary toxicity can result. These gases will only affect the fetus secondarily if severe cardiopulmonary effects occur in the mother, which is rare. Decontamination starts with removing the patient from the source, irrigation of the eyes and skin, and symptomatic treatment of respiratory symptoms. Primary attention to care of the mother will sufficiently protect the fetus.

Incapacitating Agents: The one agent usually discussed in this category is 3-quinuclidinyl benzilate (BZ). This agent causes antimuscarinic (anticholinergic) toxicity. The primary goal of this agent in warfare is to cause significant delirium in the enemy to incapacitate them. The other effects and decontamination are discussed in the appropriate chapter. Much like many of the chemical agents, treating the mother's symptoms should ensure treatment of the fetus. An antidote called physostigmine exists. Physostigmine inhibits acetylcholinesterase, therefore antagonizing the effect of the antimuscarinic blockade by increasing the amount of acetylcholine. This will reverse the toxic effects of the BZ. One must consider possible negative effects of physostigmine on the pregnant patient. Otherwise there are the usual concerns about bradycardia and bronchospasm as side effects. Most often physostigmine is not used and the patient recovers with benzodiazepines and expectant management.

Biological Agents

CDC Category A Agents

Anthrax: There are only scattered case reports about the effects of a *Bacillus anthracis* infection on the pregnant woman. The details of this infectious disease and clinical manifestations in the adult are discussed elsewhere. There are two cases of cutaneous anthrax from Turkey in which both women were infected in the third trimester. Both women delivered prematurely at 33 and 34 weeks' gestation and the neonates had no signs of infection. Two more cases involved women who died from gastrointestinal anthrax. There are no cases of perinatal transmission or inhalational anthrax in the pregnant woman in the literature. In an actively infected pregnant woman, early administration of antibiotics is most likely the most important predictor of maternal-fetal outcome. The first line treatment for cutaneous, inhalational, and gastrointestinal anthrax, recommended by the American College of Obstetrics and Gynecology and Centers for Disease Control (CDC), is intravenous ciprofloxacin if susceptible or doxycycline. Despite rare reports of arthropathy in children after receiving fluoroquinolones, it is felt that fetal malformations are unlikely and the risk of morbidity and mortality from weapons-grade anthrax is far greater.

Prophylaxis should only be done if a known inhalational exposure has occurred. Ciprofloxacin still is the first-line drug. Doxycycline can be used but maternal liver function tests must be monitored, because of hepatotoxicity. Amoxicillin can be used as prophylaxis only after 14–21 days of a fluoroquinolone or doxycycline, or when no other options are available, or hypersensitivities or contraindications to other drugs exist. The duration of therapy for all of the choices is 60 days. The same drug regimen is recommended in the breast-feeding mother. Anthrax vaccine adsorbed (AVA) is safe and effective in animal studies, providing protection against activation of inhaled anthrax spores. If it is available, this inactivated vaccine is recommended in the pregnant woman.

Plague: Plague, or *Yersinia pestis*, is a bacterium that is spread from infected fleas to humans in nature. When used as a weapon, the most likely route of infection would be inhalational. The details of this infectious disease and clinical manifestations in the adult are discussed elsewhere. Respiratory and contact isolation need to be maintained until after 48 hours of antibiotics. It is believed that fetal death is related to maternal effects and transferrence from the mother to the fetus. Prior to antibiotics maternal and fetal mortality was almost certain. In all the cases in the postantibiotic area, all the women were second trimester or farther in gestation, and suffered from bubonic plaque. They all received an aminoglycoside with or without combination with another drug. All of the mothers recovered but not without severe effects, and the neonates were largely unaffected. Because it is believed *in utero* transmission occurs or the fetus may become infected from maternal blood, prophylaxis of the neonate is recommended.

Similar to anthrax, the major determent of maternal-fetal outcome is rapid administration of antibiotics. Treatment of active pneumonic plague in the pregnant woman is gentamicin because it is very efficacious. Doxycycline and fluoroquinolones can be substituted. Chloramphenicol is recommended for meningitis. Renal function and auditory function, liver function, and bone marrow suppression have to be monitored when administering gentamicin, doxycycline, and chloramphenicol, respectively. Gentamicin is recommended for treatment of plague in the breast-feeding mother.

Prophylaxis should proceed after a known exposure. Ciprofloxacin is the first choice. Doxycycline and chloramphenicol can also be used. Sulfonamides are not recommended. Doxycycline or fluoroquinolone is recommended as prophylaxis in a breast-feeding mother. A killed bacilli vaccine was discontinued in 1999.

Botulism: Many consider botulinum toxin from the bacterium *Clostridium botulinum* the most potent toxin on earth. The details of this infectious disease and clinical manifestations in the adult are discussed elsewhere. There are a number of cases of botulism during pregnancy. In one case of food botulism, a woman at 23 weeks' gestation remained intubated for 2 months because of progressive paralysis, despite antitoxin. Fetal growth and movements were normal and the neonate was born healthy at term. Another woman at 16 weeks' gestation was admitted for weakness, received antitoxin, and was discharged after 10 days. She also delivered a healthy term infant. There are other cases of food botulism during the second trimester in which the fetus was unaffected. A case of wound botulism in a heroin abuser in the third trimester required several weeks of intensive care treatment before cesarean delivery. Unfortunately, little was reported about the newborn. It is speculated that the 150,000 Dalton botulinum toxin dose does not cross the placenta, but not enough evidence is available to be certain that in general the fetus will not suffer from botulism as well. This is another scenario in which treating the mother's symptoms should be the focus of the treatment.

Treatment consists of respiratory support until antitoxin can be administered. Antitoxin shortens the course of illness and decreases mortality, but is often ineffective if given after 72 hours in the setting of declining neurological status. The CDC distributes trivalent equine IgG and the heptavalent is only available under special protocol. The trivalent antitoxin is Pregnancy Category C. Negative effects on the fetus are unknown. At this time there is no prophylactic therapy for botulism.

Smallpox: The *Variola*, or smallpox virus, was once eradicated from earth. Now it is one of the most feared biological weapons because of its human to human transmission. It is also the most hazardous to the pregnant woman and her fetus directly. Smallpox is associated with a higher case fatality in pregnant women than nonpregnant women and men. More of the pregnant women in a case series had the severe hemorrhagic form of smallpox. Spontaneous abortion, stillbirth, and premature delivery are very common in pregnant women who have smallpox. Hemorrhagic smallpox classically occurs in the unvaccinated or remotely vaccinated women. Within 24 hours of symptoms, the women have developed ecchymoses, epistaxis, bleeding gums, erythematous rash, subconjunctival hemorrhages, vaginal bleeding, and gastrointestinal bleeding. All of these women died within 48 hours. Death results from a septic-like state with thrombocytopenia and disseminated intravascular coagulation.

Congenital smallpox occurred from 9% to 60% of deliveries during past epidemics. Physically, giant dermal pox and diffuse necrotic lesions of the viscera and placenta are seen. A variety of cases report prepartum and postpartum transmission with the range of effects from death to none, depending on vaccination/immunological status of the mother and those living with the infants. There are even cases of newborns with smallpox without clinical manifestations in the mothers. There is one report of cataracts; otherwise no teratogenicity has been reported.

Treatment of active smallpox consists of first droplet and airborne precautions with isolation for 17 days, supportive care, and vaccination. Admitting that there are certainly risks of serious morbidity and mortality resulting from the vaccine to the mother and the fetus, the vaccine is still recommended. The pregnant women can be affected by the same list of vaccine complications in the nonpregnant person. During one outbreak out of 101 pregnant women vaccinated in the first trimester, one developed encephalitis and eight others developed fever, local swelling, and lymphadenopathy. In another analysis of first trimester vaccinations in 257 women, no complications were recorded. Vaccinia virus can penetrate the placenta and was found in 3.2% of products of conception and persisted in the tissue for 30 days. The placentas were found to have hemorrhages, inflammation, and calcifications. A higher incidence of fetal loss in vaccinated versus unvaccinated women was found in another study. The effects of the vaccinia vaccine on the fetus may involve dissemination to all of the organs, placental infection, and giant pox lesions on the skin. Risk factors were primary vaccination or a delay greater than 20 years from the first vaccination in the mother. Nevertheless, a cumulative review of 8599 vaccinees and 11,104 controls in pregnancy found no increased rates of malformations or any case of fetal vaccinia, when vaccinated beyond 12 weeks of pregnancy. Therapeutic abortion is not indicated if a woman discovers she is pregnant 28 days from vaccination or anytime during her pregnancy.

Vaccinia immunoglobulin (VIG) can be administered to prevent maternal and fetal complications in high-risk patients such as first-time vaccinations or those not vaccinated within the last 3 years. One must also consider that VIG is not completely protective and its risk in pregnancy is unknown, but similar drugs have received a FDA Pregnancy Category of B. Cidofovir has been used to treat smallpox and is a FDA Pregnancy Category C drug (Table 16-1).

In general, prophylaxis of the pregnant patient with the live vaccinia virus vaccine is contraindicated. If a true exposure has occurred, the benefits of the vaccination in decreasing the spread of the smallpox outweigh the risks of the vaccine to the mother and the fetus.

Tularemia: *Francisella tularensis* is the bacterium that causes tularemia or "rabbit fever." It is an ulceroglandular infection, which is spread to humans by exposure to dead animals or bites from flies, mosquitoes, or ticks. In a biological attack, the bacteria would be aerosolized. Even less is known about tularemia infection during pregnancy than most of the Category A agents. The effects on the mother would be similar to the effects described on the nonpregnant patient in another chapter. The fetal effects are unknown.

Treatment of active tularemia in the pregnant patient should start with gentamicin or streptomycin. Alternatives are doxycycline and ciprofloxacin. Postexposure prophylaxis is recommended with ciprofloxacin or doxycycline for 14 days. Immunity is permanent and there is no person-to-person transmission. There is an experimental vaccine but its safety in pregnancy has not been established and it is not universally protective from inhalational tularemia. Therefore the vaccine is not recommended for postexposure prophylaxis.

Hemorrhagic Fever: (Arena and filoviruses) There are several families of hemorrhagic viruses, which cause a bleeding diathesis. Ebola, Marburg, Lassa, and yellow fever have been identified as possible biological weapons. This review will focus on a representative from the arenaviruses and the filoviruses. Unfortunately, the devastation of these natural viruses is well known. The Lassa fever virus is an arenavirus, which is transmitted by rodent excreta or person-to-person body fluid contact. The details of this infectious disease and clinical manifestations in the adult are discussed elsewhere. In Sierra Leone, Lassa fever accounts for 25% of the maternal deaths, and the fatality range is 30–75% in the pregnant women as compared to 1–36% in the nonpregnant women. The highest fatality rate is seen in the third trimester. Obviously, demise will be likely if there is generalized maternal hemorrhaging and hypoperfusion of the fetus. Ribavirin is an antiviral drug that is considered a FDA Pregnancy Category X (Table 16-1). Consequently, ribavirin is generally considered contraindicated in pregnancy due to its teratogenic effects. However, in the setting of severe effects from hemorrhagic fever and the possibility of reducing mortality, the Working Group on Civilian Biodefense feels the benefits of treatment outweigh the risks. Another option is delivery of the fetus or uterine evacuation. One study found this increased the mother's survival. Teratogenic effects are unknown. It appears that most likely fetal demise will be the most common fetal effect. There is no prophylaxis for this disease.

Ebola is a filovirus that is spread by aerosol. The details of this infectious disease and clinical manifestations in the adult are discussed elsewhere. Similar to the Lassa fever virus, the clinical severity is greater in the pregnant patient (96% mortality) than compared to the nonpregnant patient (77% mortality). Spontaneous abortion is reported to be 23–66%. In one outbreak, all of the infants born died within 19 days. The route on transmission is undetermined. Treatment consists of blood products and symptomatic care. The possibility of teratogenicity is unclear because the offspring do not survive long. There is no prophylaxis for this disease.

CDC Category B and C Agents

The list of these agents includes brucellosis; *Clostridium perfringens; Salmonella* species; *Escherichia coli O157:H7;*

glanders; melioidosis; psittacosis; Q fever; ricin; *Staphylococcus* enterotoxin B; typhus fever; viral encephalitis; *Vibrio cholerae, Cryptosporidium parvum*; Nipah virus; and hantavirus. All of these infectious diseases are covered in greater depth in other sections of this text. Treatment of the mother is the cornerstone of the treatment of the fetus as well. Risk and benefit to the mother and fetus will have to be determined before deciding on chemotherapeutic treatment. I will discuss two infections that are particularly pertinent to the pregnant patient and ricin.

Infection with *Coxiella burnetii* or Q fever has the potential for adverse fetal outcomes. Treatment is usually doxycycline but this is generally contraindicated in pregnancy. Because these infections are usually not a life threat and are self-limiting, treatment with trimethoprim and sulfamethoxazole is indicated throughout pregnancy, according to CDC recommendations.

The bacterium *Burkholderia pseudomallei*, which causes melioidosis, can be transferred across the placenta. A case was reported in which this occurred in a 32-week neonate delivered by cesarean section because of placenta previa. On her second day of life, she developed sepsis and respiratory distress from what later was discovered to be lung abscess. Cultures of the blood and abscess revealed *Burkholderia pseudomallei*. The neonate recovered after mechanical ventilation and antibiotic therapy. The risk for teratogenicity is unclear (melioidosis).

The toxicity of ricin in adults is discussed in depth in another chapter. Because of its disruption of ribosomes, the potential toxicity to the fetus could have serious consequences. Fetal demise should be expected if the mother is significantly toxic. Aggressive care of the mother is the only way to protect the fetus. There is not enough data at this time to predict consistent teratogenicity.

Radiation

The effects of radiation and management on the adult will be discussed in a different section of the text. Most of the knowledge about the effects of radiation on the fetus comes from the nuclear bomb attacks on Hiroshima and Nagasaki. Actively dividing cells will be affected to a greater extent, so it is logical to assume that the developing fetus will suffer negative consequences. Two Japanese researchers found that the fetal brain was most susceptible 8–25 weeks following ovulation. They proposed that the negative effects would not be seen until later tasks that are dependent on brain functioning. There also is an increased risk of cancer, especially thyroid cancer.

Decontamination guidelines for the nonpregnant patient should be followed for treatment of the pregnant patient. Antidotes for internal decontamination include diethylene triamine penta-acetic acid (DTPA, Ca, Zn), Prussian blue, potassium iodide, EDTA (Ca), penicillamine, sodium bicarbonate, aluminum hydroxide, oral phosphates, and magnesium sulfate.

Prophylactic potassium iodide can be administered after radioactive exposure to block uptake of radioactive iodine, in an effort to prevent thyroid malignancies. The FDA Pregnancy Category is listed in Table 16-1.

Explosives and Incendiaries

Evaluation of burn and traumatic injury in the pregnant woman and her fetus does present a challenge. In a third trimester woman, the body surface area of the trunk will expand. Therefore, predicting the percentage burned and fluid resuscitation will have to be upwardly adjusted. Further discussion of burns and barotrauma is continued in another section of this text. In the third trimester, fetal monitoring is recommended for 2–6 hours following trauma and obstetrical consultation should be performed. In the setting of hypotension, placing the gravid female in the left lateral decubitus position will help displace the gravid uterus off of the inferior vena cava. This will allow an increase in preload to the heart and subsequent increase in cardiac output. Open peritoneal lavage can be done safely in pregnancy but abdominal ultrasound is the least risky and can quickly evaluate the maternal abdomen, fetus, and placenta.

Cardiopulmonary resuscitation can be complicated in the pregnant woman because of difficulty ventilating the pregnant woman due to reduced rib compliance, displacement of the diaphragm because of abdominal contents, and increased oxygen demand. Cardiac compressions should be attempted on the lowest portion of the sternum. The same pharmacological, electrical, and other resuscitation therapies used in the nonpregnant patient should be used in the pregnant woman. In addition Rh-negative women will need anti-D-immune globulin within 72 hours of hemorrhage to protect against isoimmunization. Kleihauer-Betke test can confirm a mixture of maternal and fetal blood. If a laparotomy is performed, cesarean delivery of the fetus is not indicated unless the traditional indications are apparent.

Traumatic complications seen during pregnancy include uterine rupture (0.2–1.5% with one prior transverse scar; 0.0125–0.006% without a scar), abruption placentae (40–50% occurrence), and emergent cesarean delivery secondary to fetal complications. Perimortem cesarean delivery is indicated within 5 minutes of unsuccessful maternal resuscitation.

LABORATORY STUDIES

The standard laboratory studies to evaluate adults after a chemical/biological/radiological exposure are recommended. In addition, serial serum β-human chorionic gonadotrophin concentrations will be needed to monitor fetal progress, and blood type and Rh factor will have to be determined.

REFERRALS

An obstetrical consult and follow-up should be mandatory for a pregnant woman who has been exposed to a chemical, biological, explosive, or radiological attack.

TOXICOKINETICS

Toxicokinetics are not well described in the nonpregnant patient and even less is known about the pregnant patient. There are known physiological changes of a normal pregnancy that might predict changes in toxicokinetics. The decline in blood pressure may decrease perfusion to organs of metabolism and elimination such as the liver and the kidney. Gastrointestinal motility is decreased, which can allow a greater opportunity to prevent absorption by gastrointestinal decontamination. An increased glomerular filtration rate may improve elimination of toxicants. Hyperinsulinemia may complicate matters by causing hypoglycemia, and a decrease in plasma cholinesterase may make the mother more susceptible to the effects of organophosphate poisoning.

DISPOSITION

The final disposition will depend on the severity of injury, type of exposure, and gestational age of the fetus. Some stable patients can be discharged to follow up later for monitoring and laboratory tests. Many third trimester pregnant women or near-term pregnant women will need to have fetal monitoring as an inpatient, even if clinically stable. The pregnant patient with cardiovascular instability or severe pulmonary effects may need intensive care monitoring.

FORENSIC ISSUES

Forensic testing must be expanded in the pregnant patient to include analysis of fetal tissue, umbilical cord blood, placental tissue, and the standard analysis of the nonpregnant patient's body fluids.

SUGGESTED READING

Bailey B. Are there teratogenic risks associated with antidotes used in the acute management of poisoned pregnant women? *Birth Defects Res (Part A).* 2003;67:133–140.

Bailey B. Organophosphate poisoning in pregnancy. *Ann Emerg Med.* 1997;29(2):299.

Brender JD, Suarez L, Felkner M, et al. Maternal exposure to arsenic, cadmium, lead, mercury and neural tube defects in offspring. *Environ Res.* 2006;101:132–139.

Cumpston KL, Erickson TB. Maternal-fetal toxicology. In: Erickson TB, Ahrens WR, Aks SE, Baum CR, Ling LJ (eds): *Pediatric Toxicology.* New York: McGraw-Hill, 2005; p. 15.

Graeme KA, Curry SC, Bikin DS, et al. The lack of transplacental movement of the cyanide antidote thiosulfate in gravid ewes. *Anesth Analg.* 1999;89(6):1448–1452.

http://www.cdc.gov/index.htm

Infante-Rivard C. Drinking water contaminants, gene polymorphisms, and fetal growth. *Environ Health Perspect.* 2004;112(11):1213–1216.

James DC. Terrorism and the pregnant woman. *J Perinat Neonat Nurs.* 2005;19(3):226–237.

Jamieson DJ, Jernigan DB, Ellis JE, et al. Emerging infections and pregnancy: West Nile virus, monkeypox, severe acute respiratory syndrome, and bioterrorism. *Clin Perinatol.* 2005;32: 765–776.

Karalliedde L, Wheeler H, Maclehose R, et al. Review article: possible immediate and long-term health effects following exposure to chemical warfare agents. *Public Health.* 2000;114: 238–248.

Leikin JB, Paloucek FP. *Leikin & Paloucek's Poisoning Toxicology Handbook.* 3rd ed. Hudson, OH: Lexi-Comp, 2002.

McKay CA, Perez A, Goldstein R. Mercury. In: Erickson TB, Ahrens WR, Aks SE, Baum CR, Ling LJ (eds): *Pediatric Toxicology.* New York: McGraw-Hill, 2005; p. 15.

Pour-Jafari H. Congenital malformations in the progenies of Iranian chemical victims. *Vet Hum Toxicol.* 1994;36(6): 562–563.

Savitz DA, Singer PC, Herring AH, et al. Exposure to drinking water disinfection by-products and pregnancy loss. *Am J Epidemiol.* September 6, 2006:1–9.

Shannon M. Severe lead poisoning in pregnancy. *Ambul Pediatr.* Jan–Feb 2003;3(1):37–39.

Sifton DW. *PDR Guide to Biological and Chemical Warfare Response.* 1st ed. Montvale, NJ: Thomson/Physicians' Desk Reference, 2002.

Toledano MB, Nieuwenhuijsen MJ, Best N, et al. Relation of trihalomethane concentrations in public water supplies to stillbirth and birth weight in three water regions in England. *Environ Health Perspect.* 2005;113(2):225–232.

U.S. Army Medical Research Institute of Chemical Defense (USAMRICD). *Medical Management of Chemical Casualties Handbook.* 3rd ed, 2000.

von Ehrenstein OS, Guha Mazumder DN, Hira-Smith M, et al. Pregnancy outcomes, infant mortality, and arsenic in drinking water in West Bengal, India. *Am J Epidemiol.* 2006;163(7): 662–669.

Watson AP, Griffin GD. Toxicity of vesicant agents scheduled for destruction by the chemical stockpile disposal program. *Environ Health Perspect.* 1992;98:259–280.

White SR, Henretig FM, Dukes RG. Medical management of vulnerable populations and comorbid conditions of victims of bioterrorism. *Emerg Med Clin N Am.* 2002;20:365–392.

17

WOMEN'S REPRODUCTIVE ISSUES

Susan J. Piazza and Carol des Lauriers

S T A T   F A C T S

WOMEN'S REPRODUCTIVE ISSUES

- There is a linear relationship between radiation exposure and breast cancer that exists for over 10 years post exposure
- Esophageal cancer also occurs in females with increased radiation exposure
- Lewisite is present in breast milk

International history provides the information needed to learn from prior use of chemical and radiological weapons. There have been long-term health effects on women from these weapons. On August 6 and 9, 1945, two atomic bombs were used to destroy Hiroshima and Nagasaki, Japan. On April 26, 1986, the world's most serious nuclear accident occurred at the Chernobyl nuclear power station in the Soviet Union. This nuclear reactor accident resulted in global long-term medical consequences. The Semipalatinsk nuclear test site in the former Soviet Union has exposed inhabitants to fallout from nuclear weapons testing. The people (women and children) who managed to survive continue to suffer from the late health effects of radiation exposure. What is known of their health comes from systemic study and research of these and other tragic historic events.

The Radiation Effects Research Foundation (RERF), jointly funded by the governments of Japan and the United States, has reviewed and studied the late radiation-induced health effects from atomic bomb survivors. The information obtained over the 60 years aids our understanding of how radiation affects human health and in particular the health of women. Studies from the RERF show an increased incidence of ovarian and breast cancers in female atomic bomb survivors. A strongly linear relationship exists between radiation dose and incidence of female breast cancer. The increased risk for these solid tumors occurs more than 10 years after exposure and continues. The time from radiation exposure to expression of malignancy reflects the long induction interval. (In contrast, leukemia, the commonest radiation-induced cancer occurs after 3–5 years post exposure and peaks at 5–10 years.) Young girls and women (age <20) had the greatest risk. In addition to age at exposure, attained age modifies the dose-specific excess relative risk (ERR-1Sv) of female breast cancer. Site-specific cancer risk due to radiation is usually described as the excess relative risk (ERR) per sievert (Sv, unit of radiation dose), the ratio of the excess risk to the natural background risk for the cancer type. With increasing attained age, ERR-1Sv declined, the largest drop occurring around age 35. The RERF studied three breast cancer risk factors: age at first full-term pregnancy, number of deliveries, and cumulative lactation period summed over births in terms of their interactions with radiation dose. An important outcome from the study is that early age at first full-term pregnancy, multiple births, and lengthy cumulative lactation are all protective against radiation-related breast cancer. Radiation exposure also affects the incidence of benign tumors in female atomic bomb survivors. A dose-related prevalence in uterine myoma has been observed during the 28-year period, 1958–1986, and between 1991 and 1993.

Some information regarding the health effects of exposures to fallout from Soviet nuclear weapons testing comes from Semipalatinsk nuclear test site, Kazakhstan. Between 1960 and 1999, inhabitants from exposed areas were compared with inhabitants from nonexposed areas of the Semipalatinsk region. The exposed group's solid cancer

TABLE 17-1

HEALTH EFFECT ON WOMEN FROM CHEMICAL WEAPON EXPOSURE

Item	Chemical Agent	Breast Milk	Female Reproductive Health
1	Lewisite (arsenic)	Arsenic is transferred	*
2	Chloroform	Based on its physical properties, it maybe excreted in breast milk	*
3	Gasoline	Gasoline and other petroleum solvents have been found in human breast milk 3–9 days after delivery. The values were 12–18% of maternal levels	Positive association with menstrual cycle disturbances
4	Lead	Positive presence in human breast milk. Blood levels usually similar in infants and mothers. In cases of lead poisoning, breast milk levels were less	Blood lead concentrations of 3 mcg/dL were associated with decreased height and delayed puberty in African Americans and Mexican Americans
5	Phosgene oxime	†	*
6	Hydrogen cyanide	†	*
7	Cyanogen chloride	†	*
8	Berzone	†	*
9	Trihalomethanes	†	*
10	Nitric acid	†	*
11	Sulfuric acid	†	*
12	Mercury	†	*
13	Phosgene	†	*
14	Chlorine	†	*
15	Vinyl chloride	†	*
16	Vinylidine chloride	†	*

*At the time of this review, no female reproductive studies were found.

† At the time of this review, no studies regarding effect on breast feeding were found.

mortality significantly exceeded that of the comparison group. Regarding specific cancer sites in females, breast cancer and esophageal cancer occurrence trended with increasing exposure dose.

Little information is known about radiation exposure and breast milk. However, cesium has been found in breast milk after radiation exposure.

On March 16, 1988, Saddam Hussein bombarded the town of Halabja, Iraq, with a cocktail of chemical weapons. The victims of the attack included women and children; many continue to suffer from the long-term effects of their exposure. Ten years later on April 22, 1998, Dr Christine Gosden, a professor of medical genetics at the University of Liverpool in the United Kingdom, testified before the Senate Judiciary Subcommittee on Technology, Terrorism, and Government. During her testimony, she presented the type of chemical weapons used: mustard gas, sarin, tabun, and VX but emphasized the lack of systemic research on the long-term and reproductive health effects, which resulted. Breast and ovarian cancers are among the

list of long-term effects but detailed data are lacking. Despite the formation of the Halabja Post Graduate Medical Institute (HMI), a collaborative research project with the doctors and citizens of Halabja, this lack of public information exists today. More knowledge on the subject would improve our medical preparedness and response to chemical weapon exposure. The few available pieces of information regarding chemical weapon exposure as it affects breast feeding and female health are presented in Table 17-1.

Suggested Reading

Bauer S, Gusev BI, Pivina LM, et al. Radiation exposure due to local fallout from Soviet atmospheric nuclear weapons testing in Kazakhstan: solid cancer mortality in the Semipalatinsk historical cohort, 1960–1999. *Radiat Res.* 2005 Oct;164 (4 Pt 1): 409–19.

Yamada M, Wong FL, Fujiwara S, et al. Noncancer disease incidence in atomic bomb survivors, 1958–1998. *Radiat Res.* 2004;161(6):622–32.

Land CE, Tikunaga M, Koyama K, et al. Incidence of female breast cancer among atomic bomb survivors, Hiroshima and Nagasaki, 1950–1990. *Radiat Res.* 2003;160(6):707–17.

RERF: Radiation Effects Research Foundation. Late effects on the survivors: Benign tumors. 2003.

Congressional Hearings Intelligence and Security. Testimony of Dr Christine M. Gosden. April 22, 1998.

Land CE, Hayakawa N, Machado SG, et al. A case-control interview study of breast cancer among Japanese A-bomb survivors. II. Interactions with radiation dose. *Cancer Causes Control.* 1994;5(2):167–76.

Tokunaga M, Land CE, Tokuoka S, et al. Incidence of female breast cancer among atomic bomb survivors, 1950–1985. *Radiat Res.* 1994;138:209–23.

Pierce DA, Shimizu Y, Preston DL, et al. Studies of the mortality of atomic bomb survivors. Report 12, Part I Cancer: 1950–1990.

UCLA Conference. Radiation accidents and nuclear energy: medical consequences and therapy. *Ann Intern Med.* 1988;109:730–44.

Sawada H, Kodama K, Shimizu Y, et al. Adult Health Study Report 6. Results of six examination cycles, 1968–80, Hiroshima and Nagasaki. RERF Technical Report 3–86.

RERF: Tomonaga M. Late Medical Effects of Atomic bombs Still Persisting Over Sixty Years. Atomic Bomb Disease Institute, Nagasaki University graduate School of Biomedical Sciences, Nagasaki, Japan.

Ron E, Preston D, Tokuoka S, et al. *Solid Cancer Incidence among Atomic Bomb Survivors: A Second Follow-Up.* National Institute, Bethesda, MD; Hirosoft International, Eurika, CA and Radiation Effects Research Foundation, Hiroshima and Nagasaki, Japan.

Poisindex Management and Reprotext. Poisindex, editor Klasco, R.K, Thompson Micromedix, Greenwood Village, Colorado, Vol 132, June,2007.

18

HOSPITAL LABORATORY ISSUES

Robert Rosecrans

STAT FACTS

HOSPITAL LABORATORY ISSUES

- Blood lactate levels can serve as a surrogate marker for cyanide exposure.
- The sentinel laboratory must work closely with the infection control officer to determine if further investigative techniques are warranted.
- The local response network (LRN) is a procedure set up by the Centers for Disease Control (CDC) to decentralize testing thus affording a rapid response to a biological threat.

INTRODUCTION

The use of chemicals as a warfare agent dates back almost 2500 years to the Athenian and Spartan wars; however, the most extensive use of chemicals as a warfare agent goes back to World War I with the advent of mustard gas. Since World War I, military researchers have developed more potent chemical agents and isolated biological agents for warfare use. As the general public became aware of the prevalence of chemical and biological agents, concerns mounted over potential exposure to these agents due to an accidental exposure, agent transportation safety, and aging storage facilities. Newly developed is the threat that chemical and biological agents would be acquired and used by terrorist organizations. The American population felt relatively safe being protected from terrorist activity due to the geographical separation from Europe and the Middle East. This sense of security was shaken after the Oklahoma City bombing of 1991 and the horrific events at the World Trade Center in 2001. Compounding these terrorist events was the actions in 1995 by the Aum Shinrikyo cult, which released sarin gas in a

Tokyo subway killing 12 people and causing numerous casualties. Investigation of the cult discovered Aum Shinrikyo had access to biological agents and had made attempts to obtain the Ebola virus. In September 2001, anthrax filled letters were mailed in the United States; 22 people were infected by anthrax and 5 died from the exposure. The anthrax-laden letters in late 2001 created panic in the general public and there were numerous "white powder" sightings. The general public in the United States demanded protection and sought the antibiotic Cipro for prophylactics use. People demanded prescriptions from their physicians for Cipro and the antibiotic was horded in case of an anthrax exposure. The events created an environment of vulnerability and the health-care industry responded with programs to deal with potential threats. The first step in the process is to identify the threats and implement a response program. Chemical and biological agent response must be dealt with in a different manner. Agents used in a terrorist attack would likely be identified first at the local level by the health-care provider. This posed the question of laboratory readiness and the rapid response necessary so that the appropriate antidote or antibiotic could be administered. Many potential chemical and biological threats are agents not normally observed by the clinical laboratory and this presents a challenge. Potential chemicals used for terrorist activities fall into four categories: nerve gases, vesicants or blistering agents, pulmonary agents, and cyanides.

CHEMICAL AGENTS

Nerve Gases

The function or site of action for nerve gases is to inhibit the enzyme acetylcholinesterase (ACHE), the same action as organophosphate pesticides. ACHE inhibition causes increased levels of acetylcholine at the neuromuscular junction, which subsequently results in muscle fatigue and ultimate muscle failure. Nerve gases are categorized as "G" agents or "V" agents. Nerve agents designated with the code "G" (for German) are classified as nonpersistent chemicals, meaning they are readily vaporized, dissipated, and do not maintain their effectiveness. There are three "G-"coded agents: tabun or GA (ethyl-N-dimethylphosphoroamidocyanidate), sarin or GB (isopropylmethyl-phosphonofluoridate), and soman or GD (pinacolylmethyl-phosphonofluoridate). The "V" agents are persistent chemicals, meaning they will remain on clothing and because of their oily nature can be transmitted through direct contact. VX (o-ethyl S-[diisopropylamino]ethyl) methylphosphonothiate) is the prototype for the series of agents but others include VE, VG, and VM. The V series agents differ only slightly from VX. It is essential that the first responders to possible nerve gas exposure don personal protective equipment. This precaution extends to the personnel involved in the collection of blood samples and during the processing of body fluid samples. Once the human clinical sample has been obtained, the clinical laboratory can handle the specimens using the standard precautions. In a potential nerve gas exposure, the clinical laboratory will provide support care testing to the attending physician, that is, arterial blood gases, electrolytes, and complete blood count. Testing that would assist in the diagnosis of nerve gas exposure includes the measurement of serum pseudocholinesterase activity. During an ACHE inhibitor event, serum pseudocholinesterase activity decreases rapidly and is used for determining acute exposure. Cholinesterase activity is confined to the erythrocyte and reduction of RBC (red blood cells) cholinesterase is an indicator of exposure to a nerve gas or organophosphate pesticide. The measurement of pseudocholinesterase is available on a number of clinical chemistry systems. Due to the low testing volume for pseudocholinesterase at most clinical laboratory sites, the test may not be rapidly available to the attending physician. If the pseudocholinesterase is not available, it is essential that the clinical laboratory have an alternate testing site, be it a commercial reference laboratory or another hospital clinical laboratory. When setting up an offsite relationship with another laboratory, it is essential that the test turnaround time meet the clinical needs of the medical staff.

Vesicants or blistering agents cause irritation to the skin, eyes, lungs, and damage other organs after absorption. This group of agents includes sulfur mustard (2,2-dichlorodiethyl sulfide, nitrogen mustard (2,2-dichloro-N-methyldiethylamine, and Lewisite I (dichloro[2-chlorovinyl]arsine). Mustard gas was first synthesized in 1854 and was used by the German army during World War I. More recently, mustard gas was used during the 1980s by the Iraqi government against the Kurdish and Iranian populations. Stockpiles of the mustard gas vesicant likely exist around the world and the

potential for its use by a terrorist group is real. Unfortunately, there is not an effective antidote for mustard gas; therefore, the primary role of the clinical laboratory is to supply supportive care testing to the attending physician.

Lewisite I, another vesicant, was synthesized but not used by the Allied Army during World War I. The antidote for lewisite I is British Anti-Lewisite (BAL or 2,3-dimercaptopropanol). BAL is a chelating agent used against poisons containing heavy metals. As with mustard gas, the role of a routine clinical laboratory is to supply supportive care testing. There are gas chromatography mass spectrometry (GC/MS) methods available to test mustard gas and its degradation products but these methods are not generally available in the routine clinical laboratory. Mustard gas is an alkylating agent and adducts of hemoglobin, albumin, and DNA have been measured to determine human exposure to vesicants. The role of the clinical laboratory during a vesicant exposure is to provide life support testing and if not capable of measuring the nerve gas or adduct refer such testing to an alternate site.

The pulmonary chemical agents, phosgene and chlorine gas, act on the lungs ultimately causing respiratory failure. Phosgene (carbonyl chloride) was first synthesized in 1812 through the combination of carbon monoxide, chlorine, and activated charcoal. Phosgene was used by the German army against the Allied Forces during World War I causing most of the chemical-related battlefield deaths. The mechanism of action for phosgene is not understood but likely results from the production of hydrogen chloride (HCl) in the alveoli, or the production of a highly reactive molecule. Acute phosgene exposure causes a choking sensation with headache and nausea. Long-term exposure to phosgene results in respiratory failure. The mechanism of action for chlorine gas is similar to phosgene reacting with water in the alveoli to produce hydrochloric acid. The hydrochloric acid causes destruction on the alveoli capillary membrane, RBC hemolysis resulting in edema, hypoxia, respiratory failure, and death. The role of the clinical laboratory is to respond by providing rapid blood gas analysis and other supportive care testing.

Cyanides are another class of chemicals that can be used during a bioterrorist attack. Cyanogenic agents act by inhibiting mitochondrial respiratory chain cytochrome oxidase leading to anoxia. Cyanide has a high affinity for iron in its ferric state, and one competitive inhibitor strategy is to give a pool of oxidized iron. Another strategy used during cyanide exposure is to give compounds that will disassociate the cyanide from cytochrome oxidase or compete with for binding sites. Nitrites are given to victims to oxidize hemoglobin to methemoglobin; the methemoglobin will compete for the binding of the cyanogenic agents. Another strategy is giving the victims hydroxocobalamin, which binds cyanide to form cyanocobalamin or vitamin B_{12}.

Blood cyanide concentrations can be measured by either a microdiffusion method or by head space gas chromatography. These methods however are likely beyond the scope of most hospital clinical laboratories. If cyanide poisoning is suspected by the attending physician, blood lactate levels correlate with the severity of cyanide levels in blood. Since real time, cyanide level determinations are unlikely, lactate levels can be used as an indicator of tissue oxygenation and serve as a surrogate marker. A lactate level over 8 mmol/L may be helpful in identifying cyanide exposure (see Chap. 54). A limitation of lactate measurement in the metabolite is elevated in a number of disease states and cannot be used as a screen or biomarker for cyanide exposure. As with the exposure of most hazardous chemical agents, the function and role of the clinical laboratory is to provide supportive care testing.

LOCAL RESPONSE NETWORK

Biological agents are the preferred tool of terrorists because they are relatively easy to obtain and naturally occurring in the environment. Using basic microbiological techniques, the material can be isolated from the environment, grown in culture, and stored with relative ease. Biological agents can be aerosolized and after release it can take days to weeks before having its ultimate effect. The time delay factor makes it unlikely a terrorist would be caught. Some biological agents can be spread among infected individuals and not be isolated to a restricted area. Considering the mobility of the society, this factor could cause an epidemic. As if these threats were not enough, biological agents can be genetically mutated causing the emergence of resistant strains. During the anthrax threat of 2001, the terror that spread through the American society was unprecedented as the general public realized their vulnerability. All these factors make biological agents the tool of choice to send panic throughout a society and a challenge to combat.

The Centers for Disease Control (CDC) realized that if a biological threat became real, a rapid response would be necessary by the laboratory industry to at least warn of the agent. Time delays in specimen processing at the CDC in Atlanta, GA, because of physical distance from the detection site and possible work overload, the agency provided an alternate plan to protect the public. In 2000, the CDC set up a local response network (LRN) of laboratories to decentralized testing to provide for a rapid response to a biological threat. Initially the laboratories were classified as Level A, B, C, or D; however, this has changed and been condensed to three levels. At the bottom of the pyramid is the sentinel laboratory and it is responsible to perform rule out testing. In the middle of the pyramid is the reference laboratory, which performs biological confirmatory testing. At the top of the pyramid are the national laboratories that perform definitive characterization of biological agents. The sentinel laboratory consists primarily of the community-based hospital microbiology laboratories. Sentinel laboratories are the first to observe unusual bacterial strains via gram stains not indigent to the area. Their primary response is to notify a reference laboratory or the middle level LRN of unusual findings. The reference laboratories are state and public health laboratories in the area that are at a BSL-3 level (biosafety laboratory) and can perform confirmatory testing on the suspect bacteria. National laboratories are at a BSL-4 level and perform definitive testing on specimens referred by the reference laboratories.

Terrorist attacks fall into two categories: overt and covert. An overt attack is one that is announced in advance by the terrorists with the intent of causing panic. During an overt attack, the Federal Bureau of Investigation (FBI) would be involved immediately with surveillance, prevention, and protection of the general public. Likely, the local sentinel laboratory would have a limited role in the response to an overt threat but must be prepared to work with the FBI in processing specimens. A covert terrorist attack is not announced in advance and is intended to cause widespread infections and panic. Sentinel laboratories are integral in identifying the biological agent and limiting the infectious spread. Biological agents used by terrorists can be indigenous to the area or not. The sentinel laboratory does not need to identify the biological agent but rather note the suspicious nature of the isolate and bring to the attention of the appropriate personnel. The starting point of notification is the infection control officer for the hospital. The infection control officer will work with the patient's attending physician and make a determination as to the cause of infection. If there are multiple patients infected with the suspicious bacterium, this is a flag for the sentinel laboratory to contact the infection control officer. The sentinel laboratory does not make the decision that a bioterrorist attack has occurred. The infection control officer will notify the public health department and a decision will be made if an attack has occurred. The sentinel laboratory will work with the infection control officer, the public health agencies, and the federal agencies to transport any material to the health department laboratory.

Microbiology laboratories work with human specimens, therefore, they must not accept environmental samples such as food, water, powders, boxes, or animals for processing since this is beyond the scope of their care. Environmental samples should be transported directly to the local LRN reference laboratory. If the laboratory has questions concerning the transport of environmental samples, they should contact the local LRN reference laboratory for guidance.

Sentinel Laboratory "Rule Out" Guidelines

The role of the clinical microbiology laboratory does not change during a possible bioterrorist event. The microbiology laboratory must do what it is trained to do, isolate the bacteria, characterize the colonies, and identify the bacteria. The laboratory must know its limits and if suspicious colonies are noted must be brought to the attention of the infection control officer. Bacterial agents likely to be used during a bioterrorist attack include but not limited to *Bacillus anthracis*, *Brucella* species, *Francisella tularensis*, *Yersinia pestis*, and *Coxiella burnetti*. Other potential biological agents that are not as aggressive include *Burkholderia mallei*, *Salmonella* species, *Shigella dysenteriae*, *Escherichia coli* O157:H7, *Vibrio cholerae*, and *Mycobacterium tuberculosis*. The microbiology laboratory commonly works on and positively identifies agents in the second tier of potential agents. If the microbiology laboratory notices an increased prevalence of the second tier agents, it should be brought to the attention of the infection control officer for further investigation.

BIOLOGICAL AGENTS

Anthrax

Anthrax infections are a rare occurrence, however, after the 2001 letter mailings laced with *B. anthracis,* most microbiology laboratories became familiar with the characteristics of anthrax. Infections with anthrax can cause septicemia, tissue necrosis, multiple organ failure, and death. The endospores of anthrax can be found in soil and are resistant to heat, drying, ultraviolet, and γ-radiation. Exposure to the spores can occur via animal or human contact with the transmission occurring through cuts or abrasions. Contact transmission is an unlikely vehicle for bioterrorism since it is difficult to perform, inefficient, and poses a hazard to the transmitter. A more likely mode of transmission is through the aerosol inhalation of spores as was attempted in 2001. Clinical specimens will demonstrate gram-positive bacilli and the cultures will grow rapidly on sheep blood agar. *B. anthracis* colonies are catalase positive, nonmotile, and nonhemolytic. After consultation with the infectious disease officer of the sentinel laboratory, specimens fitting these criteria are suspect and should be referred to the local LRN reference laboratory.

Brucella Species

Bacteria of the genus *Brucella* primarily cause disease in domestic animals and the mode of transmission to humans has been virtually eliminated by the pasteurization of milk. Vaccines are available for cattle, sheep, and goats and these efforts have limited outbreaks of brucellosis. There are six species of *Brucella: abortus* infects cattle, *melitensis* sheep and goats, *suis* pigs, *ovis* only sheep, *canis* dogs, and *neotomae* the American wood rat. Humans contracting *Brucella species* will have influenza-like symptoms and a

fever lasting 2–4 weeks if untreated. *Brucella species* are intracellular parasites of the reticuloendothelial system and, after being phagocytized by the polymorphonucleocytes, multiply intracellularly causing bacteremia. Clinical specimens submitted to the laboratory include blood or bone marrow samples. After blood culturing, samples are subcultured to sheep blood agar. *Brucella* colonies grow as tiny gram-negative coccobacilli and are biochemically positive for catalase, oxidase, and urease. After consultation with the infectious disease officer of the sentinel laboratory, specimens fitting these criteria are suspect and should be referred to the local LRN reference laboratory.

Francisella tularensis

Tularemia or rabbit fever is a bacterial infection spread primarily through rabbits, however, other domestic animals may serve as a vehicle. Tularemia incidence is higher for adults in the early winter during hunting season and for children during the summer where ticks and deer flies can spread the bacteria. Common routes of transmission include inoculation from ticks or deer flies, handling infected animals, or ingesting undercooked rabbit meat. Patients infected from handling tainted rabbit carcass demonstrate a slow-growing ulcer at the bacterial entry and swollen lymph nodes. If the transmission occurs by inhalation, the patient will exhibit pneumonia-like symptoms. Patients who ingest infected rabbit meat have symptoms of sore throat, abdominal pain, diarrhea, and vomiting. Tularemia is not spread from person to person, so the likely mode of transmission as a bioterrorist agent is via inhalation of an aerosol or by contaminating a water source. The isolation of *F. tularensis* will be from a blood culture and will stain gram negative and appear as coccobacilli. The organism will not grow on gram-negative media and may form small colonies on sheep blood agar. Biochemically the colonies will be weakly positive or negative for catalase and positive for beta lactamase. *F. tularemia* should only be manipulated by a BSL-3 laboratory, and therefore, the institutional infection control officer should be notified immediately. After consultation, the sample should be referred to the local LRN laboratory.

Yersinia pestis

Y. pestis, the bacterium responsible for plague, is naturally occurring and can be isolated, grown in culture, and used as a bioterrorist weapon. There are two types of plague: bubonic and pneumonic. Bubonic plague is transmitted to humans through a bite from an infected flea. Pneumonic plague is transmitted through inhalation of the bacterium from an aerosolized source. The primary symptom of bubonic plague is tender lymph glands and if untreated the bacterium will spread to the lungs causing pneumonic plague. The symptoms of pneumonic plague occur

1–6 days after exposure and include shortness of breath, chest pain, cough, and bloody or watery sputum. Pneumonic plague is the likely candidate for bioterrorism since the bacterial delivery system would be through an aerosol. Symptoms would not occur for days, and the bacterium would be spread rapidly from human to human.

Y. pestis is a gram-negative bacillus with bipolar staining in which the ends of the bacillus stain darker. On sheep blood agar, the colonies are small and nonhemolytic, but after 48–72 hours the colonies develop a "fried egg" appearance. On gram-negative media, the organism grows as a small nonlactose fermenter and biochemically the colonies test as catalase positive, oxidase, indole, and urease negative. The microbiology laboratories noting such findings should contact the institutional infection control officer and after consultation be prepared to transport the specimens to the local LRN reference laboratory.

Coxiella burnetti

C. burnetti is a spore-forming gram-negative intracellular bacterium and the causative agent of Q fever. The disease was first described in 1935 as a febrile illness in Australia and has spread worldwide with the exception of New Zealand and Antarctica. The bacterium is transmitted via aerosols from infected animals; cattle, sheep, and goats are the likely sources. The possibility of aerosol bacterial spread has placed *C. burnetti* on the list of potential bioterrorist agents. Studies indicate a *Coxiella* aerosol may spread as far as 11 miles from the release point. Acute Q fever is treated with tetracyclines, quinolones, rifampicin, telithromycin, and clarithromycin and patients response well to the antibiotics; however, if left untreated Q fever causes endocarditis. In most cases, identification of *C. burnetti* is performed by serological analysis with serum samples demonstrating a fourfold or greater increase in antibody titer from the acute to convalescent samples. If *C. burnetti* has been identified in the hospital clinical laboratory, the institutional infection control officer must be notified.

SPECIMEN HANDLING

Shipping Instructions for Specimens Collected from People Exposed to Chemical and Biological Agents

The primary role of the clinical laboratory is to provide quick accurate testing results to support the attending physician in the care of a patient exposed to bioterrorist agents. Secondary to this role is the specimen transport to the CDC for agent identification. Below are the guidelines for the collection, packaging, and transport of specimens. Further information on specimen transport can be found on the CDC Web site *www.cdc.gov*

Collecting Specimens for Chemical Exposure

- Collect at least 25 mL of urine in a leak proof screw capped plastic container. The specimen should be frozen as soon as possible. It is preferable to freeze the specimen at 70°C or on dry ice. If dry ice is not available, the urine specimens may be shipped with freezer packs. For pediatric patients, collect only urine specimens, unless directed otherwise by the CDC.
- Collect three 4 mL tubes of whole blood in EDTA or four tubes of the 3 mL lavender type.
- Collect one 3 mL or larger gray top tube or one 3 mL or larger green top tube.
- Mark the first lavender top tube collected with a "1" using indelible ink. The first collection tube is used for blood metal analysis.
- For each lot of blood and urine containers used for collection, provide two empty unopened lavender top tubes, two empty unopened green top tubes, two empty unopened gray top tubes, and two empty unopened urine containers. These empty containers will serve as blanks for the analysis.
- The specimens must be labeled preferable the LIS-generated identification label. The label must include medical record number, specimen identification number, collector's initials, and date and time of collection.
- Place a single, unbroken strip of waterproof, tamper-evidence forensic tape over each specimen top but do not cover the specimen label. The tamper-evidence tape must be placed over the empty specimen container used for the blanks. The individual placing the tamper-evidence tape on the specimen container must initial the tape with indelible ink after placement.
- The laboratory must keep a log sheet indicating specimen identification, and personnel involved in the collection, packaging, and shipping of the specimens to the CDC.

Packaging

Packaging consists of three components: a leak-proof primary receptacle for blood and urine specimens, a leak-proof secondary container to protect the primary specimen collection tubes and cups, which includes absorbent material in case of leakage, and lastly, an outer container of strong corrugated cardboard with a Styrofoam lining. Multiple specimens can be placed in the secondary container but each tube must be wrapped to prevent contact. The secondary container must also contain absorbent material in the case of breakage. Lastly, the outer Styrofoam-lined box must contain absorbent material. The secondary container must be sealed with tamper-evidence tape and person sealing the bag initial the tamper-evidence tape with indelible ink.

Urine and blood samples must be transported in separate shipping boxes since the specimens require different storage temperatures. Blood samples are shipped at 4°C and packaged with cold packs in the Styrofoam-lined box. Urine samples are stored and shipped frozen and require either freezer packs or dry ice. It is important to remember that when shipping urine containers with dry ice, do not ship the specimens with large pieces of dry ice because they may scatter the urine cups in transport. To further protect the urine cups, it is a good idea to pack absorbent material between the specimens to minimize contact.

Boxes must be secured with shipping tape and mailing labels securely affixed. Place a label on the outside of the box that indicates "Exempt Human Specimens." For boxes containing dry ice, place a Class 9 (Dangerous Goods) label on the outside and indicate the amount of dry ice contained. The Class 9 sticker must be place on the side of the box along with the "Exempt Human Specimens." Ship the specimens to the CDC at 4770 Buford Hwy, Building 110 Loading Dock, Atlanta, GA, 30341. Questions concerning packaging and shipping can be directed to the CDC's National Center for Environmental Health, Division of Laboratory Sciences.

The CDC does not require the shipping laboratory send documentation of the chain of custody, but each laboratory must keep such records on file. The shipping laboratory must either have the commercial transport sign the chain of custody document or use the commercial shippers' tracking documentation.

Handling of Culture Specimens

The International Air Transport Association (IATA), a trade organization of the commercial airline industry, publishes Dangerous Goods Regulations for the packaging and shipping of biological agents. The IATA has categorized three classes of specimen type: A, B, and Exempt. Category A is the most hazardous and by list contains all the potential bioterrorist biological agents listed above. The following includes the information and procedure necessary for shipping of Category A cultures.

1. Cultures must be placed in leak-proof container made of glass, metal, or plastic and be sealed by a positive method such as heat sealing, a metal clip, or a taped screw top lid. The primary container must not exceed 50 mL or 50 g for an infectious material.
2. An absorbent material must be placed between the primary container and a solid secondary container. The secondary container must be able to withstand an internal pressure of 95 kPa or 13.8 lb/in^2 and be made of a solid rigid material.
3. A list of the contents of the primary container must be affixed to the secondary container.
4. The secondary container is placed in a shipping box made of corrugated cardboard lined with Styrofoam.

5. A Class 6 diamond-shaped label "Infectious Substance" must be affixed to the shipping container.
6. Package orientation arrows must be affixed to the shipping container indicating the top of the shipping container.
7. A Class 9 sticker indicating dangerous goods must be affixed to boxes containing dry ice.
8. A shipper's document or declaration will require an emergency response contact telephone number and therefore, the consignee's name and telephone number must be included.

CLINICAL LABORATORY CHALLENGES

Clinical Laboratory Staffing

Should a bioterrorist attack occur, would the clinical laboratory be able to respond? Clinical laboratories are facing and dealing with a workforce shortage. The average age of the clinical laboratory employee has increased and many of the medical technology schools have closed due to budgetary restraints. This formula of workforce retirement minus limited workforce entry can be defined as a negative imbalance or deficit. To respond to the workforce deficit, the industry centralizing microbiology laboratories has to take advantage of the limited personnel with experience. Fiscally this approach makes sense but presents a problem should a bioterrorist attack occur. Likely a bioterrorist attack would overwhelm the capacity of the clinical laboratory system. Many of the potential bioterrorist agents are first isolated in blood culture. The current technology uses continuous blood culture monitoring with positive detection in an incubator. After the detection, samples from the blood cultures are worked up in the traditional manual method of growth on agar plates. The challenge facing the clinical laboratory is not only one of staffing but handling the excess workload beyond the capacity of the continuous monitoring blood culture system. Does the laboratory have an adequate supply of blood culture bottles? Where can I get a supply of blood culture bottles? How many blood culture bottles are kept in inventory and not wasted due to expiration? What do I do with the specimens that do not "fit" into the continuous blood culture monitoring incubator? The sentinel laboratory must be able to address these issues and develop an implementation plan.

Personnel training must encompass not only detection of bioterrorist agents by the sentinel laboratory but general laboratory technical employees need to be prepared to process suspicious specimens and ship them either to the LRN reference laboratory or the LRN national laboratory.

CONCLUSION

The United States felt safe from enemy attacks because of distance between the continents. The events of September 11,

2001, changed all that and demonstrated an American vulnerability to terrorism. The clinical laboratory service is an integral part in the detection of agents used in a bioterrorist attack. The clinical laboratory faces many challenges in preparation for a bioterrorist event from the vantage of identification, staffing, workload, supplies, handling, and processing specimens; however, it is a challenge each laboratory must be prepared to face.

The reader is referred to the appendix regarding CDC recommendations for laboratory specimen.

Suggested Reading

Baud F, Borron SW, Megarbone, et al. Value of lactic acidosis in the assessment of acute cyanide poisoning. *Crit Care Med.* 2002;30(9):2044–50.

Biosafety in Biomedical and Microbiological Laboratories. *http://bmbl.od.nih.gov/contents.htm*

Black RM, Clark RJ, Harrison JM, et al. Biological fate of sulfur mustard: identification of valine and histidine adducts in haemoglobin from casualties of sulfur mustard poisoning. *Xenobiotica.* 1997;27:499–512.

Dangerous Goods Regulations 2006, 47th ed. *www.iata.org*

Derrick EH. "Q" fever, new fever entity: clinical features, diagnosis and laboratory investigation. *Med J Aust.* 1937;2:281–99.

Drasch G, Kretschmer E, Kauert G, et al. Concentrations of mustard gas [bis(2-chlorodiethyl sulphide] in the tissues of a victim of vesicant exposure. *J Forensic Sci.* 1987;32:1788–93.

Eckert WG. Mass deaths by gas or chemical poisoning a historical perspective. *Am J Forensic Med Pathol.* 1991;12:119–25.

Hawker JI, Ayres JG, et al. A large outbreak of Q fever in the West Midlands: wind-borne spread into metropolitan area. *Commun Dis Public Health.* 1998;1:180–87.

Hilbink F, Penrose M, Kovacova E, et al. Q fever is absent from New Zealand. *Intern J Epidemiol.* 1993;22:945–49.

Hooijschuur EW, Kinetz CE, Brinkman UA. Determination of the sulfur mustard hydrolysis product thiodiglycol by microcolumn liquid chromatography coupled on-line with sulfur flame photometric detection using large volume injections and peak compression. *J Chromatogr A.* 1999;849:433–44.

Jernigan DB, Raghunathan PL, Bell BP, et al. Investigation of bioterrorism related anthrax, United States, 2001. *Emerging Infect Dis.* 2002;8:1019–28.

Kaplan MM, Bertagna P. The geographical distribution of Q fever. *Bull WHO.* 1955;13:829–60.

Maisonneuve A, Gallebat I, Debordes L, et al. Specific and sensitive quantitation of 2,2'-dichlorodiethyl sulphide (sulfur mustard) in water, plasma and blood: application to toxicokinetic study in the rat after intravenous intoxication. *J Chromatogr A.* 1992;583:255–65.

Momeni, AZ, Ensheih S, Meghdadi M, et al. Skin manifestation of mustard gas. *Arch Dermatol.* 1992;128:775–80.

Noort D, Hulst AG, deJong LP, et al. Alkylation of human serum by sulfur mustard in vitro and in vivo: mass spectrometric analysis of a cysteine adduct as a sensitive biomarker of exposure. *Chem Res Toxicol.* 1999;12:715–21.

Odoul M, Fouillet B Nouri B, et al. Specific determination of cyanide in blood by head space chromatography. *J Anal Toxicol.* 1994;18:205–7.

Tissot-Dupont H, Torres S, Nezri M, et al. Hyperendemic focus of Q fever related to sheep and wind. *Am J Epidemiol.* 1999;150:67–74.

Troup CM, Ballantyne B, Marrs TC, (eds). *Clinical and Experimental Toxicology of Cyanide.* Bristol: IOP Publishing Limited, 1987: pp. 22–40.

van der Schans GP, Scheffer AG, et al, Immunochemical detection of sulfur mustard to DNA of calf thymus and human white blood cells. *Chem Res Toxicol.* 1994;7:408–13.

II

EMS ISSUES

INTRODUCTION

The succeeding chapters describe prehospital issues with Toxico-terrorism. Since the healthcare facility cannot expect prior or adequate notifications of such an event in advance of patient arrival, the surge capacity of the facility can easily be overwhelmed (even in a relatively small-scale event). It should be emphasized that only about 25% of patients will arrive to a healthcare facility via EMS and thus some of these prehospital principles (particularly decontumination) will apply to the hospital. With multiple individuals exposed to single (or several) agents, protecting the rescuers, prehospital substance identification and decontamination issues predominate. Communication of interventions among all responders and receivers is also an integral component.

19

CHEMPACK

Rachel Burke and Steven E. Aks

S T A T   F A C T S

CHEMPACK

- Chempack is limited to pharmaceutical agents and not PPE.
- Chempack is housed in a wire mesh/Plexiglas storage crate on wheels and weighs over 200 lb.
- Chempack contents are sufficient to adequately treat about one thousand mildly to moderate affected nerve agent exposures.

INTRODUCTION

The Strategic National Stockpile (SNS), previously known as the National Pharmaceutical Stockpile, was established in 1999 by the Department of Health and Human Services (DHHS) and the Centers for Disease Control and Prevention (CDC) in an effort to supply states with the medical resources needed to adequately respond to large scale emergencies including natural disasters and acts of bioterrorism. The SNS is controlled by the DHHS and is intended to provide states and communities with necessary supplemental medical supplies within 12 hours of a federal decision to deploy to national sites of large-scale emergencies and disasters. Materials contained in the SNS include medical supplies such as IVs and airway equipment and medications such as antibiotics and antidotes.

In the event of certain chemical emergencies or terrorist acts, specifically a nerve agent release, a 12-hour response time to deploy appropriate antidote is insufficient to adequately and effectively treat chemically exposed casualties. Nerve agent victims require timely treatment within minutes to hours of exposure for several reasons. First of all, nerve agents are extremely toxic chemicals, which can result in severe illness or death within minutes of exposure unless immediate treatment is administered. Furthermore,

antidote effectiveness may drastically decline if administration is delayed due to nerve agent aging, a process in which the bond between the nerve agent and its target, acetylcholinesterase, becomes irreversible ultimately rendering the antidote ineffective. The delayed response time required to deploy the SNS is a pitfall in the management of nerve agent mass casualty emergencies.

This potential pitfall in emergency preparedness was addressed by the CDC in 2002 with the Chempack pilot project, which was developed to determine the usefulness of more readily available stockpiles specifically for use in emergencies involving nerve agents. Chempacks are stockpiles of nerve agent antidotes, which are strategically placed throughout participating regions to expedite deployment of antidote within 6 hours in response to a nerve agent event. After the Chempack was successfully piloted in rural South Dakota, a combined urban and rural area of Washington, and urban New York City, the DHHS implemented the plan throughout the United States and the surrounding territories, including Puerto Rico and the U.S. Virgin Islands.

HISTORICAL THREAT PERSPECTIVE

Chemical agents have been used in terrorism tactics and as warfare throughout history, including the use of cyanide in ancient Greece, irritant gases and blister agents in World War I, and nerve agents in Iraq. The nerve agents were first developed for use as pesticides by the Germans in the 1930s followed by the British in the 1950s. Due to their rapid onset of action, high volatility allowing easy dispersal, and potent toxicity, nerve agents are ideal terrorism and warfare agents. Despite their mass production during World War II, they were not utilized due to fear of retaliation, and although readily available, nerve agents have not been used as warfare agents to date with the exception of the Iran-Iraq war.

Nerve agents have been utilized in several terrorist activities over the past several decades. On a small scale, the Matsumoto incident in Japan in 1994 involved a sarin release carried out by the Aum Shinrikyo sect, intended as revenge against presiding judges anticipated to rule unfavorably in a land dispute. Liquid sarin was vaporized by dripping it onto a heater and dispersing the vapor by fan toward the residential area housing the intended targets. This terrorism incident resulted in greater than 250 victims of which over 50 required hospitalization with 7 deaths.

On a larger scale, the Tokyo subway incident in 1995 also involved a sarin release carried out by the Aum Shinrikyo sect in an attempt to deter police from conducting a future raid on their chemical warfare development plant. In this incident, liquid sarin was carried onto commuter trains in plastic bags, which were then pierced with umbrella tips releasing liquid sarin into a confined space. The event was carried out during rush hour at the convergence point of several heavily populated trains located closely to the police department headquarters and several government buildings. This terrorism incident resulted in greater than 5000 people seeking medical care with 1000 mildly to moderately affected victims of which over 500 required hospitalizations and 12 died. Lack of appropriate decontamination and personal protection implementation resulted in secondary contamination of approximately 250 medical personnel.

PERSONAL PROTECTIVE EQUIPMENT AND DECONTAMINATION CONSIDERATIONS

The Chempack is limited to pharmaceutical assets and does not include personal protective equipment (PPE) or decontamination supplies. To ensure adequate preparation for a mass casualty nerve agent event, each facility will need to inventory available PPE supplies and assess available personnel trained in decontamination.

As demonstrated in the Tokyo incident, first responders and emergency personnel are at high risk for becoming casualties. Due to threat of secondary contamination, health-care providers must consider themselves potential victims and take appropriate personal protection precautions before attempting decontamination and treatment of nerve-agent-exposed victims. No decontamination or medical treatment should be rendered prior to donning appropriate PPE.

All chemically exposed patients must be appropriately decontaminated prior to entry into the treatment facility. Water irrigation is the most simple and effective initial method of decontamination. While the addition of soap or dilute bleach solution may enhance the efficacy of decontamination, attempts to obtain bleach or soap should not delay the initiation of decontamination. For further details regarding PPE and decontamination procedures in nerve agent exposure, refer to Chap. 43.

RESOURCE REQUIREMENTS

Nerve agent intoxication requires specific antidote administration and medical intervention to reverse toxicity, decrease severity of illness, and improve the likelihood of survival with a favorable outcome. Medications necessary for treatment of nerve agent toxicity include pralidoxime or 2-PAM, atropine, and diazepam. Pralidoxime supplies at most hospitals are limited and insufficient to treat large numbers of nerve agent exposures likely to be encountered in a mass casualty incident. Furthermore, certain nerve agents permanently bind acetylcholinesterase rapidly and require timely antidote intervention to reverse the binding process and prevent irreversible toxicity. Sarin, for instance, permanently binds or ages in approximately 5–6 hours.

In addition to a specific antidote requirement, nerve agent intoxication frequently requires large doses of atropine to adequately counteract the toxic effects. Although atropine is readily available in the hospital setting, a single severely exposed nerve agent casualty may require large amounts of atropine and numerous casualties could easily deplete hospital atropine stores. Urgency of administration and limited hospital supplies of nerve agent antidote and supporting medications necessitates readily accessible supplemental supplies in preparation for a mass casualty nerve agent event.

Chempack stockpiles of nerve agent antidotes are strategically placed throughout the United States for deployment in a mass casualty nerve agent event. Participation in the Chempack project is voluntary and the specific locations of the Chempack are determined by the individual participating states and regions based on hazard vulnerability analysis. In the circumstance of a special event or gathering, Chempack stockpiles can be mobilized to different locations temporarily to cover the event. Requirements for Chempack deployment include a working diagnosis of nerve agent exposure, a large-scale emergency threatening the medical security of the community, and imminent depletion of hospital supplies of medically necessary life-dependent materials.

The Chempack is housed in a wire mesh and Plexiglas storage crate on wheels that weighs over 500 lb. The contents must be kept within a certain temperature range to allow retention for use beyond their usual expiration date as sample tested and approved through the shelf life extension program (SLEP) developed by the Food and Drug Administration (FDA). The Chempack must be stored in a secure environment under lock and key and is wired with a Sensaphone device, which is directly connected to the CDC, resulting in immediate notification if the temperature goes out of range or the contents are breached.

Contents of the Chempack are sufficient supplemental resources to adequately treat approximately 1000 mildly to moderately affected nerve agent exposures with the hospital container and 454 mildly to moderately affected nerve agent exposures with the emergency medical service

TABLE 19-1
CHEMPACK

There are two containers. One is for emergency medical services (EMS) and the other is the hospital Chempack container. Below are the specific contents.			
The contents include pralidoxime chloride (2-PAM)—reactivates acetylcholine esterase (true antidote)			
Atropine sulfate blocks effects of excess acetylcholine at its site of action			
Diazepam reduces the severity of acetylcholine-induced convulsions			
Autoinjectors—nonadjustable rapid IM dosing, ideal for emergent field use			
Multidose vials—adjustable precision IV dosing, ideal for urgent hospital use and long-term care			
EMS CHEMPACK Container for 454 Casualties			
	QTY	Unit Pack	Cases
Mark 1 autoinjector	240	5	1200
Atropine sulfate 0.4 mg/mL 20 mL	100	1	100
Pralidoxime 1g inj 20 mL	276	1	276
Atropen 0.5 mg	144	1	144
Atropen 1.0 mg	144	1	144
Diazepam 5 mg/mL autoinjector	150	2	300
Diazepam 5 mg/mL vial, 10 mL	25	2	50
Sterile water for injection (SWFI) 20 cc vials	100	2	200
Sensaphone 2050	1	1	1
Satco B DEA container	1	1	1
Hospital CHEMPACK Container for 1000 Casualties			
	QTY	Unit Pack	Cases
Mark 1 autoinjector	390	240	2
Atropine sulfate 0.4 mg/mL 20 mL	850	100	9
Pralidoxime 1 g inj 20 mL	2730	276	10
Atropen 0.5 mg	144	144	1
Atropen 1.0 mg	144	144	1
Diazepam 5 mg/mL autoinjector	80	150	1
Diazepam 5 mg/mL vial, 10 mL	640	25	26
Sterile water for injection (SWFI) 20 cc vials	2760	100	23
Sensaphone 2050	1	1	1
Satco B DEA container	1	1	1

Source: The CHEMPACK Project Guidelines, CHEMPACK Project Office, Strategic National Stockpile Program, Centers for Disease Control and Prevention.

(EMS) container. Two forms of the Chempack exist: the hospital Chempack and the EMS Chempack. The EMS Chempack is intended to be field based and largely contains autoinjector forms of medications ideal for immediate use by emergency first responders. The hospital Chempack contains fewer autoinjectors and larger amounts of multidose vials for titrating medication dosages for prolonged inpatient care. (See Table 19-1.)

TOXICOKINETICS/PATHOPHYSIOLOGY

Nerve agents refer to the category of toxins that specifically inhibit the acetylcholinesterase enzyme and include GA (Tabun), GB (Sarin), GD (Soman), and VX. By inhibiting acetylcholinesterase, these agents alter the homeostatic balance of the amount of acetylcholine in the nerve terminal resulting in a state of cholinergic excess. The cholinergic effects will be manifested by the degree of action at muscarinic and nicotinic receptor sites in the nervous system. These agents are discussed in greater detail in the nerve agent chapter (Chap. 28).

CLINICAL MANIFESTATIONS/LABORATORY STUDIES

Nerve agent victims will exhibit a classic toxidrome of cholinergic signs and symptoms. Table 19-2 breaks down the symptoms into muscarinic and nicotinic effects.

The most important muscarinic effects are the excessive respiratory secretions and bronchospasm. Antidotal

TABLE 19-2

BREAKDOWN OF THE SYMPTOMS INTO MUSCARINIC
AND NICOTINIC EFFECTS

Muscarinic
Salivation
Lacrimation
Urination
Gastrointestinal distress (nausea, vomiting)
Bradycardia, bronchorrhea, bronchospasm
Abdominal cramps
Miosis
Nicotinic
Muscular fasciculations
Weakness
Tremors
Hypertension
Tachycardia

administration of atropine should be administered to overcome excessive bronchial secretions. This is the most important endpoint of treating with atropine. The nicotinic receptors are located at the neuromuscular junction, which accounts for fasciculations and weakness. There are also nicotinic receptors at the terminus of the preganglionic sympathetic nerve to the adrenal gland. This nicotinic stimulation will lead to tachycardia and hypertension, or precisely the opposite hemodynamic effect one may see after muscarinic stimulation. The degree of nicotinic versus muscarinic effects depends on the agent of exposure.

The most timely and reliable way to diagnose nerve agent exposures is toxidrome recognition on the part of the treating clinician. Appreciation of the signs and symptoms listed above will be critical to the recognition and treatment of nerve agent casualties in a (WMD) weapons of mass destruction setting. In addition to clinical recognition for the diagnosis of nerve agent toxicity, there are several detectors that may be employed by EMS or crime scene investigators to aid in the diagnosis, but communication of these results to health-care providers may be delayed.

There are two laboratory blood tests that can be obtained to confirm nerve agent exposure, the erythrocyte cholinesterase activity level and the serum or pseudo-cholinesterase activity level. Reliance on laboratory diagnosis of nerve agent toxicity is not practical because these tests will require several days for completion, and are not readily available in most clinical settings. (While the pseudocholinesterase activity level is more readily available, the erythrocyte cholinesterase level provides a more direct inference of nervous system cholinesterase activity than does the pseudocholinesterase activity. A depression of a cholinesterase activity below 10% suggests severe

poisoning, 10–20% depression suggests moderate toxicity, and 20–50% suggests mild toxicity.) Additionally, without baseline cholinesterase activity, the interpretation of these tests can be problematic.

EARLY INTERVENTIONS

Following evacuation and decontamination, nerve agent antidote should be administered as soon as possible. In severe toxicity, antidote administration may be required prior to or during the decontamination and evacuation process. Antidote administration may include self-aid, buddy aid, or third-party administration of autoinjectors, namely Mark I kits and CANA kits. Mark I kits contain two autoinjectors, a 2 mg atropine autoinjector, and a 600 mg pralidoxime autoinjector, and CANA kits contain a single 10 mg diazepam autoinjector. The atropine should be administered first followed by the pralidoxime. Nerve agent victims should be treated based on extent of exposure and severity of symptoms. Mildly symptomatic exposures should receive a single Mark I, moderately symptomatic exposures should receive two Mark I, and severe exposures should receive three Mark I doses plus a single CANA regardless of the presence or absence of seizure activity.

CONSULTATION AND REFERRAL

Presentation of numerous patients exhibiting symptoms consistent with the cholinergic syndrome should create suspicion of a possible mass casualty chemical event involving organophosphate or nerve agent poisoning. Suspicion of a mass casualty incident should trigger activation of the internal hospital disaster plan and immediate inventory of hospital supplies of pralidoxime and atropine to determine resource availability and anticipate potential supply depletion.

Imminent depletion of nerve agent antidotes and supporting pharmaceuticals should activate deployment and utilization of Chempack resources. Local protocols developed through collaboration of the department of public health (DPH), the emergency management agency (EMA), and the EMS should be followed to mobilize and access medically necessary stockpiles. Supplemental sources for nerve agent management consultation include the poison control center and CDC emergency preparedness and response Web site at *www.bt.cdc.gov*

Suggested Reading

http://en.wikipedia.org/wiki/Matsumoto_incident
http://en.wikipedia.org/wiki/Matsumoto_incident

*http://en.wikipedia.org/wiki/Sarin_gas_attack_on_the_Tokyo_
subway*

*http://en.wikipedia.org/wiki/Sarin_gas_attack_on_the_Tokyo_
subway*

*http://www.bt.cdc.gov/planning/continuationguidance/docs/chem
pack-attachj.doc*

*http://www.bt.cdc.gov/planning/continuationguidance/docs/chem
pack-attachj.doc*

http://www.bt.cdc.gov/stockpile/index.asp

*http://www.bt.cdc.gov/stockpile/index.asp. Strategic National
Stockpile. April 15, 2006-06-07*

*http://www.cbaci.org/pubs/fact_sheets/fact_sheet_2.pdf. – Matsumoto
incident*

*http://www.cbaci.org/pubs/fact_sheets/fact_sheet_2.pdf. – Matsumoto
incident*

http://www.cdc.gov/programs/php09.htm

http://www.cdc.gov/programs/php09.htm

Okumura T, Suzuki K, Fukuda Atsuhito, et al. Tokyo subway Sarin
attack: disaster management, Part 1: community emergency
response. *Acad Emerg Med.* 1998;5:613–17.

Okumura T, Suzuki K, Fukuda Atsuhito, et al. Tokyo subway
Sarin attack: disaster management, Part 2: hospital response.
Acad Emerg Med. 1998;5:618–24.

Okumura T, Suzuki K, Fukuda Atsuhito, et al. Tokyo subway
Sarin attack: disaster management, Part 3: national and international responses. *Acad Emerg Med.* 1998;5:625–28.

Okumura T, Suzuki K, Fukuda Atsuhito, et al. Tokyo subway
Sarin attack: disaster management, Part 1: community emergency response. *Acad Emerg Med.* 1998;5:613–17.

Okumura T, Suzuki K, Fukuda Atsuhito, et al. Tokyo subway
Sarin attack: disaster management, Part 2: hospital response.
Acad Emerg Med. 1998;5:618–24.

Okumura T, Suzuki K, Fukuda Atsuhito, et al. Tokyo subway
Sarin attack: disaster management, Part 3: national and international responses. *Acad Emerg Med.* 1998;5:625–28.

Strategic National Stockpile. April 15, 2006-06-07. A more appropriate citation for the above reference is *http://www.bt.cdc.
gov/stockpile* CDC Emergency Preparedness and Response.
Strategic National Stockpile. April 14, 2005.

The working draft of the WHO publication *Health Aspects of
Biological and Chemical Weapons.* 2nd ed., due for publication in December 2001.

World Health Organization. *Public Health Response to Biological
and Chemical Weapons: WHO Guidance.* 2nd ed. World Heath
Organization, Geneva, 2004. *www.who.int/csr/delibepidemics/
biochemguide/en/index.html*

20

APPROACH TO DISASTER AND MASS CASUALTY INCIDENTS

J. Marc Liu and D. Robert Rodgers

S T A T   F A C T S

APPROACH TO DISASTER AND MASS CASUALTY INCIDENTS

Disaster Planning—Key Concepts

- Know the hospital plan. The best plan is useless if no one is familiar with it.
- Know the enemy. Be armed with current medical knowledge. Know what is more likely to happen.
- Know yourself. Be familiar with personnel and equipment. Know what they can and cannot do.
- Practice, practice, practice! Hold frequent drills of different types to maintain proficiency.
- Be prepared to improvise. This can only be done if one has fulfilled the preceding steps.

Disaster Response—Key Concepts

- Consider activating a disaster plan for any internal or external event that may overwhelm the normal ED capacity.
- Appoint an experienced command staff. Such persons must be easily identifiable.
- Clear the ED before the patients arrive.
- Most patients will have relatively minor injuries and will be self-referred. They will not have had any on-scene evaluation or decontamination.

- Triage is the most important part of a mass casualty response. Therefore, the triage officer should be the most experienced clinician available.
- Keep the ED clear by maintaining forward patient flow. Only the lifesaving/stabilizing care is to be provided in the ED. Patients are moved as rapidly as possible to other areas of the hospital for further testing and definitive management.
- The goal is to provide the greatest good for the greatest number.

Disaster Recovery—Key Concepts

- Stay alert for psychological and stress-related problems in patients, employees, and oneself. Seek help when needed.
- Be prepared for above average patient volume for days or even weeks after an incident.
- Analyze what went right and what went wrong in the response. Apply this experience to the next event.

INTRODUCTION

Recent world events have increased the salience of mass casualty and disaster medicine in the consciousness of health-care providers and the general public. Rare and always unexpected, mass casualty events can take many forms. Emergency departments (EDs) are more frequently being called upon to respond to events as varied in scope as terrorist attacks, high-rise fires, or hurricanes. Despite the need for capable care in these situations, few physicians have been trained in mass casualty care, and fewer still have ever been exposed to a real disaster. Education is often limited in scope, with didactics and rehearsal abbreviated by lack of time, lack of funding, the need to focus on "day-to-day" issues, and general apathy. The result is that many misconceptions about disaster medicine are perpetuated.

This chapter will provide a practical overview for physicians in the ED. It will highlight the major concepts in disaster and mass casualty medicine, and propose new strategies applicable to many situations.

PREPARING FOR THE UNEXPECTED— DISASTER PLANNING

Webster's Dictionary defines a *disaster* as "an event causing great loss, hardship, or suffering to many people." In medical terms, a disaster is any event that results in injuries that cannot be adequately cared for by the medical resources of the community involved. A *mass casualty* event results in a number of patients that exceed a specific facility's ability to care for them. In order to have an effective response to a mass casualty incident, it is important to have an organized approach. Thus, disaster response actually begins long before any damage is incurred, with thought and preplanning to develop such organization.

Around 350 BC, the Chinese strategist Sun Tzu wrote, "Know the enemy and know yourself; in a hundred battles you will never be in peril." From this statement are derived the main elements of emergency preparedness. A proper approach to disaster planning consists of knowledge of what can happen ("knowing the enemy") and being familiar with the resources one has available to respond ("knowing yourself").

"Knowing the enemy" first involves maintaining the fund of medical knowledge and skills required to treat patients. Common problems in managing a large number of patients will occur regardless of the specific nature of the incident. Triage, patient flow, security, and communications become issues that need organized resolution.

Recognition of the importance of these areas resulted in the development of HICS (the Hospital Incident Command System), an administrative framework designed to manage hospital resources during disruptions of normal functions. HICS is now the federally mandated system for hospital emergency planning. It uses a multidisciplinary/ departmental strategy to avoid the pitfall of delineating a separate response for every conceivable crisis.

"Knowing yourself" first includes a formal disaster plan. A disaster plan is developed with input from all hospital departments and services. It defines what is considered a disaster, and how the facility would respond. A written plan alone, though, is not sufficient, as one can develop the "paper plan syndrome"—the false sense of security engendered by the mere existence of a written document.

Emergency physicians are both required and assumed to be well-versed in the disaster protocols of the hospital.

"Knowing yourself" also entails being aware of the resources that can be applied to a disaster. An effective response requires efficient use of the finite amount of resources, including which personnel are available and their types of training. A stressful situation like a mass casualty incident is the worst time to attempt to perform something new. Whenever possible, personnel should be given roles utilizing skills that are known to them. Supplies and physical space are also resources that are actively managed, even on routine days.

Training and rehearsal are essential for true preparedness. They help combat the loss of knowledge and skills that occur with infrequency of use. ED physicians should consider such training as part of their practice, and willingly assume the role of leader and teacher in their department and hospital. The individual physician must maintain his or her own procedural skills, medical knowledge, and familiarity with the disaster plan. Effective leadership and implementation of an organized educational program based on the hospital plan is the cornerstone of preparedness.

The last step in planning is the disaster drill, which is the only controlled way to gain experience. Drills serve a valuable purpose in testing the adequacy of a disaster plan, as well as personnel's knowledge of the plan. Unfortunately, most institutions rarely, if ever, perform drills. Rehearsals acclimatize people to the mass casualty situation, and can help decrease the stress of an actual event. They also help in identifying deficiencies in planning and training. Drills can take many forms, from "tabletop" paper exercises to full-scale drills involving the entire hospital. A comprehensive schedule of drills would include a mix of the different types. This includes separate drills for different services (e.g., administration, security, housekeeping, nursing). Service-specific rehearsals help personnel learn and practice emergency protocols without the distractions of a full-scale drill. This method also has the benefit of being less costly and time-consuming, allowing it to be done more frequently.

A solid comprehension of potential threats, the disaster plan, and the resources available allows an organized approach to a real event. It also allows one to tailor a response to the particulars of a situation, called "planned improvisation." Every situation has unique challenges that may not be foreseen in even the best of plans. Only through an understanding of what is and is not feasible can a physician skillfully counter the inevitable unexpected problem.

UNTO THE BREACH—DISASTER RESPONSE

Activating the Plan

When one receives word of a possible disaster, the first step is to obtain as much information as possible. However, in the confusion of an event, early accurate information will not be available. The physician must determine whether the predicted number and severity of injuries is beyond the current capabilities of the ED and hospital, based on the information available. If this is the case, then the mass casualty plan should be activated to mobilize additional resources. Different hospitals have defined different levels of activation based on the nature of the event, so physicians must have a clear understanding of specific plans used by their facility.

Appointing the Command Staff and Allocating Personnel

A unified and clear chain of command is necessary for efficient functioning. The first and most critical action is to identify the physician in charge of the ED's entire response. This ED commander/supervisor is responsible for ensuring the rapid and appropriate treatment of patients, selecting team leaders, and coordinating requests for resources with other departments and services in the hospital.

It is important to consider the skills and experience of each person when assigning particular duties. People work best when given tasks familiar to them. Early and effective delineation of responsibilities will minimize later confusion as the response develops.

Communications

For an organized response, all parties need an effective method to communicate with each other. However, in almost every disaster, communications become a problem.

Two-way radios provide portable, real-time voice communications and are the preferred system, but nonetheless have drawbacks. They require charged batteries, require personnel to know the devices and frequencies, and are subject to interference. If no other system is available, one can use people as runners/couriers to physically deliver messages.

A frequent problem is the overuse of communication. Too many messages can be as bad as too few. Messages should be as concise as possible, conveying the necessary information without jargon or slang that can be misunderstood.

Security and Access

Maintaining security is a major portion of any mass casualty incident. Part of the physician's role is to coordinate with security personnel to maintain a safe and efficient environment for patient care.

Only 688 of over 4000 patients in the Tokyo sarin attack arrived via emergency medical services (EMS). The rest arrived by foot or private vehicle, flooding into hospitals in any way possible. Victims and families, who are in distress, may become impatient or hostile, and may attempt to enter a facility without proper triage or decontamination. All access to the hospital and ED must be locked or guarded, with additional security stationed at triage and every treatment area. The ED supervisor will rely on the security officer to accomplish this vital mission.

Patient Flow and Treatment Areas

A functional hospital plan has predesignated spaces for the treatment of each level of injury. All personnel, especially the ED physician, should be aware of the designated areas and routes for moving patients. A critical aspect of ensuring overall efficiency is to maintain forward patient flow. A patient never moves backwards in the system. Once patients leave the triage area, they proceed directly to a treatment area. Once they leave a treatment area they do not return, proceeding to an end destination.

The ED is the only space in the hospital equipped to handle a large amount of patients at one time. Therefore, the ED must open as many beds as possible within minutes. The staff determines who can be discharged and who is stable enough for transport, whether to a temporary holding area or an assigned inpatient bed. The main goal is to clear the emergency room in order to make space for the expected patients.

The Patient Population

While preparations are being made to receive victims, the wise physician is already anticipating what types and numbers of injuries will present. A common misconception concerning mass casualty incidents is that a hospital will quickly receive a sudden influx of ambulances arriving with a large number of critically wounded victims. Analysis of multiple disasters has shown this is usually not the case.

A mass casualty incident can range anywhere from a handful of patients to thousands. There have only been seven United States civilian disasters with more than 1000 fatalities. On average, there are 10–15 incidents a year with more than 40 injuries. Most large disasters will produce 100–200 casualties.

The overwhelming majority of patients have minor injuries. A review of over two dozen mass casualty incidents by the Disaster Research Center determined that fewer than 10% of victims would meet criteria for hospital admission in normal circumstances, and many stayed less than 24 hours. After Hurricane Hugo in 1989, almost half of patients seen in one area of North Carolina were for wounds and insect stings.

In most cases, the initial wave of patients arriving at the ED will be ambulatory with injuries of low acuity. These patients are able to move relatively quickly to the hospital. More critical patients, who are often unable to refer themselves, usually begin arriving later. This "second wave" phenomenon has been observed in numerous incidents. Minor injuries must be quickly triaged and moved to a definitive care area in order to keep beds available for more serious injuries.

The majority of patients will not arrive via EMS transport. In the Oklahoma City bombing, 56% of the patients seen in area hospitals arrived by privately owned vehicles. Patients and bystanders will go to the closest hospital as quickly as possible, often bypassing on-scene triage and aid stations. The physician can expect a large number of victims who will not have had any evaluation, triage, or intervention by EMS. There can also be a risk in hazardous materials (hazmat) incidents, where patients may arrive at the hospital without having received any on-scene decontamination. Security and medical personnel must cooperate to route all patients through the triage process. Self-referral also implies that one cannot expect EMS to equally distribute casualties between local hospitals. This problem is often compounded by the natural tendency for rescue workers to transport to the nearest hospital. The Disaster Research Center study found that two-thirds of patients in each event were seen by one hospital. Workers in a hospital geographically closest to an incident can expect to bear the brunt of the response.

Triage

Triage is the process of prioritizing medical care by severity of injury. The single most important clinical role that the emergency physician can undertake is that of the triage officer. Rapid and accurate triage is essential to a successful emergency response. For this reason, selection of the triage officer and team is one of the supervisor's most important duties. The triage officer is traditionally the most experienced physician available.

The key concept of mass casualty triage is to obtain the maximal benefit to the largest number of people using the limited resources available. In a mass casualty incident, the fundamental focus on the individual patient has to be altered to a focus on the whole patient population. These triage principles conflict with the normal medical principle to do everything possible in each individual. Triage personnel must be able to shift the mindset away from the patient and toward the group as a whole, and must be willing to accept greater levels of morbidity and mortality than in usual practice.

There are numerous scoring systems that have been developed to aid in classifying patients. Each system uses its own combination of mechanism of injury, vital signs, and physical examination criteria to triage patients. Although many of these systems are able to accurately predict mortality, they are less accurate at differentiating between levels of acuity. Almost all were tested primarily on trauma patients. To date, there have been no data to show that any one scoring system is superior. Comparisons of selected triage systems and criteria are shown in Tables 20-1 through 20-4.

Triage scoring systems can serve as guidelines to help classify victims. However, "there is no substitute for good judgment, sound experience, and attention to the principles of triage." The triage team's priority is to classify, and *not* to treat, patients. Interventions at triage are kept to minimum, lifesaving measures. Once triaged, a patient is moved to the appropriate treatment area.

Triage is a dynamic process. Patients should be reassessed frequently to look for changes in their status. If necessary, patients can be reassigned to another category and transferred to the appropriate treatment area.

As one of the most critical aspects of mass casualty care, triage is discussed in depth in Chaps. 25 and 52.

Patient Assessment and Treatment

The goal of treatment areas in a mass casualty incident is to perform assessment and interventions necessary for stabilization. To ensure the most efficient care possible for a large number of patients, patient flow out of the ED must be maintained at a maximum. The physician assigned to a treatment area performs a more thorough evaluation than at triage, though the priority remains to minimize interventions and tests to lifesaving measures. The physician must rapidly decide whether the patient requires admission, and, if so, to what location. Only tests needed to stabilize and disposition the patient should be done. Extensive diagnostic testing is performed in other areas of the hospital, and not in the emergency room. Once patients leave a treatment area, they do not return to that area.

Hazardous Materials and Decontamination

Hazardous materials incidents present special challenges to the emergency provider. Every hospital is required to have procedures in place to handle patients contaminated with biologic, chemical, or radioactive substances.

With hazmat incidents, the two main issues are to stop ongoing injury to patients, and to prevent secondary contamination of the caregivers and facility. In 1995, 110 of 472 hospital workers in Tokyo reported symptoms possibly due to secondary exposure to sarin gas. The majority of these providers were not using any sort of protective equipment. There are little data to form recommendations on the levels of protection used by hospitals. An emergency physician must be familiar with the type of protective equipment available at the hospital, and the limitations of such equipment. All personnel who may come in contact with contaminated patients must wear protective gear.

Removing all clothing can remove 85–90% of contamination, and rinsing with soap and copious amounts of water is usually successful in removing the rest. After decontamination is complete, any participating personnel then undergo decontamination, and are examined for any signs or symptoms of exposure that may require medical attention.

TABLE 20-1

SUMMARY OF SELECTED TRIAGE SYSTEMS

Scoring System	Variables Considered	Features
Trauma index	Body region, type of injury, cardiovascular status, central nervous system status, respiratory status	Useful to nonphysicians; lacks predictive sensitivity and specificity
Triage index	Respiratory expansion, capillary refill, eye opening, verbal response, motor response	Maximum score, 16; patients with scores greater than 4 should be triaged to trauma facility
Trauma score	Respiratory effort, respiratory rate, systolic blood pressure, capillary refill, eye opening, verbal response, motor response	Score of 14 may indicate need for trauma facility; sum not calculated in field by prehospital personnel, difficulty in judging capillary refill and respiratory expansion at night
CRAMS score	Circulation, respiration, abdominal findings, motor ability, speech	Each component graded 0–2; score of 8 or less denotes major trauma; score not calculated initially by prehospital personnel; triage decisions not based on score
Revised trauma score	Glasgow Coma Scale (GCS), systolic blood pressure, respiratory rate	Respiratory expansion and capillary refill excluded; improved assessment for head injuries
Prehospital index	Systolic blood pressure, pulse, respiratory rate, level of consciousness	Only physiologic components used; sum calculated by emergency staff after receiving information from prehospital personnel
Trauma triage rule	Systolic blood pressure less than 85 mm Hg, motor component of GCS less than 5, penetrating trauma to head, neck, or trunk	Claimed 92% sensitivity, 92% specificity; concern that physiologic derangements may not have occurred at the time of triage
Anatomic factors	Penetrating wounds to chest and abdomen, traumatic amputation, comorbid factors	May decrease undertriage rate, but at expense of increased overtriage rate
Mechanism of injury	Falls greater than 20 feet, motor vehicle accident with death of occupant in same compartment, ejection from vehicle, high-speed impact	Requires accurate prehospital information; may be hampered by time, environment factors, expertise of health-care providers, and need to provide care

Source: Modified from Kennedy et al. Triage: techniques and applications in decision making. Ann Emerg Med. 1996;28:136–144. With permission from the American College of Emergency Physicians.

TABLE 20-2

SENSITIVITY AND SPECIFICITY OF PHYSIOLOGIC VARIABLES USED IN MASS CASUALTY TRIAGE

Variable	Sensitivity, %	Specificity, %
Respiratory rate >29 breaths/min	14.8	95.3
Respiratory rate <10 or >29 breaths/min	25.2	95.3
Glasgow Coma Scale—Motor Response score <6	72.6	96.2
Systolic blood pressure <80 mm Hg	30.4	99.2
Capillary refill >2 seconds	36.3	93.2
Heart rate >120 beats/min	33.3	91.8

Source: From Garner et al. Comparative analysis of multiple-casualty incident triage algorithms. Ann Emerg Med. 2001;38:541–548. With permission from the American College of Emergency Physicians.

Documentation and Record-Keeping

During the frenzied process of treating large numbers of patients, record-keeping often becomes a low priority. There is a fine line between inadequate documentation that provides no useful information, and excessive documentation, which can slow care. Documentation is necessary for identifying and locating victims. It can also be used for legal and scientific purposes. Members of the medical records staff must be part of disaster drills, and be assigned to all triage and treatment units. At triage, patients must receive some form of identifier on a card, tag, or wristband. Registration personnel at every triage and treatment area must keep an accurate, up-to-date list of all patient admissions, discharges, and destinations to and from the area. There also needs to be a simple chart to record important details of medical history, physical examination, and care received. The HICS model includes a suggested medical record format.

TABLE 20-3

PREDICTIVE VALUE OF FACTORS FOR SEVERE INJURY

Predictors	Odds Ratio (95% CI)	Jackknife Adjusted Odds Ratio (95% CI)
Model 1		
Respiratory rate (≥30 vs. <30 breaths/min)	2.24 (0.82–6.11)	2.35 (0.99–5.61)
Glasgow Coma Scale—Motor Response score (≤5 vs. 6)	75.49 (42.67–133.53)	72.81 (39.98–132.62)
Systolic blood pressure (<80 vs. >80 mm Hg)	32.47 (11.38–92.67)	31.73 (9.18–109.71)
Capillary refill (>2 vs. ≤2 s)	3.56 (1.64–7.71)	3.56 (1.31–9.67)
Heart rate (>120 vs. ≤120 beats/min)	2.63 (1.03–6.69)	2.53 (1.15–5.60)

Source: From Garner et al. Comparative analysis of multiple-casualty incident triage algorithms. Ann Emerg Med. 2001;38:541–548. With permission from the American College of Emergency Physicians.

Volunteers

Hospitals have to be prepared to deal with the large number of well-meaning volunteers that inevitably arrive. Contrary to popular wisdom, many people do not remain stunned and confused after an incident, but will instead rush to see what assistance they can provide. Volunteers should be required to present proof of their identity and skills. If utilized, volunteers should be assigned, based on their skills and experience, to augment existing teams/units, and never independently. If the use of volunteers would hinder the response, then they should be politely and firmly turned away.

The Media and Public Information

The physician may also find him or herself asked to deal with members of the media, as well as concerned relatives and friends. Any questions should be directed to a member of the hospital's media relations staff, rather than healthcare providers. Members of the press cannot be allowed into triage or treatment areas, where they may serve as a distraction to personnel and may violate patient privacy. If one must speak to the press, it is a wise precaution to have a member of the media relations staff present.

EX POST FACTO—DISASTER RECOVERY

Once the incident commander and ED supervisor determines that all casualties have been triaged, assessed, and have arrived at their end destinations for definitive care, the incident can enter the recovery phase. This, though, does not mean operations instantly return to normal. The hospital must still provide services for the large number of patients and the personnel mobilized to care for them. The ED must remain ready to receive patients that come in after the event. These patients may be injured in the course of cleaning up afterward. Also, in a large disaster, people may be unable to access their usual medical care, and may go to the emergency room.

All involved personnel should participate in an incident debriefing. Incident debriefing serves two main functions. First, it is a way to identify successful and unsuccessful techniques in the emergency response. Second, it provides an opportunity for all to receive information about formal psychological and stress management counseling. Past incidents have shown that responders and victims are at risk for posttraumatic stress disorder, depression, and substance abuse. Physicians should encourage patients and coworkers (and themselves) to utilize support resources.

TABLE 20-4

COMPARISON OF SELECTED TRIAGE SYSTEMS

Triage Algorithm	Sensitivity, % (95% CI)	Specificity, % (95% CI)	Odds Ratio (95% CI)
Simple triage and rapid treatment (capillary refill)	85 (78–90)	86 (84–88)	35 (21–61)
Modified simple triage and rapid treatment (palpable radial pulse)	84 (76–89)	91 (89–93)	52 (31–90)
Triage sieve (capillary refill)	45 (37–54)	89 (87–91)	7 (4–10)
Triage sieve (heart rate)	45 (37–54)	88 (86–90)	6 (4–10)
CareFlight triage	82 (75–88)	96 (94–97)	99 (56–176)

Source: From Garner et al. Comparative analysis of multiple-casualty incident triage algorithms. Ann Emerg Med. 2001;38:541–548. With permission from the American College of Emergency Physicians.

CONCLUSION

Disasters and mass casualty incidents are among the most intimidating occurrences a physician can face. Adding to their inherent difficult nature is the fact that they are always unexpected. In such an event, the ED becomes the center of patient care as well as community support. The physician will frequently be placed in a leadership role. Proper handling of a large-scale event requires a fluency in the principles of disaster and mass casualty medicine, as well as a familiarity with available assets. With knowledge, preparation, and good judgment, one can deliver quality medical care even in the most trying times.

Suggested Reading

Auf der Heide E. Disaster planning, part II: disaster problems, issues, and challenges identified in the research literature. *Emerg Med Clin North Am.* 1996;14:453–480.

Brewer RD, Morris PD, Cole TB. Hurricane-related emergency department visits in an inland area: an analysis of the public health impact of Hurricane Hugo in North Carolina. *Ann Emerg Med.* 1994;23:731–736.

Burkle FM, Sanner PH, Wolcott BW (eds). *Disaster Medicine: Application for the Immediate Management and Triage of Civilian and Military Disaster Victims.* New Hyde Park, NY: Medical Examination Publishing Co. 1984.

Cayne B (ed). *New Webster's Dictionary and Thesaurus of the English Language.* Danbury, CT: Lexicon Publications. 1993.

Committee of Trauma, American College of Surgeons. *Advanced Trauma Life Support for Doctors.* Chicago, IL: American College of Surgeons. 1997.

Cox RD. Decontamination and management of hazardous materials exposure victims in the emergency department. *Ann Emerg Med.* 1994;23:761–770.

Dacey MJ. Tragedy and response—the Rhode Island nightclub fire. *N Engl J Med.* 2003;349:1990–1992.

Gans L. Disaster planning and management. In: Harwood-Nuss A (ed). *The Clinical Practice of Emergency Medicine.* 3rd ed. Philadelphia, PA: Lippincott Williams & Wilkins. 2001.

Garner A, Lee A, Harrison K, et al. Comparative analysis of multiple-casualty incident triage algorithms. *Ann Emerg Med.* 2001;38:541–548.

Hick JL, Hanfling D, Burstein JL, et al. Protective equipment for health care facility decontamination personnel: regulations, risks, and recommendations. *Ann Emerg Med.* 2003;42:370–380.

Hogan DE, Waeckerle JF, Dire DJ, et al. Emergency department impact of the Oklahoma City terrorist bombing. *Ann Emerg Med.* 1999;34:160–167.

Horton DK, Berkowitz Z, Kaye WE. Secondary contamination of ED personnel from hazardous materials event, 1995–2001. *Am J Emerg Med.* 2003;21:199–204.

Kaji AH, Waeckerle JF. Disaster medicine and the emergency medicine resident. *Ann Emerg Med.* 2003;41:865–870.

Kales SN, Christiani DC. Acute chemical emergencies. *N Engl J Med.* 2004;350:800–808.

Kennedy K, Aghababian RV, Gans L, et al. Triage: techniques and applications in decisionmaking. *Ann Emerg Med.* 1996;28:136–144.

Lai TI, Shih FY, Chiang WC, et al. Strategies of disaster response in the health care system for tropical cyclones: experiences following typhoon Nari in Taipei City. *Acad Emerg Med.* 2003;10:1109–1112.

Lanoix R, Wiener DE, Zayas VD. Concepts in disaster triage in the wake of the World Trade Center terrorist attack. *Top Emerg Med.* 2002;24:60–71.

Lovejoy JC. Initial approach to patient management after large-scale disasters. *Clin Ped Emerg Med.* 2002;3:217–223.

Macintyre AG, Christopher GW, Eitzen E, et al. Weapons of mass destruction events with contaminated casualties: effective planning for health care facilities. *JAMA.* 2000;283:242–249.

North CS, Tivis L, Mcmillen JC, et al. Coping, functioning, and adjustment of rescue workers after the Oklahoma City bombing. *J Trauma Stress.* 2002;15:171–175.

Okumura T, Suzuki K, Atsuhiro F, et al. The Tokyo subway sarin attack: disaster management, part 1: community emergency response. *Acad Emerg Med.* 1998;5:613–617.

Okumura T, Suzuki K, Fukada A, et al. The Tokyo subway sarin attack: disaster management, part 2: healthcare facility response. *Acad Emerg Med.* 1998;5:618–624.

San Mateo County Health Services Agency. *HEICS The Hospital Emergency Incident Command System.* San Mateo, CA: San Mateo County Health Services Agency. Available at: *http://www.heics.com* Accessed January 19, 2004.

Tzu S. *The Art of War.* London, UK: Oxford University Press. 1963.

Waeckerle JF, Seamans S, Whiteside M, et al. Executive summary: developing objectives, content, and competencies for the training of emergency medical technicians, emergency physicians, and emergency nurses to care for casualties resulting from nuclear, biological, or chemical (NBC) incidents. *Ann Emerg Med.* 2001;37:587–601.

Waeckerle JF. Disaster planning and response. *N Engl J Med.* 1991;324:815–821.

21

HAZARDOUS MATERIALS (HAZMAT) EMERGENCIES

Richard G. Thomas and Frank G. Walter

STAT FACTS

HAZARDOUS MATERIALS (HAZMAT) EMERGENCIES

- A vast majority of agents involve gases or vapors with inhalation being the most common route of exposure.
- Regional poison centers should be contacted in hazardous substance exposure incidents.
- Water-soluble compounds can be decontaminated dermally with water ("like dissolves like").
- Fit-testing must occur prior to respirator use.

INTRODUCTION

A hazardous materials emergency involves the uncontrolled or unexpected release of a hazardous material that produces an actual or potential exposure to the environment including humans and animals. The release of these materials may be the result of an industrial accident or an act of terrorism. Regardless of the cause, the medical response to a hazmat incident focuses on the care of patients exposed to these hazardous materials. The general principles of toxicology apply whether a patient is at the site of the release, in a prehospital triage and treatment area, or in a hospital emergency department (ED) or intensive care unit. Although patient-care resources vary among these treatment settings, the fundamental principles of patient care remain the same.

Because the number of hazardous materials is so large, it is efficient to group hazardous materials according to their toxicological characteristics. Various classification systems have been devised. Individual hazmat studies commonly utilize their own classification systems, emphasizing the toxicodynamic effects of hazardous materials such as systemic asphyxiants or highlighting individual chemicals such as ammonia or chlorine or general classes of chemicals such as acids, bases, or volatile organic compounds (VOCs).

EPIDEMIOLOGY

Although hazardous materials incidents are not a new phenomena, a systematic study of these events has only begun in recent years. Three sources of information provide a better but limited picture of these events. These sources are the U.S. Department of Transportation (U.S. DOT), the Agency for Toxic Substances and Disease Registry (ATSDR), part of the National Institute of Environmental Health (NIEH) at the Centers for Disease Control (CDC), and articles from the medical literature involving small case series and anecdotal reports.

Because U.S. DOT regulates transportation of hazardous materials, it has been collecting data on hazmat incidents since 1971. During the period of 1990–1998, there was a 72% increase in the number of transportation incidents involving hazardous materials with more than 16,000 incidents occurring in 1994. During this same time, the average annual number of serious incidents was 407, deaths averaged 11 per year and more than 17,000 people were evacuated annually due to hazardous materials transportation accidents.

Utilizing the Hazardous Substances Emergency Events Surveillance (HSEES) database, ATSDR reported its data from 13 states from both transportation and fixed facility-based incidents. These data show that the vast majority of hazmat incidents do not result in human injury. Of 53,142 hazmat incidents, only 4413 incidents (9%) produced toxic exposures. Hazardous material releases are often depicted as causing morbidity and mortality in a large number of victims. The HSEES data show that 60% of incidents involve only one victim and 72% of incidents involve only one to two victims.

The vast majority of these victims do not require hospital admission. Of 8126 total victims, 24% were treated on scene and released, 3% were transported to a hospital, observed and released without treatment; 51% were transported, received treatment in the emergency room and then discharged; 8% were transported and subsequently admitted to a hospital; and 6% were never seen at a hospital but rather went to their private physicians' offices within 24 hours of the incident.

Hazmat incidents can result in fatalities as well as injuries. The HSEES data for 4413 patient-producing hazmat incidents resulted in 17,743 patients, of whom 244 (1%) died. For the period of 1993–1997, there were 63 deaths in 36 fatal incidents. The majority of these incidents, 26 of 36 (72%) occurred at fixed facilities, with 10 of 36 (28%) being transportation-related. Among the 63 total fatalities, 6% were responding rescue personnel. Explosions killed 16 of the 63 victims (25%). Rescue personnel and health-care providers must focus on the whole patient and not just poisoning because hazmat victims can also have injuries caused by vehicular crashes, explosions, or thermal burns.

The substances most commonly encountered at hazmat incidents vary from one locale to another and are predominately determined by the major industries in a particular area. For example, pesticides are the most commonly encountered class of hazardous materials in Fresno County, located in the California Central Valley, where the major industry is agribusiness. The HSEES data show that the top categories of agents for fixed facilities (FF) and transportation (T) incidents include VOCs (FF-21%, T-16%), inorganics (FF-27%, T-12%), acids (FF-7%, T-14%), pesticides (T-8%), ammonia (FF-7%), bases (T-7%), and mixtures (FF-12%). Of particular significance was the finding that regardless of the site of release, 85% of hazardous material exposures are due to a single agent.

The vast majority of these agents are released as gases or vapors. One study reported that inhalation was the most common route of exposure at hazmat incidents and was the route of exposure at 73% of the hazmat incidents, accounting for 76% of the exposed patients. This finding is important for two reasons. The first is that most victims will need respiratory-related treatments instead of other types of therapy. The second is that gases do not cause percutaneous absorption and therefore victims do not require decontamination with water. It is estimated that 80% of residual vapors are trapped in the victim's clothes and hair. Therefore the risk of secondary contamination to rescuers and health-care workers from gas or vapor exposure victims is small and can usually be eliminated by the removal of the victim's clothing. (See Primary and Secondary Contamination below.)

This conclusion is supported by the HSEES data that showed that through 2001 in 2562 HSEES events where victims were transported to a hospital, only 0.2% or approximately 50 incidents resulted in ED personnel being affected by secondary exposure. In every instance, none of the ED personnel injured wore any form of respiratory protection at the time of their exposure. Respiratory tract and eye irritation were the primary symptoms and no employees required hospitalization.

Substance Identification

Once a hazardous materials emergency has been recognized, responders must know what the material is and its potential health effects. Obviously, exact identification is desirable but not always possible. Information with regard to the site of the hazmat incident, the type of business, laboratory, or vehicle involved allows hazmat responders to safely search for and identify essential placards or documents. Fixed facility placards, vehicular placards, material safety data sheets (MSDSs), bills of lading, shipping documents, inventory sheets, verbal information from employees and management are potential sources of information.

HAZARDOUS MATERIALS AND HAZMAT RESPONSE

Chemical Names and Numbers

Chemical compounds may be known by several names, including the chemical, common, generic, or brand (proprietary) name. A chemical may be the sole substance in a given hazardous material or one of several compounds in a mixture.

The Chemical Abstracts Service (CAS) of the American Chemical Society (ACS) numbers chemicals to overcome the confusion regarding multiple names for a single chemical. The CAS assigns a unique CAS registry number (CAS#) to atoms, molecules, and mixtures. For example, the CAS# of methanol is 67–56–1. These numbers provide a unique identification for chemicals as well as a means for cross-checking chemical names. Identifying a chemical by name and CAS# is critical because one must be as specific as possible about the hazardous material in question. Trade or brand names can be misleading. The MSDS describing a product usually lists the chemical name, the CAS#, and the brand name.

Vehicular Placarding: United Nations Numbers, North America Numbers, and Product Identification Numbers

Substances in each hazard class of the International Hazard Classification System (IHCS) are assigned four-digit identification numbers, which are known as United

Nations (UN), North American (NA), or Product Identification Numbers (PIN) and are displayed on characteristic vehicular placards. This system is used by the U.S. DOT in the *Emergency Response Guidebook*. The IHCS assigns a chemical to a hazard class based on its most dangerous physical characteristic, such as explosiveness or flammability. Other potential hazards of an agent, such as its ability to cause cancer or birth defects, are not considered. This system provides very little guidance in treating poisonings caused by hazardous materials.

National Fire Protection Association 704 System for Fixed Facility Placarding

Fixed facilities such as hospitals or laboratories use a placarding system that is different from the vehicular placarding system. The National Fire Protection Association (NFPA) 704 system is used at most fixed facilities. The NFPA system uses a diamond-shaped sign that is divided into four color-coded quadrants: red, yellow, white, and blue. This system gives hazmat responders information about the flammability, reactivity, health effects, and also other information, such as the water reactivity, oxidizing activity, or radioactivity.

The red quadrant on top indicates flammability, the blue quadrant on the left indicates health hazard, the yellow quadrant on the right indicates reactivity, and the white quadrant on the bottom is for other information, such as OXY for an oxidizing product, W for a product that has unusual reactivity with water, and the standard radioactive symbol for radioactive substances.

Numbers in the red, blue, and yellow quadrants indicate the degree of hazard: numbers range from 0, which is minimal, to 4, which is severe and indicate specific levels of hazard.

Like all placarding systems, this one also has limitations. It does not name the specific hazardous substances in the facility and gives no information about the quantities or locations of the materials.

HAZARDOUS SUBSTANCE INFORMATION INCLUDING TOXIC EFFECTS

If the name of the substance is known before arrival at the scene, then research can begin en route with reviews of the physical, chemical, and toxicologic properties of the material. If the chemical is not known before arrival at the scene, efforts to obtain this information should begin as soon as safely possible. Responder safety is a priority.

A regional poison control center is an extremely valuable resource in the assessment and management of hazardous materials incidents involving human exposures. Poison control centers are staffed 24/7 by health professionals trained and experienced in identifying products and their ingredients, assessing the clinical symptoms of the victims and providing toxicologic and treatment information.

Poison control centers are linked by a national toll-free number, 1-800-222-1222, which routes calls to the closest center from the incident.

CHEMTREC is a service of the Chemical Manufacturers Association. It has information about shippers, products, and manufacturers. CHEMTREC can be reached at 1–800–424–9300. The Internet address for CHEMTREC is *http://www.chemtrec.org*. CHEMTREC provides information at no charge, 24 hours a day. Details of an incident are relayed to the shipper's or manufacturer's 24-hour emergency contacts, and they, in turn, are linked to hazmat incident responders. Technical data are available on handling the substance(s) involved, including the physical characteristics, transportation, and disposal.

Other information sources include local and state health departments, the American Conference of Governmental and Industrial Hygienists (ACGIH), the Occupational Safety and Health Administration (OSHA), National Institutes of Occupational Safety and Health (NIOSH), Agency for Toxic Substances and Disease Registry (ATSDR), and the Centers for Disease Control and Prevention (CDC).

Even if the exact identity of the toxic material is not known, hazmat responders may be able to classify the hazardous material into one of several major toxicologic classes by identifying a hazmat toxidrome that allows them to reasonably treat the patient and protect themselves and others; for example, do patients have irritation of the mucous membranes and upper airway caused by a highly water-soluble irritant gas? Do the patients exhibit signs of asphyxia with major central nervous system and/or cardiopulmonary signs and symptoms? Do patients exhibit signs of cholinergic excess caused by organic phosphorus compounds or carbamate poisoning? Do patients exhibit chemical burns compatible with corrosives? Do patients have the odor of solvents with signs of CNS depression and cardiac irritability, compatible with exposure to hydrocarbons or halogenated hydrocarbons?

PHYSICAL PROPERTIES OF A HAZARDOUS MATERIAL

Physical State

Even when the exact identity of the hazardous material is not known, what is usually known is the physical state of the material, that is, solid, liquid, or gas. Airborne toxicants potentially mean many more victims. Airborne toxicants include not only gases and vapors but also the liquid suspensions, fog and mists, and the solid suspensions, smoke, fumes, and dusts. The physical state of a material determines how it will spread through the environment and gives clues to the potential route(s) of exposure for the material.

Unless moved by physical means such as wind, ventilation systems or people, solids will usually stay in one area.

Solids can cause exposures by inhalation of dusts, by ingestion, or rarely by absorption through skin and mucous membranes. Solids that undergo sublimation, changing directly from a solid into a gas without passing through the liquid state, can give off vapors that can cause airborne exposure. Only two commonly encountered solids sublime, dry ice and naphthalene. A vapor is defined as a gaseous dispersion of the molecules of a substance that is normally a liquid or a solid at standard temperature and pressure (STP), that is, 0°C (32°F = 273 K) and 1 atm (760 torr = 760 mm Hg = 14.7 psi). Uncontained liquids will spread over surfaces and flow downhill. Liquids can evaporate, creating a vapor hazard.

Vapor Pressure

The vapor pressure (VP) is useful to estimate whether enough of a solid or liquid will be released in the gaseous state to pose an inhalation risk. VP is defined essentially as the quantity of the gaseous state overlying an evaporating liquid or a subliming solid. The lower the VP, the less likely the chemical will volatilize and generate a respirable gas. Conversely, the higher the VP of a chemical, the more likely it will volatilize or generate a respirable gas. Water has a VP of approximately 20 mm Hg at 70°F (21°C), and acetone has a VP of 250 mm Hg at the same temperature. Therefore, acetone evaporates more rapidly than water and poses more of an inhalation risk. Standard reference texts (*NIOSH Pocket Guide to Chemical Hazards Merck Index*) list VPs for commonly encountered chemicals.

Water Solubility

The water solubility of a hazardous material determines whether water alone is sufficient for skin decontamination or whether a detergent must also be used. The general rule regarding solubility is that "like dissolves like." In other words, a polar solvent, such as water, will dissolve polar substances such as salts. For example, the herbicide paraquat is actually a salt, paraquat dichloride, that is, miscible in water. Therefore, if a patient's skin is contaminated with paraquat, copious water irrigation is sufficient for skin decontamination. A mild liquid detergent is acceptable but is not necessary. On the other hand, a nonpolar solvent, such as toluene, is not water-soluble and is immiscible. Therefore, if a patient's skin is contaminated with toluene, water irrigation alone may be insufficient for decontamination, and a mild liquid detergent is also necessary.

CONTAMINATION AND DECONTAMINATION

Primary and Secondary Contamination

Understanding the physical properties of a hazardous material can help health-care providers determine whether the hazardous material presents a significant risk of secondary contamination and whether decontamination of the skin and mucous membranes is necessary.

Primary contamination is defined as contamination of people or equipment caused by direct contact with the initial release of a hazardous material at its source of release. Primary contamination can occur whether the hazardous material is a solid, a liquid, or a gas.

Secondary contamination is defined as contamination of health-care personnel or equipment caused by exposure to a patient or equipment that experienced primary contamination and has been removed from the source of the hazardous material release. Secondary contamination generally occurs only with solids or liquids although off-gassing can possibly cause secondary contamination and exposure.

DECONTAMINATION

Contamination is the act or process of rendering something harmful or unsuitable for use. Harmful means injurious to health (toxic) or able to cause physical or psychological damage. Unsuitable means unable to be used or adapted for a particular purpose. Decontamination is then employed to prevent or limit the toxic, physical or psychological injury from a hazardous material, as well make physical objects available for use. There are three primary purposes for decontamination:

- To prevent injury or further harm to a person by terminating their exposure to a hazardous substance.
- To avoid injury or harm to the unexposed by preventing an exposure from taking place.
- To make objects suitable for use again (e.g., equipment, etc).

Patients or equipment with primary contamination to solids in the form of dusts or powders should be decontaminated before transportation to prevent secondary contamination of health-care providers and equipment. Primary contamination from dusts and powders can occur in a variety of situations including exposure to aerosols. Aerosols are airborne toxicants that are not gases. Aerosols are suspensions of solids or liquids in air, such as solid dusts or nonvolatile liquid sprays or mists. Often the amounts that result in dermal exposures are exceedingly small because of the large dilution factor of the air. However depending on the substance, even small amounts may present a risk of secondary contamination, for example, radioactive substances, anthrax spores, and so forth. These patients will require decontamination with water and perhaps soap.

Another instance where decontamination may be appropriate occurs when there is exposure to high concentrations of a highly water-soluble irritant gas in a patient who has had sweaty skin at the time of the exposure. Gases such as ammonia and chlorine mix with the water in sweat to produce corrosive ammonium hydroxide and hydrochloric acid, respectively. In these cases, victims will usually complain of burning or irritated skin. Decontamination with water is appropriate treatment of the patient's skin irritation or chemical burns.

Hazmat Scene Control Zones

Scene management is a fundamental feature at a hazmat incident. It is almost always necessary to isolate the scene, deny access to the public and the media, and limit access to emergency response personnel in order to prevent needless contamination and exposure. Three control zones are established around a scene and are described either by "temperature," "color," or "explanatory terminology." NIOSH, the U.S. Environmental Protection Agency (EPA), and most American prehospital and hospital health-care professionals use the temperature terminology system.

The *hot zone* is the area immediately surrounding a hazardous materials incident. It extends far enough to prevent the primary contamination of people and materials outside this zone. Primary contamination can occur to those who enter this zone. In general, evacuation, but no decontamination or patient care, is carried out in this zone, except for opening the airway and placing the patient on a backboard with spine precautions. This is because rescuers are generally hazmat technicians who wear level A suits that severely limit visibility and dexterity.

The *warm zone* is the area surrounding the hot zone and contains the decontamination or access corridor where victims, the hazmat entry team members, and their equipment are decontaminated. It includes two control points for the access corridor.

The *cold zone* is the area beyond the warm zone. Contaminated victims and hazmat responders should be decontaminated before entering this area from the warm zone. Equipment and personnel are not expected to become contaminated in this zone. This is the area where resources are assembled to support the hazmat emergency response. The incident command center is usually located in the cold zone, and definitive patient care is conducted here. This zone includes the primary survey and resuscitation with management of airway (with cervical spine control), breathing, circulation, disability, and exposure with evaluation for toxicity and trauma. Definitive care also includes antidotal treatment for specific poisonings.

PERSONAL PROTECTIVE EQUIPMENT

A critical goal of hazmat emergency responders is protecting themselves as well as the public. Safeguarding hazmat responders includes wearing appropriate personal protective equipment (PPE) to (1) prevent exposure to the hazard and (2) prevent injury to the wearer from incorrect use of or malfunction of the PPE equipment.

PPE can create significant health hazards, including loss of cooling by evaporation, heat stress, physical stress, psychological stress, impaired vision, impaired mobility, and impaired communication. Because of these risks, individuals involved in hazmat emergency response must be trained regarding the appropriate use, decontamination, maintenance, and storage of PPE. This training includes instruction regarding the risk of permeation, penetration, and degradation of PPE. PPE with a self-contained breathing apparatus (SCBA) has a fixed supply of air that significantly limits the amount of time the wearer can operate in the hot zone, usually about 20 minutes.

Levels of Protection

The EPA defines four levels of protection for PPE, levels A (highest) through D (lowest). The different levels of PPE are designed to provide a choice of PPE, depending on the hazards at a specific hazmat incident. *Level A* provides the highest level of both respiratory and skin (clothing) protection and provides vapor protection to the respiratory tract, mucous membranes, and the skin. This level of PPE is airtight, and the breathing apparatus must be worn under the suit. *Level B* provides the highest level of respiratory protection but less skin protection. Level B provides skin splash protection by using chemical-resistant clothing. *Level C* protection should be used when the type of airborne substance is known, when its concentration can be measured, when the criteria for using air-purifying respirators are met, and when skin and eye exposures are unlikely. Level C provides skin splash protection, the same as level B; however, level C has a lower level of respiratory protection than either level A or B. *Level D* is basically a regular work uniform. It should not be worn when significant chemical respiratory or skin hazards exist. It provides no respiratory protection and minimal skin protection.

Respiratory Protection

Personnel must be fit-tested before using any respirator. A tiny space between the edge of the respirator and the face of the hazmat responder could permit exposure to an airborne hazard. Contact lenses cannot be worn with any respiratory protective equipment. Corrective eyeglass lenses must be mounted inside the face mask of the PPE. The only exception to these general rules are the use of hooded level C powered air purifying respirators (PAPRs) that do not require fit-testing and allow individuals to wear their own eyeglasses within the hooded PAPR.

HAZMAT INCIDENT RESPONSE RULES AND STANDARDS

The U.S. Labor Department's OSHA and the nonprofit standards setting organization, the NFPA, have developed, respectively, rules and guidelines regarding hazmat incident response. OSHA rules are mandated as law and must be followed. Meeting NFPA guidelines will ensure OSHA compliance.

The Superfund Amendments and Reauthorization Act of 1986, known as SARA, required OSHA to develop and implement standards to protect employees responding to hazardous materials emergencies. This resulted in the "Hazardous Waste Operations and Emergency Response" standard, 29 CFR 1910.120, or HAZWOPER. This regulation defines the various levels of training those responders to hazardous material incidents should receive. There are three levels: awareness, operational, and hazmat technician.

NFPA 471, "Recommended Practice for Responding to Hazardous Materials Incidents," outlines the following tactical objectives: incident response planning, communication procedures, response levels, site safety, control zones, PPE, incident mitigation, decontamination, and medical monitoring.

NFPA 472, "Standard on Professional Competence of Responders to Hazardous Materials Incidents," helps define the minimum skills, knowledge, and standards for training outlined in HAZWOPER for the following three types of responders.

ADVANCED HAZMAT COMPONENTS

Advanced Hazmat Providers

Paramedics are trained in the recognition of signs and symptoms caused by exposure to hazardous materials, and the delivery of antidotal therapy to victims of hazmat poisonings. The inclusion of such training into a department's hazmat response team is beneficial, not only for the needs of the public but also to protect hazmat technicians who make entry into hazardous atmospheres. Ideally, hazmat technician entry into hazardous atmospheres should not be performed, unless appropriately trained paramedics are standing by, on scene, with resuscitative equipment in place, including a drug box containing essential antidotes for specific hazardous materials.

Medical Control

Obtaining medical control should begin early in the development of the hazmat team. Incidents involving hazardous materials can have far-reaching community implications. The ideal medical director for a hazardous materials team should be board certified in medical toxicology and should be familiar with the operations and logistics of functioning in the prehospital environment. This physician should be consulted in all aspects of planning for a hazmat response. In addition to developing training curricula and treatment plans for toxic exposures, this physician can work with emergency responders and hospitals to help integrate emergency personnel into the incident command structure and assist with the logistics of decontamination and hospital preparedness for victims of hazmat incidents.

Online, direct medical control plays an important role in caring for hazmat victims. Contact with medical control should be established as soon as possible after deciding that hot zone entry is necessary. This prealert notification allows the physician and hospital staff to be prepared to institute contingency plans when patients are identified who may require transport to a receiving facility.

Medical control should also include consultation with a regional poison control center, if possible. Field personnel should be familiar with how to access information through the poison center. Medical toxicologists and poison information specialists should be available at the poison center. Similarly, the poison center should be familiar with the level of training of responding EMS personnel.

Patient-Care Responsibilities of the Prehospital Decontamination Team and the Hazmat Entry Team

Hazmat responders should identify the entry and exit areas by controlling points for the access corridor (decontamination corridor) from the hot zone, through the warm zone, to the cold zone. This corridor should be upwind, uphill, and upstream from the hot zone, if possible. Hazmat technician entry team members should remove victims from the contaminated hot zone and deliver patients to the inner control point of the access (decontamination) corridor. Hazmat decontamination team members decontaminate patients in the decontamination (access) corridor of the contamination reduction (warm) zone. After decontamination, hazmat responders deliver patients to paramedics in the cold zone.

The primary responsibility of the *prehospital hazmat medical sector* is the protection of the hazmat entry team personnel. This is accomplished by researching and recording clinically pertinent information about the hazardous material remaining available on scene for medical treatment, and assessing individuals before entry into, and on exit from, a hazardous environment. Documentation of each assessment should be recorded on a prepared form and compared to the exclusion criteria defined by NFPA 471. A position in the hazmat medical sector should be held by advanced hazmat-trained individuals, preferably with operational level responder competency and ideally with hazmat technician level competency.

Patient-Care Responsibilities of EMS Paramedics at Hazmat Incidents

EMS paramedics who are not part of the hazmat team should report to the incident staging area and await direction from the incident commander. They should approach the site from upwind, uphill, and upstream, if possible.

EMS paramedics should remain in the cold zone until properly protected hazmat incident responders arrive, decontaminate, and deliver patients to them for further triage. Then, paramedics should evaluate each patient, direct patients without complaints to the occupant staging area, and take patients with complaints to the patient staging area. A paramedic should stay with the patients in the occupant staging area to continually reevaluate these asymptomatic victims and transfer them to the patient staging area if they do become symptomatic. Patients leaving the occupant staging area should receive instructions regarding potential signs and symptoms that may develop that will necessitate their subsequent evaluation at a health-care facility.

Initial EMS patient care takes place in the cold zone's patient staging area, including medical management of hazmat victims. Decontamination should not be necessary because EMS paramedics in the cold zone should care only for decontaminated patients or patients who did not have skin contamination.

Transportation of patients from the hazmat incident is ultimately under the control of the incident commander but is usually delegated to the prehospital medical sector and EMS paramedics in consultation with a base hospital physician. In general, no victim with skin contamination should be transported from the hazmat site without being properly decontaminated. Before transportation, EMS should notify the base hospital of the number of victims being transported, as well as their toxicological history, patient assessments, and treatment rendered. The base hospital physician may have additional orders, either before or after consultation with the poison control center and/or a medical toxicologist. If a patient is to be transported to a hospital other than the base hospital, the receiving hospital should be contacted.

EMERGENCY DEPARTMENT RESPONSIBILITIES FOR HAZMAT VICTIMS

It is critical that hospitals be involved with community hazmat planning to ensure that there is a coordinated response to these incidents in the event that there are human victims. Since 2001, many, but not all, hospitals and EDs have dramatically improved their decontamination equipment, and their ability to use PPE. OSHA recently provided specific guidance for hospitals in the document, *OSHA Best Practices for Hospital Based First Receivers of Victims from Mass Casualty Incidents Involving the Release of Hazardous Substances*. However, given the infrequency with which these events occur and the small number of victims from a typical incident, it is an ongoing challenge for hospitals to maintain a state of readiness. In addition, mass casualty hazmat incidents occur so rarely that most hospitals will never have the need to decontaminate more than one to two victims.

In those singular events when there is a large number of victims from a chemical release, it should be the goal to perform field decontamination for all hazmat victims when decontamination is necessary. However, it is very likely that in these incidents where there are numerous victims, as many as 80% will self-evacuate from the scene and deliver themselves to the nearest hospital without the benefit of decontamination. Whether it is a few victims or many, all hospitals should have established protocols by which designated hospital staff members triage victims for life-saving treatment and decontaminate them. Patients without life-threatening problems but who carry a significant risk of secondary contamination should be denied entry to the ED until decontamination is accomplished by a properly trained and equipped hospital response team. The emergency physician or some other predesignated staff member will determine when any patient is safe to enter the ED.

Hospital Decontamination

Exposures solely to gases or vapors, such as simple asphyxiants, low concentrations of irritant gasses or VOCs, generally require no skin or mucous membrane decontamination with water to prevent secondary contamination of others. These victims may need no decontamination or may undergo "dry" decontamination where they simply disrobe to their under clothing, put on a disposable or washable outer garment, and their clothing is bagged and tagged for later disposition.

When indicated by the presence of dusts, powders, or liquids on a patient, "wet" decontamination of the skin with water should be performed in an area outside the ED if weather conditions permit or in a well-ventilated room that does not share air circulation with the rest of the hospital. This type of decontamination is a multistep procedure and applies to both ambulatory and nonambulatory patients. After placing the victim in an area where modesty can be protected, all personal effects such as jewelry, wallets, car keys, etc. should be removed and placed in a bag and tagged with the patient's name. These personal possessions can later be returned to the victim after they are decontaminated or it is determined that decontamination is unnecessary. All clothing should be placed in another, larger bag, sealed and tagged for later disposition. Next the victim should wash with water and a mild liquid detergent if the adherent solids or liquids are not water-soluble or if the identity of the material is unknown. Most decontamination solutions are made for equipment, not people. Do not use these potentially irritating solutions on people. Pay close attention to all exposed skin and in particular the skin folds, the axillae, the genital area, and the feet. Use lukewarm water with gentle water pressure to reduce the risk of hypothermia.

Exposed, symptomatic eyes should be continuously irrigated with water throughout the patient contact, including transport, if possible. Remember to check for and remove contact lenses. Use of therapeutic lenses is the most efficient method to decontaminate a patient's eyes, but this requires using an ocular topical anesthetic such as proparacaine.

In contrast to the scene of a hazardous material release where there are three functional areas, there are only two functional areas at a hospital receiving hazardous material–exposed patients. The hospital decontamination zone includes any areas where the type and quantity of hazardous substance is unknown and where contaminated victims, contaminated equipment, or contaminated waste may be present. It is in this area that it can be reasonably anticipated that employees might have exposure to contaminated victims, their belongings, equipment, or waste. In the hospital decontamination zone, patients will receive their initial triage and/or medical stabilization, be staged in predecontamination waiting/staging areas for victims, and be decontaminated. This area will typically end at the ED door. This area corresponds to the "warm zone" in the prehospital setting. The hospital postdecontamination zone is an area that is considered uncontaminated. Equipment and personnel are not expected to become contaminated here. At a hospital receiving contaminated victims, the hospital postdecontamination zone includes the ED (unless contaminated). This zone corresponds to the "cold zone" in hazardous material incidents.

SUMMARY

In summary, hazmat incident response is an integrated, interdisciplinary approach involving prehospital, hospital, poison center, and public health professionals. Incidents may occur at fixed facilities or in transportation accidents. Most patients from a hazardous material release are exposed through inhalation of a gas or vapor. The general principles of toxicology apply regardless of whether a patient is at the scene of a hazmat incident or in the hospital setting. Although patient-care resources vary among these treatment settings, the fundamental principles of patient care remain the same. All patients should receive a primary survey and resuscitation, emphasizing airway, breathing, circulation. Prehospital and hospital personnel must use appropriate PPE when caring for patients that have not been decontaminated. Decontamination is critical to alter absorption for the patient and to prevent secondary contamination of downstream health-care providers and equipment.

Suggested Reading

Agency for Toxic Substances and Disease Registry: Web page *www.atsdr.cdc.gov*

Berkowitz Z, Haugh GS, Orr MF, et al. Releases of hazardous substances in schools: data from Hazardous Substances Emergency Events Surveillance system, 1993–1998. *J Environ Health.* 2002;65:20–27.

Berkowitz Z, Orr MF, Kay WE, et al. Hazardous substances emergency events in the agricultural industry and related services in four mid-western states. *J Occup Environ Med.* 2002;44:714–723.

Berkowitz Z, Barnhart HX, Kaye WE. Factors associated with severity of injury resulting from acute releases of hazardous substances in the manufacturing industry. *J Occup Environ Med.* 2003;45:734–742.

Burgess JL, Blackmon GM, Brodkin CA, et al. Hospital preparedness for hazardous materials incidents and treatment of contaminated patients. *West J Med.* 1997;167:387–391.

Burgess JL. Hospital evacuations due to hazardous materials incidents. *Am J Emerg Med.* 1999;17(1)50–52.

Burgess JL, Kovalchick DF, Harter L, et al. Hazardous materials events: an industrial comparison. *J Occup Environ Med.* 2000;42:546–553.

Cox RD. Decontamination and management of hazardous materials exposure victims in the emergency department. *Ann Emerg Med.* 1994;23:761–770.

Hall HI, Haugh GS, Price-Green PA, et al. Risk factors for hazardous substance releases that result in injuries and evacuations: data from 9 states. *Am J Public Health.* 1996;86:855–857.

Horton KD, Berkowitz Z, Kaye WE. Secondary contamination of ED personnel from hazardous materials events, 1995–2001. *Am J Emerg Med.* 2003;21:199–204.

Horton DK, Berkowitz Z, Kaye WE. Surveillance of hazardous materials events in 17 states, 1993–2001: a report from the hazardous substances emergency events surveillance (HSEES) system. *Am J Ind Med.* 2004;45:539–548.

Kirk MA, Cisek J, Rose SR. Emergency department response to hazardous materials incidents. *Emerg Med Clin North Am.* 1994;12(2):461–481.

National Institute of Occupational Safety and Health. Web page: *www.cdc.gov/niosh*

OSHA. Web page: *www.osha.gov.* Notes available by phone: 1–202–693–1999.

Walter FG, Bates G, Criss EA, et al. Hazardous materials incidents in a mid-sized metropolitan area. *Prehosp Emerg Care.* 2003;7:214–218.

22

ENHANCING HOSPITAL EMERGENCY PREPAREDNESS

Christina L. Catlett

S T A T   F A C T S

ENHANCING HOSPITAL EMERGENCY PREPAREDNESS

- The EMP should be based on incident command and compliant with Joint Commission and federal standards.
- Hospitals must plan for hazmat response, contagious disease outbreaks, and surge capacity.
- Health-care workers should be educated regarding the emergency operations plan and personal preparedness.

INTRODUCTION

Hospital emergency management programs (EMPs) have been evolving over the last several decades. Originally, hospital disaster plans were designed for natural and man-made disasters, such as earthquakes and transportation accidents, which are typically acute events with a finite number of victims. However, terrorism and emerging infectious diseases have changed the response paradigm and entered us into a new era of preparedness. A more comprehensive approach to disaster planning has evolved, one that looks beyond the emergency department (ED) or even the hospital and into the resources of the entire health-care system.

For years, the health-care industry has experienced significant obstacles to preparedness, not the least of which is fiscal constraints. The business model of just-in-time purchasing has led to minimal reserves of equipment, supplies, and medications. Hospital surge capacity is limited by downsizing of beds and staffing. Compensation for preparedness and response efforts is not guaranteed. Despite these challenges, most hospitals clearly acknowledge the need for a

robust EMP and are devoting significant resources to improving emergency preparedness. The following recent events have provided impetus for such planning:

- 2001—The terrorist attacks of September 11 and subsequent anthrax attacks;
- 2003—The Rhode Island nightclub fire, the New York City blackout, and the emergence of severe acute respiratory syndrome (SARS);
- 2004—The Madrid train bombing and Asian tsunami;
- 2005—The London subway bombing, Hurricanes Katrina and Rita, the Pakistani earthquake, and the emergence of avian influenza; and,
- 2006—The Mumbai (Bombay) train bombing.

THE EMERGENCY MANAGEMENT PROGRAM

A hospital's EMP encompasses all aspects of emergency management, as mandated by the Joint Commission:

- *Mitigation*: Activities that lessen the impact of an emergency, including performance of a risk assessment and implementing strategies that address vulnerabilities.
- *Preparedness*: Activities that allow the hospital to manage the effects of an emergency, such as building a disaster resource database, developing and maintaining a robust emergency operations plan (EOP), and staff training and education.
- *Response*: Actions that include both staff and management responsibilities during an emergency.
- *Recovery*: Activities that allow the hospital to restore and resume normal operations as soon as possible following an event.

Most hospitals have an emergency management committee, a multidisciplinary group charged with understanding, reviewing, and improving the EMP. The EMP manager coordinates EMP activities, but ultimately senior hospital managers have the responsibility for development, implementation, and maintenance of the hospital's EMP.

Development and Maintenance of an Emergency Operations Plan

The EOP describes the hospital's response to both external and internal (within the hospital campus) events, including activation and implementation of emergency procedures and coordination with outside agencies. Its goal is to provide the best possible care for victims while protecting its staff and patients and maintaining the integrity of the facility.

Performance of a Hazard and Vulnerability Analysis

The Joint Commission requires that hospitals develop a hazard and vulnerability analysis to identify potential emergencies that could affect its operations, such as natural disasters, an accident or man-made disaster, or an intentional act of malice. The estimated probability of occurrence of one of these events may be plotted on a grid against the magnitude of impact that the event would have on the business operations of the hospital (Table 22-1). The resulting risk assessment matrix may be used as a planning platform for the health-care facility in the setting of limited resources and preparedness funding.

Performing an effective risk assessment may require input from local and regional experts, such as law enforcement, fire and emergency medical services (EMS), the military, the Federal Bureau of Investigation, the state's Emergency Management Agency, the Local Emergency Preparedness Committee, local and state public health agencies, and weapons of mass destruction experts. New information, world events, improved response capabilities, improved terrorist capabilities, and countermeasures at the federal, state, and local levels may change the likelihood of a disaster or attack occurring and/or its consequences; therefore, the risk assessment matrix must be frequently reassessed.

Adoption of an Incident Command System

The Joint Commission also requires the use of an identifiable management structure. The Hospital Incident Command System (HICS) is one command structure commonly used by the medical community (*www.emsa.ca.gov/hics/hics.asp*). HICS is an efficient and effective tool for hospital emergency response, providing a predictable chain of management, prioritized checklists for each position in the command structure (accountability), and language common to external response agencies to promote ease of communication and collaboration with other entities such as police, fire, and EMS. The implementation of an incident command system facilitates information management and effective decision-making and promotes a more organized response during emergency situations.

NIMS Compliance

In 2003, President Bush issued Homeland Security Presidential Directive-5 (HSPD-5), which directed the Department of Homeland Security (DHS) to develop and manage a National Incident Management System (NIMS). The purpose of NIMS is to provide a national template to allow all government, private-sector, and nongovernmental organizations to work together to manage any domestic incident, regardless of size or complexity. It is a flexible organizational framework that defines the requirements for processes, procedures, and systems to improve interoperability between responding entities.

HSPD-5 mandates state and local adoption of NIMS as a requirement for receipt of federal preparedness assistance funding. For example, in order to receive National Bioterrorism Hospital Preparedness Program funding from the Healthcare Resources and Services Administration (HRSA), awardees agree to adopt and implement the NIMS principles and policies, including the use of an incident command system such as HICS. It is important that those responsible for emergency preparedness at the hospital complete the required NIMS courses (located online at *http://training.fema.gov/EMIWeb/IS/crslist.asp*) and ensure that the emergency preparedness program is NIMS compliant.

STRATEGIES TO ENHANCE THE EMERGENCY MANAGEMENT PROGRAM

Building Redundant Communications Systems

In disaster literature, the most common issue raised in after-action reports of both disaster drills and actual disasters is communication. The problems are traditionally twofold: both communications device failure and lack of information sharing.

Building a robust and redundant communications infrastructure is imperative. Important factors to consider include cost effectiveness, ease of use of technology, dependability during a system overload, dependence on electrical power, and interoperability with existing communication systems. Whatever systems hospitals decide to use (see Table 22-2), multiple layers of redundancy ensure a backup means of communications when one or more technologies fail. The assistance of a systems engineer may be required to perform an analysis of available technology and a cost-benefit analysis of communications augmentation.

Possession of robust and redundant technology is only part of the equation. Efficient sharing of information and effective communication with hospital staff, patients, the

TABLE 22-1

PERFORMING A HAZARD VULNERABILITY ANALYSIS

Potential Threats to Hospital Operations

Internal Hazards

- Fire
- Structural failure
- Utility failure
- IT failure
- Hazardous materials

Natural Disasters

- Extreme heat/cold
- Severe weather incident (hurricane, tornado, blizzard, etc.)
- Flood
- Wildfire
- Soil movement
- Earthquake
- Natural epidemic

Man-Made Disasters

- Utility failure
- Major transportation accident
- Building fire/collapse
- Violent crime incident

- Hazmat accident
- Civil disturbance, riots
- Prison incident

Terrorist Attack

- Conventional explosive device
- Suicide bomber, other explosive attacks
- Aviation attack
- Noncontagious biological attack
- Contagious biological attack
- Chemical attack
- Dirty bomb/radiological dispersion device
- Critical infrastructure attack (e.g., water reservoir, power grid, telecommunications, cyber attack)
- Hospital attack
- Nuclear power plant attack
- Nuclear weapon attack
- Food contamination incident
- Attack on a chemical facility or chemical tanker
- Port attack

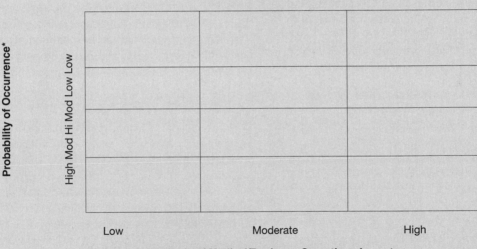

HAZARD VULNERABILITY ANALYSIS

Probability of Occurrence* — High Mod Hi Mod Low Low

Low   Moderate   High

Magnitude of Medical/Business Operations Impact

*Suggested guidance for determining probability

	Natural Disaster	*Man-made Disaster*	*Terrorist Attack*
High Probability	Occurs multiple times/ year in region	Occurs multiple times/year	Has occurred in the United States in last year
Mod High Probability	Occurs about once every 1–2 years	Occurs about once every 1–2 years	Has occurred in the United States (or to one of its allies) in last 10 years
Mod Low Probability	Occurs once every 10 years	Occurs once every 10 years	Has occurred in the United States or world in last 25 years
Low Probability	Does not typically occur in region	Does not typically occur in region	Unlikely to occur due to difficulty of attack

TABLE 22-2

SAMPLE COMMUNICATIONS MODALITIES

- Telephone (landlines and cellular)
- Blackberry devices
- Text pagers
- Fax machines
- Overhead announcements
- Handheld radios
- Internet (e-mail, Web sites, web-based disaster management software)
- Media: television and radio
- Runners
- Bullhorns
- Satellite phones
- Ham radios

general public, and other responding agencies are equally important but beyond the scope of this chapter.

Creation of a Resource Database

An inventory of critical resources allows for rapid location and deployment of hospital equipment, supplies, and personnel in disasters. The database should identify resource type, amount available, location, and contact information. It also allows key decision-makers to identify potential inadequacies or shortages during the planning phase. See Table 22-3 for an example of key resources to be considered for the database.

Developing Hospital Action Items for National Alert Level Changes

In the wake of September 11, DHS initiated the *Homeland Security Advisory System*, a color-coded threat level system used to communicate with public safety officials

TABLE 22-3

ITEMS FOR A RESOURCE DATABASE

- Total number of physical beds, stretchers, cots, reclining chairs, and wheelchairs in the hospital
- Number/type of medical and nonmedical personnel
- Major medical equipment (e.g., ventilators, dialysis machines, portable x-ray machines, etc.)
- Stockpiled medications, such as antibiotics, antidotes, and vaccines
- Communications capability
- Blood products
- Number/type/location of transportation vehicles
- Names and contact information of regional experts on topics such as hazardous materials, radiation, infectious disease
- Address, phone numbers, and key contacts of all regional response agencies
- Location and type of all surge capacity supplies
- Amenities of each possible alternate care site

TABLE 22-4

EXAMPLES OF HOSPITAL ACTION ITEMS FOR NATIONAL ALERT LEVEL CHANGES

Elevated (Yellow—Significant risk of terrorist attacks)
- Confirm employee contact numbers quarterly
- Managers conduct monthly reviews of disaster procedures
- Conduct weekly tests of communications systems
- Increase security monitoring

High (Orange—High risk of terrorist attacks)
- Test employee call-down lists
- Test communications with outside agencies
- All personnel to review disaster response plan
- Begin active education campaign for employees about threat if explicit
- Physicians preidentify dischargeable patients
- Prestage key disaster response supplies
- Increase security measures

and the general public so that certain protective measures can be implemented when specific information is received.

An increase in the national alert level, while concerning, does not directly translate into a change in operations for hospitals (unless accompanied by a Homeland Security Threat Advisory with actionable information). Hospitals can identify specific actions to correspond with each alert level, allowing a graded, organized response to an evolving situation. See Table 22-4 for an example of this strategy.

Emphasis on Personal Preparedness

Most experts agree that hospitals will lose some portion of their staff if a significant event occurs. Health-care workers and other staff are much more likely to remain on the job or show up for work during a major catastrophe if they know their loved ones are safe and cared for. Personal preparedness planning allows providers to function more effectively during a crisis and should be strongly encouraged and actively promoted by hospital leadership as a mitigation strategy.

Basic principles of personal preparedness include:

1. A family communications plan
2. A family care plan
3. A preparedness kit, placed in an inner windowless room for shelter-in-place

For more information on personal preparedness planning, see *www.ready.gov www.redcross.org/services/disaster/* and *www.fema.gov/areyouready/*

ENHANCING THE EMERGENCY OPERATIONS PLAN

Conventional EOPs work well for natural and man-made disasters, such as fires, floods, transportation accidents, and structural collapses. However, catastrophes due to weapons of mass destruction or epidemics resulting from current or emerging infectious diseases have introduced new complexities and challenges to disaster responses, which are not well-addressed by traditional disaster plans, such as the need for decontamination, specialized personal protective equipment, medication and antidote stockpiling, prophylaxis of staff, and surge capacity.

Most experts advocate an "all-hazards" approach to disaster planning in which the EOP describes the standard operating procedures for response, with some incident-specific modifications included as annexes to the EOP. Hospitals should plan in advance the response to more complicated emergencies such as a hazardous materials event, a contagious disease outbreak, and a mass casualty event (MCE) that completely overwhelms the health-care system.

Hazardous Materials Event Planning

Plausible hazmat scenarios include a transportation or industrial accident involving a chemical spill or radioactive materials, a chemical terrorist attack, an explosion tainted with radioactive material ("dirty bomb"), a mass exposure to radioactive material, an attack on a nuclear plant, or detonation of a nuclear weapon. Hospitals must assume that many victims of a hazmat event will present independently to the facility without in-field decontamination. Therefore, regardless of whether or not a hospital is considered an Occupational Health and Safety Administration (OSHA)–certified decontamination facility, it must have the capability of performing full-body decontamination quickly and effectively.

Hazardous materials event contingency planning should describe

- Preparation of the decontamination equipment, emergency department, and hospital to receive victims of a hazmat event;
- decontamination procedures;
- definitive care of victims; and
- the measures that must be undertaken to maintain the integrity of the facility and to prevent hospital employees from becoming victims themselves while caring for patients.

Decontamination Equipment

Decontamination systems may be fixed (built-in showers) or portable (e.g., tents, trailers). The type of decontamination system a facility chooses may be dependent on community population and existing community decon resources. The decontamination area must be activated quickly at the onset of an event.

Security Issues

Maintenance of the integrity of the hospital is paramount; therefore, all entrances/egresses must be immediately secured to prevent contaminated victims from entering the facility.

Personal Protective Equipment

All personnel involved in triage and decontamination (including security) must don Class C personal protective equipment (PPE): chemical-resistant clothing with a powered air-purifying respirator (PAPR) or full-face respirator with appropriate cartridges. Donning and doffing of PPE must be supervised by an individual trained and certified in the use of Level C equipment.

Personnel Monitoring

To ensure safety of personnel, a mechanism must be in place to monitor the health and well-being of all staff in PPE during the hazmat disaster. Depending on weather conditions, personnel may be required to rotate out of the decontamination area frequently (every 10–20 minutes) to avoid PPE-induced heat exhaustion or dehydration. If applicable, the safety officer may utilize air-monitoring equipment to ensure safety of the work environment.

Other Considerations

Planning should take into consideration icy conditions and areas of standing water. Hospitals must be in compliance with state regulations on the handling of runoff decontamination water.

Additional Planning for a Radiation Event

Initial management of a radiation event is similar to that of other hazmat events; however, pre- and postdecontamination radiation monitoring of victims can be added. Radiation exposure monitoring for personnel must occur with individual sensors. An area of the ED (and the OR if needed) must also be prepped to receive casualties that cannot be completely decontaminated due to inhalation of radioactive materials or implantation into wounds.

Contagious Disease Outbreak Planning

Contagious disease outbreaks may result from a natural pandemic of a current or emerging infectious disease or from a biological attack with a contagious agent. Due to the prolonged disaster response required and the need for patient isolation, some logistics of a response to a contagious disease outbreak are unique; therefore, additional planning is required to support the core functions of the EOP. Many of the lessons learned on this topic come from the experiences of Singapore and Toronto during the SARS epidemic. Contagious disease outbreak planning has become even more urgent recently with the emergence of avian influenza and the threat of an influenza pandemic.

Establishment of an External Patient Triage Site

During a contagious disease outbreak, it is important to minimize exposure of staff and other patients to potentially infectious patients. Initial screening prior to entry into the facility allows for early identification of potentially infectious patients and immediate isolation and geographical separation from patients with other medical problems.

Patient Isolation and Cohorting

Health-care facilities have limited negative pressure isolation capacity, so considerations must be made early for measures to be implemented once that isolation capacity is exceeded, both in the emergency department and on inpatient units. Ideally, all hospitals would increase their baseline isolation capacity through permanent building construction; however, this is usually cost-prohibitive. One alternative is the use of temporary negative pressure equipment, such as portable high efficiency particulate air (HEPA) filters and anterooms. Another alternative is the concept of cohorting, or placement of patients with the contagious illness in an area of the emergency department or hospital that is geographically separated from other patients (and preferably with its own air-handling system) to minimize the spread of illness through the droplet or airborne route. As a caveat, patient care staff should also be cohorted to prevent health-care providers from going back and forth between the rooms of infectious and noninfectious patients.

Employee Health and Safety

Because staff can be exposed to infection during an outbreak, every effort must be made to protect and monitor staff during the event if they are to feel safe and confident in their work environment. Appropriate and adequate respiratory PPE (e.g., N95 masks or PAPRs) must be available to staff. If immunizations or medications are available for prophylaxis, they must be obtained and administered as soon as possible (see below).

There are several methods for monitoring employee health during the outbreak. In self-monitoring, employees check their temperatures three times a day and report to a central location if they develop fever and/or concerning symptoms. Alternatively, monitoring can be done daily through a fever check site upon arrival at the hospital for a shift. Ill or febrile employees should undergo further evaluation.

Mass Prophylaxis Planning

Mass prophylaxis involves the distribution of antibiotics, antivirals, or immunizations to a select population. While generally the responsibility of the department of health, it is not inconceivable that hospitals will play a role, in addition to providing prophylaxis to its own staff. During the anthrax attacks of 2001, one District of Columbia hospital provided antibiotic prophylaxis to approximately 800 exposures in 1 day.

Mass prophylaxis planning should describe an appropriate location for prophylaxis distribution, staffing of the site, equipment and supplies needed, and preprinted forms for screening, evaluation, and disposition. It is useful to develop a database of the hospital's stockpiled medications along with preprinted medication information sheets.

Other Considerations

During a contagious disease outbreak, it is imperative that each hospital works with other hospitals in the area, the city and state departments of health, and the Centers for Disease Control (CDC) to establish guidelines and standards for hospitals during the event, such as level of personal protective equipment for staff, antibiotics to be used for ill patients, and handling of exposures.

Surge Capacity Planning

The health-care system of the twenty-first century has reached critical mass. In today's milieu, MCEs threaten to overwhelm the entire health-care system. In the post-9/11 era, hospitals must have the capacity to respond to an acute surge in demand for resources until local, state, and federal assets are available.

Security

A large scale disaster will cause the hospital to become rapidly inundated with victims, psychological casualties, press, onlookers, family members, and friends. Security measures are paramount to allow the hospital to function efficiently. If not included in its standard EOP functions, hospital security must immediately initiate crowd and traffic control measures, including:

- Securing of all entrances/egresses to the hospital to prevent patients from entering the hospital without undergoing triage.
- Traffic diversion, if appropriate, using traffic cones, traffic barrels, barricades, and so on.
- Crowd and pedestrian traffic control at the entrance to the triage area. Flagged rope and stanchions may be used to establish patient waiting lines. Bullhorns can be used for verbal crowd control.
- If needed, deputizing of auxiliary security staff to assist with immediate security issues.
- Communicating with the local police department to request additional resources.

Mass Triage

Past disasters have demonstrated that approximately 80–90% of victims arriving at the hospital will be psychological casualties and/or have minor trauma. Lower acuity victims frequently overwhelm the ED and consume vital resources needed for more critical victims requiring extrication and transport by EMS. Therefore, it is important that the triage team identifies patients who can receive delayed or supportive care initially and divert them to another care location (see below).

Mass triage is usually accomplished external to the hospital (e.g., on the ambulance ramp or in a parking lot) by a triage team in appropriate PPE. The MASS triage model (standing for Move, Assess, Sort, and Send) taught in Advanced Disaster Life Support is one technique that may be employed by the triage team to quickly and effectively sort low-acuity patients from those with higher acuity.

Outpatient Surge Capacity Planning

Until community resources are activated, the hospital may choose to identify its own alternative care site (ACS) to which patients with a "green" or "minimal" triage tag may be diverted for their care. See Table 22-5 for a list of considerations when identifying an appropriate ACS. Planning must consider staffing, security issues, patient tracking, and documentation. If the site chosen is not normally a patient care facility (e.g., a gymnasium), the hospital must have additional supplies available for the facility, such as cots, linens, and basic first aid supplies.

Inpatient Surge Capacity Planning

Inpatient surge capacity planning describes measures to increase the number of inpatient beds available for MCE victims requiring hospitalization. The most common strategies are expedited patient discharges, cancellation of elective procedures and admissions, and opening unstaffed beds. Repurposing of treatment areas used for gastrointestinal, cardiac and pulmonary procedures, and creative use of unlicensed patient care spaces (such as lobbies and meeting rooms) can also increase surge capacity. See Table 22-6.

Staffing for Surge Capacity

Staffing during prolonged MCEs is perhaps the biggest challenge facing the health-care, system. A 25–30% staff

TABLE 22-5

FACTORS TO CONSIDER FOR ALTERNATIVE CARE SITES*

• Ability to house large numbers of patients and staff
• Communications and IT infrastructure
• Proximity to hospital
• Beds or cots available
• Handicap accessible
• Backup generator capability
• Food service capability
• Toilet, shower, and laundry capability
• Facility security
• Parking
• Electricity, water, and climate control
• Storage areas
• Loading dock
• Space for auxiliary services (treatment, lab, mental health, religious support, etc.)

Source: *www.ahrq.gov/research/altsites/index.html*

TABLE 22-6

STRATEGIES FOR INCREASING INPATIENT SURGE CAPACITY

• Immediately discharge all appropriate patients.
• Cancel elective procedures and admissions.
• Identify all patients that may be placed in the home care program.
• Convert single rooms to double rooms with an additional bed (e.g., hospital bed or temporizing "bed" such as a stretcher, cot, or reclining chair).
• Convert large double rooms to triple rooms with an additional bed.
• Convert the post-anesthesia care unit to an intensive care unit.
• Convert outpatient procedure beds (e.g., endoscopy suite, outpatient surgery suites, and sleep study unit, etc.) to patient care areas.
• Convert open spaces to treatment areas (e.g., meeting rooms, auditorium).
• Transfer patients to rehabilitation hospitals and nursing homes.

absenteeism rate is anticipated by many experts. First and foremost, hospitals must consider strategies for staff retention, such as prophylaxis distribution if available and comfortable rest areas with beds or cots, food services, technology for communications with family, and childcare if appropriate and feasible. To backfill gaps in staffing during an MCE, hospitals should consider maintaining a database of "alternative" providers, such as health-care workers in retirement or in research labs and allied health professionals such as dentists, veterinarians, and public health specialists. If credentialing of volunteers will not be handled by the hospital, it should be well-versed in community agencies to/from which it may send or draw volunteers.

Outstanding Issues

There are many critical issues still being defined involving health care during an MCE. Intra- and interstate credentialing of health-care professionals is in its infant stages. Hospitals still need definitive guidance on the graceful degradation of care (e.g., increased patient care ratios), emergency standard of care versus gold standard of care, and end-of-life decisions when critical care resources are strained.

THE IMPORTANCE OF TRAINING AND EDUCATION

Training and education in disaster topics and response procedures is vital to a successful emergency preparedness program. Educational programs should be competency based and address knowledge, skills, and/or behaviors needed to perform tasks specific to that individual's role in emergency response.

There are multiple levels of training for hospital employees:

- General orientation to the EOP—usually accomplished during employment and hospital orientation; a laminated pocket card with key components of response is a useful adjunct.
- Focused training for specific departments or position roles—could focus on general disaster response, the pertinent part of the EOP, and/or training in specific HICS job action sheets.
- Skills training—may be accomplished through skill-specific workshops, training videos, etc. (e.g., donning/doffing of PPE, mass triage, infection control procedures).
- Training to meet local, state, and federal training requirements—such as training in NIMS, the Hazardous Waste Operations and Emergency Response Standard (HAZWOPER), etc.
- Full-scale training
  - Curriculum-based medical training courses such as Advanced Trauma Life Support and Advanced Disaster Life Support: combines didactics with skills training and exercises or training scenarios.
  - Facility exercises: allow key decision makers to activate and assess the EOP and to identify weaknesses or deficiencies in response; may be accomplished with tabletop exercises, games or simulations, and operations-based exercises including drills, functional exercises, and full-scale exercises.
  - Citywide or regional disaster drills with other hospitals, first responders, the department of health, the regional emergency management agency, and other civilian and military assets.

Other potential venues for training include

- An employee disaster education Web site
- A disaster education publication for employees

THE IMPORTANCE OF REGIONAL COLLABORATION

Perhaps one of the most important components of hospital preparedness is regional collaboration. In the post-9/11 era, horizontal and vertical integration of response plans and resources is the only logical strategy for effective regional preparedness.

Many regions now have preestablished mutual aid agreements between hospitals allowing the sharing of important resources including personnel, equipment, and facilities during crisis times. These memorandums of understanding should address issues such as credentialing, compensation, liability, and procedures for transfer of patients.

There are many response agencies at the local, state, and federal level. The hospital's liaison officer must be able to identify pertinent response agencies by acronym and have a solid understanding of the role of each agency, the resources that each agency has to offer and who the contact person(s) are and how to reach them. Hospital leadership should have a solid understanding of the NIMS and the role that the health-care facility plays in regional response. Finally, the hospital must understand how to access local, regional, and federal resources such as the National Disaster Medical System and the CDC's Strategic National Stockpile.

CONCLUSION

Hospitals have begun to upgrade and enhance their EMPs in the face of increasingly sophisticated terrorist attacks, overwhelming natural disasters such as Hurricane Katrina, and the threat of an influenza pandemic. Improved preparedness allows health-care facilities to respond to and recover from MCEs more effectively.

Suggested Reading

Altered Standards of Care in Mass Casualty Events. Prepared by Health Systems Research Inc. under Contract No. 290-04-0010. AHRQ Publication No. 05-0043. Rockville, MD: Agency for Healthcare Research and Quality. April 2005.

Health Care Planning. PandemicFlu.gov. Available at *www.pandemicflu.gov/plan/tab6.html*

Hick JL, Hanfling D, Burstein JL, et al. Health care facility and community strategies for patient care surge capacity. *Ann Emerg Med*. 2004 Sep;44(3):253–61.

JA Barbera, AG Macintyre. *Jane's Mass Casualty Handbook: Hospital Emergency Preparedness and Response, First Edition*. Surrey, UK: Jane's Information Group, Ltd, 2003.

Managing Radiation Emergencies: Guidance for Hospital Medical Management. Radiation Emergency Assistance Center/Training Site (REAC/TS). Available at *www.orau.gov/reacts/emergency.htm*

Medical Surge Capacity and Capability: A Management System for Integrating Medical and Health Resources During Large-Scale Emergencies. Prepared by the CNA Corporation under Contract #233-03-0028 for the Department of Health and Human Services. August 2004.

OSHA Best Practices for Hospital-Based First Receivers of Victims from Mass Casualty Incidents Involving the Release of Hazardous Substances. Occupational Safety and Health Administration. January 2005. Available at *http://www.osha.gov/dts/osta/bestpractices/firstreceivers_hospital.html*

Rocky Mountain Regional Care Model for Bioterrorist Events: Locate Alternate Care Sites During an Emergency. Rockville, MD: Agency for Healthcare Research and Quality. September 2004. Available at *http://www.ahrq.gov/research/altsites*

23

EMS-ED CONSIDERATIONS

J. Marc Liu, Brigham Temple, and Jack Whitney

STAT FACTS

EMS-ED CONSIDERATIONS

- Seamless EMS-ED interactions are essential to a successful response to a disaster or mass casualty incident.
- Emergency department staff needs to be well-versed in basic principles of prehospital care, as well as the specifics of the local EMS system.
- ED and EMS personnel should train together to improve skills and knowledge, and to build rapport.
- Communication of information between field and hospital providers improves the chances of successfully recognizing and responding to an event.
- In the event of a disaster, the ED must be prepared to provide direct and indirect medical oversight for the EMS system.

INTRODUCTION

Under routine circumstances, the integration of emergency medical services (EMS) and emergency departments (EDs) is important for ensuring quality medical care. The EMS system and local EDs form the first line of defense in any mass casualty or disaster incident. Thus, a mutually supportive EMS-ED interaction is even more crucial in the event of a large-scale incident. As with any other aspect of emergency preparedness, effective execution requires forethought and rehearsal. This chapter will highlight major issues involved in EMS-ED coordination.

MEDICAL OVERSIGHT

Medical oversight (also referred to as medical direction or medical control) is the system in which physicians oversee the care provided by EMS personnel in order to maintain a standard of care. This encompasses many areas, including system design, standardized protocols and policies, training and education, quality assurance, and real-time decisions on individual patients. While an in-depth discussion of medical oversight is beyond the scope of this textbook, this chapter will briefly review general principles.

Medical oversight can be divided into two general categories: direct and indirect. Direct (or "online") medical oversight occurs when a physician provides real-time orders to EMS field personnel on a specific patient. The physician is communicating directly with EMS by radio, phone, or being physically present at the scene. The advantage of direct medical control is that the physician can provide immediate decisions and feedback based on prehospital information. However, a disaster situation is the worst time to attempt to learn the idiosyncrasies of an EMS system. Thus, any physician authorized to provide direct medical oversight should have completed a training course designed to familiarize them with general EMS principles, as well as the specific system policies and protocols used in their area.

Indirect (also "offline") medical oversight is a broad category. The simplest definition is that it covers all areas of medical direction that is not direct oversight. Because of the frequency of encounters with EMS, the ED staff becomes an important resource. Disaster preparedness is a part of indirect medical control. ED personnel involved with medical direction must ensure that the EMS system has policies and protocols in place to handle mass casualty, disaster, and hazardous materials (hazmat) situations. Often, ED clinicians will be consulted to help write these protocols. Such protocols must be clear, concise, and consistent with accepted, cost-effective, evidence-based medical practice. They also must take into account available equipment, provider levels of training, and limitations of delivering care in the field. All ED staff should be familiar with the

TABLE 23-1

SAMPLE BURN PROTOCOL

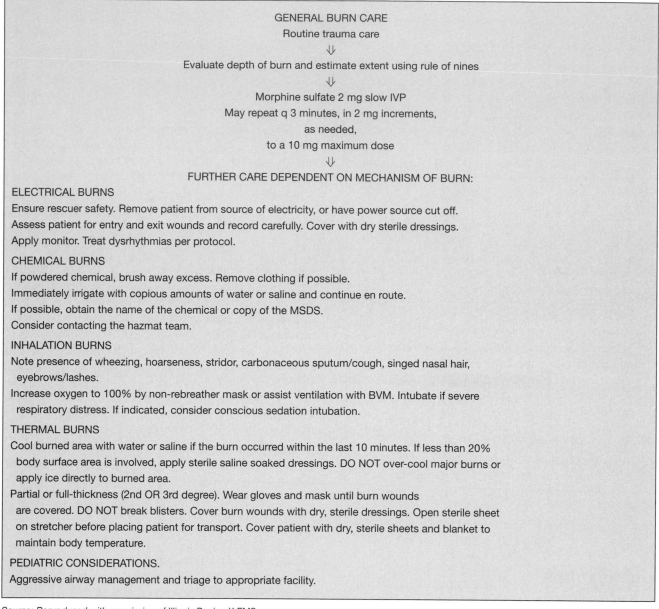

GENERAL BURN CARE

Routine trauma care

⇓

Evaluate depth of burn and estimate extent using rule of nines

⇓

Morphine sulfate 2 mg slow IVP

May repeat q 3 minutes, in 2 mg increments,

as needed,

to a 10 mg maximum dose

⇓

FURTHER CARE DEPENDENT ON MECHANISM OF BURN:

ELECTRICAL BURNS

Ensure rescuer safety. Remove patient from source of electricity, or have power source cut off.

Assess patient for entry and exit wounds and record carefully. Cover with dry sterile dressings.

Apply monitor. Treat dysrhythmias per protocol.

CHEMICAL BURNS

If powdered chemical, brush away excess. Remove clothing if possible.

Immediately irrigate with copious amounts of water or saline and continue en route.

If possible, obtain the name of the chemical or copy of the MSDS.

Consider contacting the hazmat team.

INHALATION BURNS

Note presence of wheezing, hoarseness, stridor, carbonaceous sputum/cough, singed nasal hair,
  eyebrows/lashes.

Increase oxygen to 100% by non-rebreather mask or assist ventilation with BVM. Intubate if severe
  respiratory distress. If indicated, consider conscious sedation intubation.

THERMAL BURNS

Cool burned area with water or saline if the burn occurred within the last 10 minutes. If less than 20%
  body surface area is involved, apply sterile saline soaked dressings. DO NOT over-cool major burns or
  apply ice directly to burned area.

Partial or full-thickness (2nd OR 3rd degree). Wear gloves and mask until burn wounds
  are covered. DO NOT break blisters. Cover burn wounds with dry, sterile dressings. Open sterile sheet
  on stretcher before placing patient for transport. Cover patient with dry, sterile sheets and blanket to
  maintain body temperature.

PEDIATRIC CONSIDERATIONS.

Aggressive airway management and triage to appropriate facility.

Source: Reproduced with permission of Illinois Region X EMS.

capabilities of their local EMS system. Examples of EMS protocols are shown in Tables 23-1and 23-2, and Fig. 23-1.

EDs should also actively encourage and participate in the education and training of EMS providers. Regular training not only improves knowledge of disaster and mass casualty medicine, but also promotes cooperation between the ED and EMS system. Sending representatives to training sessions conveys the message that the ED is a partner with EMS in disaster preparedness. EDs should participate in full-scale drills with the EMS system and rest of the hospital. ED personnel may also be asked to develop a didactic program for EMS providers. Anyone developing lectures or

drills should remember the military aphorism, "Train as you fight, and fight as you train." Realistic rehearsals, coupled with organized instruction, are necessary to maintain readiness. Working together in the planning stages can reduce confusion during the stress of an actual event.

EMS-ED INTERACTIONS DURING AN EVENT

Maintaining a line of communication between the EDs and EMS is important for an effective response to any disaster. When a large-scale event occurs, the affected community

TABLE 23-2

SAMPLE TREATMENT PROTOCOL FOR CHEMICAL NERVE AGENTS

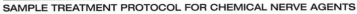

Antidotes for Organophosphate/Carbamate Poisoning (Chemical Nerve Agents)

BLS

1. Oxygen NR
2. Assist ventilation, if needed.
3. Monitor pulse oximetry, if available.
4. If available, may administer one (1) **MARK I** kit consisting of Atropine 2 mg and **2-PAMCL** 600 mg autoinjectors. Administer one (1) additional **MARK I** for moderate respiratory distress, or two (2) additional **MARK I** kits for severe intoxication (gasping respirations, twitching, seizures).
5. Decontaminate patient as indicated based on extent and type of exposure.
6. Request ALS, if available.

ALS

7. Place on cardiac monitor, if available.
8. Establish IV access.
9. If patient exhibits signs/symptoms of miosis (for a vapor exposure), and at least one of the **SLUDGE** symptoms or altered mentation, administer **Atropine** 2 mg IV/IM.
10. May repeat **Atropine** dose every 5 minutes as necessary to reduce secretions and ventilatory resistance.

    NOTE: If available and not previously administered, may administer one (1) **MARK I** kit consisting of **Atropine** 2 mg and **2-PAMCL** 600 mg autoinjectors. Administer one (1) additional **MARK I** for moderate respiratory distress, or two (2) additional **MARK I** kits for severe intoxication (gasping respirations, twitching, seizures).

11. Administer **Diazepam (Valium)** 10 mg IV/IM for severe intoxication or seizures.
12. May repeat **Diazepam (Valium)** dose every 15 minutes as necessary to control seizures, to a maximum of 30 mg.

Source: Reproduced with permission of the Protective Medicine Branch, Federal Protective Service and the Casualty Care Research Center, Uniformed Services University of the Health Sciences.

may not initially be aware of it. Sudden disasters such as tornados or explosions are obvious. Such events as a chemical terrorist attack or infectious epidemic may not be apparent for hours or even days. Free flow of information between first responders and local hospitals can lead to a more complete appraisal of the overall situation, which will lead to improved care for each patient. EMS personnel can provide critical information, which allows the ED and hospital to mobilize the appropriate resources. The ED can give recommendations to EMS as to how to best treat patients and protect personnel in the field.

The ED will often assume a crucial coordinating role in a disaster situation. When faced with a potential disaster or mass casualty incident, the ED should attempt to gather as much information as possible from the scene, keeping in mind that EMS providers will have their hands full and will have limited time. Ideally, the on-scene responders will have established an incident command system, although this may not always be the case. If incident command has been established, the ED should communicate solely with the designated EMS officer to avoid unnecessary distractions to the scene. Based on the initial information, the

ED staff must decide whether to activate hospital disaster procedures. The department may consider instituting its own incident command structure, which may include designating a specific person to act as a liaison with the EMS system. It is also important to consider whether other agencies will need to be alerted (e.g., fire department, law enforcement, public health, ED/hospital administration).

The ED serves as a source of medical information for prehospital providers. It can bring to bear the medical expertise of its staff, as well as the use of available medical references. Since disaster events will fall outside of day-to-day operations, the ED can offer guidance on how best to care for victims. Clinicians can issue online orders to responders treating patients in the field. Online support is best provided by experienced ED personnel knowledgeable in EMS, as any medical decision must consider the system capabilities. ED staff should never respond to a scene unless specifically requested by the EMS agency. Even then, personnel should only be sent if they are trained and experienced in prehospital care.

In addition to assisting with patient care, ED staff can play an important role in maintaining the safety of EMS

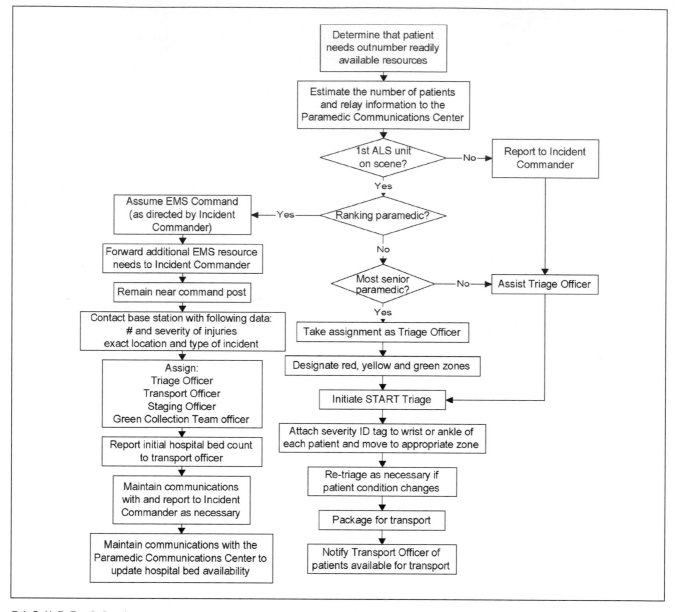

FIGURE 23-1

EXAMPLE OF A MASS CASUALTY ALGORITHM
Source: Reproduced with permission of Milwaukee County EMS.

personnel. In the confusion of a large-scale emergency, first responders occasionally set aside their own well-being in order to assist the victims. ED staff should remind EMS personnel to utilize appropriate basic precautions and personal protective equipment. This is especially important in nuclear, biological, and chemical incidents. The ED should also monitor providers for symptoms and signs of illness, injury, or overexertion, and intervene accordingly.

In some instances, an ED may be asked to furnish EMS units with additional medications or supplies for patient care. Needed materials can be provided, but caution must be exercised in order to retain enough supplies to treat

patients brought to the ED. A formal agreement between the hospital and EMS system addressing reimbursement issues with a prearranged method for resupply are prudent measures to take before any incident occurs.

If an ED acts as medical control for the EMS system, it may be asked to assume the responsibility of allocating casualties to area hospitals. This requires an integrated knowledge of hospital and EMS capabilities and triage, along with attention to detail. It also necessitates communication between the scene, the control ED, and other receiving hospitals. Patients should be transported to area EDs based on severity, transport times, and hospital resources. More severely injured patients should be sent to closer hospitals that are capable of managing their injuries. Less critical casualties that are less time-sensitive can be moved to hospitals further from the scene. The ED staff responsible for directing EMS must also remember that up to 80% of patients do not arrive via EMS, but instead by foot or private vehicle. Therefore, the closest hospital will usually receive the bulk of the casualties. Patients should be divided among hospitals to reduce the probability that any one hospital is overwhelmed.

CONCLUSION

Successful management of a mass casualty incident can only be accomplished with smooth coordination between all personnel and agencies involved. The interface between the ED and EMS system is a complementary one. A mutually supportive environment is built on a foundation of shared insights, knowledge, and daily interactions. By working together, ED and EMS personnel become the community's best defense in troubling times.

Suggested Reading

Elliott SK, Atkins JM. ED interaction with prehospital providers. In: Kuehl AE (ed). *Prehospital Systems and Medical Oversight*. 3rd ed. Dubuque, IA: Kendall/Hunt Publishing, 2002; pp 449–451.

Gluckman WA, Oster NS, Holecek N. Emergency departments and EMS. In: Brennan JA, Krohmer JR (eds). *Principles of EMS Systems*. 3rd ed. Sudbury, MA: Jones and Bartlett Publishers, 2006; pp 59–62.

Kuehl AE, Baker EF. Medical oversight. In: Kuehl AE (ed). *Prehospital Systems and Medical Oversight*. 3rd ed. Dubuque, IA: Kendall/Hunt Publishing, 2002; pp 301–307.

Murphy MF. Emergency medical services in disaster. In: Hogan DE, Burstein JL (eds). *Disaster Medicine*. Philadelphia, PA: Lippincott Williams & Wilkins, 2002; pp 90–103.

Okumura T, Suzuki K, Atsuhiro F, et al. The Tokyo subway sarin attack: disaster management, part 1: community emergency response. *Acad Emerg Med.* 1998;5:613–617.

Weiss SB, Dworsky PI, Gluckman WA. Disaster response, In: Brennan JA, Krohmer JR (eds). *Principles of EMS Systems*. 3rd ed. Sudbury, MA: Jones and Bartlett Publishers, 2006; pp 200–217.

24

FIELD IDENTIFICATION AND DECONTAMINATION OF TOXINS

Chad Tameling and Bijan Saeedi

FIELD IDENTIFICATION AND DECONTAMINATION OF TOXINS

- Three categories of toxin identification: Natural characteristics, field characterization, and mobile laboratory identification.
- Natural characteristics are most applicable to chemical agents.
- Field characterization should be associated with personal protection equipment and an established decontamination system.
- Spectroscopy and polymerase chain reaction technologies are the primary modalities utilized in mobile laboratories.
- Standard decontamination plans should be addressed and adjusted to site-specific situations before entering a hazardous environment.

INTRODUCTION

Hazardous materials emergency responders are faced with the challenge of identifying toxins in the field (biological, radiological, chemical) and cleaning them off of people, buildings, and the environment in as quick and efficient manner possible. Ramifications of not correctly identifying and decontaminating toxins could be life-threatening as well as monetarily damaging.

Over the years, SET Environmental, Inc. has developed an operating procedure to achieve the goals of (1) quickly and accurately identifying the toxin and (2) effectively decontaminating people, property, and environment in a time-sensitive manner.

Basic theory of hazardous materials emergency response dictates that when responders arrive on the scene, prior to "going to work," they must know the identity of the toxin. Protective equipment selection, decontamination, remediation, and disposal technologies are dictated by toxin identification. Unfortunately, the luxury of knowing toxin identity is not always the case.

There are three categories of toxin identification methods SET implements in hazardous materials emergency response: (1) natural characteristics, (2) field characterization, and (3) mobile laboratory identification.

NATURAL CHARACTERISTICS

This is the quickest (and most crude) method of toxin identification, and is mostly applicable to chemical agents. Employing two of the five senses (sight, smell), emergency responders are sometimes able to get an idea of toxin identity. Please note if an emergency responder is close enough to the scene to smell an unknown toxic release, he is too close! However, there are many instances when an incidental odor may be a telltale sign of toxin identity. Many chemical agents have characteristic odors (freshly mowed straw smell of phosgene, pungent choking odor of corrosives, sweet-smelling odor of aromatic compounds, garlic-like odor of arsine gas) that may lead to a tentative identification or general categorization of an unknown toxin.

Many chemicals have characteristic colors in their sedentary state or when they are reacting. When an emergency responder pulls up to the scene, he may observe brown smoke (nitrogen dioxide gas from reacting nitric acid) or see a bright yellow/orange powder (potential explosive compounds) or a green vapor cloud (chlorine gas leak) and be able to tentatively identify or categorize the unknown toxin. Although the natural characteristic method is simple and sometimes effective, it is not always conclusive. That is why the modern emergency responder employs field characterization techniques.

FIELD CHARACTERIZATION

This method employs a combination of wet chemistry and real-time direct read instrumentation to identify the unknown toxin. Please note if an emergency responder is close enough to the unknown toxin to employ field characterization, he should be donned in appropriate personal protection equipment (PPE) and have a decontamination system established (see later sections). A well-equipped hazardous materials emergency response team should have a compliment of direct read instrumentation including, but not limited to the following:

- Radiation survey meters (α-, β- and γ-radiation at a minimum)
- Organic vapor analyzers (PID, FID)
- 4- or 5-gas meters (for oxygen, % flammability and toxic gas readings)
- Mercury vapor analyzer
- Inorganic gas (chlorine) detector

Direct read instrumentation is complemented with wet chemistry. When responders are able to approach an unknown toxin, they can also use wet chemistry techniques to identify chemical families or characteristics of the material. In the past 2 years, with the recent focus on weapons of mass destruction (WMD) and terrorism, there have been many manufacturers of "test kits" that can claim to positively identify unknown chemical agents. These test kits are still in the developmental stage, and have many false readings and/or interferences. There are other test kits on the market that test for a particular agent (VX, botulism). These kits are more accurate, however, they have a shelf-life and a responder could fill a 12-foot straight truck just with test kits if he had to get every agent-specific kit on the market. SET's approach is to employ simpler tests and use these findings, in conjunction with a solid understanding of chemistry, to characterize or identify unknown chemical toxins.

SET responds with the following wet chemistry field tests:

- pH
- Oxidizer potential
- Flammability
- Cyanide
- Sulfide
- Water solubility
- Sugar
- Chlorine
- Nitrate/nitrite/nitrogen

While these methods are sound and effective, they do not address today's threat of biological or natural occurring toxins. To meet this challenge, SET had to incorporate instrumentation for identification of unknown toxins.

INSTRUMENTATION IDENTIFICATION

For many years prior to the WMD phenomenon, SET utilized Fourier transform infrared spectroscopy (FT-IR) and gas chromatograph/mass spectroscopy (GC/MS) as primary tools in positively identifying inorganic and organic solids, liquids, and gases. FT-IR spectra is used for identification of functional groups such as alcohols, amines, esters, and so on. The fingerprint portion of FT-IR spectrum is used to exactly identify a compound. The spectrum of an unknown compound can be searched against libraries of thousands of spectrums within seconds using a fast computer. Sometimes the size of a sample is so small that a good spectrum cannot be obtained using conventional FT-IR spectroscopy. FT-IR microscope equipped with nitrogen-cooled mercury cadmium telluride (MCT) detector is capable of giving a good spectrum of a sample as small as few microns (see Fig. 24-1).

GC-MS is used for complex mixtures. In GC-MS, compounds are separated and identified by their mass fragments (mass spectrum). Figure 24-2 depicts an example of the mass spectrum of chloropicrin (trichloronitromethane).

A graphic example of FT-IR spectrum obtained with microscope follows.

This instrumentation, combined with wet chemistry tests and other information obtained during the field survey, has enabled emergency responders to positively identify toxins in the field or in the laboratory setting for years.

Immediately following the World Trade Center attacks, the anthrax epidemic heightened the public awareness and concern about the threat of biological agents. The standard practice of preparing a sample, culturing, and growing it for 2–3 weeks was not acceptable. Businesses faced with the possibility of a bioagent attack in their factories or offices stood to lose tens of thousands of dollars each hour they were shut down!

SET responded by utilizing polymerase chain reaction (PCR) technology. Rapid replication of an unknown sample's DNA allowed to test against positive controls for well-known bioterrorist agents within hours rather than weeks. PCR testing in the field is relatively new, and there are a limited number of bioagent tests available, but it is the quickest, most accurate method available today. The positive result needs to be verified by conventional culture growth in the laboratory.

An example may help illustrate SET's methodology. The first example was recent news in the Chicago area when police arrested Dr Chaos for storing sodium cyanide in the Chicago Metro train tunnels. The FBI had already obtained the sample. The sample originally thought to be cocaine came to SET as an unknown white powder. The following tests were administered:

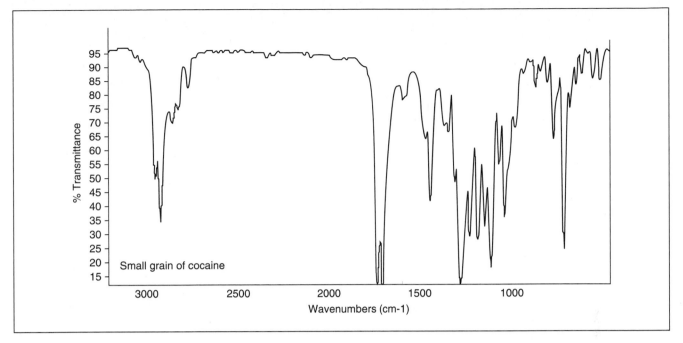

FIGURE 24-1

SAMPLE SPECTRUM OF A SMALL GRAIN OF COCAINE

- Water-soluble.
- pH of the material is around 8, not corrosive.
- FTIR spectra presented key functional group peak of cyanide at 2088 wavenumber (see Fig. 24-3) identifying cyanide. In addition to cyanide, the sample contained sodium carbonate.
- Flame test of material presented bright orange flame identifying sodium salt.
- Wet chemistry test using pyridine barbituric acid confirmed the presence of cyanide.
- Unknown toxin is identified as sodium cyanide.

NONINTRUSIVE IDENTIFICATION OF COMPOUNDS

Sometimes a suspicious container is too dangerous to open for sampling; in this case, other methods may be employed.

To identify a substance through a metal shell, a method such as isotopic neutron spectroscopy (INS) is used. The metal shell is emitted by a neutron source (isotope of californium 252) then the emitting ray from chemical contents is detected with a sensitive detector such as nitrogen-cooled germanium detector.

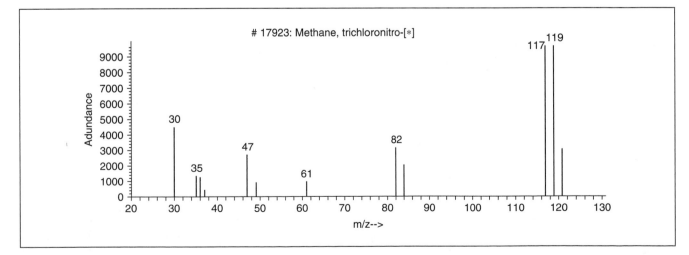

FIGURE 24-2

MASS SPECTRUM OF CHLOROPICRIN (TRICHLORNITROMETHANE)

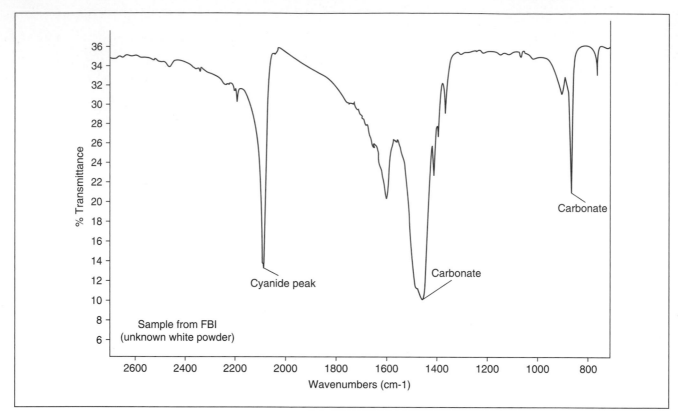

FIGURE 24-3

FTIR SPECTRA OF CYANIDE

For nonintrusive sampling through glass or plastic or even a powder in medical gel capsule, FT-Raman spectroscopy may be used (see Fig. 24-4).

Field Decontamination

Hazardous materials emergency response operations mandate a decontamination plan in accordance with 29 CFR 1910.120(q). Emergency responders should have a standard decontamination plan that can be adjusted to site-specific situations prior to entering a hazardous environment. The basis of the plan should encompass the following:

1. What type of equipment will be needed to implement the decontamination?
2. What type of decontamination and decontamination agent will be effective against the toxin?
3. How many decontamination stations are appropriate for the situation?
4. Considerations when setting up a decontamination site.

Decontamination Equipment Selection

There are many brands and suppliers of decontamination equipment such as showers and absorbent pads. Emergency responders should have the following equipment:

- 6-mL polysheeting for staging areas and ground cover
- Decon pools (plastic pools from Kmart work well)

- Absorbent pads (universal and hydrocarbon)
- Low-pressure hand sprayers with wands
- Scrub brushes (soft/stiff bristle)
- Hand scrapers and putty knives
- Drums (55-gallon and 5-gallon poly and steel)
- 55-gallon capacity 2 mL poly bags (to hold contaminated personal effects)
- Duct tape (lots of it)
- Decon showers (make your own or buy online)
- Hose (garden hose, fire hose)
- Fittings for various water supplies (garden hose, Chicago, fire hydrant Cam lock, NPT)
- Chemical decontamination agents (hypochlorite, citric acid, bicarbonate, surfactant)
- Collapsible bladders for holding decon rinse
- Submersible pumps for pumping decon rinse out of decon stations
- Stretchers/back boards/foldable cots for nonambulatory patients

Types of Decontamination and Decontamination Agents

There are two basic methods of decontamination: physical removal and chemical removal. There are many suggestions by OSHA, NIOSH, and EPA about gas/vapor sterilization, halogen stripping, thermal degradation, and so on,

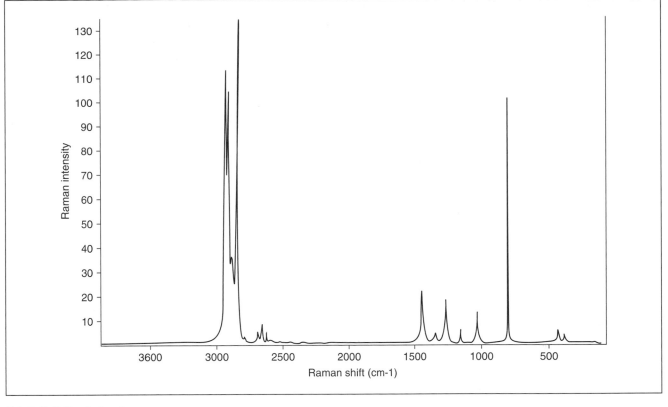

FIGURE 24-4

FT RAMAN SPECTRUM OF CYCLOHEXANE

but many of these methods are not practical from a time and money standpoint.

Physical decontamination (mechanically removing contaminant) is most applicable for gross decontamination of gooey tar-like material. High-volume water streams from a fog nozzle or pressure wash tip may mechanically remove material but produce overspray and lots of runoff to be managed. Typical physical decontamination consists of

- Scraping off goop with a tongue depressor or putty knife
- Wiping areas with absorbent pads
- Doffing contaminated clothing or PPE

Drums should be staged on 6-mL polysheeting at the decontamination station. Contaminated PPE, clothes, and absorbent pads should be placed in the drums and sealed for proper disposal.

Chemical decontamination (inactivate contaminants by chemical detoxification or disinfect ion) is most applicable for highly soluble contaminants. The most readily available material (and probably most widely effective) is hypochlorite solution. The military uses two different concentrations of chlorine solution in decontamination procedures. A 0.5% solution is used for skin decontamination, and a 5% solution is used for equipment. Examples of other chemical decontamination agents are

- Surfactants (ionic or nonionic)
- Detergents
- Citric acid solution
- Sodium bicarbonate solution
- Kerosene/light fuel oils
- D-Limonene/α-pinene solution

Chemical decontamination solutions can be administered via hand sprayers or showers at appropriate stations. Showers produce much more runoff than hand sprayers and will require much more chemical since it is applied at a faster rate. Do not let victims freeze if outside temperatures are cold. Also, cold water from a fire hydrant can cause hypothermia in victims even in warm weather.

How Many Decontamination Stations Are Appropriate for the Situation?

In the mid-1980s and early 1990s, emergency responders would try to establish decontamination as described by OHSA 29CFR 1910.120(q)(2)(vii) and spend 4–6 hours setting up decon pools, drop pads, and safety showers before any work in the hot zone occurred (see Fig. 24-5). In today's post-9/11 terrorism era, the 19-step decontamination stations are too cumbersome for time-sensitive situations where protecting life and property is critical.

EPA has a suggested minimum decontamination layout, which is more applicable to the emergency responder (see Fig. 24-6).

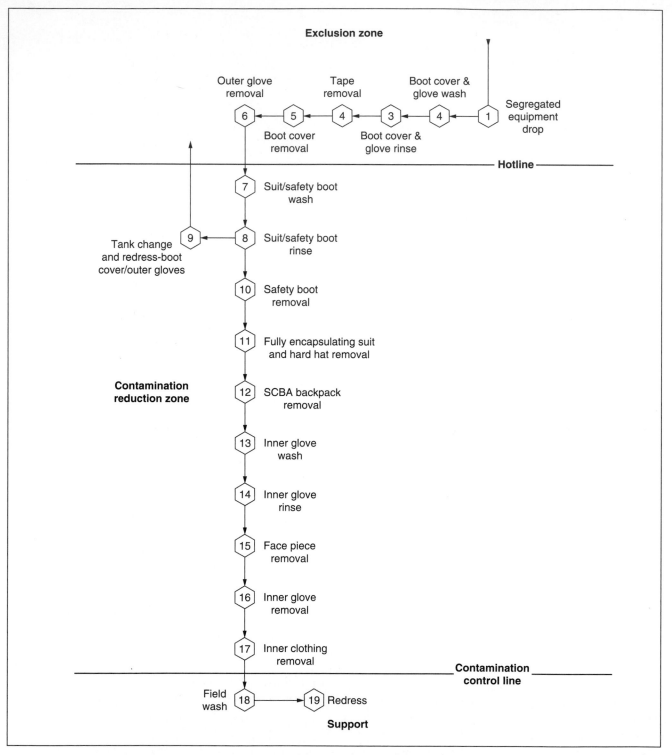

Exclusion zone

Outer glove removal — Tape removal — Boot cover & glove wash

6 ← 5 ← 4 ← 3 ← 4 ← 1   Segregated equipment drop

Boot cover removal   Boot cover & glove rinse

——— **Hotline** ———

7   Suit/safety boot wash

9 ← 8   Suit/safety boot rinse

Tank change and redress-boot cover/outer gloves

10   Safety boot removal

11   Fully encapsulating suit and hard hat removal

Contamination reduction zone

12   SCBA backpack removal

13   Inner glove wash

14   Inner glove rinse

15   Face piece removal

16   Inner glove removal

17   Inner clothing removal

——— **Contamination control line** ———

Field wash   18 → 19   Redress

Support

FIGURE 24-5

EPA SUGGESTED MAXIMUM DECONTAMINATION LAYOUT FOR LEVEL A PROTECTION

Experience and cost-benefit analysis of spending time to decontaminate protective suits for reuse versus doffing protective suits and disposing of them has proven that disposable suits made much more sense on a time and money basis. For that reason, SET Environ-mental, Inc. has used a modified version of the EPA minimum decontamination layout. This modified decontamination layout works on the principle of "keeping it simple" and working with a 3-step process (see Fig. 24-7).

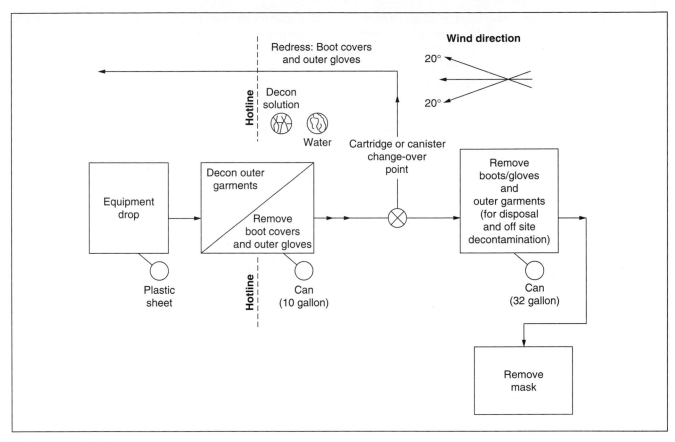

FIGURE 24-6

MINIMUM LAYOUT FOR LEVEL C PROTECTION

3-Step Process

1. Equipment drop and gross mechanical decontamination.
2. Quick physical decon by doffing suits and placing them in 55-gallon drums to be sealed and sent for off-site disposal.

3. Remove breathing apparatus (SCBA or APR) and place on 6-mL poly for staging, and finally remove inner gloves. Breathing apparatus can be decontaminated for reuse, and the inner glove drum shall be sealed and sent for offsite disposal.

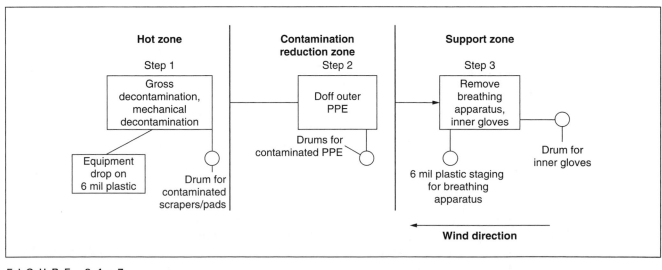

FIGURE 24-7

THE 3-STEP PROCESS

If necessary, Step 1 can be modified by adding a chemical decontamination stage. Sludge-like materials or acutely toxic materials may require dissolving/detoxification/neutralization before the responder should attempt to doff his suit. Chemical decontamination agents are applied with hand sprayers, collected and pumped into portable tanks or drums for offsite disposal.

Emergency responders are able to progress through this decontamination scenario with little or no help from "decon techs" who traditionally had to be at each station to support decon operations. This allows more trained personnel to work the incident rather than man decon stations (see Fig. 24-8).

The 3-step process can be adapted for emergency responders decontaminating nonambulatory patients as well.

1. Gross decontamination/physical decontamination (remove clothes).
2. Chemical decontamination, addition of detoxification/neutralization chemicals to patients using hand sprayers.
3. Final rinse, using walk through decontamination showers, which allow emergency responders to carry a litter/gurney/backboard with a patient on it.

This scenario requires "decon techs" at each station, and also requires personnel to carry patients on stretchers through the system.

Considerations for Setting up a Decontamination Site

Rule number one in emergency response is to stage uphill and upwind of a hazardous materials incident.

1. The decontamination pad should be a safe distance from any potential hazardous exposures, secondary devices, or structural collapse.

2. Consider the topography of the location for natural drainage patterns or natural pools that could be used for runoff collection.
3. Are there buildings (parking garages, car washes) that could be used as shelters or triage/staging areas for incoming patients?
4. The closest utilities, such as water and electric, should be identified for potential use.
5. Establish staging area for additional resources (vehicles, ambulance) that coordinate with traffic flow patterns to and from the site.

Verification of Decontamination

In an emergency situation, people are moving quickly, working long hours, fatigued, and may not completely decontaminate absolutely everything. This poses the threat that a residual hazard may be present. A rule of thumb is the more porous the material, the harder it is to decontaminate. Nonporous material (plastics, metal, enamel) can be readily cleaned. Materials like leather are going to readily absorb chemicals and slowly leach vapors over time. Equipment should be tested prior to being put back in service:

1. Articles should be placed in 2 mL plastic bags and sealed and allowed to sit in the sun and heat for at least 30 minutes.
2. After 30 minutes, the bags should be slightly opened and an air monitor placed in the bags to read vapors in the bag. Wipe samples can be taken for certain contaminants and sent to a lab for analysis.
3. If residual contamination is found, the materials should be disposed of, or if the materials are critical, additional decontamination can be performed.
4. Porous materials (leather, canvas) can be additionally decontaminated by being soaked in water heated to 122°F to 131°F for 4–6 hours and then air-dried without excess heat.
5. Metal or plastic can be decontaminated with a bleach slurry or hot soapy water. After 30 minutes, flush with water and aerate the item outdoors for several hours.

Suggested Reading

Emergency Response to Terrorism Job Aid, by Federal Emergency Management Agency, United States Fire Administration, National Fire Academy, and United States Department of Justice Office of Justice Programs, May 2000, 1st ed.

Illinois Emergency Management Agency Chem-Bio Handbook, 1998, Jane's Information Group.

NIOSH/OSHA/USGC/EPA Occupational Safety and Health Guidance Manual for Hazardous Waste Site Activities, October 1985.

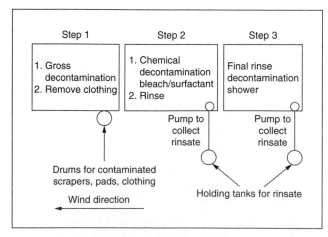

FIGURE 24-8

MODIFIED 3-STEP PROCESS

SECTION

III

EMERGENCY DEPARTMENT PREPAREDNESS

INTRODUCTION

With the Emergency Department acting as the "gateway" to the medical system, the approach to Toxico-terrorism events involve triage, drug preparedness and hospital staff response. The Emergency Department should be considered "the first receiver" from the event and thus becomes the focus for the incident command, pharmacy, security, media and communications systems. These chapters should serve as a basis for integration with the rest of this text in responding to such an event.

25

TRIAGE IN THE EMERGENCY DEPARTMENT

Deborah A. Hassman

INTRODUCTION

Rapid response to a bioterrorism outbreak is essential to reduce the incidence of dissemination of infectious agents to the community. The local emergency department will be the focal point for recognition, treatment, communication, and data collection related to a bioterrorist event. The triage area will serve as a discovery phase for a bioterrorist event. Health-care professionals will sort, screen, and prioritize victims in the triage area. Triage is the first principle in mass casualty care. The triage practitioners' role requires that several victims be assessed and prioritized quickly to ensure that the victim gets the appropriate treatment. The purpose of this chapter is to show the necessary triage steps in order to be prepared and rapidly triage and treat the patients exposed to biological or chemical agents of bioterrorism.

TRIAGE PROCESS

Discovery Phase of the Triage Process

A bioterrorist disaster is an intentional epidemic, and may be suspected when increasing numbers of otherwise healthy persons with similar symptoms seek treatment, or will be known due to the mass numbers of people exposed to chemicals or toxins. Outcomes will depend on how rapidly victims can be triaged based on the recognition and identification of high-risk syndromes (i.e., typical combination of clinical features of the illness at presentation), in order to reduce transmission of disease.

The word triage describes a medical decision-making process, which determines what is a priority that needs immediate action. In a disaster situation, it is a tool to divide an unmanageable task into manageable components, by sorting casualties to determine the priority of medical treatment.

Most of the time the desired terrorist bioagent is an airborne virus or bacteria; the virus or bacteria travels through respiratory droplets, and is highly contagious. Since it takes time to truly detect an outbreak from laboratory testing, surveillance, and reporting techniques, initial identification must rely on presenting signs and symptoms. Therefore, knowledge of these symptoms by triage personnel establishes the basis for detecting bioterrorism.

Basic Triage Rules

If patients walk into the department, and the triage practitioner notices similar illness patterns, triage the patients in a primary area, and consider a possible bioterrorism event has occurred. Follow an appropriate clinical pathway to determine emergency department placement. (See Fig. 25-1.)

If a known bioterrorism event has occurred, there will be several patients to categorize. Triage will be a process involving repeated reassessment, at various stages during the victims care. Initial assessment should begin with a START (Simple Triage and Rapid Treatment) triage

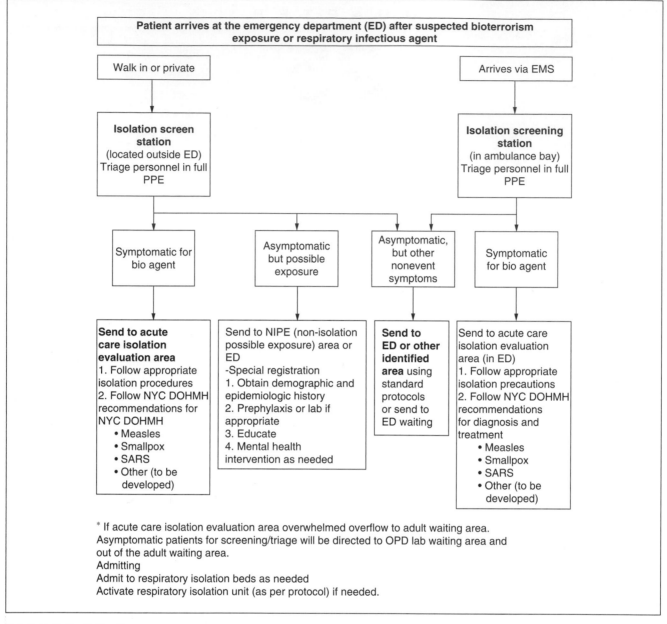

FIGURE 25-1

EMERGENCY DEPARTMENT PROTOCOL
Source: Retrieved from http://www.hscbklyn.edu/emergency_medicine/pdf.docs/uhbsection06a.pdf

protocol. (See Figs. 25-2 and 25-3). This is the protocol used by EMS in the field and it is important to keep consistency. The patients should be quickly assessed, less than 30 seconds per person. Staff should first clear the walking wounded, tag them as minor, and direct them to the appropriate area. The goal of START triage is to help identify those patients, who are the most critically ill or injured, as quickly as possible. Also to determine how well the patient is able to utilize their own resources to deal with their injuries. Thirdly, which conditions will benefit the most from expenditure of the limited available resources?

- **Red:** Critical patients in need of immediate life-saving care
- **Yellow:** Relatively stable patients in need of prompt medical attention
- **Green:** Minor injuries that can wait for appropriate treatment
- **Black:** Deceased patients or those who have no chance of survival

The triage assessment is based on the RPM method: respiration, perfusion, and mental status. Respiration:

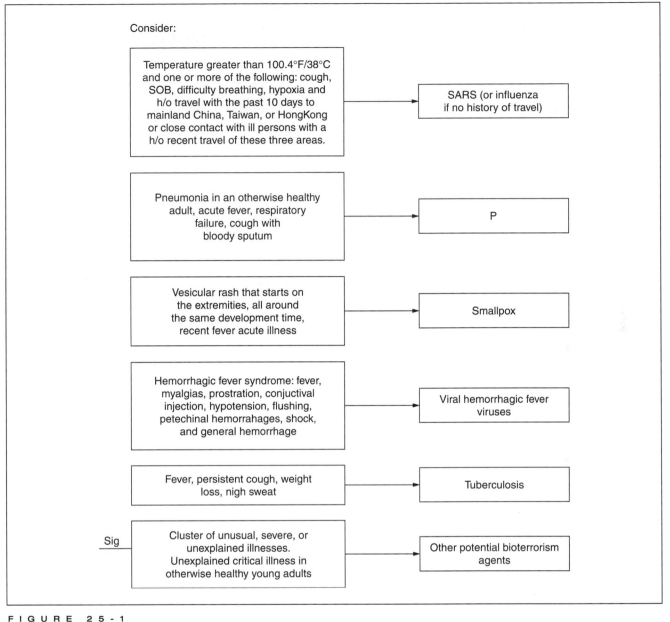

Consider:

Temperature greater than 100.4°F/38°C and one or more of the following: cough, SOB, difficulty breathing, hypoxia and h/o travel with the past 10 days to mainland China, Taiwan, or HongKong or close contact with ill persons with a h/o recent travel of these three areas. → SARS (or influenza if no history of travel)

Pneumonia in an otherwise healthy adult, acute fever, respiratory failure, cough with bloody sputum → P

Vesicular rash that starts on the extremities, all around the same development time, recent fever acute illness → Smallpox

Hemorrhagic fever syndrome: fever, myalgias, prostration, conjuctival injection, hypotension, flushing, petechinal hemorrahages, shock, and general hemorrhage → Viral hemorrhagic fever viruses

Fever, persistent cough, weight loss, nigh sweat → Tuberculosis

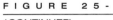 Sig — Cluster of unusual, severe, or unexplained illnesses. Unexplained critical illness in otherwise healthy young adults → Other potential bioterrorism agents

FIGURE 25-1

(*CONTINUED*)

determine breathing rate, if it is greater than 30/min tag the patient red. This is the primary sign of shock. If the patient is not adequately breathing, perform airway maneuvers. Perfusion is checked by obtaining a radial pulse for at least 10 seconds, if it is abnormal or not present, tag the patient red. Mental status can be checked by assessing three simple commands. Have the patient open their eyes, smile, and squeeze a hand. If they have adequate airway and circulation and can follow commands, tag the patient delayed or yellow. If the patient is unresponsive or not following commands, tag the patient red.

Once a bioterrorism event has been identified, several patients will present to the emergency department. It is going to be the triage practitioner's role to separate those with illness and injury from the worried well. This will help to determine individual victim disposition, and will help to identify the evolving epidemic.

Triage Goals

Triage goals should be to rapidly treat patients with likelihood of success with available resources. If the bioterrorism agent is considered highly transmittable, triage should be directed at preventing secondary infections. Therefore strict barrier protection needs to be in place. Another triage goal is to utilize communication. It is important, once a

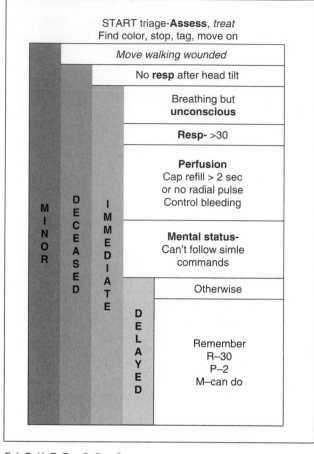

FIGURE 25-2

START TRIAGE

Source: From www.citmt.org/start Used by permission of Lou E.
Romig, MD, FAAP, FACEP.

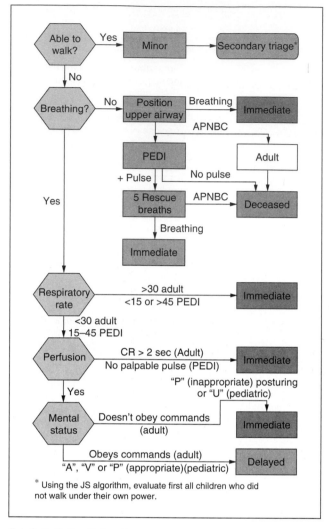

FIGURE 25-3

COMBINED START/JUMPSTART TRIAGE ALGORITHM
Source: From: www.jumpstarttriage.com Used by permission
of Lou E. Romig, MD, FAAP, FACEP.

bioterrorism event has been identified, to communicate within the hospital, and have the disaster plan initialized, based on the institutions protocols. Disaster plans must be coordinated across regional health-care facilities. Triage is the cornerstone in medical management of a disaster or mass-casualty type response. Therefore triage efforts and protocols should be standardized across the region, to help ensure the greatest number of survivors.

Health-care professionals should be trained in the basic principles of disaster management, especially in relation to the triage process. There must be a clear understanding of the role of the triage officer, the principles of triage, and management of resources. Institutions should educate staff on current protocols in place in the event of a disaster, and undergo regular training to keep skills up-to-date.

Also to ensure that the susceptible worried well group of individuals does not overwhelm health-care facilities. A critical action should be in providing information and education to the public about the bioterrorism event.

DETECTING BIOTERRORISM CASE STUDY

It is a busy evening in the emergency department, you are the nurse in triage. A 32-year-old male presents to the emergency department with complaint of 5 days of fever up to 104°F, vomiting, headache, backache, and lethargy. The patient also complains of acne-like pustules on the soles of the feet and palms that developed the previous day afternoon, he first noted it on his face. He also complains of ulcerations in his mouth. He took ibuprofen 2 hours ago for the fever and body aches. He appears acutely ill, and uncomfortable. His vital signs are BP 142/86, RR 22, HR 126, temperature 102.8°F orally. He notes he works at a local hospital in environmental services, and approximately 2 weeks ago he had been cleaning rooms, on a floor where some of the patients have had adult-onset chicken pox recently. However, he was assigned to those rooms because he was aware that he had chicken pox as a child. Which of his symptoms lead you to think about a bioterrorism exposure?

EPIDEMIOLOGIC SYNDROME RECOGNITION

Epidemiologic Features Related to High-Risk Syndrome Criteria

In the emergency department triage setting, epidemiologic principles should be used to alert health-care providers to the possibility of a bioterrorism-related outbreak.

Bioterrorism attacks are likely to present with acute outbreaks of unusual symptoms, or an outbreak of an illness in the wrong season or geographic area. The triage nurse wants to think about terrorism when there is an overt attack (known bomb, blast, agent), or a covert attack (>2 people with similar symptoms).

If you see patients with any of the following syndromes that are acute in onset, and occur in young, immunologically intact, healthy individuals consider a bioterrorist event. Some of the most likely Category A pathogens are anthrax, smallpox, pneumonic plague, botulism, and SARS. (See Fig. 25-1 and Table 25-1.)

TABLE 25-1

TEXT-BASED SYNDROME CASE DEFINITIONS AND ASSOCIATED CATEGORY A CONDITIONS

Syndrome	Definition	Category A Condition
Botulism-like	ACUTE condition that may represent exposure to botulinum toxin	Botulism
	ACUTE paralytic conditions consistent with botulism: cranial nerve VI (lateral rectus) palsy, ptosis, dilated pupils, decreased gag reflex, media rectus palsy	
	ACUTE descending motor paralysis (including muscles of respiration)	
	ACUTE symptoms consistent with botulism: diplopia, dry mouth, dysphagia, difficulty focusing to a near point	
Hemorrhagic illness	SPECIFIC diagnosis of any virus that causes viral hemorrhagic fever (VHF): yellow fever, dengue, Rift Valley fever, Crimean-Congo HF, Kyasanur Forest disease, Omsk HF, Hantaan, Junin, Machupo, Lassa, Marburg, Ebola	VHF
	ACUTE condition with multiple organ involvement that may be consistent with exposure to any virus that causes VHF	
	ACUTE blood abnormalities consistent with VHF: leukopenia, neutropenia, thrombocytopenia, decreased clotting factors, albuminuria	
Lymphadenitis	ACUTE regional lymph node swelling and/ or infection (painful bubo—particularly in groin, axilla, or neck)	Plague (bubonic)
Localized cutaneous lesion	SPECIFIC diagnosis of localized cutaneous lesion/ulcer consistent with cutaneous anthrax or tularemia	Anthrax (cutaneous) tularemia
	ACUTE localized edema and/ or cutaneous lesion/vesicle, ulcer, eschar that may be consistent with cutaneous anthrax or tularemia	
	INCLUDES insect bites	
	EXCLUDES any lesion disseminated over the body or generalized rash	
	EXCLUDES diabetic ulcer and ulcer associated with peripheral vascular disease	
Gastrointestinal	ACUTE infection of the upper and/ or lower gastrointestinal (GI) tract	Anthrax (gastrointestinal)
	SPECIFIC diagnosis of acute GI distress such as Salmonella gastroenteritis	
	ACUTE nonspecific symptoms of GI distress such as nausea, vomiting, or diarrhea	
	EXCLUDES any chronic conditions such as inflammatory bowel syndrome	
Respiratory	ACUTE infection of the upper and/or lower respiratory tract (from the oropharynx to the lungs, includes otitis media)	Anthrax (inhalational) tularemia plague (pneumonic)
	SPECIFIC diagnosis of acute respiratory tract infection (RTI) such as pneumonia due to parainfluenza virus	
	ACUTE nonspecific diagnosis of RTI such as sinusitis, pharyngitis, laryngitis	
	ACUTE nonspecific symptoms of RTI such as cough, stridor, shortness of breath, throat pain	
	EXCLUDES chronic conditions such as chronic bronchitis, asthma without acute exacerbation, chronic sinusitis, allergic conditions (Note: Include *acute exacerbation* of chronic illnesses.)	

TABLE 25-1

TEXT-BASED SYNDROME CASE DEFINITIONS AND ASSOCIATED CATEGORY A CONDITIONS (*CONTINUED*)

Syndrome	Definition	Category A Condition
Neurological	ACUTE neurological infection of the central nervous system (CNS) SPECIFIC diagnosis of acute CNS infection such as pneumococcal meningitis, viral encephalitis ACUTE nonspecific diagnosis of CNS infection such as meningitis not otherwise specified (NOS), encephalitis NOS, encephalopathy NOS ACUTE nonspecific symptoms of CNS infection such as meningismus, delirium EXCLUDES any chronic, hereditary or degenerative conditions of the CNS such as obstructive hydrocephalus, Parkinson's, Alzheimer's	Not applicable
Rash	ACUTE condition that may present as consistent with smallpox (macules, papules, vesicles predominantly of face/arms/legs) SPECIFIC diagnosis of acute rash such as chicken pox in person > XX years of age (base age cutoff on data interpretation) or smallpox ACUTE nonspecific diagnosis of rash compatible with infectious disease, such as viral exanthem EXCLUDES allergic or inflammatory skin conditions such as contact or seborrheic dermatitis, rosacea EXCLUDES rash NOS, rash due to poison ivy, sunburn, and eczema	Smallpox
Specific infection	ACUTE infection of known cause not covered in other syndrome groups, usually has more generalized symptoms (i.e., not just respiratory or gastrointestinal) INCLUDES septicemia from known bacteria INCLUDES other febrile illnesses such as scarlet fever	Not applicable
Fever	ACUTE potentially febrile illness of origin not specified INCLUDES fever and septicemia not otherwise specified INCLUDES unspecified viral illness even though unknown if fever is present EXCLUDE entry in this syndrome category if more specific diagnostic code is present allowing same patient visit to be categorized as respiratory, neurological, or gastrointestinal illness syndrome	Not applicable
Severe illness or death potentially due to infectious disease	ACUTE onset of shock or coma from potentially infectious causes EXCLUDES shock from trauma INCLUDES sudden death, death in emergency room, intrauterine deaths, fetal death, spontaneous abortion, and still births EXCLUDES induced fetal abortions, deaths of unknown cause, and unattended deaths	Not applicable

Source: From Department of Defense, Global Emerging Infections System. ESSENCE: Electronic Surveillance System for the Early Notification of Community-based Epidemics. Available at http://www.geis.fhp.osd.mil/GEIS/Surveillance/Activities/ESSENCE/SyndrSurvDefnICD9CM%20codeweb101403.doc.

Some identifiers are

1. Acute respiratory distress
2. Acute onset of neurologic symptoms with obtundation or mental status changes
3. Unexplained rash with fever
4. Fever with bleeding from mucous membranes
5. Unexplained acute icteric syndromes
6. Massive diarrhea with dehydration

Some other key identifiers are

- A rapidly increasing disease incidence within hours or days in a healthy population of individuals.
- Unusual clinical presentation.

- Unusual increase in the number of people seeking care, with fever, respiratory or gastrointestinal complaints.
- A cluster of previously healthy individuals with similar symptoms who live, work, or recreate in the same geographical area.
- Same age distribution or were at the same public event.
- Lower incidence in those persons who are protected (confined indoors, or are not exposed to crowds).
- An increased number of patients who expire within 72 hours after hospital admission.
- Any person with history of recent travel (2–4 weeks) to a foreign country who presents with symptoms of

TABLE 25-2

CLINICAL PRESENTATIONS AND SYNDROMIC DIFFERENTIAL DIAGNOSIS OF SELECTED AGENTS OF BIOTERRORISM

If Patient Has:	Consider	In Addition To:
Few days of nonspecific "flu-like" symptoms with nausea, emesis, cough ± chest discomfort, without coryza or rhinorrhea→ abrupt onset of respiratory distress ± shock ± mental status changes, with CXR abnormalities (wide mediastinum, infiltrates, pleural effusions)	Inhalational anthrax	Bacterial mediastinitis, tularemia, ruptured aortic aneurysm, SVC syndrome, histoplasmosis, coccidioidomycosis, Q fever, psittacosis, Legionnaires' disease, influenza, sarcoidosis
Pruritic, painless papule→vesicle(s)→ulcer→edematous black eschar ± massive edema and regional adenopathy, ± fever, evolving over 3–7 days	Cutaneous anthrax	Recluse spider bite, atypical Lyme disease, staphylococcal lesion, Orf, glanders, tularemia, rat-bite fever, ecthyma gangrenosum, plague, rickettsialpox, atypical mycobacteria, diphtheria
Cough, fever, dyspnea, hemoptysis, lung consolidation ± shock	Pneumonic plague	Severe bacterial or viral pneumonia, inhalational anthrax, pulmonary infarct, pulmonary hemorrhage
Sepsis, DIC, purpura, acral gangrene	Primary septicemic plague	Meningococcemia; gram-negative, streptococcal, pneumococcal or staphylococcal bacteremia with shock; overwhelming postsplenectomy sepsis, acute leukemia
Synchronous, progressive papular→vesicular→pustular rash on face, extremities>>trunk→generalization ± hemorrhagic component, with systemic toxicity	Smallpox	Atypical varicella, drug eruption, Stevens-Johnson syndrome, atypical measles, secondary syphilis, erythema multiforme, meningococcemia, monkeypox (with African travel history)
Acute febrile illness with pleuropneumonitis, bronchiolitis ± hilar lymphadenopathy, variable progression to respiratory failure	Inhalational tularemia	Inhalational anthrax, influenza, mycoplasma pneumonia, Legionnaire's disease, Q fever, plague
Acute onset of afebrile, symmetric, descending flaccid paralysis that begins in bulbar muscles, dilated pupils, dry mucous membranes with normal mental status and absence of sensory changes	Botulism	Brain stem CVA, polio, myasthenia gravis, Guillain-Barre syndrome, tick paralysis, chemical intoxication

Source: Reprinted with permission from the Infectious Diseases Society of America.

high fever, rigors, delirium, rash, extreme myalgias, shock, diffuse hemorrhagic lesions or petechiae, or extreme dehydration due to vomiting or diarrhea without blood loss.
• Greater number of ill or dead animals.

Immediate Care of Mr S

Mr S had a mask placed over his mouth and nose in triage, and is placed into a private isolation room with negative pressure in the emergency department. The triage nurse informs the doctor that the patient appears acutely ill, and she is concerned about the patient's symptoms. She alerts the doctor about the patient's fever, lethargy, and myalgias, and that Mr S's rash appears to be all pustules and is in the same stage of development, mostly on his face and extremities. She also alerts the doctor of his exposure to "adult-onset chicken pox" even though he previously has had chicken pox. She knows to use standard precautions, and that airborne and contact precautions should be utilized for

chicken pox, or in case this is an outbreak of smallpox. (See Table 25-2.)

Once a biological agent has been identified, it is important to contain the disease from spreading. All patients in healthcare facilities with suspected or confirmed bioterrorism-related illnesses should be managed using standard precautions. Additional precautions may be needed for certain syndromes.

CHEMICAL AGENTS AND BIOTERRORISM

Patient triage for chemical agents should be down having staff protected with PPE equipment. Patients should be separated into three categories:

1. The degree of injury is very severe, and deemed irreversible. Care is focused on comfort of the patient.
2. The second group consists of casualties who require immediate intervention for survival. Treat the ABCs and give necessary antidotes.

3. The third group of people consists of those who have injuries that place them in no immediate danger. They are stable with minor injuries.

The following is an overview of possible chemical agents that could be expected in an incident related to bioterrorism.

- Nerve agents—Tabun, sarin, soman, VX, organophosphates
- Blood agents—Hydrogen cyanide, cyanogen chloride
- Choking agents—Phosgene, chlorine, ammonia
- Blister agents—Mustard, lewisite
- Riot agents—Mace, pepper spray

(See Tables 25-3, 25-4, and 25-5.)

If bioterrorism is expected via a chemical agent, hazardous materials (hazmat) team should be notified and decontamination protocols should be initiated.

DECONTAMINATION

Preparation for Chemical Exposure and Decontamination from Stanford Hospital Chemical Exposure

1. Contact the hazmat response team.
2. Break out personal protection equipment, decon supplies, antidotes, and so on.

TABLE 25-3

CATEGORIES FOR TRIAGE OF CHEMICAL CASUALTIES

	Immediate	Delayed	Minimal	Expectant
Nerve agent	Talking, not walking (severe distress with dyspnea, twitching, and/or nausea, vomiting); moderate-to-severe effects in two or more systems (e.g., respiratory, GI, muscular); circulation intact Not talking (unconscious), not walking; circulation intact Not talking, not walking; circulation not intact (if treatment facilities are available; if not, classify as expectant)	Recovering from severe exposure, antidotes, or both	Casualty walking and talking; capable of self-aid; imminent return to duty	Not talking; circulation failed (with adequate treatment resources, classify as immediate)
Cyanide	Severe distress (unconscious, convulsing, or postictal, with or without apnea) with circulation intact	Recovering; has survived more than 15 minutes after vapor exposure		Circulation failed
Vesicant	Airway injury; classify as immediate if help obtainable (rare)	Skin injury on greater than 5% but less than 50% (liquid exposure) of body surface area; any body surface area burn (vapor exposure); most eye injuries; airway problems beginning more than 4 hours after exposure	Skin injury on less than 5% of body surface area in noncritical areas; minor eye injuries; minor upper airway injury	Greater than 50% body surface area skin injury from liquid; moderate-to-severe airway injury, particularly with early onset (<4 hours after exposure)
Phosgene	Acute airway injury: classify as immediate if resources available	Onset of symptoms more than 4 hours postexposure		Moderate-to-severe injury with early onset (<4 hours, resource dependent)

Source: From: http://www.emedicine.com/emerg/topic892.htm

TABLE 25-4
BIOLOGICAL WARFARE

BIOTERRORIST AGENTS

WATCH FOR THESE SYMPTOMS

Disease	Signs & Symptoms	Incubation Time (Range)	Person-to-Person Transmission	Isolation	Diagnosis	Postexposure Prophylaxis for Adults	Treatment for Adults
Anthrax Bacillus anthracis A. Inhalation	Flu-like symptoms (fever, fatigue, muscle aches, dyspnea, nonproductive cough, headache), chest pain; possible 1-2 day improvement then rapid respiratory failure and shock. Meningitis may develop.	1 to 6 days (up to 6 wks)	None	Standard Precautions	Chest x-ray evidence of widening mediastinum; obtain sputum and blood culture. Sensitivity and specificity of nasal swabs unknown – do not rely on for diagnosis	Prophylaxis for 60 days: Ciprofloxacin* 500 mg PO q 12h Or Doxycycline 100 mg q 12h Alternative (if strain susceptible and above contraindicated): Amoxicillin 500 mg PO q 8h *In vitro studies suggest that Levofloxacin 500 mg PO q 24h Or Gatifloxacin 400 mg PO q 24h Or Moxifloxacin 400 mg PO q 24h could be substituted	Inhalation anthrax Combined IV/PO therapy for 60d Ciprofloxacin 500 mg q 12h Or Doxycycline 100 mg q 12h, AND 1 or 2 additional drugs (vancomycin, rifampin, imipenem clindamycin, chloramphenicol, clarithromycin, and if susceptible penicillin or ampicillin Cutaneous anthrax Ciprofloxacin 500 mg PO q 12h Or Doxycycline 100 mg PO q 12h
B. Cutaneous	Intense itching followed by painless papular lesions, then vesicular lesions, developing into eschar surrounded by edema.	1 to 12 days	Direct contact with skin lesions may result in cutane-ous infection.	Contact Precautions	Peripheral blood smear may demonstrate gram positive bacilli on unspun smear with sepsis.		
C. Gastrointestinal (GI)	Abdominal pain, nausea and vomiting, severe diarrhea, GI bleeding, and fever.	1 to 7 days	None	Standard Precautions	Culture blood and stool.	Recommendations same for pregnant women and immunocompromised persons	Recommendations same for pregnant women and immunocompromised persons
Botulism botulinum toxin	Afebrile, excess mucus in throat, dysphagia, dry mouth and throat, dizziness, then difficulty moving eyes, mild pupillary dilation and nystagmus, intermittent ptosis, indistinct speech, unsteady gait, extreme symmetric descending weakness, flaccid paralysis, generally normal mental status.	Inhalation: 12-80 hours Foodborne: 12-72 hours (2-8 days)	None	Standard Precautions	Laboratory tests available from CDC or Public Health Dept; obtain serum, stool, gastric aspirate and suspect foods prior to administering antitoxin. Differential diagnosis includes polio, Guillain Barre, myasthenia, tick paralysis, CVA, meningococcal meningitis.	Pentavalent toxoid (types A, B, C, D, E) 0.5 ml SQ may be available as investigational product from USAMRIID.	Botulism antitoxins from public health authorities. Supportive care and ventilatory support. Avoid clindamycin and aminoglycosides.
Pneumonic Plague Yersinia pestis	High fever, cough, hemoptysis, chest pain, nausea and vomiting, headache. Advanced disease: purpuric skin lesions, copious watery or purulent sputum production; respiratory failure in 1 to 6 days.	2-3 days (2-6 days)	Yes, droplet aerosols	Droplet Precautions until 48 hrs of effective antibiotic therapy	A presumptive diagnosis may be made by Gram, Wayson or Wright stain of lymph node aspirates, sputum, or cerebrospinal fluid with gram negative bacilli with bipolar (safety pin) staining.	Doxycycline 100 mg PO q 12h Or Ciprofloxacin 500 mg PO q 12h	Streptomycin 1 gm IM q 12h; Or Gentamicin 2 mg/kg, then 1.0 to 1.7 mg/kg IV q 8h Alternatives: Doxycycline 200 mg PO load, then 100 PO mg q 12h Or Ciprofloxacin 400 mg IV q 12h
Smallpox variola virus	Prodromal period: malaise, fever, rigors, vomiting, headache, and backache. After 2-4 days, skin lesions appear and progress uniformly from macules to papules to vesicles and pustules, mostly on face, neck, palms, soles, and subsequently progress to trunk.	12-14 days (7-17 days)	Yes, airborne droplet nuclei or direct contact with skin lesions or secretions until all scabs separate and fall off (3 to 4 weeks)	Airborne (includes N95 mask) and Contact Precautions	Swab culture of vesicular fluid or scab, send to BL-4 laboratory. All lesions similar in appearance and develop synchronously as opposed to chickenpox. Electron microscopy can differentiate variola virus from varicella.	Early vaccine critical (in less than 4 days). Call CDC for vaccinia. Vaccinia immune globulin in special cases - call USAMRIID 301-619-2833.	Supportive care. Previous vaccination against smallpox does not confer lifelong immunity. Potential role for Cidofovir.

(Continued)

BIOLOGICAL WARFARE (*CONTINUED*)

Photo Credits: Anthrax A and C - JAMA 1999;281:1737-8 ; Anthrax B - CDC; Botulism - JAMA 2001;285:1062 Copyrighted 2001 American Medical Association; Plague - JAMA 2000;283:2283; Smallpox - CDC

References:
- Amon SS, Schechter R, Inglesby TV, et al. for the Working Group on Civilian Biodefense. Botulinum toxin as a biological weapon: medical and public health management. JAMA 2001;285:1059-1070.
- Centers for Disease Control and Prevention. Chemical/Biological Survival Cards for Civilians. 2000.
- Chin J, ed. Control of Communicable Diseases Manual. 17th edition. Washington, DC: American Public Health Association. 2000.
- Henderson DA, Inglesby TV, Bartlett JG, et al. for the Working Group on Civilian Biodefense. Smallpox as a biological weapon: medical and public health management. JAMA 1999;281:2127-2137.
- Inglesby TV, Henderson DA, Bartlett JG, et al. for the Working Group on Civilian Biodefense. Anthrax as a biological weapon: medical and public health management. JAMA 2002;287:2236-2252.
- Inglesby TV, Dennis DT, Henderson DA, et al. for the Working Group on Civilian Biodefense. Plague as a biological weapon: medical and public health management. JAMA 2000;283:2281-2290.
- U.S. Army Medical Research Institute of Infectious Diseases. USAMRIID's Medical Management of Biological Casualties Handbook. 4th ed. Fort Detrick, Frederick, Maryland. 2001.
- Update: Investigation of Bioterrorism-Related Anthrax and Interim Guidelines for Clinical Evaluation of Persons with Possible Anthrax. MMWR 2001;50:941-948.

NOTIFICATION PROCEDURES IN THE EVENT OF A BIOTERRORIST INCIDENT	DECONTAMINATION FOR ALL OF THESE AGENTS
1. First call the Public Health Officer at your local health department; after hours contact local Health Director via 911. 2. If criminal activity is suspected, call your local law enforcement and the FBI in your state. **FOR MORE INFORMATION ON BIOTERRORISM:** CDC - Centers for Disease Control and Prevention www.bt.cdc.gov/ APIC - Association for Professionals in Infection Control & Epidemiology www.apic.org/bioterror/ SPICE - North Carolina Statewide Program for Infection Control and Epidemiology www.unc.edu/depts/spice/ 919-966-3242 USAMRIID's Medical Management of Biological Casualties Handbook www.usamriid.army.mil/education/bluebook.html	1. Place clothing from suspected victims in airtight impervious (e.g., plastic) bags and save for law authorities (e.g., FBI, SBI). 2. Use soap and water for washing victim. 3. For environmental disinfection for all of the above, use bleach (standard 6.0% - 6.15% sodium hypochlorite) in a 0.6% concentration (1 part bleach to 9 parts water). For botulism, plague and smallpox an alternative is to use an EPA-approved germicidal detergent. 4. For smallpox, all bedding and clothing must be autoclaved or laundered in hot water and bleach. 5. Healthcare worker should wear PPE (gowns, gloves and mask) during decontamination of anthrax, plague, and smallpox. **DETECTION OF OUTBREAKS** **Epidemiologic Strategies** • A rapidly increasing disease incidence • An unusual increase in the number of people seeking care, especially with fever, respiratory, or gastrointestinal symptoms • An endemic disease rapidly emerging at an uncharacteristic time or in an unusual pattern • Lower attack rate among persons who had been indoors • Clusters of patients arriving from a single locale • Large numbers of rapidly fatal cases • Any patient presenting with a disease that is relatively uncommon and has bioterrorism potential

Chart developed by:	
North Carolina Statewide Program for Infection Control and Epidemiology (SPICE) email: spice@unc.edu KK Hoffmann, DJ Weber, EP Clontz, WA Rutala	**Support provided by:** The North Carolina Institute for Public Health and The North Carolina Center for Public Health Preparedness, in the School of Public Health at The University of North Carolina at Chapel Hill

Source: Used with permission from the North Carolina Statewide Program for Infection Control and Epidemiology (SPICE). http://www.emedicinehealth.com/images/4453/4453-15666-15704-25709.pdf

TABLE 25-5

PROTOCOLS FOR CHEMICAL AGENTS

A.   NERVE AGENT PROTOCOL

1. Severe respiratory distress?

YES: Intubate and ventilate

ATROPINE

Adults: 6 mg IM or IV

Inf/ped: 0.05 mg/kg IV

2-PAM C1

Adults: 600–1000 mg IM or slow IV

Inf/ped: 15 mg/kg slow IV

2. Major secondary symptoms?

NO: Go to 6

YES: *ATROPINE*

Adults: 4 mg IM or IV

Inf/ped: 0.02–0.05 mg/kg IV

2-PAM C1

Adults: 600–1000 mg IM or slow IV

Inf/ped: 15 mg/kg

OPEN IV LINE

3. Repeat atropine as needed until secretions decrease

and breathing easier

Adults: 2 mg IV or IM

Inf/ped: 0.02–0.05 mg/kg IV

4. Repeat 2-PAM C1 as needed

Adults: 1 g IV over 20–30 minutes Repeat q lh x 3 prn

Inf/ped: 15 mg/kg slow IV

5. Convulsions?

NO: Go to 6

YES: DIAZEPAM 10 mg slow IV

Inf/ped: 0.2 mg/kg IV

6. Reevaluate q 3–5 minutes

IF SIGNS WORSEN, repeat from 3

B.   CHLORINE PROTOCOL

1. Dyspnea?

- Try bronchodilators

- Admit

- Oxygen by mask

- Chest x-ray

2. Treat other problems and reevaluate (consider phosgene)

3. Respiratory system OK?

YES: Go to 5

4. Is phosgene poisoning possible?

YES: Go to PHOSGENE PROTOCOL

5. Give supportive therapy; treat other problems or discharge

C.   LEWISITE PROTOCOL

1. Survey extent of injury

2. Treat affected skin with British Anti-Lewisite (BAL) oint-

ment (if available)

3. Treat affected eyes with BAL ophthalmic ointment

(if available)

4. Treat pulmonary/severe effects

- BAL in oil, 0.5 mL/25 lb body wt. deep IM to max of 4.0

ml. Repeat q 4 h x 3 (at 4, 8, and 12 hours) Morphine

prn

5. Severe poisoning?

YES: Shorten interval for BAL injections to q 2 h

D.   MUSTARD PROTOCOL

1. Airway obstruction?

YES: Tracheostomy

2. If there are large burns:

- Establish IV line—do not push fluids as for thermal

burns

- Drain vesicles—unroof large blisters and irrigate area

with tropical antibiotics

3. Treat other symptoms appropriately:

- Antibiotic eye ointment/sterile precautions

prn/morphine prn

E.   PHOSGENE PROTOCOL

1. Restrict fluids, chest x-ray, blood gases

- Results consistent with phosgene poisoning?

YES: Go to 4

2. Dyspnea?

YES: OXYGEN, positive end-expiratory pressure

3. Observe closely for at least 6 hours

IF SEVERE DYSPNEA develops, go to 4

IF MILD DYSPNEA develops after several hours, go to 1

4. Severe dyspnea develops or x-ray or blood gases consis-

tent with phosgene poisoning-

- Admit/oxygen under positive end-expiratory

pressure/restrict fluids/chest x-ray/blood

gases/seriously ill list

F.   CYANIDE PROTOCOL

1. Immediate casualty (within minutes of exposure) with

apnea and/or convulsions?

YES

- 300 mg of sodium nitrite injected IV over 2–4 minutes

followed by 12.5 g sodium thiosulfate injected IV

2. Minimal casualty (mild symptoms: dizziness, nausea, vom-

iting, headache)

YES

- Consider treatment for immediate casualty—may

alleviate symptoms

- Once removed from cyanide source, progression of

symptoms unlikely

- Generally, a casualty who has had inhalation exposure

and survives long enough to reach medical care will

need little care

TABLE 25-6

STANFORD HOSPITAL'S CHEMICAL EXPOSURE FLOWCHART DESCRIBING PREPARATION FOR CHEMICAL EXPOSURE AND DECONTAMINATION

When victim arrives

(Note: A contaminated patient may present at an emergency room without prior warning.)

6. Does chemical hazard exist?

- Known release/exposure (including late notification)
- Liquid on victim's skin or clothing
- Symptoms in victim, EMTs, others
- Odor
- Mustard gas—garlic, onion, or mustard smell
- Lewisite—geraniums
- Phosgene—freshly cut grass or hay
- Chlorine—chlorine odor
- Cyanide—bitter almonds

YES: Go to 7

NO: Handle victim routinely

7. Hold victim outside until preparations are completed (don personal protective equipment to assist EMTs as necessary)

8. If patient is grossly contaminated (liquid on skin) *or* if there is any suspicion of contamination, decontaminate patient before entry into building

Decontamination (coordinated by hazmat team):

- Provide adequate ventilation and oxygenation
- Removal of all exposed clothing—double bag
- Extensive water wash in shower (5 minutes for low suspicion or vapor exposure, 10 minutes for liquid or powder exposure). Liquid detergent (Joy) should be applied as well
- Once patient has been decontaminated, there is little risk of injury to HCPs
- Note for patients with C-spine precautions or unconscious patients, hazmat team will require physician supervision—physicians will need to don Level C PPE and assist with these patients

3. Set up hotline (dedicated line). (Plan on contacting county, state health departments, CDC, and army.)
4. Hazmat team will
   a. Coordinate clearing and securing all areas, which could become contaminated and secure hospital entrances and grounds.
   b. Notify local emergency management authorities if needed.
   c. If the chemical is a military agent and army has not been informed, call them.
5. If an organophosphate (nerve agent) is involved, notify hospital pharmacy that large amounts of atropine and 2-PAM may be needed.

(See Table 25-6 for a flowchart describing procedures to follow when the victim arrives and Table 25-7 for a flowchart describing procedures to follow for initial treatment and identification of the chemical agent.)

CONCLUSION

The threat of a bioterrorism event is real, and therefore emergency departments must be prepared to receive patients exposed to biological or chemical agents. Triage is an integral part in dealing with a bioterrorist event. Triage is cornerstone of defense against bioterrorism. It is important for emergency departments to establish set protocols in order to streamline care in the event of a bioterrorist event or mass casualty disaster. Communication should be established through each institution, as well as throughout the region. All hospital personnel should be trained to recognize and identify high-risk syndromes related to potential biologic agent outbreak, and be aware of chemical agents and decontamination procedures. By having staff educated and protocols in place, it will ensure that the maximal amount of care will be provided if an event was to occur.

TABLE 25-7

STANFORD HOSPITAL'S INITIAL TREATMENT AND IDENTIFICATION OF THE CHEMICAL AGENT

1. Establish airway if necessary
2. Give artificial respiration if not breathing
3. Control bleeding if hemorrhaging
4. Symptoms of cholinesterase poisoning?
   - Pinpoint pupils
   - Difficulty breathing (wheezing, gasping, etc.)
   - Local or generalized sweating
   - Fasciculations
   - Copious secretions
   - Nausea, vomiting, diarrhea
   - Convulsions
   - Coma

YES: Go to NERVE AGENT PROTOCOL (Table 25-5)

5. History of chlorine poisoning?

YES: Go to CHLORINE PROTOCOL (Table 25-5)

6. Burns that began within minutes of poisoning?

YES: Go to 7

NO: Go to 8

7. Thermal burn?

YES: Go to 9

NO: Go to LEWISITE PROTOCOL (Table 25-5)

8. Burns or eye irritation beginning 2–12 hours after exposure?

YES: Go to MUSTARD PROTOCOL (Table 25-5)

NO: Go to 9

9. Is phosgene exposure possible?
   - Known exposure to phosgene
   - Known exposure to hot chlorinated hydrocarbons
   - Respiratory discomfort beginning a few hours after exposure

YES: Go to PHOSGENE PROTOCOL (Table 25-5)

10. Is cyanide exposure possible?
    - Known exposure to cyanide
    - Smell of bitter almonds (only 50% can detect cyanide by odor)

YES: Go to CYANIDE PROTOCOL (Table 25-5)

11. Check other possible chemical exposures:
    - Known exposure
    - Decreased level of consciousness without head trauma
    - Odor on clothes or breath
    - Specific signs or symptoms

Suggested Reading

Berger ME, Leonard RB, Ricks RC, et al. Hospital Triage in the First 24 hours after a Nuclear or Radiological Disaster. ORISE: Oak Ridge Institute for Science and Education. Available at *http: www.orise.orace.gov/reacts/files/triage.pdf*

Bioterrorism and Emergency Preparedness for hospitals and professionals, 1/09/2002. Retrieved 12/21/05 *http://www.stanfordhospital.com/forPhysiciansOthers/bioterrorism/bioterrorism*

Burkle FM. Mass casualty management of a large scale bioterrrorist event: an epidemiological approach that shapes triage decisions. *Emergency Med Clin North Am.* May 2002;20(2): 409–436.

Department of Defense, Global Emerging Infections System. ESSENCE: Electronic Surveillance System for the Early Notification of Community-based Epidemics. Available at *http://www.geis.fhp.osd.mil/GEIS/Surveillance/Activities/ESSENCE/SyndrSurvDefnICD9CM%20codeweb101403.doc*

Department of Defense, Global Emerging Infections System. ESSENCE: Electronic Surveillance System for the Early

Notification of Community-based Epidemics. Available at *http://www.geis.fhp.osd.mil/GEIS/SurveillanceActivities/ESS-ENCE/SyndrSurvDefnlCD9CM%20codeweb101403.doc*

Detecting Bioterrorism: The Clinician's Role (Stanford). Retrieved on January 4, 2006. *http://www.stanfordhospital.com/PDF/bioterrorism/CliniciansRole.pdf*

English JF, Cundiff MY, Malone JD, et al. Bioterrorism readiness plan: a template for healthcare facilities. April 13, 1999. Retrieved November 11, 2005, *http://www.cdc.gov/ncidod/dhqp/pdf/bt/13apr99apic-cdcbioterrorism.pdf*

Hazardous materials, chemical, and radiation exposure decontamination protocol. Retrieved January 29, 2006. *http://www.emedicine.com/ emerg/topic892.htm*

Hoffmann KK, Weber DJ, Clontz EP, et al. Bioterrorist agents. North Carolina Statewide Program for Infection Control and Epidemiology. June 2002. *http://www.emedicinehealth.com/images/4453/4453-15666-15704-25709.pdf* Retrieved January 9, 2006.

http://www.hscbklyn.edu/emergency_medicine/pdf.docs/UHBSection06a.pdf

http://www.idsociety.org/Template.cfm?Section=Home&CONTENTID=6612&TEMPLATE=/ContentManagement/ContentDisplay.cfm Table 3. Retrieved January 27, 2006.

Jagminas L, Erdman DP. CBRNE-Evaluation of a chemical warfare victim. September 15, 2004. Retrieved from emedicine January 29, 2006.

Johnson SE. Isolation guidelines. Revised by Saint Louis University, Institute for Biosecurity. June 2004. Retrieved December 29, 2005. *http://www.bioterrorism.slu.edu/ bt/quick/Isolation.pdf*

Lanoix R, Wiener DE, Zayas VD. Concepts in disaster triage in the wake of the world trade center terrorist attack. *Topics Emergency Medicine.* 2002;24(2):60–71.

Romig LE. JumpSTART Pediatric Multiple Casualty Incident Triage. *www.jumpstarttriage.com* Retrieved January 27, 2006.

Simple Triage and Rapid Assessment: *http://www.cert-la.com/triage/ start.htm*

Stanford University Hospital Preliminary Chemical Agent Response Protocol. *http://www.stanfordhospital.com/PDF/bioterrorism/chemProtocolFlowchart3.pdf* Retrieved January 4, 2006.

26

PHARMACY PREPAREDNESS FOR INCIDENTS INVOLVING NUCLEAR, BIOLOGICAL, OR CHEMICAL WEAPONS

Anthony M. Burda and Todd Sigg

STAT FACTS

PHARMACY PREPAREDNESS FOR INCIDENTS INVOLVING NUCLEAR, BIOLOGICAL, OR CHEMICAL WEAPONS

- Until delivery of large amounts of medical supplies from the Strategic National Stockpile (SNS) and other state emergency agencies, hospitals should be prepared to treat mass casualties for 4–24 hours using in-house inventory and/or supplies rapidly procurable from other institutions and pharmaceutical suppliers.
- Nerve agent antidotes, such as injectable atropine sulfate, in various sizes, pralidoxime chloride in 1-g vials, and injectable diazepam, are available through pharmaceutical manufacturers and wholesalers. Hospitals and government emergency agencies may now obtain military-style autoinjectors of these antidotes. Some hospitals have chosen to participate in the Chempack Program, which prepositions large amounts of nerve agent antidotes on site.
- The cyanide antidote kit containing amyl nitrite pearls and injectable sodium nitrite and sodium thiosulfate is manufactured by one U.S. company. Hydroxycobalamin is currently under investigation as a cyanide antidote and may offer an improved safety and efficacy profile.

- Pharmaceuticals used for exposures to radioactive isotopes, e.g., Ca-DTPA/Zn-DTPA, Prussian blue, and potassium iodide, are not typically stocked in hospital pharmacy inventories. They may be obtained through the SNS, state emergency agencies or Radiation Emergency Assistance Center/Training Site (REAC/TS), and their manufacturer.
- Many local, state, and federal domestic preparedness agencies are stockpiling antibiotics, for example, ciprofloxacin and doxycycline, for the treatment and prophylaxis of large numbers of patients, health-care workers, and emergency personnel. These antibiotics will protect against many strains of anthrax, pneumonic plague, and other biological threats.
- The Centers for Disease Control and Prevention (CDC) controls the supply and distribution of smallpox vaccines and vaccinia immune globulin.
- The CDC controls the supply and distribution of botulinum antitoxin. Currently, there are no vaccines or antitoxins for other biotoxins such as ricin, abrin, staphylococcus enterotoxin B, and trichothecene mycotoxins.

INTRODUCTION

Events such as the sarin gas attack in a Tokyo subway station in March 1995, the September 11, 2001, attacks, several anthrax hoaxes, and the actual anthrax and ricin letters in the United States have heightened concern among public health and law enforcement agencies that a real nuclear, biological, or chemical (NBC) attack may occur in this nation. The potential for a terrorist attack using a chemical or biological agent has many individuals involved in public health and safety equipping themselves with information, contingency plans, and procedures to cope with such threats. Information concerning preparedness for a terrorist attack involving NBC weapons is available from various governmental agencies and other organizations. Instruction in this area is available via journal articles, Web sites, and on-site and Internet training programs, seminars, and conferences. Most references will provide practical discussion on issues such as local and statewide planning, on-site and hospital decontamination procedures, recognition and detection of NBC agents, diagnosis and pathophysiology of disease states, protocols for first responders, and a variety of other public health issues.

The objective of this article[1] is to provide the practitioner a concise summary and description of the types of pharmaceutical products that a health-care facility pharmacy may be asked to provide as part of an overall response to an incident involving weapons of mass destruction (WMD). These products include antidotes, antibiotics, antitoxins, and other agents used in the symptomatic and supportive care of the poisoned patient. Pharmacy managers are urged to check inventory for these products, and know where the nearest supplier (e.g., wholesaler, pharmaceutical manufacturer, etc.) is located for each agent. It is important to know how supplies can be obtained quickly in emergencies; many health-care facilities are unprepared for poisoning emergencies. Small nonurban hospitals are more likely to have fewer antidotes in stock than larger urban, tertiary care facilities. In addition to monitoring inventory, pharmacy managers and pharmacy and therapeutics (P&T) committee members should be aware of their local or state governmental agencies that may support a depot of some pharmaceuticals. Often this information is classified and not readily available to individuals not serving on WMD readiness task forces or committees.

The Nunn-Lugar-Domenici Domestic Preparedness Act of 1996 established a $250,000,000 program to train 120 cities in the United States in the preparedness of emergency and medical response to chemical and biological agents. Headed by the Department of Homeland Security (DHS), federal agencies involved with domestic preparedness programs include the Department of Energy (DOE), Federal Bureau of Investigation (FBI), Federal Emergency Management Agency (FEMA), Environmental Protection Agency (EPA), and Centers for Disease Control and Prevention (CDC). Local government bodies created metropolitan medical response systems (MMRS), whose mission is to create a multiple level, technically diverse, professional response to any deliberate or accidental act involving an NBC agent within that jurisdiction. Antidote caches funded by federal grants to MMRS will be intended for use by Emergency Medical System (EMS) first responders for self-administration, to treat a number of casualties at the site of the NBC incident, and to provide pharmaceuticals to treat large numbers of hospitalized patients and asymptomatic outpatients. The first 4–12 hours of emergency response will need to be managed by local resources prior to the arrival of the DHS and other federal assistance, such as delivery and distribution of the Strategic National Stockpile (SNS) formerly known as the National Pharmaceutical Stockpile (NPS). Two primary missions of the Homeland Security Act of 2002 are to reduce the vulnerability of the United States to terrorism, and to minimize the damage and assist in the recovery from terrorist attacks that do occur within the United States.

Strategic National Stockpile

The CDC, in consultation with other partners in chem/biopreparedness, has developed a stockpile to respond to biological or chemical terrorism emergencies. To determine and review the composition of the SNS, CDC considers many factors, such as current biological and/or chemical threats, the availability of medical materiel, and the ease of dissemination of pharmaceuticals. One of the most significant factors in determining SNS composition, however, is the medical vulnerability of the U.S. civilian population. SNS depots are stored at strategic locations throughout the United States to assure the most rapid response possible. CDC ensures that the medical materiel in these SNS storage facilities is rotated and kept within potency shelf life limits.

More information about the SNS program is available at *www.bt.cdc.gov/stockpile*, or by calling the SNS operations center at 404-639-7120.

The Veteran's Administration (VA) is a part of the National Disaster Medical System and can be asked to aid local civilian responders. The VA has a role in maintaining the SNS. VA procures pharmaceuticals for the CDC and manages contracts for the storage, rotation, security, and transportation of these items. It is also responsible for the deployment of up to five "push packages" of pharmaceuticals in an emergency. VA has stockpiled four packages of pharmaceuticals and medical surgical supplies for the National Disaster Medical System and has a fifth package that is placed on site at high-risk national events such as a presidential inauguration.

---

[1]Revised and updated, originally published in the Journal of Pharmacy Practice, April 2000, 13(2):141–55, Copyright 2000 by Sage Publications, Inc. Reprinted by Permission of Sage Publications, Inc.

Chempack Project

In 2003, the DHS/CDC Strategic National Stockpile Program began pilot testing a project that "forward" positions nerve agent antidote and symptomatic treatments at the local hospital and EMS level. The Chempack Project is a sustainable resource that would enhance local response to nerve agent attacks. As a cost-avoiding measure, the Chempack pharmaceuticals are kept fresh with respect to expiration dating via participation in the Food and Drug Administration Shelf-Life Extension Program (FDA SLE). It is projected that FDA SLE participation will deliver $97 million of cost savings to taxpayers over 10 years; the alternative being outright replacement of product when it reaches the expiration date. Hospitals and EMS participation in this project was voluntary. The pilot test was successful, demonstrating project implementation and maintenance procedures to be feasible. The project expanded throughout 2004, with SNS selecting more localities nationwide to position Chempacks. Where Chempacks have been positioned, hospital pharmacists play a lead role, working with SNS and the local health department to receive, secure, and maintain these assets.

Every hospital should have a WMD plan as part of their disaster readiness. The U.S. Army Edgewood Chemical Biological Center and the Army Corps Department of Justice (DoJ) Office of Domestic Preparedness offers training and technical assistance to jurisdictions to help them respond to, and mitigate the consequences of, domestic terrorism.

CHEMICAL AGENTS

As defined by the U.S. Army, a chemical warfare agent is a "chemical substance intended for use in military operations to kill or seriously injure or incapacitate humans or animals through its toxicologic effects." Terrorists would find chemical agents attractive to use for several reasons, such as they are extremely toxic and readily available or easily synthesized. In many respects, emergency response systems and health-care facilities need to respond to a WMD chemical attack in the same fashion as a hazardous materials incident. The same principles regarding triage, decontamination, and allocation of resources that shape disaster plans related to hazardous materials go into action during a WMD chemical attack.

Chemical agents are generally classified into several groups: blood agents, nerve agents, choking agents, and blistering agents. Each agent has been designated its own North Atlantic Treaty Organization (NATO) designation symbol (a military symbol), which is not its chemical formula. This may be confusing at times. For instance, the NATO designation symbol for cyanide is AC, while its chemical formula is CN. Whereas, the NATO designation symbol for Mace is CN.

An important principle to recognize concerning chemical agents is that the onset of symptoms is very rapid, typically within minutes. Therefore, prompt initiation of rescue, decontamination, medical attention, and antidotal therapy is critical in minimizing casualties. The Chemical and Biological Hotline (1-800-424-8802) based in Aberdeen, MD, serves as an emergency resource to all health-care providers for technical assistance. Much of the following information has been adapted from the U.S. Army handbook, *USAMRIID's Medical Management of Chemical Casualties Handbook*. This reference is located online at *www.usamriid.army.mil*

CYANIDE

In the form of an NBC agent, cyanide would most likely be encountered as hydrogen cyanide (AC), cyanogen chloride (CK), and cyanogen bromide or cyanogen iodide gases. An explosion of an industrial storage tank containing acetonitrile or acrylonitrile would pose a high risk of delayed cyanide toxicity. Cyanide toxicity is characterized by a rapid onset of dizziness, confusion, dyspnea, tachycardia, and hypertension followed by coma, convulsions, bradycardia, hypotension, arrhythmias, and metabolic acidosis. Death may occur within minutes following significant exposures. Cyanide is classified as a blood agent by some WMD references. A cyanide antidote kit containing amyl nitrite pearls, injectable sodium nitrite, and sodium thiosulfate is available. Nitrites in this kit convert RBC hemoglobin into methemoglobin. Methemoglobin combines with cyanide to form cyanmethemoglobin which theoretically decreases the amount of free cyanide available. In synergism with 100% oxygen, thiosulfate combines with cyanide via the rhodanese enzyme to form less toxic thiocyanate, which is eliminated in the urine. Two other pharmaceuticals, which serve as adjunctive therapy for cyanide poisoning, are injectable sodium bicarbonate to correct metabolic acidosis and benzodiazepines (e.g., diazepam or lorazepam) as anticonvulsants. Their availability is discussed later in the article. Hydroxocobalamin (Vitamin $B_{12}A$) is a promising cyanide antidote; and just became available in the United States trials. This chemical binds with cyanide in vivo to form nontoxic cyanocobalamin (Vitamin B_{12}). Hydroxocobalamin (Cyanokit ® Dey Pharmaceuticals) was FDA approved in June 2006. It is given (over 15 minutes) in an intravenous dose of five grams (70 mg/kg in pediatric patients) which may be repeated, It can be obtained through Dey L.P. (800-755-5560). It should be noted that sodium thiosulfate is not compatable with hydroxocobalamin and if required, should be administered through a separate intravenous line. Skin and bodily fluids may turn orange-red for a few days after administration. It is supplied in vials contained 2,5 grams of the lypholized product. Another antidote, cobalt edentate (Celocyanor), is used in Great Britain and France. A more rapid methemoglobin inducer, 4-dimethylaminophenol (4-DMAP), is used in some European countries. Stroma-free methemoglobin has been studied in animals and is not available for human use.

Eli Lilly & Company no longer manufactures the cyanide antidote package. It is now available from Akorn, Inc. Each package contains 12 amyl nitrite pearls, two 10 mL vials of 3% sodium nitrite for injection, and two 50 mL vials of 25% sodium thiosulfate for injection. Akorn, Inc. is located at 2500 Millbrook Drive, Buffalo Grove, IL, 60089. The phone number to the company is (800) 535-7155. Its Web site address is *www.akorn.com* The price of the kit is $274.56 and has a shelf life of 24 months.

Three percent sodium nitrite for injection (300 mg/10 mL vials) is available from Hope Pharmaceuticals, located at 8260 East Gelding, Suite 104, Scottsdale, AZ, 85260. The phone number to the company is (800) 755-9595. Its Web site address is *www.hopepharm.com* This product costs $42.48 and has a shelf life of 24 months.

Packages of 12 amyl nitrite pearls (0.18 mL or 0.3 mL) are available from James Alexander Corporation, located at 845 Route 94, Blairstown, NJ, 07825. The phone number to the company is (908) 362-9266. Its Web site address is *www.james-alexander.com* The product costs $3.96 and has a shelf life of 4 years (refrigerated).

This product also is available from Pharma-Tek, Inc., P.O. Box 1920, Huntington, NY, 11743-0568. The phone number to the company is (800) 645-6655. Its Web site address is *www.pharmatek.com* Please note that for maximum product stability, amyl nitrite inhalant should be packaged in unit dose containers wrapped loosely in gauze or other suitable material and stored at 2°C to 15°C.

Sodium nitrite powder USP can be used to extemporaneously prepare 3% sodium nitrite solution for injection, although no referenced source could be found for compounding instructions. Suppliers will add additional charges for special packaging and shipping. Sodium nitrite powder USP is available from Spectrum Chemicals and Laboratory Products, located at 14422 South San Pedro Street, Gardena, CA, 90248. The phone number to the company is (800) 813-1514. Its Web site address is *www.spectrumchemical.com* The product costs $21.00/50 g or $72.00/2500 g, and has a shelf life of 3–5 years.

The product also is available from Integra Chemical Company, located at 710 Thomas Avenue SW, Renton, WA, 98055. The phone number to the company is (800) 322-6646. Its Web site address is *www.integrachemical.com* The product costs $21.00/500 g or $72.00/2500 g.

The product also is available from Ruger Chemical Company, Inc., P.O. Box 806, Hillside, NJ, 07205. The phone number to the company is (800) 274-7843. Its Web site address is *www.rugerchemical.com* The cost of the product is $3.50–7.00/lb in bulk. Fifty (50) mL vials of 25% sodium thiosulfate solution for injection are available from American Regent Laboratories, Inc., a subsidiary of Luitpold Pharmaceuticals Inc. The company is located at One Luitpold Drive, Shirley, NY, 11967. The phone number

to the company is (800) 645-1706. Its Web site address is *www.luitpold.com* The cost of the product is $22.50/vial and has a shelf life of 36 months.

NERVE AGENTS

Nerve agents are organophosphates, which are potent inhibitors of acetylcholinesterase enzymes. Some examples of this group are sarin (GB), soman (GD), tabun (GA), GF, and VX. Signs and symptoms of nerve agent or organophosphate poisonings include muscarinic, nicotinic, and CNS findings. Muscarinic symptoms include SLUDGE BAM: salivation, lacrimation, urination, defecation, gastric secretions, emesis, bronchospasm, bronchorrhea, bradycardia, abdominal cramping, and miosis. Nicotinic symptoms may include tachycardia, mydriasis, hypertension, muscle weakness, fasciculations, and respiratory paralysis. CNS symptoms range from blurred vision, restlessness, anxiety, and headaches to seizures and coma. Serious poisonings are managed with three antidotal agents. Atropine sulfate blocks muscarinic receptor sites, thus reversing all SLUDGE BAM complications. Glycopyrrolate (Robinul), a quaternary ammonium anticholinergic medication, has been proposed as an adjunctive agent in the management of organophosphate insecticide poisoning; however, it is not routinely administered. Pralidoxime chloride (Protopam), also known as 2-PAM, regenerates cholinesterase enzyme activity. Administration of 2-PAM reverses nicotinic complications and works synergistically with atropine sulfate to correct muscarinic and CNS symptomatology. Obidoxime dichloride (Toxogonin, LUH6) is an alternative agent to pralidoxime chloride that is available in some European countries but is not FDA approved for use in the United States. HI-6 (asoxime chloride) is an oxime also currently under investigation. It is important to note that both atropine sulfate and pralidoxime chloride must be stocked for adequate antidote preparedness; atropine sulfate alone will correct muscarinic signs and symptoms, but 2-PAM is necessary to correct nicotinic signs and symptoms. Diazepam, lorazepam, and other benzodiazepines as anticonvulsants are adjunctive measures to treat nerve-agent-induced seizures. Barbiturates (e.g., Phenobarbital) may be considered for seizures refractory to benzodiazepines. Topical ocular homatropine or atropine can relieve miosis, pain, dim vision, and nausea. Pyridostigmine bromide (Mestinon) dosed at 30 mg orally every 8 hours serves as a "prophylactic antidote" or "antidote enhancement." Based on animal studies, pretreatment provides some protection against nerve agents, especially soman, which demonstrates rapid ageing of the cholinesterase enzyme. On February 5, 2003, the FDA approved the use of pyridostigmine bromide to increase survival after exposure to soman nerve agent poisoning. Pyridostigmine bromide binds reversibly to 30% of the cholinesterase enzymes, thus, temporally protecting the enzyme from the nerve agent. Tablets are provided to military personnel in combat zones; pyridostigmine stockpiling in civilian hospitals is unnecessary and not recommended.

Pralidoxime chloride was previously available from Wyeth, but as of August 2003, this product was sold to Baxter, Inc. Baxter, Inc. is located at 95 Spring Street, New Providence, NJ, 07974. The phone number to the company is (908) 286-7000. Its Web site address is *www.baxter.com* The cost of the product is $108.38/vial and has a shelf life of 5 years.

Atropine sulfate for injection is available as a generic product from a variety of manufacturers. Some common forms are 0.4 mg/mL, 20 mL multidose vials (8 mg/vial) with a shelf life of 24–36 months; syringe sizes (0.1 mg/mL, 5 mL or 10 mL syringes); and 1 mg/mL, 1 mL single-dose vials.

Stability of expired injectable atropine sulfate solutions was addressed in one study. The authors tested several samples ranging from in date to 12 years beyond expiration. They noted high concentrations of atropine sulfate in clear colorless solutions along with an absence of breakdown products in the test samples. These findings suggest their potential utility in times of emergency.

Note: Readers are advised to refer to the *Drug Topics Red Book* or nearest pharmacy wholesaler for a complete list of drugs.

Atropine sulfate USP powder is available from several suppliers. This pharmaceutical grade powder may be used to prepare atropine sulfate for injection extemporaneously in large amounts. Two references were identified that give instructions for preparing intravenous (IV) solutions extemporaneously. The manufacturers of this pharmaceutical grade chemical have provided no shelf life guidelines. One study of extemporaneously prepared atropine sulfate 1 mg/1 mL in 100 mL multidose bags demonstrated stability of over 95% at controlled temperatures of 22.2°C (72°F) and 37.8°C (100°F) for periods of up to 72 hours. When ordering product, additional charges are added for special packaging and shipping. The product is available from Ruger Chemical Company, located at 83 Cordier Street, Irvington, NJ, 07111. The phone number to the company is (800) 274-2636; fax (973) 926-4921. Its Web site address is *www.rugerchemical.com* The cost of the product is $11.20/5 g or $44.80/125 g. The product is also available from Spectrum Chemicals and Laboratory Products, located at 14422 South San Pedro Street,

Gardena, CA, 90248. The phone number to the company is (800) 772-8786. Its Web site address is *www.spectrumchemical.com* The cost of the product is $20.45/5 g or $80.60/25 g.

The Letco Companies also has the product available. The company is located at 1316 Commerce Drive NW, Decatur, AL, 35601. The phone number to the company is (800) 239-5288; fax (256) 353-7237. Its Web site address is *www.letcoinc.com* The cost of the product is $16.00/25 g or $415/1 kg.

Diazepam for injection is available as a generic product from a variety of manufacturers. Some common forms are 5 mg/mL, 2 mL prefilled syringes (10 mg/syringe) with a shelf life of 24 months; 5 mg/mL, 2 mL ampoules (10 mg/amp); and 5 mg/mL, 10 mL multidose vial (50 mg/vial).

Lorazepam for injection is available as a generic product from a variety of manufacturers. Some common forms are 2 mg/mL, 1 mL single-dose vial (2 mg/vial) with a shelf life of 18–24 months; 2 mg/mL, 10 mL multidose vial (20 mg/vial); 4 mg/mL, 1 mL single-dose vial (4 mg/vial); and 4 mg/mL, 10 mL multidose vial (40 mg/vial).

Military style autoinjectors containing atropine sulfate, pralidoxime chloride, and diazepam are available from Meridian Medical Technologies, Inc., the only FDA-approved manufacturer in the United States (see Table 26-1). These autoinjectors are manufactured in large quantities of 25,000 and 40,000. Smaller orders may be filled if the product is in company inventory; however, the shelf life may be shorter. In 2003, the FDA approved the marketing of infant and pediatric strength AtroPen autoinjectors; atropine sulfate 1 mg/0.7 mL, 0.5 mg/0.7 mL, and 0.25 mg/0.3 mL. The doses approved for use in children and adolescents with mild symptoms of nerve agent poisoning include: 0.25 mg for infants weighing less than 15 lbs (generally less than 6 months), 0.5 mg for children weighing between 15 and 40 lbs (generally 6 months to 4 years), 1 mg for children weighing between 40 and 90 lbs (generally 4 to 10 years of age), and 2 mg doses for adults and children weighing over 90 lbs (generally over 10 years of age). For infants and children with symptoms of severe nerve agent poisoning, doses up to three times these doses may be given.

Each Mark I Kit (Nerve Agent Antidote Kit) contains one AtroPen (atropine sulfate; 2 mg/0.7 mL) and one ComboPen (pralidoxime chloride; 600 mg/2 mL).

TABLE 26-1

NERVE AGENT AUTOINJECTORS BY MERIDIAN MEDICAL TECHNOLOGIES

Autoinjectors	Item Number	Shelf Life	Units per Box	Price per Box	Unit Price
Mark I Kit (NAAK)	NSN 6505-01-174-9919	5 years	30	$916.50	$30.55
AtroPen 2 mg	NDC 11704-106-01	3 years	12	$201.84	$16.82
AtroPen 1 mg	NDC 11704-105-01	3 years	12	$201.84	$16.82
AtroPen 0.5 mg	NDC 11704-104-01	3 years	12	$201.84	$16.82
AtroPen 0.25 mg	NDC 11704-107-01	3 years	12	$241.20	$20.10
ComboPen (2-PAM Cl) 600 mg	NSN 6505-01-125-3248	5 years	100	$2175.00	$21.75
Diazepam (CANA) 10 mg, C-IV	NSN 6505-01-274-0951	4 years	15	$375.00	$25.00

The diazepam autoinjector contains 10 mg diazepam in 2 mL. Both the Mark I Kit and the diazepam autoinjector are available from Meridian Medical Technology, Inc., located at 10240 Old Columbia Road, Columbia, MD, 21046. The phone number to the company is (800) 638-8093; fax (443) 259-7801. Its Web site address is *www.meridianmeds.com* Per Meridian Medical Technologies (MMT): "Please note that MMT requires the following information to accompany a purchase order (PO), excluding the training kits which do not contain drugs: a physician's prescription for all items; a copy of the DEA registration certificate is required if the PO includes the diazepam auto-injector; the PO must include the following wording: 'We certify that the items purchased under PO # .... will be used only by ....{company name}. The material will not be sold to a third party, distributed or used for any other purpose.'"

As of February 2004, Bound Tree Medical, Inc. became the exclusive distributor of all Meridian autoinjector products to hospital pharmacies. Bound Tree Medical, Inc. is located at 6106 Bausch Road, Galloway, OH, 43119; and can be reached at (800) 533-0523 or by fax at (800) 257-5713. Their web address is *www.boundtree.com*

Diomed in Istanbul, Turkey, manufactures DIO-ATRO, an autoinjector containing atropine sulfate 2 mg and pralidoxime chloride 600 mg and has a NATO stock #6515-27-013-3995.

PULMONARY OR CHOKING AGENTS

Chlorine (Cl), phosgene (CG), diphosgene (DP), and chloropicrin act primarily as pulmonary irritants causing cough, shortness of breath, and dyspnea. However, it may be several hours before serious complications become evident (e.g., pulmonary edema). No specific antidote is available for treatment of these exposures. Symptomatic and supportive care may include administration of oxygen, ventilatory support, and bronchodilators such as albuterol sulfate. Nebulized 3.75% sodium bicarbonate has provided dramatic symptomatic improvement in chlorine exposures, as noted in several anecdotal case reports. This may be prepared by mixing 2 mL of 7.5% sodium bicarbonate for injection with 2 mL of sterile 0.9% sodium chloride. Antibiotics should be reserved for those patients with an infectious process documented by sputum gram staining and culture. Parenteral steroids may be indicated in those patients demonstrating latent or overt reactive airway disease. Ipratropium bromide (Atrovent) may be used adjunctively following chloropicrin exposure.

Albuterol sulfate is available as a generic product in a variety of forms such as a solution for nebulization, 0.09 mg/inhalation (17 g) with a shelf life of 18–36 months; a solution for inhalation, 0.083% 3 mL vials; and a solution for inhalation, 0.5% 20 mL multidose vial. Sodium bicarbonate for injection is available in concentrations of 4.2%, 7.5%, and 8.4% in syringes and vials in sizes of 10 or 50 mL, and has a shelf life of 18 months.

Methylprednisolone acetate for injection is available as a generic product in several concentrations, including 20 mg/mL, 10 mL vials (200 mg/vial) with a shelf life of 24–36 months; 40 mg/mL, 5 mL vials (200 mg/vial); and 80 mg/mL, 5 mL vials (400 mg/vial).

BLISTER AGENTS

A number of potent alkylating agents may be used as chemical warfare agents. Examples include nitrogen mustard (HS), distilled mustard (HD), mustard gas, phosgene oxime (CX), and Lewisite (L). Toxicity produced by these agents includes blisters, vesiculations, eye injury, airway damage, vomiting and diarrhea, and bone marrow stem cell suppression. Blisters may form several hours after contact with the skin. Erythema may be treated with calamine or other soothing lotion or cream. Denuded skin areas should be treated with topical antibiotics such as silver sulfadiazine or mafenide acetate. Systemic analgesics should be used liberally. For eye exposures, 2.5% sodium thiosulfate irrigations, homatropine ophthalmic ointment (or other mydriatics), topical antibiotics, and topical steroids may be indicated depending on the severity of injury. Atropine or other anticholinergic agents or antiemetics should control the early nausea and vomiting. Antibiotics are necessary to treat infections, which are usually the cause of death. Colony stimulating factors (e.g., filgrastim [Neupogen], sargramostim [Leukine]) may be considered for patients demonstrating serious cytopenia. Lewisite is the only blistering agent for which an antidote may be useful since it is an arsenic derivative. The antidote dimercaprol (British anti-Lewisite, BAL) is a chelating agent for arsenicals and other heavy metals. BAL administration may reduce systemic toxicity of Lewisite. Although not commercially available, 5% BAL skin and eye ointments may reduce the severity of lesions when applied soon after decontamination. Since BAL is formulated in peanut oil, it must be given intramuscularly (IM). BAL is available as 300 mg/3 mL vials in quantities of 10 from Akorn, Inc., located at 2500 Millbrook Drive, Buffalo Grove, IL, 60089. The phone number to the company is (800) 535-7155. Its Web site address is *www.akorn.com* The cost of the product is $716.45 and has a shelf life of 5 years.

Dimercaptosuccinic acid (DMSA, succimer, Chemet) has been used experimentally in animals for the treatment of Lewisite exposures. It may be preferred in the treatment of multiple exposures because it is administered orally and exhibits fewer adverse reactions. Chemet is supplied in 100 mg capsules and is available in quantities of 100 from Ovation Pharmaceuticals, Inc., located at Four Parkway North, Deerfield, IL, 60015. The phone number to the company is (847) 282-1000; fax (847) 282-1001. Their Web site address is *www.ovationpharma.com* The average wholesale price of the product is $663.21 and has a shelf life of 24 months.

DMPS, which is the sodium salt of 2,3-dimercapto-1-propanesulfonic acid, is a chelating agent available in Europe demonstrating some efficacy in treating Lewisite-exposed experimental animals.

The colony stimulating factors are available as (1) Leukine in 250 mcg/mL, 1 mL, multidose vial ($154.91) and 500 mcg/mL, 1 mL, multidose vial ($309.82). This product is available from Berlex Laboratories, Inc., located at 1191 Second Avenue, Seattle, WA, 98101-2120. The phone number to the company is (888) 237-5394. Its Web site address is *www.berlex.com* The shelf life is 18 months for the liquid product, and 36 months for the powder product; and (2) Neupogen in 300 mcg/0.5mL ($236.28), 480 mcg/0.8mL ($376.44), and 480 mcg/1.6mL ($343.20). These products are available from Amgen, Inc., located at One Amgen Center Drive, Thousand Oaks, CA, 91320. The phone number to the company is (805) 447-1000. Its Web site address is *www.amgen.com* The product has a shelf life of 24 months.

Based on experimental studies, it has been proposed that administration of sodium thiosulfate 12.5 g may act as a "mustard scavenger" following exposure to mustard agents. Potential benefits of sodium thiosulfate therapy following mustard agent exposure are not known. See cyanide section for suppliers of sodium thiosulfate.

INCAPACITATING AGENTS

BZ, also known as QNB, (3-quinuclidinyl benzilate) and Agent 15 (the Iraqi equivalent of BZ) are anticholinergic agents, which incapacitate victims by causing delirium and hallucinations. BZ and related anticholinergic compounds can be synthesized in clandestine laboratories. Patients demonstrate anticholinergic signs and symptoms (e.g., mydriasis, tachycardia, dry flushed skin, urinary retention, etc). Symptoms of agitation and hallucinations may be managed with benzodiazepines. Serious symptoms may be reversed by IV physostigmine salicylate (Antilirium), a reversible carbamate cholinesterase inhibitor. Neostigmine methylsulfate (Prostigmin) and pyridostigmine bromide (Mestinon) are quaternary amines that do not cross the blood-brain barrier, and therefore, will not reverse CNS symptomatology caused by these agents. Antilirium is available in 2 mL vials (1 mg/mL) in quantities of 10 vials from Akorn, Inc., located at 2500 Millbrook Drive, Buffalo Grove, IL, 60089. The phone number to the company is (800) 535-7155. Its Web site address is *www.akorn.com* The cost of the product is $48.60 and has a shelf life of 24 months.

On October 26, 2002, the Russian government used aerosolized fentanyl as an incapacitating agent during a terrorist attack in a Moscow theater. This incident resulted in the death of over 100 hostages and terrorists and critically injured many more. Fentanyl is a very potent opiate narcotic with significant exposures causing sedation, miosis, bradycardia, hypotension, and respiratory depression leading to coma and respiratory arrest. Fentanyl toxicity may be completely reversed by adequate doses of the opiate antagonists naloxone (Narcan) or nalmefene (Revex). Injectable naloxone is available generically in 0.4 mg/1 mL ampoules, 0.4 mg/1 mL syringes, 1, 2, and 10 mg vials, and 1 mg/1 mL in 2 mL ampoules. Nalmefene is available in ampoules of 1 mg/2 mL and 0.1 mg/1 mL from Baxter, Inc.

RIOT CONTROL AGENTS

These agents are commonly known as CN (alpha-chloroacetophenone, Mace), CS (ortho-chlorobenzylidene malononitrile), or CR (dibenoxazepine) tear gas. Diphenyl-aminochloroarsine (adamsite) and diphenylchloroarsine are riot control/vomiting agents that are organic arsenicals; however, they do not cause systemic arsenic poisoning. Some "pepper spray" products contain hot pepper extracts such as oleoresin capsicum. Usually, the exposure effects of these agents are self-limiting. They include burning, itching, and watering of the eyes, burning and tingling of the skin, and respiratory discomfort. In most cases, no specific therapy is indicated other than basic measures such as movement of the patient to fresh air, eye irrigation with water, and skin washing. More pronounced symptoms such as bronchospasm and pulmonary edema are possible with significant exposures (i.e., in enclosed spaces). Symptomatic patients may require supplemental oxygen, ventilatory support, and inhaled β-agonist with or without systemic steroids.

NUCLEAR AGENTS

Although the detonation of a nuclear weapon is a concern with respect to global and international conflicts, it is considered to be very difficult for a terrorist group to obtain, build, conceal, or deliver such a weapon. It is believed that a "dirty bomb" is more likely to be deployed. "Dirty bombs" are conventional explosives combined with radioactive material and are designed to frighten the populace and cause a major hazardous material cleanup rather than many injuries.

Radiation emitted by radioactive materials can be characterized into three types: α-particles, β-particles, and γ-rays. The health hazards of radiation are divided into acute or chronic exposure risks. Chronic exposures (i.e., a low dose over a long period of time) increase the risk of cancers; while acute exposures (with γ irradiation) produce nausea, vomiting, blood dyscrasias, and death. Since α- and β-particles do not travel great distances, materials such as protective clothing easily block them. Inhalation or ingestion of radioactive materials pose the greatest potential for harm because their radiations can continue to cause tissue damage long after the acute event. γ-Rays travel great distances and require dense materials, such as lead, to block penetration of tissues.

Internal contamination with radioactive materials may require, treatment with either a chelator or a radionuclide blocker. Chelating agents for radionuclides are available through Radiation Emergency Assistance Center/Training Site (REAC/TS). Insoluble Prussian blue (ferric hexacyanoferrate) is indicated for cesium and thallium chelation therapy. Prussian blue is a pharmaceutical grade product obtained from Germany under the brand name Radiogardase. It is available in 500 mg capsules, manufactured by Heyl GmbH, located in Berlin, Germany. On October 2, 2003, the FDA approved a New Drug Application for Radiogardase to treat patients exposed to harmful levels of radioactive cesium or radioactive and nonradioactive thallium. Prussian blue is now a component of the SNS. Zinc-diethylenetriamine pentaacetic acid (Zn-DTPA), also known as pentetate zinc trisodium, and calcium-DTPA (Ca-DTPA) also known as pentetate calcium trisodium, are chelators for radioactive transuranic elements (see Table 26-2). On May 20, 2005, Ca-DTPA and Zn-DTPA were approved by the FDA for treatment of individuals with known or suspected internal contamination with plutonium, americium, or curium to increase rates of elimination. They are currently available to hospitals and state and local health agencies through Akorn, Inc. at *www.akorn.com* Both of these drugs are supplied as 200 mg/mL 5 mL, 1 g ampoules.

REAC/TS trains, consults, and assists in the response to all types of radiation accidents or incidents. The center utilizes physicians, nurses, health physicists, and emergency coordinators to provide 24-hour assistance at the local, national, or international level.

Other pharmaceutical chelators may be used for a variety of radionucleotide exposures and would be found in any well-stocked hospital pharmacy. These include d-penicillamine (Cuprimine), calcium disodium EDTA (Versenate), dimercaprol (BAL), succimer (Chemet), and deferoxamine (Desferal).

Colony stimulating factors, filgrastim (Neupogen) and sargramostin (Leukine), may be considered in patients experiencing significant bone marrow suppression. See blister agents section for suppliers of colony stimulating factors.

Radionuclide blocking agents saturate tissues with a nonradioactive element, which reduces the uptake of radioactive iodine. The most commonly used agents are potassium iodide (KI) tablets (130 mg and 65 mg), saturated solution of potassium iodide (SSKI) (300 mg/0.3 mL), and Lugol's solution (10% potassium iodide, 5% iodine), which reduce uptake of I into the thyroid tissue. Most states with departments of nuclear safety will stock enough quantity of KI tablets to protect workers and emergency personnel involved in a nuclear reactor incident. Some states offer supplies of KI to the general public residing in areas close to nuclear reactors. Sodium iodide (NaI) can theoretically be used instead of KI; however, no such pharmaceutical product is available in the United States. Sodium iodide USP powder is available from several sources listed in the *2005 Drug Topics Red Book*. ThyroShield is a recently approved KI solution for ease and use in pediatric administration; it is available in 30 mL bottles, in a concentration of 65 mg/mL. Several other examples of substances employed as radionuclide blockers include sodium alginate for strontium; chlorthalidone for rubidium; and Lugol's solution, for technetium.

Table 26-3 is provided by the U.S. FDA, Center for Drug Evaluation and Research (*www.fda.gov/cder/guidance/4825fnl.htm*). It gives the recommended doses of KI for various age and risk groups.

Lugol's solution and SSKI are available from several suppliers; they have shelf lives of two to five years; see *2005 Drug Topics Red Book*. FDA-approved manufacturers of KI tablets are (1) Anbex, Inc., located at 15 West 75th Street, New York, NY, 10023, which manufactures Iosat. The phone number to the company is (212) 580-2810. Its Web site address is *www.anbex.com* The product is available as 130 mg tablets with 14 tablets to a package. The cost of the product is $10.00/package and has a shelf life of 4–5 years; (2) Medpointe, Inc. (*www.nitro-pak.com* or *www.medpointeinc.com*) manufactures Thyro-Block, which is distributed by Nitro-Pak, Inc.; their phone number is (800) 866-4876. The phone number to the manufacturer is (732) 564-2200. Thyro-Block is available as 130 mg tablets with 14 tablets in a bottle; a case is 100 bottles. The cost of a single bottle is $9.95; a case of 100 bottles costs $799. Medpointe, Inc. markets potassium iodide tablets directly to nuclear power plants and utility companies; (3) Reciep AB (*www.thyrosafe.com*) manufactures and distributes Thyrosafe. The phone number to the company is (866) 849-7672. The product is available as 65 mg tablets with 20 tablets per package. The cost of the product is $9.95 per

TABLE 26-2

CHELATING AGENTS FOR RADIONUCLEOTIDES

Chelating Agent	Radionucleotide
Calcium and Zinc-DTPA	Americium (^{243}Am), Californium, Cesium, Curium, Lanthanum, Lutetium, Plutonium, Promethium, Scandium, Uranium, Yttrium, Zinc, and rare earth metals
Calcium Disodium EDTA	Copper, Lead, and Uranium
D-Penicillamine	Copper, Lead, and Mercury (^{203}Hg)
Deferoxamine mesylate	Iron
Dimercaprol	Copper, Mercury, and Polonium
Succimer/DMSA	Lead and Mercury

TABLE 26-3

THRESHOLD THYROID RADIOACTIVE EXPOSURES AND RECOMMENDED DOSES OF KI FOR DIFFERENT RISK GROUPS

	Predicted Thyroid Exposure(cGy)	KI Dose (mg)	# of 130 mg Tablets	# of 65 mg Tablets
Adults over 40 years	≥500	130	1	2
Adults over 18 through 40 years	≥10			
Pregnant or lactating women	≥5			
Adolescents over 12 through 18 years*		65	1/2	1
Children over 3 through 12 years				
Over 1 month through 3 years		32	1/4	1/2
Birth through 1 month		16	1/8	1/4

*Adolescents approaching adult size (≥70 kg) should receive the full adult dose (130 mg).

Note: KI from tablets (either whole or fractions) or a fresh saturated KI solution may be diluted in milk, formula or water, and the appropriate volume administered to babies. A home preparation procedure for emergency administration of KI tablets to infants and small children using water, milk, juice, syrup, or soda pop can be found at www.fda.gov/cder/drugprepare/kiprep.htm. The KI prepared in these liquids will keep for up to 7 days in the refrigerator. The FDA recommends that the KI drink mixtures be prepared weekly; unused portions should be discarded.

package; (4) Fleming & Company Pharmaceuticals, 1733 Gilsinn Lane, Fenton, MO, 63026, manufactures and distributes ThyroShield liquid. The phone number to the company is (636) 343-8200, fax (636) 343-8203. The cost is $13.25 per one ounce bottle with a shelf life of 5 years.

For immediate assistance regarding a nuclear or radiological agent incident, contact the REAC/TS, located at P.O. Box 117, MS-39, Oak Ridge, TN, 37831-0117. Their phone number is (865) 576-3131 (business hours); (865) 576-1005 (24-hour emergency line). Also contact the Department of Nuclear Safety—for the state in which the incident occurred—and the health physicists affiliated with hospital nuclear medicine departments, who can serve as expert consultants for radiation incidents.

BIOLOGICAL AGENTS

As NBC terrorist weapons, biological agents may be encountered as bacteria (e.g., anthrax), viruses (e.g., smallpox), or toxins (e.g., botulinum or ricin). This fact will explain the striking differences in the manner which victims present to health-care facilities. A catastrophe caused by detonation of a chemical weapon (e.g., nerve agent or cyanide) would be characterized by immediate death or severe disablement of individuals at the site of the attack. First responders to such an incident would be paramedics, police, and other emergency personnel.

In contrast, with respect to biological agents, there is a delayed onset of signs and symptoms since incubation may take days. Emergency department clinicians and primary care practitioners would be the first to recognize and manage exposed patients. Knowing what medical and pharmaceutical interventions may be requested in a mass casualty event is crucial. It is beyond the scope of this chapter to delineate all the diagnostic clues, pathophysiology,

laboratory monitoring, infectious disease control, guidelines for patient isolation, epidemiologic procedures, and public health ramifications of a bioterrorism event. Clinicians, however, should take note of this extensive list of pharmaceuticals (both oral and parenteral) that may be required in extraordinarily large amounts during an outbreak involving a biological weapon. Additionally, the duration of illness may be weeks to months, thus creating an additional stress on the health-care infrastructure. Once the cause of illness in a large number of patients has been identified as a biological agent, prompt availability and distribution of appropriate medication can greatly mitigate the destructive impact of the act of terrorism. It should be noted that special products, uncommonly used vaccines, and antitoxins would be provided via federal government storage and distribution programs. Pharmacist and public health personnel in the drug delivery system must be aware that it may require 24–48 hours or more for material in the SNS, to be transported, broken down, and delivered to local distribution centers. See discussion of the SNS in the introduction section. Adjunctive medications such as analgesics and antipyretics should be readily available to manage symptoms such as headache, fever, and myalgias. New therapies are under development. Detailed information on diagnosis, patient management, vaccines, and so on, may be obtained through Commander U.S. Army Medical Research Institute of Infectious Diseases (USAMRIID) at (301) 619-2833 during business hours, or at (888) USA-RIID, 24 hours a day. In the event of an emergency, contact the National Response Center at (800) 424-8802. Also, contact the CDC emergency operations center at (770) 488-7100.

The following information is a very brief synopsis of 14 possible threats as biological agents. Much of this information has been adapted from an article in *JAMA:* "Clinical Recognition and Management of Patients

Exposed to Biological Warfare Agents," and USAMRIID's *Medical Management of Biological Casualties Handbook,* 6th edition, April 2005.

BACTERIA

Anthrax

The etiologic agent causing anthrax is *Bacillus anthracis*, a gram-positive spore-forming bacillus. As a biological weapon, the spores of these bacteria would be aerosolized, with inhalation being the primary route of exposure. The clinical course is characterized by a necrotizing hemorrhagic mediastinitis. Initially, symptoms may resemble a flu-like illness with fever, fatigue, malaise, vague chest pain, and nonproductive cough. Initial symptoms are followed by abrupt progression to dyspnea, stridor, diaphoresis, and cyanosis. Systemic complications of sepsis, shock, and meningitis may occur in up to half of the cases. Unfortunately, once symptoms occur, treatment is usually ineffective. Intravenous ciprofloxacin should be initiated at the earliest sign of anthrax. Other fluoroquinolones may be substituted; however, no animal studies exist for quinolones other than ciprofloxacin. All natural strains of anthrax have been found to be sensitive to erythromycin, chloramphenicol, and gentamicin. Historically, penicillin G has been the drug of choice for anthrax. An alternative regimen is doxycycline and one or two other antibiotics with in vitro activity against *B. anthracis*, such as rifampin, vancomycin, penicillin, ampicillin, chloramphenicol, imipenem, clindamycin, and clarithromycin. Ampicillin and penicillin should not be used alone because of possible β-lactamase production. Chemoprophylaxis with oral ciprofloxacin, doxycycline, or amoxicillin, if the strain of *B. anthracis* is proven susceptible in exposed individuals, should be initiated and continued for at least 60 days or until three doses of anthrax vaccine are administered. A licensed attenuated vaccine, anthrax vaccine adsorbed (BioThrax) in 5 mL multidose vials, is available for prophylaxis. This vaccine stock is owned by the Department of Defense. In order to obtain it, contact USAMRIID at (301) 619-2833. It is manufactured by BioPort Corporation, located at 3500 North Martin Luther King Jr. Boulevard, Lansing, MI, 48906. The phone number to the company is (517) 327-1500. Its Web site address is *www.bioport.com* The cost of 5 mL (10 doses) of the product is $1,331.19 and has a shelf life of 18 months. The product must be stored between 2°C to 8°C. Per BioPort Corporation, as of February 2006, the only way one could obtain BioThrax was by writing a letter describing the reason for the request, the number of people to be vaccinated, and contact information. Once this letter is received, it would go through an approval process at the Department of Defense. Depending on the level of risk, they would either accept or reject the request.

BioPort Corporation currently has vaccine available for civilian personnel and is very close to signing a domestic distributor for the management of the sale of BioThrax. Once this becomes official, a physician will be able to contact the distributor to find out if he/she is eligible to receive the vaccine. The supply of the vaccine is still low in comparison to the very high demand, but BioPort will be selling the vaccine to those civilian markets most at risk and most vital to our country.

Brucellosis

Human infection may be caused by four species of *Brucella*, which is a nonspore-forming gram-negative aerobic coccobacillus. Clinical manifestations include fever, chills, and malaise, which may lead to cough and pleuritic chest pain. Other complications may include osteomyelitis, genitourinary infection, hepatitis, endocarditis, and CNS infections. To prevent the possibility of relapse, combination therapy is advised. Various antibiotic regimens have been proposed from the following list of antimicrobials: doxycycline, gentamicin, streptomycin, rifamin, ofloxacin, sulfamethoxazole/trimethoprim (SMZ/TMP). There are no approved vaccines or chemoprophylaxis treatments.

Cholera

This infection is caused by *Vibrio cholerae*, a gram-negative nonspore-forming bacillus. Clinical manifestations include vomiting, abdominal distention, and pain, with little or no fever, followed rapidly by diarrhea. Fluid losses may be excessive with death caused by dehydration and shock. Antibiotic treatment may include tetracycline, ampicillin, and SMZ/TMP. Intravenous fluid/electrolyte solutions are necessary to treat dehydration. At the present time, the manufacture and sale of the only licensed cholera vaccine in the United States (Wyeth-Ayerst) has been discontinued. Two recently developed vaccines for cholera are licensed and available in other countries (Dukoral, Biotec AB [*www.activebiotech.com*] and Mutacol, Berna [*www.berna. org*]); however, neither of these two vaccines are available in the United States.

Glanders

Glanders and melioidosis are caused by *Burkholderia mallei* and *Burkholderia pseudomallei,* respectively. Both are gram-negative bacilli with a safety pin appearance on microscopic examination. Both pathogens affect animals (e.g., horses, mules, donkeys) and human beings. Symptoms of inhalation exposure include high fever, rigors, sweating, myalgias, headache, pleuritic chest pain, cervical adenopathy, hepatosplenomegaly, and generalized papular/pustular eruptions. Pulmonary disease may progress to potentially fatal bacteremia and septicemia. Oral antibiotic regimens include amoxicillin/clavulanate, tetracycline, or sulfamethoxazole/trimethoprim given for 60–150 days. For serious systemic disease, administer parental Ceftazidime and SMZ/TMP for 2 weeks followed by oral therapy for 6 months. There are currently no available vaccines for human use. Chemoprophylaxis may be considered using SMZ/TMP.

Pneumonic Plague

The gram-negative, nonspore-forming bacillus, *Yersinia pestis,* is responsible for both pneumonic and bubonic plague. Patients exposed to pneumonic plague as a biological weapon will present with high fever, chills, malaise, cough with bloody sputum, headache, myalgia, and sepsis. Late in the course of illness, dyspnea, cyanosis, and respiratory failure may be noted. Effective antibiotic therapy includes streptomycin or gentamicin. Alternative drugs are ciprofloxacin, chloramphenicol, and doxycycline. In the United States, a licensed, killed, whole bacilli vaccine was discontinued by its manufacturer in 1999, and is no longer available. Exposed individuals may be treated with doxycycline, ciprofloxacin, or chloramphenicol for 7 days for chemoprophylaxis.

Q Fever

Q fever is a rickettsial disease caused by *Coxiella burnetii*. The most common symptoms of Q fever are fever, chills, headache, fatigue, diaphoresis, malaise, anorexia, and myalgias. In some cases, cough with chest pain may be noted. Rare complications include hepatomegaly, splenomegaly, and jaundice. Effective therapies for Q fever include tetracycline or doxycycline for 15–21 days; alternatives are ofloxacin or pefloxacin. Hydroxychloroquine added to antibiotic therapy has increased the effectiveness of therapy; especially in patients with chronic Q fever endocarditis. There is currently no commercially available Q fever vaccine in the United States. One vaccine, Q-VAX, has been successfully tested and is commercially available for use in humans in Australia. Tetracycline or doxycycline may be given as chemoprophylaxis to exposed patients.

Tularemia

Tularemia is caused by *Francisella tularensis*, a gram-negative aerobic coccobacillus. It is known as "rabbit fever" or "deer fly fever." Inhalation of tularemia organisms produces a typhoidal tularemia. Patients present with fever, weight loss, substernal discomfort, and nonproductive cough. The drug of choice is streptomycin. Other treatment options include gentamicin, fluoroquinolones (ciprofloxacin, norfloxacin), tetracycline, and chloramphenicol; however, high relapse rates are associated with these treatment options. Although

not commercially available, a live attenuated vaccine is available under Investigational New Drug (IND) status for prophylaxis (available through USARMIID). Doxycycline or tetracycline may be used for chemoprophylaxis.

VIRUSES

Smallpox

The etiologic agent that causes smallpox is the variola major virus. Smallpox was declared eradicated by the World Health Organization in 1980. Much concern exists regarding the stockpiling of this infectious agent as a weapon of bioterrorism due to its high morbidity and mortality. Patients infected with variola present with fever, malaise, rigors, vomiting, headache, and backache. Dermal manifestations include appearance of a rash followed by lesions, which appear as macules, then papules, then eventually form pustular vesicles. By the second week, scabs form, which leave depigmented scars upon healing. Patients are contagious until all scabs are healed. All patients exposed to variola virus must be immediately vaccinated. Those U.S. citizens who were vaccinated against smallpox in the 1950s and the 1960s are no longer protected against the virus. The only smallpox vaccines available in the United States are Dryvax (Wyeth Laboratories, Inc.) and WetVax (Aventis Pharmaceuticals, Inc.), available by calling the CDC at (404) 639-2888. Both smallpox vaccine products are components of the SNS. The CDC has contracted with Acambis to develop a new smallpox vaccine (ACAM 2000), which may have a more acceptable safety profile. In early 2003, the CDC made smallpox vaccine available through state health departments to civilian health-care workers on a voluntary basis. Dryvax is available as one vial of dried smallpox vaccine and one container of diluent (0.25 mL) with 100 sterile bifurcated needles. The manufacture of Dryvax was discontinued in 1981. The U.S. Army and the CDC maintain a supply of vaccinia immune globulin (VIG), which is used for the treatment of complications due to the vaccinia vaccination. Limited data suggest that VIG may be of value in postexposure prophylaxis of smallpox when given within the first week following exposure, and concurrently with vaccination. Contact the CDC at (800) CDC-INFO or USARMRIID at 301-619-2833 to obtain VIG. There is currently no chemotherapeutic agent proven effective against smallpox. Cidofovir (Vistide) is not a licensed treatment for smallpox; however, it is being studied under an FDA investigational protocol. Cidofovir is a nucleoside analog DNA polymerase inhibitor, which has been demonstrated in in vitro studies to inhibit poxvirus replication and cell lysis. Cidofovir is currently licensed for the treatment of CMV retinitis and has demonstrated antiviral activity against poxviruses in vitro, and against cowpox and vaccinia viruses in mice. However, its use for the treatment of vaccinia adverse reactions is restricted under an IND protocol. Under the IND, cidofovir would only be used when VIG was not efficacious. Renal toxicity is a known adverse reaction of cidofovir. Although the CDC makes no recommendations for the use of antivirals at this time, it is recommended that health-care providers continue to consult the CDC at 800-CDC-INFO to obtain updated information regarding treatment options for serious vaccine complications. Many states have surveyed hospital pharmacies to identify local sources of this product if a smallpox outbreak is suspected.

Cidofovir is available from Gilead Sciences, located at 333 Lakeside Drive, Foster City, CA, 94404. The phone number to the company is (800) 445-3235. Its Web site address is *www.gilead.com* The product is available as 75 mg/mL, 5mg vial for $888.00. It has a shelf life of 3 years.

Venezuelan Equine Encephalitis

Members of the alpha virus genus of the Togaviridae family produce this encephalopathic syndrome. The usual mode of transmission is mosquitoes; however, aerosolization makes those pathogens a very effective WMD. Alpha virus will produce neurologic syndromes noted by fever, headaches, confusion, drowsiness, seizures, dysphasia, ataxia, myoclonus, cranial nerve palsies, photophobia, myalgias, and vomiting. No specific chemotherapeutic agents are indicated. Treatment is symptomatic and supportive care. Antipyretics and anticonvulsants may be used in severe cases. A live attenuated vaccine for VEE TC-83 is available for prophylaxis, while inactivated vaccines are under IND status. A monoclonal antibody has been developed and is in the animal test phase for protection against infection and disease when given before or up to 24 hours after an airborne challenge with virulent virus.

Viral Hemorrhagic Fevers

The most widely known examples of this group are the Ebola and Marburg viruses; these belong to the family Filoviridae, which are enveloped, nonsegmented, negative-stranded RNA viruses. Common features of VHF are myalgias, fever, and prostration. Mild symptoms include conjunctival injection, mild hypotension, flushing, and petechial hemorrhaging that may progress to shock. More severe symptoms include mucous membrane hemorrhage with maculopapular rashes and disseminated intravascular coagulation (DIC). Other VHF agents include Crimean Congo hemorrhagic fever (Bunyaviridae family), Hanta virus (Bunyaviridae family), and Lassa fever (Arenaviridae family). No specific antiviral agents are effective against Ebola or Marburg viruses. Other related strains (e.g., Crimean Congo, Lassa) may respond to ribavirin. Postexposure prophylaxis may be considered with oral ribavirin. Many different pharmaceutical agents may need

to be employed in the supportive management of hypotension, shock, and DIC. No vaccines or medicinals exist to protect against these viral illnesses.

Ribavirin (Virazole) is available from ICN Pharmaceuticals, Inc., located at 3300 Hyland Avenue, Costa Mesa, CA, 92626. The phone number to the company is (800) 548-5100. Its Web site address is *www.valeant.com* The product is available as 6 g vials of lyophilized powder for $1,573.80. It has a shelf life of 5 years.

Ribavirin (Rebetol) is available from Schering Plough Corporation, located at 2000 Galloping Hill Road, Kenilworth, NJ, 07033. The phone number to the company is (800) 222-7579. Its Web site address is *www.schering-plough.com* It markets 200 mg capsules, available in bottles of 42, 56, 70, and 84, which cost $10.60/tablet. Its shelf life is "proprietary information."

TOXINS

Botulinum

Botulinum toxin is a protein exotoxin produced by *Clostridium botulinum*, an anaerobic gram-positive bacillus. There are seven types of botulism neurotoxins known as types A-G. Botulism poisonings are more commonly associated with improperly processed or canned foods. As a WMD, botulinum toxin may be inhaled from an aerosol or ingested in the form of sabotaged food. These toxins are the most toxic of all the NBC weapons. Clinical manifestations include blurred vision, mydriasis, diplopia, ptosis, photophobia, dysarthria, dysphonia, and dysphasia. Skeletal muscle paralysis follows, which presents as a symmetrical and descending progressive weakness resulting in respiratory failure. Patients are typically awake, alert, and afebrile. A trivalent equine antitoxin (types A, B, and E) for food-borne botulism is available from the CDC at eight urban quarantine sites: Atlanta, Chicago, Honolulu, Los Angeles, Miami, New York City, San Francisco, and Seattle. To obtain these antitoxins, contact the CDC 24 hours a day at (404) 639-2888 or during business hours at (404) 639-2206. Connaught Laboratories, Ltd., one of only three suppliers in the world, manufactures this antitoxin for the CDC. A despeciated equine heptavalent antitoxin against all seven types was prepared and is under IND status. It should be noted that all horse serum-based antitoxins pose the risk of anaphylaxis and serum sickness; therefore, skin testing is advised. A pentavalent (types A-E) toxoid also is available under IND status.

Ricin/Abrin

Ricin is a biological toxin derived from the plant *Ricinus communis*, commonly known as the castor bean. After inhalation exposure, victims may experience fever, weakness, cough, necrosis of upper and lower airway, and pulmonary edema followed by hypotension and cardiovascular collapse. Ingestion of castor beans or ricin may cause esophagitis, abdominal pain, nausea, vomiting, profuse bloody diarrhea, shock, and delayed cytotoxic effects to the liver, kidney, CNS, and adrenal glands. Abrin is a similar biotoxin which is found in the seeds of the *Abris precatorius*, commonly known as the jequirity bean or rosary pea. There are no available antitoxins for either ricin or abrin. Treatment is supportive care only. Also, there are no commercially available vaccines or other chemoprophylactic agents; however, candidate vaccines for ricin are under development that are immunogenic and confer protection against lethal aerosol exposures in animals. The most promising of these is RiVax, which has successfully completed an FDA Phase 1 clinical trial. This vaccine is manufactured by DOR BioPharma, Inc., located at 1691 Michigan Ave. Suite 435, Miami, FL, 33139. The phone number to the company is (305) 534-3383. Its Web site address is *www.dorbiopharma.com*

Staphylococcus Enterotoxin B(SEB)

SEB is an exotoxin produced by *Staphylococcus aureus*, a gram-positive coccus. SEB is most commonly recognized as a cause of food poisoning as it is produced by bacterial growth in improperly handled foods. Inhalation of SEB in a biological warfare scenario may rapidly incapacitate its victims. Signs of exposure may include fever, chills, headache, myalgias, and nonproductive cough with severe problems including dyspnea, retrosternal chest pain, vomiting, and diarrhea. No specific antitoxin is available. Supportive therapies are directed towards adequate oxygenation and hydration. Antipyretics and antitussives may provide symptomatic relief. The value of steroids is unknown. No vaccines for SEB are currently available; however, several vaccine candidates are in development.

Trichothecene (T-2) Mycotoxins

Fungi of the genera *Fusarium*, *Myrotecium*, *Trichoderma*, and *Stachybotrys* produce these compounds. Clinical manifestations of exposure include skin irritation, pruritus, redness, vesicles, necrosis, sloughing of the epidermis, nose and throat pain, nasal discharge, fever, cough, dyspnea, chest pain, and hemoptysis. Serious cases are associated with prostration, weakness, shock, and death. There is no antidote or antitoxin. Treatment is supportive care. No vaccine or chemoprophylactic agent exists for T-2 mycotoxins.

The following are some of the aforementioned pharmaceutical products available for the treatment of patients exposed to biological warfare agents. If a variety of sizes and formulations are available for a particular pharmaceutical product, only the largest dose forms are listed. (Readers are advised to refer to the *2005 Drug Topics Red Book* or nearest pharmacy wholesaler for a complete list of companies that manufacture or distribute the following products.)

Ciprofloxacin is available in several different oral and parenteral dosage forms.

Doxycycline hyclate is available from a number of generic suppliers in 100 mg tablets or capsules.

Erythromycin is available in a large variety of salt forms and strengths: 500 mg tablets or capsules.

Penicillin V and G are available in a variety of formulations, both oral and parenteral: 500 mg tablets, 10 million unit vials.

Gentamicin sulfate is a powerful aminoglycoside antibiotic that is only used for systemic infections. It is available in a variety of formulations: 40 mg/mL, 20 mL multidose vials (800 mg/vial); 40 mg/mL, 2 mL single-use vials (80 mg/vial).

Streptomycin is a rarely used antibiotic; however, it has efficacy against several of the biological warfare agents. It is supplied in 1 g vials for injection. Streptomycin is available from X-Gen Pharmaceuticals, Inc., P.O. Box 445, Big Flats, NY, 14814. The phone number to the company is (607) 732-4411; fax (607) 732-2900. The cost of the product is $9.10/vial, available in units of 10 vials. It has a shelf life of 24 months.

Chloramphenicol is another rarely used antibiotic. Smaller quantities can be obtained in vials and larger quantities may be obtained in powdered form. This may be required to treat a large number of casualties: 1000 mg vial, 25 g USP powder.

SMZ/TMP is another antibiotic that has efficacy against several of the biological warfare agents. The most commonly used formulation contains 800 mg of sulfamethoxazole and 160 mg of trimethoprim (Bactrim DS): SMZ/TMP (800/160 tablets).

Rifampin is available in 300 mg capsules or in large quantities in powdered form, 300 mg capsules, 500 grams USP powder.

Tetracycline is available in 500 mg capsules or also in powdered form, 500 mg capsules, 100 g USP powder.

CONCLUSION

With the increasing probability of an incident involving a WMD agent, many local, state, and federal agencies have initiated plans for appropriate and effective emergency medical response. Experts in the area of EMS, emergency medicine, infectious disease, and public health are becoming trained in the medical management of exposure to NBC agents.

Any large mass casualty scenario will demand the expertise and professional services of a hospital pharmacy. Therefore, clinicians should equip themselves with knowledge of antidotes, antibiotics, antitoxins, and other supportive agents used to treat casualties, and how they may be obtained quickly in the event of an act of terrorism. Currently, there are no guidelines mandating minimum hospital inventory of the pharmaceutical products that may be needed. Pharmacy managers, poison center personnel and pharmacy, and therapeutics committee members are urged to participate in, or at least be familiar with, plans coordinated through local domestic preparedness programs.

Suggested Reading

CDER KI Taskforce. Guidance Potassium Iodide as a Thyroid Blocking Agent in Radiation Emergencies. U.S. Department of Health and Human Services Food and Drug Administration Center for Drug Evaluation and Research (CDER), 2001. *http://www.fda.gov/cder/guidance/index.htm* and *http:// fda.gov/cder/drugprepare/kiprep.htm*

The Centers for Disease Control <http://cdc.gov> Guide B – Vaccination Guidelines for State & Local Health Agencies, November 2002. *http://www.bt.cdc.gov/agent/smallpox/response-plan/ index.asp*

The Centers for Disease control *http://cdc.gov* Strategic National Stockpile, December 2002. *http://www.bt.cdc.gov/stockpile*

Franz DR, Jahrling PB, Friedlander AM, et al. Clinical recognition and management of patients exposed to biological warfare agents. *JAMA.* 1997;278(5):399–411.

Hendee W, Palmer R, Hall AH, et al. *Poisindex, Radiation [monograph on CD-ROM].* Englewood, CO: Micromedex Healthcare Series, Vol 127, 2006.

Inglesby TB, Henderson DA, Bartlett JG, et al. Anthrax as a biological weapon: medical and public health management: working group on civilian biodefense. *JAMA.* 1999;281(18): 1735–45.

Kales SN, Christiani DC. Acute chemical emergencies. *N Engl J Med.* 2004;350(8):800–8.

Lawrence D.T., Kirk MA; Chemical Terrorism Attacks: Update on Antidotes. *Emerg Med Clin N. Am* 2007:25:567–595.

Ricks RC, Lowry PC, Townsend RD. *Radiogardase-Cs Insoluble Prussian Blue (Ferric Hexacyanoferrate, $Fe_4 [Fe (CN)_6]_3$), Ca-DTPA (Trisodium Calcium Diethylenetriaminepentaacetate), Zn-DTPA (Trisodium Zinc Diethylenetriaminepentaacetate).* Oak Ridge, TN: Radiation Emergency Assistance Center/ Training Site, November 2002. *www.usamriid.army.mil/*

USAMRIID's Medical Management of Biological Casualties Handbook. 6th ed. Fort Detrick, MD: Operational Medicine Department. USAMRIID, 2005. *http://www.usamriid.army.mil/*

USAMRIID's Medical Management of Chemical Casualties Handbook, 4th ed. Fort Detrick, MD: Chemical Casualty Care Division, USAMRIID, 2001.

27

HOSPITAL STAFF ISSUES

Jorge del Castillo

INTRODUCTION

It is essential that hospitals be fully prepared for any type of disaster. Unfortunately, most hospitals are not completely prepared for a bioterrorism event in many ways. There are many obstacles facing hospitals these days among which are a decrease in workforce, regulatory burdens, and the constant pressure that the different payment systems bring to bear upon these institutions. Additionally, in an effort to cut costs, most hospitals have taken a JIT (just in time) approach for obtaining supplies and have little surge capacity for any potential disaster. The Joint Commission requires hospitals to prepare for mass casualty events, including those caused by bioterrorism. Since most hospitals adhere to the Joint Commission requirements, it is expected that they will be ready for any type of disaster facing the communities they serve.

Hospitals are the sites of significant intervention and community support and are required to establish and maintain links with local law enforcement, prehospital response teams, and hazardous materials (hazmat) units. These links will be essential to the proper functioning of the entire system. Finally, rural hospitals have a similar but yet different set of obstacles that regulatory agencies will

need to address to ensure the success of these institutions if faced with a bioterrorism event.

In short, hospitals need to improve their response and communications systems as well as the competency of their staff to recognize and effectively respond to the needs of their communities in the event of a mass casualty/biological disaster.

HISTORICAL PERSPECTIVE

During the 1970s, as the specialty of emergency medicine developed, a number of hospitals began designing formal "disaster plans." These morphed into more sophisticated plans assuming the name of emergency preparedness in the 1980s.

The early plans prepared for a range of natural and man-made disasters, but did not include any preparation for mass casualties due to terrorism.

In the 1990s, the Federal Emergency Management Agency (FEMA) and the Department of Health and Human Services (HHS) required that hospital preparedness plans follow a broad and uniformly national approach to emergency preparedness.

The Joint Commission a not-for-profit organization, is the nation's predominant agency in the setting of standards and accreditation in health care.

Prior to 9/11, the Joint Commission standards were focused on emergency preparedness management plans, security management plans, hazardous materials and waste management plans, and emergency preparedness drills.

In January 2001, Environment of Care (EC) standards that address emergency preparedness were revised by the Joint Commission. They required hospitals to do the following:

- Have an emergency management plan integrated with the community it serves
- A vulnerability and risk assessment of the facility be conducted
- The personnel participating in these responses be properly trained and oriented (especially to personal protective equipment)
- Drills be conducted regularly to test emergency management response and the validity of recommended training

According to the revised Joint Commission standard EC 1.4, "The emergency management plan must comprehensively describe the organization's approach to responding to emergencies within the organization or in its community that would suddenly and significantly affect the need for the organization's services, or its ability to provide those services."

The plan must address the four phases of a disaster:

- Mitigation
- Preparedness
- Response
- Recovery

In a survey conducted by the American Hospital Association (AHA) in 2002, approximately 78% of the 5000 hospitals included indicated that the absence of financial resources limited their ability to establish additional safeguards for preparation against bioterrorism attacks. This resulted in the government issuing grants to all states to prepare for any eventuality related to bioterrorism.

GOVERNMENT SUPPORT

In 2002, the federal government issued grants totaling $205 million to the 50 states and closely followed this up by the release of an additional $747 million. The goal of this grant funding was to achieve "17 critical benchmarks for bioterrorism preparedness planning." Fourteen benchmarks were related to public health preparedness, while the remaining three were related to hospital preparedness.

Hospitals were directed to

- designate a coordinator for bioterrorism hospital preparedness planning
- establish a hospital preparedness planning committee
- devise a plan for a potential epidemic in each state or region

The FY 2006 Labor-HHS-Education Appropriations Bill approved by the Senate Appropriations Committee provided $550 million for the Health Resources and Services Administration's (HRSA) Bioterrorism Hospital Preparedness program, which is $50 million more than included in the House-passed version of the bill. In FY 2005, the program received $514.6 million. The National Bioterrorism Hospital Preparedness program sponsored by

HRSA has several requirements for the disbursement of funds and identified six priority areas in 2005. It is useful to be familiar with these requirements so that those institutions seeking funding may submit a complete and successful application.

HRSA Priority Area #1: Administration Financial Accountability

Develop and maintain a financial system capable of tracking expenditures by priority area, by critical benchmark, and by funds allocated to hospitals and other health-care entities. A minimum of 75% of the award must be used for implementation.

HRSA Priority Area #2: Surge Capacity

1. **Hospital bed capacity**
   The system must provide triage treatment and initial stabilization, above the current daily staffed bed capacity, for adult and pediatric patients requiring hospitalization within 3 hours in the wake of a terrorism incident or other disaster.
2. **Isolation capacity**
   All participating hospitals should have the capacity to maintain, in negative pressure isolation, at least one suspected case of a highly infectious disease (e.g., smallpox, pneumonic plague, SARS, influenza, and hemorrhagic fevers).
3. **Surge capacity: health-care personnel**
   Establish a response system that allows the immediate deployment of additional health-care personnel in support of surge bed capacity noted in critical benchmark # 2-1. The number of health-care personnel must be linked to already established patient care ratios noted by the institution's Patient Care Practice Acts based on 24-hour operations. This benchmark must describe how these personnel are recruited, received, processed, and managed through the incident.
4. **Emergency system for advance registration of volunteer health professionals**
   Develop a system that allows for the advance registration and credentialing of clinicians needed to augment a hospital or other medical facility to meet patient/victim care and increased surge capacity needs.
5. **Pharmaceutical caches**
   Establish a regional system that ensures a sufficient supply of pharmaceuticals to provide prophylaxis for 3 days to hospital personnel (medical and ancillary staff), hospital-based emergency first responders and their families—in the wake of a terrorist-induced outbreak of anthrax or other disease for which such countermeasures are appropriate.
6. **Personal protection and decontamination**
   Adequate personal protective equipment (PPE) per defined region, to protect current and additional

health-care personnel, during an incident. This benchmark is tied directly to the number of health-care personnel the institution must provide to support surge capacity for beds.

7. **Decontamination**

Ensure that adequate portable or fixed decontamination systems exist for managing adult and pediatric patients as well as health-care personnel, who have been exposed during a chemical, biological, radiological, or explosive incident in accordance with their numbers.

8. **Mental health**

Enhance the networking capacity and training of health-care professionals to be able to recognize, treat, and coordinate care related to the behavioral health consequences of bioterrorism or other public health emergencies.

9. **Surge capacity: trauma and burn care**

Enhance statewide trauma and burn care capacity to be able to respond to a mass casualty incident due to terrorism. This plan should ensure the capability of providing trauma care to at least 50 severely injured adult and pediatric patients per million of population.

10. **Communication and information technology**

Establish a secure and redundant communications system that ensures connectivity during a terrorist incident or other public health emergency between health-care facilities and state and local health departments, emergency medical services, emergency management agencies, public safety agencies, neighboring jurisdictions, and federal public health officials.

HRSA Priority Area #3: Emergency Medical Services (EMS)

Enhance the statewide mutual aid plan to deploy EMS units in jurisdictions/regions they do not normally cover, in response to a mass casualty incident due to terrorism.

HRSA Priority Area #4: Linkages to Public Health Departments

1. **Hospital laboratories**

Implement a hospital laboratory program that is coordinated with currently funded CDC laboratory capacity efforts, and which provides rapid and effective hospital laboratory services in response to terrorism and other public health emergencies.

2. **Surveillance and patient tracking**

Enhance the capability of rural and urban hospitals, clinics, EMS systems, and poison control centers to report syndromic and diagnostic data that is suggestive of terrorism or other highly infectious disease to their associated local and state health departments on a 24-hour-a-day, 7-day-a-week basis.

HRSA Priority Area #5: Education and Preparedness Training

Staff must participate in competency-based education and training programs for adult and pediatric prehospital, hospital, and outpatient health-care personnel responding to a terrorist incident or other public health emergency.

HRSA Priority Area #6: Terrorism Preparedness Exercises

As part of the state or jurisdiction's bioterrorism hospital preparedness plan, functional exercises will be conducted.

These exercises/drills should encompass, if possible, at least one biological agent. The inclusion of scenarios involving radiological and chemical agents as well as explosives may be included as part of the exercises/drills.

ACTIONS WHEN AN EMERGENCY OCCURS

A number of decisions must be made by hospital administration along with designated medical staff. These decisions will impact the management and throughput of patients during periods of high influx due to a bioterrorism event.

First and foremost would be the decision to implement the institution's bioterrorism-management plan once a threat is recognized. Table 27-1 shows some of the other decisions that are critical to successfully deal with such an event.

HOSPITAL PREPARATION CHECKLIST

The Agency for Healthcare Research and Quality commissioned Booz-Allen and Hamilton to prepare a questionnaire that would facilitate the assessment of preparedness and capacity of individual hospitals to respond to and treat victims of a biological incident (see Fig. 27-1).

TABLE 27-1

DECISIONS NECESSARY FOR HIGH INFLUX OF PATIENTS

- Determining whether an off-site facility is necessary
- Determining the number of staff and supplies necessary to sustain the off-site facility
- Canceling elective procedures
- Clearing the hospital by discharging and/or transferring patients to other facilities
- Securing PPE and medications (antibiotics) from stock supplies or communicating with designated agencies that can effect prompt delivery
- Determining when it will be safe to discharge patients identified with communicable diseases
- Assessing the maximum capacity of the hospital morgue

BIOTERRORISM QUESTIONNAIRE

Bioterrorism Emergency
Planning and Preparedness Questionnaire
for
Healthcare Facilities

Name of Hospital: _____

Hospital Address: _____

_____

Name and Title of Person(s) Completing Form: _____

_____

_____

Contact Information:

Phone:	(___) _____
Pager:	(___) _____
Fax:	(___) _____
Email:	_____

Healthcare facilities play a vital role in the detection of and response to biological emergencies, including new emerging infections, influenza outbreaks, and terrorist use of biological weapons. The information and data obtained from this questionnaire will be used to help assess the preparedness and capacity of your hospital to respond to and treat victims of a biological incident. Many of the questions only require yes, no, or don't know (DK) responses. Others will require some research.

Thank you for taking the time to complete this questionnaire.

F I G U R E   2 7 – 1

BIOTERRORISM QUESTIONNAIRE
(Developed by Booz-Annel & Hamilton under Contract No. 290-00-0019 ("Understanding Needs for Health System Preparedness and Capacity for Bioterrorist Attacks") from the Agency for Healthcare Research and Quality. This document is in the public domain and may be reproduced without permission.)

| **I.** | **Biological Weapons Training for Hospital Personnel** |

1. Does your hospital conduct in-service training on biological weapons? ❑ Yes ❑ No ❑ DK
   If yes:

   a) When was the last training provided? _____

   b) Who is being trained?   c) Is training mandatory?

Medical Staff	❑ Yes ❑ No ❑ DK	❑ Yes ❑ No ❑ DK
Nursing Staff	❑ Yes ❑ No ❑ DK	❑ Yes ❑ No ❑ DK
Medical/Nursing Students	❑ Yes ❑ No ❑ DK	❑ Yes ❑ No ❑ DK
Residents	❑ Yes ❑ No ❑ DK	❑ Yes ❑ No ❑ DK
Administration	❑ Yes ❑ No ❑ DK	❑ Yes ❑ No ❑ DK
Laboratory Personnel	❑ Yes ❑ No ❑ DK	❑ Yes ❑ No ❑ DK
Security Personnel	❑ Yes ❑ No ❑ DK	❑ Yes ❑ No ❑ DK

   d) How often is in-service training on biological weapons provided?

   - ❑ Quarterly
   - ❑ Biannually
   - ❑ Annually
   - ❑ Other
   - ❑ Don't Know

   e) Who provides the biological weapons training to your hospital staff?

   - ❑ In-house instructor (please list) _____
   - ❑ Outside consultant (please list) _____
   - ❑ Other (please list) _____
   - ❑ Don't Know

   f) What type of training was provided (check all that apply)?

   - ❑ Classroom/seminar training
   - ❑ Home study manuals (i.e., self-study)
   - ❑ Computer based training
   - ❑ Satellite broadcast
   - ❑ Video
   - ❑ Other, please specify _____

2. Does your hospital send staff to Bioterrorism training seminars offered outside of the hospital?

   ❑ Yes ❑ No ❑ DK

| Ver. 1.0 | 2 | March 10, 2002 |

FIGURE 27-1

(CONTINUED)

II. General Hospital & Emergency Preparedness Information

1. What is your average daily inpatient census (averaged over the 2000 calendar year)?

_____

2. Approximately how many people work at your hospital? _____

3. Please indicate your licensed, operational, and surge bed capacity below:

Bed capacity in the following areas	Licensed Beds *(Under Certificate of Need)*	Staffed Beds *(Operational Capacity)*	Approximate Surge Bed Capacity* *(Estimated maximum number of additional staffed beds created in 6 & 12 hours)*
Adult medical & surgical			/
Pediatric medical & surgical			/
Adult ICU (*all units including CCU*)			/
Adult Intermediate Care Ward (Progressive Care Unit)			/
Pediatric ICU (*including NICU*)			/
Pediatric Intermediate Care Ward (Progressive Care Unit)			/
Emergency department beds			/
OB/GYN			/
Psychiatry			/
Substance Abuse			/
Transitional Care (*e.g., short-term care facility, rehabilitation*)			/
All other departments (*including outpatient surgical areas*)			/
TOTAL			/

* Surge bed capacity: In the event of an emergency, what is the maximum number of additional staffed beds that your institution can create in 6 hours and in 12 hours for the treatment of mass casualties? (e.g., beds made available by opening up closed wards/units; beds made available by canceling elective surgeries; beds obtained from associated clinics; endoscopy suites; outpatient surgical areas; etc.)

4. How many times a month does your hospital reach 100% of operational capacity (i.e., staffed beds)?

_____

5. Has your hospital implemented the Incident Command or Management System facility-wide?

❏ Yes ❏ No ❏ DK

6. Does your hospital's emergency preparedness plan address mass casualty incidents involving biological agents (i.e., influenza epidemics, new emerging infections, or terrorist use of biological agents)?

❏ Yes ❏ No ❏ DK

If yes:

a) How frequently is this facet of your plan exercised and updated? _____

b) What was the date of your last exercise involving biological agents? _____

Ver. 1.0	3	March 10, 2002

FIGURE 27-1

(*CONTINUED*)

c) How is your bio-plan initiated?

_____

d) How are hospital personnel and medical staff within the hospital notified about the plan's initiation?

_____

e) How is affiliated medical staff notified about the plan's initiation? _____

_____

g) How does the hospital monitor staff's knowledge of the plan? _____

_____

7. Does your hospital have a coordinator designated to oversee all preparedness efforts as it relates to your hospital's bioterrorism preparedness efforts?   ❑ Yes ❑ No ❑ DK

8. Does your hospital have a medical director that oversees all training and preparedness efforts as it relates to your hospital's bioterrorism preparedness efforts?   ❑ Yes ❑ No ❑ DK

9. Does your hospital's emergency preparedness plan address expanding staff availability?   ❑ Yes ❑ No ❑ DK

If yes:

a) Where would you access additional staff (please check all that apply)?

    ❑ Local registry (agency)?

    ❑ Change shift length from 8 to 12 hours?

    ❑ Change nursing/patient ratios?

    ❑ Offer services to keep staff at the hospital (e.g., babysitting, elderly care)?

    ❑ Does your hospital's emergency preparedness plan address requesting state or federal resources for assistance?   ❑ Yes ❑ No ❑ DK

b) Does your hospital participate in multiple facility credentialing procedures to permit rapid recognition of credentialed staff from other facilities or hospitals?   ❑ Yes ❑ No ❑ DK

10. Does your hospital experience problems staffing your ED, general medical, pediatrics, and surgical floors with nurses employed by the hospital?   ❑ Yes ❑ No ❑ DK
If yes:

a) During calendar year 2000, how many shifts per week (on average) are you short of nurses for:

_____ General medical

_____ Pediatrics

_____ Surgery (post-surgical care)

_____ ICU

_____ ED

b) Does your hospital have an on-call nursing policy for the following areas (i.e., where nurses are on call and will come in when additional staff is required)?

General medical   ❑ Yes ❑ No ❑ DK

Pediatrics   ❑ Yes ❑ No ❑ DK

Surgery (post-surgical care)   ❑ Yes ❑ No ❑ DK

ICU   ❑ Yes ❑ No ❑ DK

ED   ❑ Yes ❑ No ❑ DK

FIGURE 27-1

(CONTINUED)

11. Does your hospital's emergency preparedness plan address increasing operational (staffed-bed) capacity by at least:

    a) 10%   ❑ Yes ❑ No ❑ DK

    b) 15%   ❑ Yes ❑ No ❑ DK

    c) 20%   ❑ Yes ❑ No ❑ DK

12. Does your hospital's emergency preparedness plan address canceling elective surgeries in order to make additional beds available for inpatient use?   ❑ Yes ❑ No ❑ DK

13. Does your hospital's emergency preparedness plan address early inpatient discharge protocols to create additional beds?   ❑ Yes ❑ No ❑ DK

    If yes:

    a) Who decides which patients can be discharged early? _____

    b) Is this a voluntary policy with your medical staff?   ❑ Yes ❑ No ❑ DK

    c) Is there a staff member involved in early discharge planning?   ❑ Yes ❑ No ❑ DK

14. Are you able to utilize hallways as short-term inpatient care areas in the event of a declared disaster?   ❑ Yes ❑ No ❑ DK

    If yes:

    a) How many additional inpatient beds can be opened using the hallways during a declared disaster?

         _____

    b) Can your hospital's computer process orders for patients not residing in traditional patient care areas (i.e., residing in the hallways)?   ❑ Yes ❑ No ❑ DK

    c) Do you have a mechanism to provide privacy to patients residing in the hallway?   ❑ Yes ❑ No ❑ DK

15. Do you have other areas of the hospital designated for emergency overflow of patients (e.g., an auditorium, lobby) in the event of a declared disaster?   ❑ Yes ❑ No ❑ DK

    a) If yes:

        i.   Where are these areas located? _____

        ii.   Do you have beds or cots available onsite for these alternative patient care areas?   ❑ Yes ❑ No ❑ DK

        iii. Do you have a mechanism to provide privacy to these patients?   ❑ Yes ❑ No ❑ DK

        iv. Do these overflow patient care areas have ready access to:

            Supplemental oxygen source   ❑ Yes ❑ No ❑ DK

            Running water   ❑ Yes ❑ No ❑ DK

            Pharmaceuticals   ❑ Yes ❑ No ❑ DK

            Bath/showers   ❑ Yes ❑ No ❑ DK

            Toilets   ❑ Yes ❑ No ❑ DK

            Suction   ❑ Yes ❑ No ❑ DK

            Supplies   ❑ Yes ❑ No ❑ DK

            Monitoring units   ❑ Yes ❑ No ❑ DK

Ver. 1.0   5   March 10, 2002

FIGURE 27-1

(CONTINUED)

Computer access   ❏ Yes ❏ No ❏ DK
Hand washing areas   ❏ Yes ❏ No ❏ DK
Food and drink   ❏ Yes ❏ No ❏ DK
Telephone   ❏ Yes ❏ No ❏ DK

    v. In the past five years, have you ever had to expand your bed capacity beyond your licensed number of beds?   ❏ Yes ❏ No ❏ DK

16. Does your hospital have a memorandum of agreement (MOA) with nearby extended care facilities (ECF) or rehabilitation hospitals to accept patients during a declared disaster that can be discharged early from the affected hospital but still require nursing care?   ❏ Yes ❏ No ❏ DK

17. Does your hospital have a memorandum of agreement (MOA) with outlying hospitals to accept inpatients during a declared disaster?   ❏ Yes ❏ No ❏ DK

18. Does your hospital's emergency preparedness plan address processes to increase inpatient treatment capacity within the city?   ❏ Yes ❏ No ❏ DK

19. Does your hospital's emergency preparedness plan address extending outpatient clinic hours (on and off-campus) beyond normal scheduled hours?   ❏ Yes ❏ No ❏ DK

If yes:

a) How do you staff these extended hours? _____

b) Has there ever been a need to extend clinic hours during a disaster situation?   ❏ Yes ❏ No ❏ DK

20. Does your hospital's emergency preparedness plan address processes to increase outpatient treatment capacity within the city?   ❏ Yes ❏ No ❏ DK

21. Does your hospital's emergency preparedness plan address the provision of the following services if staff had to return to work during a community disaster (check all that apply)?

Provided

❏ Yes ❏ No ❏ DK   Day (night) care for their children?
❏ Yes ❏ No ❏ DK   Day (night) care for their dependent adults?
❏ Yes ❏ No ❏ DK   Day (night) care for their pets?
❏ Yes ❏ No ❏ DK   Sleeping quarters?
❏ Yes ❏ No ❏ DK   Nourishment?
❏ Yes ❏ No ❏ DK   Distribution of medication prophylaxis?

22. Does your hospital have policies concerning emergency department diversion?   ❏ Yes ❏ No ❏ DK

If yes:

a) What are your hospital's criteria to go on diversion? _____
_____

b) Who is delegated within the hospital to make the decision to go on diversion? _____
_____

c) List who needs to be notified about your diversion policy outside the hospital? _____
_____

Ver. 1.0   6   March 10, 2002

FIGURE 27-1
(*CONTINUED*)

d) In general, how many times a year does your hospital go on diversion? _____
_____

23. What is the approximate number of functioning on-site ventilators that belong to your institution? ____

  a) How many ventilators, if any, can be mobilized from associated long-term care, rehab facilities, or other satellite clinic facilities? _____

  b) How many additional ventilators does your institution rent weekly (average over the past year)?
  _____

  c) Do you have access to ventilators that can be rented on an emergency basis? ❑ Yes ❑ No ❑ DK
  If yes:
  _____ How many can be obtained?
  How long does it take your hospital to obtain these additional ventilators?

  d) Is there a regional plan to provide extra ventilators if needed?   ❑ Yes ❑ No ❑ DK

  If yes:

  _____ How many additional ventilators can you access within 4 hours?
  _____ How many additional ventilators can you access within 8 hours?
  Do other hospitals in your area access ventilators from the same vendor?
                                                          ❑ Yes ❑ No ❑ DK

24. Does your hospital have an information system that provides the following:

  a) Inpatient staffing?   ❑ Yes ❑ No ❑ DK

  b) Hospital bed availability?   ❑ Yes ❑ No ❑ DK

  c) Diversion status of other hospitals in the area or region?   ❑ Yes ❑ No ❑ DK

  d) Bed availability of other hospitals in the area or region?   ❑ Yes ❑ No ❑ DK

  e) Information on biological agents and the management of infectious patients?
                                                          ❑ Yes ❑ No ❑ DK

  f) Internet access?   ❑ Yes ❑ No ❑ DK

25. Does your hospital's emergency preparedness plan address stockpiling antibiotics and supplies?
                                                          ❑ Yes ❑ No ❑ DK
  If yes:

  a) Does your hospital currently maintain a separate cache of antibiotics to treat hospital staff in the event of a bioterrorist incident?   ❑ Yes ❑ No ❑ DK
  If yes:

    i. What antibiotics are cached (check all that apply)?

                    Name   **Unit Doses**
          ❑   Doxycycline   _____
          ❑   Tetracycline   _____
          ❑   Ciprofloxin   _____
          ❑   Levaquin   _____
          ❑   Gentamicin   _____
          ❑   Tobramycin   _____

FIGURE 27-1

(CONTINUED)

    ii.   How quickly can supplies be accessed? _____

    iii. Where are these supplies stored? _____

26. How many days supply of antibiotics does your pharmacy maintain (based on current average daily usage)? _____

27. Does your hospital stockpile or have 12-hour access to antibiotics (doxycycline, ciprofloxacin) in order to provide community prophylaxis?   ❏ Yes ❏ No ❏ DK

28. During an average 24-hour period, how many additional orders (based on standard dosing) for the following antibiotics would exhaust your current **in-hospital** pharmaceutical supply (inventory):

    _____ Doxycycline i.v.

    _____ Doxycycline p.o.

    _____ Ciprofloxacin i.v.

    _____ Ciprofloxacin p.o.

    _____ Levofloxacin i.v.

    _____ Levofloxacin p.o.

    _____ Gentamycin i.v.

    _____ Tobramycin i.v.

    a) How long would it take you to replenish these supplies? _____

    b) How would you obtain these supplies? _____

    _____

    c) Do other hospitals in your area access these drugs in the same manner and from the same source?   ❏ Yes ❏ No ❏ DK

29. During an average 24-hour period, how many prescriptions for the following antibiotics (based on standard dosing) would exhaust your current **outpatient** pharmaceutical supply (inventory):

    _____ Doxycycline p.o.

    _____ Tetracycline p.o.

    _____ Ciprofloxacin p.o.

    _____ Levofloxacin p.o.

    a) How long would it take you to replenish these supplies? _____

    b) How would you obtain these supplies? _____

    c) Who do you obtain these supplies from? _____

    d) Do other hospitals in your area access these drugs in the same manner and from the same source?   ❏ Yes ❏ No ❏ DK

30. Has your hospital ever participated in a community or regional pharmaceutical stockpile?   ❏ Yes ❏ No ❏ DK

31. Is your hospital's emergency preparedness plan integrated into the city emergency preparedness plan?   ❏ Yes ❏ No ❏ DK

32. Does your hospital's emergency preparedness address the following:

    a) Designating mental health services (Critical Incident Stress Management - CISM) to care for emergency workers, victims and their families, and others in the community who need special assistance coping with the consequences of a disaster?   ❏ Yes ❏ No ❏ DK

    b) Provisions to provide for the proper examination, care, and disposition of deceased?   ❏ Yes ❏ No ❏ DK

    c) Mass immunization/prophylaxis?   ❏ Yes ❏ No ❏ DK

FIGURE 27-1

(*CONTINUED*)

d) Mass fatality management?   ❑ Yes ❑ No ❑ DK

   If yes, does the plan address the following:

   i.   Augmenting morgue facility and staff   ❑ Yes ❑ No ❑ DK

   ii. Expanding morgue capacity   ❑ Yes ❑ No ❑ DK

   iii. Procedures for decontamination/isolation of human remains   ❑ Yes ❑ No ❑ DK

   iv. Backup isolation procedures when morgue capacity is exceeded   ❑ Yes ❑ No ❑ DK

   v.   Environmental surety   ❑ Yes ❑ No ❑ DK

e) Ensuring adequate bio-protection (universal precautions) gear for hospital/clinic personnel?
                                                                           ❑ Yes ❑ No ❑ DK

f) Ensuring adequate supplies (including food, linens & patient care items) are available from local or
   regional suppliers, or that plans are in place to obtain them in a timely manner in order to be self-
   sufficient for 48 hours?   ❑ Yes ❑ No ❑ DK

g) Access to portable cots, sheets, blankets, and pillows?   ❑ Yes ❑ No ❑ DK

h) Triage of mass casualties?   ❑ Yes ❑ No ❑ DK

i) Enhancing hospital security by utilizing community law enforcement assets? ❑ Yes ❑ No ❑ DK

j) Tracking expenses incurred during an emergency?   ❑ Yes ❑ No ❑ DK

k) Coordination with state or local public health authorities?   ❑ Yes ❑ No ❑ DK

l) Creating additional isolation beds?   ❑ Yes ❑ No ❑ DK

33. Does your hospital have an internal health surveillance system in place that tracks patients presenting
problems or complaints?   ❑ Yes ❑ No ❑ DK

If yes:

a) Does your hospital's surveillance system track the following (please check all that apply):

   ❑   ED visits

   ❑   Hospital admissions (total numbers and patterns)

   ❑   Presenting patients' complaints

   ❑   Influenza-like illness monitoring

   ❑   Increased antibiotic prescription rate

b) Is this information gathered automatically electronically or done manually? _____

c) When is this information gathered? _____

d) Who gathers this information? _____

e) Who (and how – phone, fax, etc.) does the ED notify when unusual clusters of illnesses present
   and can they be notified 24 hours per day (check all that apply)?

	24-hour Notification	How Contacted
❑ Hospital infection control personnel	❑ Yes ❑ No ❑ DK	_____
❑ Other designated (resource) in-house personnel	❑ Yes ❑ No ❑ DK	_____
❑ Local Health Department	❑ Yes ❑ No ❑ DK	_____
❑ State Health Department	❑ Yes ❑ No ❑ DK	_____
❑ Other, please specify_____	❑ Yes ❑ No ❑ DK	_____

FIGURE 27–1

(CONTINUED)

34. Is your in-patient laboratory staffed 24 hours a day, 7 days a week?   ❏ Yes ❏ No ❏ DK

35. What diagnostic capability does your in-patient laboratory have? (Check all that apply.)

    ❏ Minimal identification of agents

    ❏ Identification, confirmation, and susceptibility testing

    ❏ Advanced laboratory capacity with some molecular testing

36. What is the highest Biosafety Level (BSL) capability of your in-patient lab?

    ❏ BSL 1 (basic level of containment for minimal potential hazards)

    ❏ BSL 2 (primary containment practices for moderate potential hazards)

    ❏ BSL 3 (primary and secondary containment practices for potentially lethal agents)

37. What is the current volume of culture specimens that can be processed in your in-patient lab on a daily basis?

    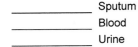
    _____ Sputum
    _____ Blood
    _____ Urine

38. What is the estimated maximum volume of culture specimens that can be processed in your in-patient lab on a daily basis?

    _____ Sputum
    _____ Blood
    _____ Urine

39. Does your hospital have protocols or procedures for the handling of laboratory specimens in the event of a biological terrorism incident?   ❏ Yes ❏ No ❏ DK

    If yes, do these protocols or procedures address the following (please check all that apply):

    ❏ Collection

    ❏ Labeling

    ❏ Chain of custody (similar to rape packages)

    ❏ Secure storage

    ❏ Processing

    ❏ Transportation to secondary laboratory

    ❏ Storage

    ❏ Referral to Public Health Department (PHD) lab

    ❏ Contacting the CDC

    ❏ Contacting local law enforcement

    ❏ Contacting the FBI

    ❏ Decontamination of biohazardous waste

    ❏ Safe disposal of waste

40. Please check the appropriate box to describe your hospital's in-patient laboratory capacity with regard to the following organisms (check all that apply):

Ver. 1.0   10   March 10, 2002

FIGURE 27-1

(CONTINUED)

Anthrax	Culture	Rule Out	Confirm*	None**
Plague	Culture	Rule Out	Confirm*	None**
Tularemia	Culture	Rule Out	Confirm*	None**
Brucellosis	Culture	Rule Out	Confirm*	None**
Q-Fever	Culture	Rule Out	Confirm*	None**
Smallpox	Culture	Rule Out	Confirm*	None**

* If checked, please indicate how your lab confirms the organism's identification. _____

** *Checking none means your hospital laboratory does not have the capacity to culture, rule out, or confirm the listed organism.*

41. How would you rate your laboratory's ability to identify specimens of biological terrorism?

❑ Very poor

❑ Poor

❑ Fair

❑ Good

❑ Very good

42. How would you rate your hospital's ability to manage victims of biological terrorism?

❑ Very poor

❑ Poor

❑ Fair

❑ Good

❑ Very good

Sources: Questions 1, 2, 3, and 23 in Section II of this questionnaire were adapted from New York City Department of Health, institutional surge capacity questions 1-6 in "Biological, Chemical, and Radiological Emergency Planning/Preparedness Capabilities Survey," dated 11/13/2000. The following documents were also consulted: Marasco Newton Group Ltd., "Hospital Weapons of Mass Destruction Needs and Resource Assessment urvey," dated 2/8/2000; Booz-Allen & Hamilton, WMD Checklist; Institute of Medicine, 2000 MMRS Evaluation Instrument in "Preparing for Terrorism: Tools for Evaluating the Metropolitan Medical Response System"; American Hospital Association, Chemical and Bioterrorism Preparedness Checklist; Disaster Preparedness International, "Hospital Capability to Respond to Pandemic Influenza, Bioterrorism, and Emerging Infectious Disease Outbreaks," dated 12/11/2001.

Ver. 1.0   11   March 10, 2002

FIGURE 27-1

(*CONTINUED*)

DILEMMAS FACING HOSPITALS IN BIOTERRORISM PREPAREDNESS

Preparedness for a potential terrorist attack involving biologicals is expensive and hospitals are reluctant to create capacity that is not needed on a routine basis and may indeed never be used. Therefore, terrorism events earn a low-priority rank in virtually all hospital vulnerability assessments. As a result of HRSA funding and the continued efforts of the federal government in promoting the need for readiness, hospital administrators are beginning to recognize that their facilities are an essential component of terrorism preparedness. They have therefore become more proactive in the planning and training of staff to increase response capacity within their institutions.

Despite the efforts and funding by the government, a large percentage of hospitals are still only in the planning stages of preparation for mass casualty incidents. During disaster training, many institutions have identified recurring issues that to date have yet to be corrected:

1. Lack of specific directives from state bioterrorism preparedness planner

    A coordinated response requires a high level of preparation among first responders and emergency personnel to be effective. In most instances, one hopes that a coordinated local response will be sufficient for community recovery. In worst-case scenarios, the coordinated response would be statewide, regional, or even national. In some areas communication among state and national agencies continue to be inadequate.

2. Communications

    Remain poor among neighboring institutions not to mention the lack of connectivity that exists between hospitals and state as well as national disaster control areas. Some institutions rely on landline communications that may be quickly lost should the local electric and phone companies become disabled.

3. Hospital security

    It appears that in general, security staff is poorly trained and lacking in numbers sufficient to safeguard their respective institutions. Lockdown criteria and specific plans are often random and poorly executed.

4. Decontamination procedures, equipment, and training

    Most hospitals still lack equipment, medical stockpiles, and isolation facilities for even a small-scale response. Even more ominous is the expense potentially incurred in preparation for events that may never occur. Finally, the ongoing costs of storing equipment and the costs of training personnel throughout the entire institution remain significant.

ISSUES OF RURAL HOSPITALS

Although it appears that most hospitals are making progress in preparing for a potential bioterrorism attack, rural hospitals are significantly behind in their readiness for such a situation. Unlike their urban counterparts who can avail themselves of a larger workforce and a wider range of resources, rural hospitals face the following obstacles:

1. Availability of personnel and reserve capacity

    Rural hospitals do not have the availability of personnel found in urban areas. Employees of rural hospitals may also hold positions in nearby urban hospitals, which will make it difficult during times of crisis for the smaller institutions to call on their reserve capacity. Additionally, a good number of rural hospital employees wear many hats due to the lack of available personnel in this setting. This makes it difficult for them to obtain the necessary training and potentially taxes their resources during a crisis.

    Therefore, not only are these individuals assuming a significant burden when asked to prepare their institutions for bioterrorism attacks, but they will also bear the brunt of the many positions they hold in a time of crisis.

2. Training

    Providing proper training for the staff of rural hospitals can be a challenge. The lack of available workforce with any type of experience is generally lacking. Attending training meeting that are usually at great distances from the rural institutions cuts significantly into the daily duties of the staff. Hence, a 1-day training session becomes a 3-day absence for an already poorly staffed institution. Finally, ancillary staffs such as housekeeping, food services, and other clerical personnel almost never receive any type of training since this is usually reserved for the professional component of the institution.

3. Storage capacity and resources

    National guidelines regarding supplies and stockpiling are directed at urban settings and are not generally feasible for hospitals in rural communities. Other issues involve setting up distribution channels to obtain needed pharmaceuticals and other medical supplies during a catastrophic event. Therefore, it behooves rural hospitals to create some contingency with local transport companies to be part of the plan to serve as emergent transport during a national/state crisis.

4. Lack of coordination and communication among rural hospitals and their state agencies

    This is not entirely an issue pertinent to rural hospitals. However, due to their size, location, and lack of political clout, rural hospitals are usually at the end of the line when it comes to coordination and communication efforts with their state agencies. Moreover, the lack of personnel and the lack of time by personnel responsible for the daily operations of the institution becomes an obstacle to the completion of the required "all hazards" plan.

As a result of their size and geography, rural hospitals operate in a different way than urban hospitals. The funding requirements set forth by federal agencies are not practical for rural hospitals. Consequently these institutions go unfunded as a result of their inability to comply with mandates structured for urban institutions. Therefore, federal agencies must modify their rules as applied to rural hospitals so they can be part of the preparation for catastrophic events without burdening their staffs, budgets, and communities.

SUMMARY

Hospitals must step up their readiness and hone their preparedness plans to conform to current requirements. Funding has been made available by the federal government in an effort to enable hospitals to meet the requirements for the creation and maintenance of an effective disaster program. It is essential that rapid recognition of any syndromic trends be noted and that plans be activated promptly. Excess influx of patients must be promptly identified so that alternate site facilities can be made available, staffed with critical personnel, and supplied with necessary equipment and medications.

Communication among local health departments and hospitals is essential for the prompt deployment of necessary personnel and resources required in a crisis.

Suggested Reading

Aldridge J, Launt P. *Are Hospitals our Weakest Link: Policy Analysis Brief.* Walsh Center for Rural Health Analysis. W series No. 4, April 2004.

Bentley JD. *Hospital Preparedness for Bioterrorism.* Public Health Reports. Vol. 116, supplement 2, 2001.

Darling RG, Mothershead JL, Waeckerle JF, et al. *Emergency Medicine Clinics of North America: Bioterrorism.* Philadelphia: W.B. Saunders Company, May 2002.

General Accounting Office Report to Congressional Committees: Hospital Preparedness; Most Urban Hospitals Have Emergency Plans but Lack Certain Capacities for Bioterrorism Response; August 2003.

JCAHO. Emergency management in the new millennium. *Jt Comm Perspect.* December 200;21(12):1–27

JCAHO. Emergency Management Standards EC.1.4 and EC.2.9.1. Comprehensive Accreditation Manual for Hospitals, 2002.

U.S. Department of Health and Human Services: HHS Awards $498 Million to States to Improve Hospitals' Response to Bioterrorism and Other Disasters. May 2004.

IV

SPECIFIC CHEMICAL AGENT: TOXINS/TOXICANTS

INTRODUCTION

Chemical agent exposure to a mass population presents an interesting challenge to the first responder and emergency physician. The general principles of basic poison management (i.e., decontamination, toxidrome recognition, antidotal administration) apply to the management of this entity. Furthermore, these principles are focused on the dose-effect relationship premise articulated by Paracelsius several hundred years ago.

The first responder must utilize these tenets within several minutes upon recognition that such an event has occurred. The clinician must primarily utilize the history and physical examination to determine a therapeutic regimen because the hospital based laboratory (utilizing biological specimens) will be of limited usefulness in the initial hours. Infield laboratory analysis (as described in a previous chapter of the same name) could be the most productive methodology in identifying the causative agent.

Basically, the approach to chemical agent exposure can be summarized into two categories: mucosal irritants and systemic effects. Riot control agents and most pulmonary agents are examples of mucosal irritants while nerve agents and most of the heavy metals cause systemic effects with little mucosal irritation warning. The succeeding chapters will focus on the particular application of these principles.

28

NERVE AGENTS

Jerrold B. Leikin and Frank Walter

NERVE AGENTS

- Nerve agents were originally derived from organophosphate insecticides and inhibit acetyl cholinesterase
- Sarin, soman, and tabun are volatile liquids while VX is a persistent oily liquid, which is well-absorbed dermally
- Pre-entry considerations include Level A PPE
- Volatile nerve agents can cause immediate symptoms on inhalation exposure while VX exposure can cause delayed onset of symptoms after dermal absorption
- Clinical manifestations include cholinergic excess (miosis, bronchoconstriction, fasciculations, weakness, etc)
- Plasma or red blood cell cholinesterase depression can help confirm exposure
- Atropine, pralidoxime, and diazepam are the essential antidotes

INTRODUCTION

Nerve agents were developed in Germany during the 1930s as potential insecticides of the organophosphate family. The agents are traditionally divided into two classes, the G and V agents (Table 28-1). The first G agent was synthesized in Germany in 1936 by a group of chemists at IG Farbenindustrie. The V agents were first synthesized in the United Kingdom in 1954. The G agents are typified by the compounds known as tabun (GA), sarin (GB), and soman (GD). Only two V compounds have been produced in large quantities, VX and the V-gas, which is the Russian equivalent of VX. The V agents are roughly 10 times more toxic than G agents, but are less volatile than the G agents.

PROPERTIES

The properties of the nerve agents are summarized in Table 28-2. The nerve agents are esters of phosphoric acid, known as organophosphates. Their general structure is shown in Fig. 28-1.

At normal temperatures, the nerve agents are liquids. Thickening agents, such as acrylates, can be added to some nerve agents. This alters some of the physical properties of the resultant mixture thus increasing its persistency in the environment.

Sarin (Fig. 28-2) is mixable with water (capable of mixing in any ratio without separating into two phases) and hydrolyzed by water to produce a relatively nontoxic product resulting from removal of fluorine. Soman is moderately water-soluble, but readily soluble in organic solvents. Tabun is moderately water-soluble, but readily soluble in organic solvents. Tabun is also hydrolyzed by water. VX is only slightly water-soluble at room temperature, but is miscible in cold water and organic solvents.

The G agents are slowly hydrolyzed at neutral and acidic pHs, but are rapidly hydrolyzed at alkaline pHs. Hydrolysis of soman and tabun produces hydrogen fluoride and hydrogen cyanide respectively. This alkaline hydrolysis is exploited by decontaminating surfaces with alkaline, dilute, household bleach solutions (0.5% sodium hypochlorite). The environmental half-life of sarin in water, with a pH of 7, is 5.4 hours, versus a half-life of 15 minutes at a pH of 9.

Although the vapor pressures of the nerve agents are not high, they are significant. Sarin is most volatile, with a vapor pressure of 2.9 mm Hg at 77°F (Table 28-3). The most volatile agent, sarin, has a vapor pressure that is more than 400 times that of the least volatile agent, VX. Water,

TABLE 28-1

NAMES, NUMBERS, AND SOURCES OF EXPOSURE FOR NERVE AGENTS

Common Name	Synonym	CAS#	Sources of Exposure
Sarin	GB	107-44-8	U.S. and other military chemical weapons depots. Illicit manufacturing by terrorists
Soman	GD	96-64-0	Illicit manufacturing by terrorists
Cyclohexyl Sarin	GF or CMPE	329-99-7	U.S. and other military chemical weapons depots. Illicit manufacturing by terrorists
Tabun	GA	77-81-6	Illicit manufacturing by terrorists
VX	None	50782-69-9	U.S. and other military chemical weapons depots. Illicit manufacturing by terrorists
Russian VX	R-VX or VR-55	159939-87-4	Russian/Illicit manufacture by terrorists

Source: Adapted with permission from: Thomas RG. Chemoterrorism: nerve agents. Walter FB, Klein R, Thomas RG. Advanced Hazmat Life Support Provider Manual. 3rd ed. Tucson, AZ: Arizona Board of Regents; 2003: 295–314.

by comparison, is more volatile, with a vapor pressure of 23.8 mm Hg at 77°F. Most importantly, the volatility of the nerve agents (vapor concentration in mg/m^3) exceeds their recommended control limits for workers exposed to these agents at U.S. Department of Defense facilities (Table 28-3).

The volatility of the nerve agents and their rates of vaporization are key physical properties that are responsible for the greatest hazard from these agents, a lethal dose by inhalation (Table 28-3). Primary vaporization of nerve agents can occur from the heat of an explosive device or from the vaporization of droplets that have been dispersed (aerosolized) by a sprayer, etc. Secondary vaporization can occur from the ground or other surfaces that have been coated with the liquid or droplets. The persistence of a nerve agent is inversely related to its volatility, for example, VX is the least volatile but the most environmentally persistent nerve agent (Table 28-3).

TOXICOKINETICS

Routes of Exposure

Inhalation

The three G agents, GA (tabun), GB (sarin), and GD (soman), are volatile liquids at normal ambient temperatures. As can be seen in Table 28-3, the G agents are significantly more volatile than VX, which has the consistency of motor oil. Consequently, the most likely route of exposure with the G agents is inhalation. GF can be absorbed by both inhalation and dermal routes. It has about equal the potency of soman with a hyman LD$_{50}$ of 30 mg/kg. Inhalation of VX can occur, but is much less likely because of its low vapor pressure.

Absorption of a nerve agent by inhalation occurs within seconds. However, several factors influence the inhaled dose of vaporized (gaseous) nerve agents. For

TABLE 28-2

CHEMICAL PROPERTIES OF NERVE AGENTS

Chemical	State	Color	Odor/ Irritation	Water Solubility	Boiling Point (°F)	Molecular Weight	Flash Point (°F)
Sarin (GB)	Liquid	Colorless	Odorless	Miscible	297	140.1	NR
Soman (GD)	Liquid	Colorless	Fruity	2.1%	333	182.2	250
Tabun (GA)	Liquid	Colorless to brown	Fruity, like bitter almonds	7.2%	464	162.1	172
VX	Liquid	Colorless to straw	Odorless	Miscible if <49°F	568	267.4	318

Unless noted, properties are determined at 68°F and an atmospheric pressure of 760 mm Hg (1 atm). NR: Not reported

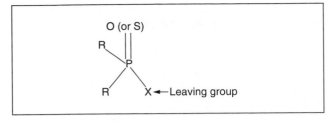

FIGURE 28-1
ORGANOPHOSPHATE STRUCTURE

An organophosphate's rate of reactivity with acetylcholinesterase and its degree of toxicity depend on which compounds are substituted for the X and the two R substituents. Extreme toxicity results when strongly electronegative groups, such as the halides (e.g., chlorine, fluorine), cyanide, or thiocyanate, are the leaving group. The X substituent for sarin is thiocyanate. The formula of sarin is shown in Fig. 28-2. The V agents are sulfur-containing organophosphates.

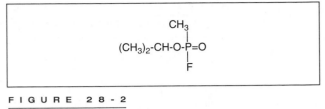

FIGURE 28-2
STRUCTURE OF SARIN (GB)

comparative purposes, the concentration time function (Ct) is used to describe the amount of a nerve gas to which a victim is exposed. This term, expressed as Ct, is equal to the concentration in the air (C), in mg/m^3, times the exposure time (t), in minutes. The LCt_{50} is the Ct that kills 50% of exposed victims. ICt_{50} is the Ct that incapacitates 50% of the exposed victims. MCt_{50} is the Ct that produces miosis (pinpoint pupils) in 50% of exposed victims. Table 28-4 compares these various Ct values in $mg-min/m^3$.

Note the very small exposure concentration times to produce miosis and the small differences between the LCt_{50} and ICt_{50} values. This means only a slight increase in either the time of exposure or the concentration can result in a potentially lethal exposure, rather than an incapacitating exposure.

Skin and Mucous Membranes

All the nerve agents can be absorbed through the skin. However the more volatile the agent, the larger the topical dose required to produce toxicity. Tabun and sarin generally evaporate before skin penetration can occur. Skin

exposure to tabun vapors (2.5 to 5 times the LCt_{50}), either by limbs in chambers or by whole body exposures with respiratory protection, produced no signs or symptoms of tabun toxicity.

VX is a persistent agent and is well-absorbed through the skin after minimal contact time. The dermal LD_{50} (the dose applied to the skin required to kill 50% of the victims exposed), for contact with liquid VX, for a 70 kg adult human, is only approximately 6 mg. In comparison, the dermal LD_{50} for contact with liquid tabun, sarin, and soman are approximately 1610 mg, 1960 mg, and 1260 mg, respectively.

Clothing that has been sprayed with a nerve agent can either offer a protective barrier that prevents skin contact or it can promote continued absorption when wetted sufficiently and allowed to remain in contact with the skin.

Even if skin decontamination has taken place, continued absorption from the inner layers of the skin can result in a delayed onset of symptoms. The onset of symptoms from dermal exposure to small amounts of nerve agent liquid has occurred as long as 18 hours after exposure. The symptoms have usually been minor. As a general rule, the longer the time interval between the exposure and the onset of symptoms, the less severe the effects will be. In other words, the time interval between the exposure and the onset of symptoms is inversely proportional to the severity of the signs and symptoms. Large liquid dermal exposures can result in onset of symptoms within 1 to 30 minutes. Disabling signs and symptoms from a dermal exposure can occur abruptly with little, if any, warning. For example, respiratory distress can rapidly ensue, in

TABLE 28-3

VAPOR DATA AND ENVIRONMENTAL PERSISTENCE OF THE NERVE AGENTS

Name	Synonym	Vapor Density (Relative to Air, Equal to 1)	Vapor Pressure (mm Hg)	Volatility (mg/m^3 at 77°F)	Recommended Control Limit (mg/m^3 at 68°F)	Environmental Persistence
Sarin	GB	4.9	2.9 at 77°F	22,000	0.0001	No
Soman	GD	6.3	0.4 at 77°F	3900	NR	No
Tabun	GA	5.6	0.04 at 68°F	610	0.0001	No
VX	None	9.2	0.007 at 68°F	10.5	0.00001	Yes

NR: Not reported.

Source: Adapted with permission from: Thomas RG. Chemoterrorism: nerve agents. Walter FB, Klein R, Thomas RG. Advanced Hazmat Life Support Provider Manual. 3rd ed. Tucson, AZ: Arizona Board of Regents; 2003: 295–314.

HUMAN LETHAL, INCAPACITATING, AND MIOSIS CONCENTRATION-TIME PRODUCTS

Nerve Agent	LCt_{50} (Human)	ICt_{50} (Human)	MCt_{50} (Human)
Sarin (GB)	100	75	3
Soman (GD)	70	Unknown	<1
Tabun (GA)	400	300	2–3
VX	50	35	0.04

Source: Adapted from *Medical Management of Chemical Casualties Handbook*, 3rd ed, July 2000, US Army Medical Research Institute of Chemical Defense, Public Domain.

spite of a lack of miosis that usually is the first sign after nerve agent vapor exposure.

The location of dermal exposure can also play an important role. Maximal skin absorption appears to occur in the head/neck region followed by the extremities and then the torso.

Ambient temperature also affects skin absorption. Decreased absorption occurs at lower temperatures and increased absorption occurs at higher temperatures. In fact, decontamination procedures at typical room temperatures, after exposures at very low temperatures (e.g., 0°F to 36°F), resulted in enhanced absorption.

PATHOPHYSIOLOGY

Acetylcholinesterase is a member of a family of enzymes that hydrolyzes esters. An ester is an alcohol connected (covalently bonded) to an acid. Choline is an alcohol and acetic acid is an acid. Acetylcholinesterase hydrolyzes acetylcholine into its constituents, choline and acetic acid. At physiologic pH, that is, at the normal blood pH of 7.4, acetic acid (CH_3COOH) is ionized and exists mainly as acetate (CH_3COO^-) and the hydrogen ion (H^+) in aqueous solution.

The acetylcholinesterase enzyme found in the nervous system is only one type of cholinesterase. Cholinesterases are also found in other organ systems. For example, red blood cells (RBCs) have cholinesterase activity that is very similar to that in the nervous system. The cholinesterase that is found in the plasma (EC 3.1.1.8), also called plasma cholinesterase, butyryl cholinesterase, or pseudo-cholinesterase, can be measured relatively easily (because it is a blood test), in contradistinction to measuring nervous system acetylcholinesterase activity that requires a nerve or brain biopsy. However, RBC cholinesterase activity correlates better with nervous system cholinesterase activity than plasma cholinesterase. Symptoms do not always correlate exactly with RBC cholinesterase inhibition; unless activity is reduced to 50%, or lower, even minor symptoms might not be present.

Organophosphates and carbamates are cholinesterase inhibitors. Cholinesterase inhibitors block the activity of the enzyme acetylcholinesterase resulting in acetylcholine accumulation at all cholinergic receptors. This causes continued receptor stimulation, thereby producing the cholinergic toxidrome (Table 28-5).

Acetylcholine binds at muscarinic receptors and nicotinic receptors. Muscarinic receptors are located in the central nervous system (CNS), and in the peripheral nervous system (PNS) at neuroeffector junctions (the connection between a nerve cell and a muscle, a gland, etc.) of the parasympathetic portion of the autonomic nervous system. Nicotinic receptors are located in the CNS, in the PNS sympathetic and parasympathetic ganglia, and in the neuromuscular junction. Cholinesterase inhibitors act at all these sites, that is, they act in the CNS and PNS, at both muscarinic and nicotinic sites. Therefore, the signs and symptoms caused by cholinesterase inhibitor pesticide poisoning consist not only of the typically remembered PNS muscarinic signs and symptoms (SLUDGE: salivation, lacrimation, urination, defecation, gastroenteritis, and emesis) but also PNS nicotinic signs and symptoms (MTWHF: mydriasis, tachycardia, weakness, hypertension, and fasciculations), and CNS nicotinic and muscarinic signs and symptoms (Table 28-5). The preferred muscarinic mnemonic is DUMBELS because it contains the "killer bees," that is, those effects that can be fatal (bradycardia, bronchorrhea, and bronchospasm). The wide distribution of acetylcholinesterase, at both nicotinic and muscarinic receptors throughout the PNS and CNS, can result in seemingly contradictory signs and symptoms.

Clinically, nicotinic signs often predominate early in the course of cholinesterase inhibitor poisoning. However, concurrent nicotinic and muscarinic signs and symptoms are often present in both the PNS and CNS. Later in the course of cholinesterase inhibitor poisoning, muscarinic signs and symptoms predominate. Severely poisoned patients can suffer the nicotinic effect of depolarizing neuromuscular blockade (fasciculations followed by flaccid [floppy] paralysis), muscarinic PNS effects such as bradycardia, and CNS effects such as coma. Acute respiratory insufficiency is the primary cause of death in acute poisonings.

Organophosphates will bind irreversibly to acetylcholinesterase, unless the patient receives the antidote

TABLE 28-5

SIGNS AND SYMPTOMS OF POISONING CAUSED BY CHOLINESTERASE INHIBITORS

Peripheral Nervous System (PNS)		Central Nervous System (CNS)
Muscarinic	**Nicotinic**	
Diarrhea	Mydriasis	Confusion
Urination	Tachycardia	Convulsions
Miosis	Weakness	Coma
Bradycardia, Bronchorrhea	Hypertension	
Bronchospasm	Hyperglycemia	
Emesis	Fasciculations	
Lacrimation		
Salivation, Secretion		
Sweating		

Source: Adapted with permission from: Thomas RG. Chemoterrorism: nerve agents. Walter FB, Klein R, Thomas RG. Advanced Hazmat Life Support Provider Manual. 3rd ed. Tucson, AZ: Arizona Board of Regents; 2003: 295–314.

pralidoxime before "aging" occurs. "Aging" is the average time required for irreversible binding to occur between organophosphates and acetylcholinesterase. "Aging" can occur within minutes for soman or can take up to days for some commercial organophosphate pesticides (Table 28-6). Aging is discussed further with regards to Pralidoxine administration in the treatment section.

CLINICAL MANIFESTATIONS

The accumulation of acetylcholine at the muscarinic and nicotinic receptor sites produces a predictable clinical syndrome, a cholinergic toxidrome. Initial symptoms can actually be the result of local effects and not from systemic toxicity. Because the dose that produces minimal effects is often only a little less than that capable of causing death, the presence or absence of various signs and symptoms can be misleading as to the correct diagnosis and prognosis.

TABLE 28-6

CHOLINESTERASE "AGING" HALF-TIMES FOR NERVE AGENTS

Name	Synonym	"Aging" Half-Time
Sarin	GB	~5 hours
Soman	GD	~2 minutes
Tabun	GA	>40 hours
VX	None	>40 hours

Source: Adapted with permission from: Thomas RG. Chemoterrorism: nerve agents. Walter FB, Klein R, Thomas RG. Advanced Hazmat Life Support Provider Manual. 3rd ed. Tucson, AZ: Arizona Board of Regents; 2003: 295–314.

OCULAR SYSTEM

Nerve agents may have variable effects on the eye, depending on the agent and route of exposure. Vapor exposure usually causes miosis, ocular pain, and dimmed or blurred vision. These are local effects and do not correlate with RBC cholinesterase activity, unless there has also been inhalational exposure. The duration of miosis is variable, ranging from several days to regain normal dilatory activity in indoor lighting to as long as 9 weeks to regain maximal dilation in total darkness. Pain sometimes accompanies the miosis and is probably because of ciliary spasm. The discomfort can be characterized as a sharp or aching ocular pain and be associated with a mild to severe headache. Sometimes the pain is accompanied by nausea and vomiting. Dermal or gastrointestinal absorption of nerve agents, particularly VX, can produce moderate signs and symptoms, but not usually miosis. Thus the presence or absence of miosis does not provide good prognostic information.

Impaired visual acuity is a common effect from vapor exposure to nerve agents. The duration of effect, like that of miosis, can be variable, with normal vision returning within 2 to 35 days. The duration of effect, like that of miosis can be variable, with normal vision returning in 48 hours or taking as long as 35 days. Tearing is not a reliable sign of early exposure to nerve agent vapor. Some eyes can have a bloodshot appearance caused by subconjunctival vascular dilation.

RESPIRATORY SYSTEM

Rhinorrhea is generally considered a local effect after a vapor exposure, but can be a manifestation of systemic toxicity. The rhinorrhea is often copious, much worse than nasal secretions from a cold or hay fever; the severity is dose dependent.

Depending on the dose, respiratory symptoms range from local effects (e.g., increased secretions or bronchoconstriction) to systemic effects (e.g., ventilatory muscle paralysis with apnea). Large exposures to nerve agent vapors can result in immediate severe bronchiolar smooth muscle constriction, wheezing, copious secretions (bronchorrhea), and ventilatory failure. Although the ventilatory failure is caused, in part, by flaccid paralysis of ventilatory muscles, there is also greatly diminished respiratory drive from the CNS.

CARDIOVASCULAR SYSTEM

Excessive levels of acetylcholine can have a profound effect on cardiac activity. The expected effect on the heart would be increased vagal tone with bradycardia and atrioventricular (AV) heart blocks, even third degree AV block. In fact, the heart rate can actually increase because of increased sympathetic tone from acetylcholine accumulating in sympathetic ganglia and at the adrenal medulla. Sidell described heart rate effects in 199 patients with mild-to-moderate nerve agent exposures who were treated at the Edgewood Arsenal Toxic Exposure Aid Station. Only 6.5% had heart rates less than 64 beats per minute (bpm), while 35% had heart rates greater than 90 bpm. Ventricular arrhythmias are uncommon. Torsades de pointes (with prolonged QT interval) was reported in a dog study using sarin and in case reports of humans following organophosphate poisonings.

NERVOUS SYSTEM

Dermal exposures often produce local neuromuscular effects, including sweating and subjacent muscle fasciculations. Higher doses can cause muscle weakness, fatigue, and even flaccid paralysis. After a large exposure, generalized fasciculations are common and can continue for some time after other acute signs have decreased.

The cardinal CNS signs and symptoms after exposure to large amounts of nerve agents are seizures, coma, and apnea. Depending on the dose and route, these conditions can develop within 1 to 30 minutes after an initially asymptomatic period. Seizures can develop suddenly, last briefly, and resolve spontaneously, or seizures can be prolonged, with status epilepticus. Children may be more prone to seizures than adults. Apnea can also be abrupt in onset and does not resolve without antidotal therapy.

Exposure to small amounts of nerve agents can produce several, nonspecific CNS effects. Victims of low-dose nerve agent exposures have complained of forgetfulness, insomnia, irritability, depression, impaired judgment, bad dreams, and inability to concentrate. These symptoms can occur in the absence of physical signs. Survivors of large-dose exposures can also develop these symptoms. Recovery can take 4–6 weeks.

SKIN AND MUCOUS MEMBRANES

Dermal application of a liquid nerve agent can produce localized sweating and fasciculations of the underlying muscle. Generalized sweating is a common systemic effect following prolonged or extensive dermal exposure, or after inhalation. Localized sweating can last as long as 1 month following topical exposure to the forearms from sarin.

GASTROINTESTINAL SYSTEM

Excess acetylcholine increases gastrointestinal motility and secretions. Nausea and vomiting are common after inhalation and dermal exposures. Nausea and vomiting are among the first effects after dermal exposure. Paradoxically, diarrhea is an infrequent finding for all routes of exposure. Of 111 patients who survived the Tokyo subway sarin attack and were treated at St. Luke's Hospital, because of moderate to severe poisoning, only six (5.4%) had diarrhea. In contrast nausea occurred in 60.4%, and vomiting in 36.9%.

GENITOURINARY SYSTEM

After large dermal exposures and after the inhalation of significant amounts of vapors, micturition can occur. However no cases were reported in either of the two sarin terrorist attacks in Japan or in the cases previously reported by Sidell.

Tables 28-7 and 28-8 summarize the clinical signs and symptoms associated with nerve agent exposures by the two primary routes of exposure, inhalation and dermal.

PERSONAL PROTECTION EQUIPMENT

Level B will not protect skin from vapor exposures. Positive-pressure self-contained breathing apparatus (SCBA) with Level A protection is necessary; secondary contamination potential is especially high for VX. Chemical protective clothing, chemical goggles, face shields, and butyl rubber gloves are recommended.

DECONTAMINATION

There are few well-designed studies on the efficacy of various decontamination protocols in the medical literature. Although generalizations can be made, pragmatic decisions will need to be made. Severe weather conditions could override theoretical considerations because the risk of prolonged hypothermia might be greater than the worst possible effect

SIGNS AND SYMPTOMS AFTER ACUTE INHALATION EXPOSURE TO NERVE AGENTS

Low-Dose with Mild Effects:
- The eyes and nose are most affected by exposure.
- Miosis with eye or head pain
- Dim or blurred vision
- Conjunctival injection
- Rhinorrhea
- Bronchoconstriction with tightness in chest
- Mild bronchosecretions

Medium-Dose with Moderate Effects:
- Shortness of breath (moderate to marked dyspnea)
- Coughing
- Wheezing
- Nausea
- Vomiting
- Fasciculations
- Generalized feelings of weakness

High-Dose with Severe Effects:
- Loss of consciousness
- Seizures
- Apnea
- Flaccid paralysis
- Death usually occurs within minutes

of the chemical. Mass victim incidents will limit the amount of time and resources available to treat any one patient. In these situations, self- or buddy assistance will be necessary. The recommended duration of decontamination suggested

TABLE 28-8

SIGNS AND SYMPTOMS AFTER ACUTE DERMAL EXPOSURE TO NERVE AGENTS

Low-Dose with Mild Effects:
- Localized sweating at the exposure site
- Fine muscle fasciculations at the exposure site
- Miosis is *not* an early sign after dermal liquid contact and may not be present at all

Medium-Dose with Moderate Effects:
- Nausea
- Vomiting
- Severe headache
- Generalized fasciculations
- Feelings of weakness
- *Beware, no respiratory signs or symptoms are present, yet*

High-Dose with Severe Effects:
- Sudden loss of consciousness
- Seizures
- Flaccid paralysis
- Apnea
- Death

below could be drastically lessened in order to provide rapid decontamination of multiple victims in the field. Realizing that the delay to decontamination could be more critical than the length of decontamination, it is plausible that with large numbers of victims a 1-minute rinse, after removal of contaminated garments, might be acceptable decontamination for 15 people, in 15 minutes, rather than a "thorough" decontamination of only 1 person for 15 minutes. Most of the contamination from solids or liquids is removed by taking off all garments and by a brief decontamination. The exact benefits of longer decontamination are intuitive, but have not been proven in the medical literature. The potential toxicity of the agent should also be considered, especially for chemicals that are absorbable through the skin, such as the nerve agents. A major goal of adequate decontamination is to prevent secondary contamination of downstream health-care workers who will come into contact with the nerve agent victim.

Decontamination of the respiratory system is accomplished by removing the patient from the source of the airborne exposure. The most important method of decontamination is adequate ventilation. Therefore, ensure adequate ventilation and oxygenation.

Skin decontamination is not necessary, if the exposure has been to *vapor only*. However, clothing exposed to nerve agent vapor can carry minute amounts of the agent and can cause minor secondary contamination. The medical staff of St. Luke's Hospital in Tokyo was minimally affected by the condensed sarin vapor on victims' clothing. Medical staff complained only of symptoms, and manifested no verifiable signs or laboratory abnormalities such as cholinesterase inhibition. Once victims have been removed from the vapor source, their clothing should be removed and double bagged; this is generally sufficient decontamination for *vapor* exposures.

Because of the volatility of the G agents, it is unlikely that liquid skin exposures will result in a significant amount of nerve agent on the skin when the victim reaches medical attention. In other words, exposed patients pose a relatively low risk of secondary contamination to rescuers. However, liquid nerve agents should be removed from the skin immediately to alter the absorption for the exposed patient. Since the nerve agents are inactivated by alkaline solutions, a neutralizing agent such as 0.5% sodium hypochlorite solution, (1 part household bleach plus 9 parts water) is currently recommended by the U.S. Army. Continued contact with a nerve agent, from wet clothing or hair, requires that the clothing be removed and the hair washed as soon as possible. After contact with nerve agents, both the skin and the hair should be washed with dilute bleach solution. If an isolated area of the skin has been exposed and local symptoms are evident, a pad soaked in 0.5% hypochlorite should be applied to the area for approximately 20 minutes and then the area should be washed with water.

Eye contact with liquid nerve agents should be decontaminated by irrigating with large quantities of water or sterile saline solution. Irrigation of the conjunctival sac should continue throughout patient contact and during prehospital transport, if possible. If continuous decontamination of the eyes is not possible, decontaminate at the scene prior to ambulance transport, for at least 20 minutes. Use of Morgan lenses with an ophthalmic local anesthetic, such as proparacaine, can make decontaminating the patient's eyes easier for the patient and the health-care provider.

The assessment of a nerve agent victim should focus on the patient's clinical condition and the route of exposure. Vapor exposure usually causes immediate symptoms. Symptom onset can be significantly delayed after dermal exposure; these patients should be observed for many hours. No minimum, safe duration of observations has yet been established, because of lack of clinical experience and clinical studies.

Resuscitation must begin immediately following a significant inhalational exposure. Life-threatening symptoms can begin less than 5 minutes after exposure and death can occur within 5 minutes after the onset of seizures and respiratory arrest. Atropine and pralidoxime are essential antidotes for the resuscitation and treatment of victims of nerve agent poisoning.

LABORATORY

Laboratory analysis should focus on plasma and RBC cholinesterase activity. Immunoassay can rapidly measure cholinesterase depression, but the preferred method is gas chromatography coupled with mass spectrometry (GC-MS). Chemical and electron-impact ionization, followed by tandem MS, has also been utilized. Plasma cholinesterase activity appears to be a sensitive assay for exposure with over 50% depression of activity correlated with symptoms and over 70% activity depression associated with severe symptoms. Toxicity appears to correlate better with RBC cholinesterase depression than with plasma cholinesterase depression. Miosis does not correlate with cholinesterase depression. Plasma choline-sterase usually recovers within about 1 week, while RBC cholinesterase takes about 3 months to recover. Alkylmethylphosphonic acids can be analyzed in serum or urine by high-performance liquid chromatography, capillary electrophoresis, LC-mass spectrometry or GC-MS-MS with derivatization to convert the polar compounds to substances for gas chromatography. The latter method can be performed within an hour with a limit of detection of 0.3–0.9 ug/L in the urine. In the Tokyo subway exposure, serum levels of GB acid (sarin metabolic) were between 2 and 135 ng/L. Field detection technologies may include potentiometric sensor, ion-sensitive field-effect transistors and reversed osmotic capillary flow, and electrophoresis. The latter has a detection limit of 75 ug/L. Anti-VX monoclonal antibodies have also been developed and have a detection limit of 4 ug/L.

TREATMENT

Atropine

Atropine is a symptomatic antidote for the muscarinic signs and symptoms of nerve agent poisonings. Atropine is a competitive antagonist at muscarinic receptors only, and thus blocks the effects of acetylcholine at muscarinic receptors in the PNS and CNS. Therefore, atropine is a parasympatholytic. Atropine works only at the muscarinic receptors and cannot counteract acetylcholine's effects at nicotinic receptors in the PNS or CNS. Therefore, atropine cannot counteract fasciculations, weakness, flaccid paralysis, or respiratory arrest caused by neuromuscular blockade at nicotinic receptors. Atropine does not regenerate the poisoned acetylcholinesterase, that is, it does not reactivate the inactivated acetylcholinesterase, and thus, it is not curative.

The total doses of atropine for nerve agent poisoning are often much smaller than those usually required to treat organophosphate *insecticide* poisoning. Organophosphate insecticides are more slowly metabolized and more lipid-soluble. Consequently, they are cleared much more slowly from the body; therefore, the cumulative dose of atropine can reach much higher totals.

Atropine should be reserved to treat moderate to severe systematic symptoms of nerve agent poisoning. Mild exposures resulting only in miosis do not require atropine because atropine does not reverse miosis, and it can cause other problems due to its anticholinergic effects. Miosis and ciliary spasm with severe eye pain can be treated with topical homatropine ophthalmic drops, if necessary. Rhinorrhea generally does not merit atropine administration, unless it is severe and interferes with patient management.

Patients with mild respiratory distress can be observed for 15–30 minutes to see if these effects diminish after removal from the source of exposure. If respiratory symptoms don't improve, then atropine, 1–2 mg IV or IM, can be given. IV administration is preferable. IM is reserved for the prehospital, multicasualty setting or when IV access cannot be obtained. Moderate airway discomfort from bronchospasm and increased secretions should be treated with atropine, 1–2 mg IV or IM, and repeated, as needed, every 5–10 minutes, until ventilation is easy. Dried secretions are not necessarily the endpoint of therapy in mild to moderate poisoning. In severe cases of nerve agent poisoning, atropine can be given as an initial dose up to 6 mg IV or IM, and then 2 mg IV or IM, every 5–10 minutes, until ventilation is easy and secretions have dried.

The indications to treat children with atropine are the same as those in adults. Children's dosing of atropine must be adjusted for weight and age. The U.S. Office of the Surgeon General recommends the following doses for children.

Infant (<2 years old): 0.5 mg maximum single dose, repeated as clinically indicated

Child (2–10 years old): 1 mg maximum single dose, repeated as clinically indicated

Adolescent: 2 mg maximum single dose, repeated as clinically indicated. A cumulative dose of approximately 10–20 mg of atropine in the first 2–3 hours postexposure may be needed to adequately control the symptoms

Atropine is available in a variety of different injectable dosage forms, including single and multidose vials, prefilled syringes, and autoinjectors. The U.S. Armed Forces use AtroPen autoinjectors containing 2 mg of atropine in 0.7 mL of fluid. These atropine autoinjectors are packaged with another autoinjector containing pralidoxime in units called Mark I kits. These kits and the single autoinjectors are being made available, on a limited basis, to the civilian community as part of the Chemical Stockpile Emergency Preparedness Program (CSEPP). These Mark I kits are available to some of the federal domestic preparedness programs such as the Metropolitan Medical Response System (MMRS).

It has been recommended that hospitals stock at least 150 mg of atropine. In the event that atropine doses are depleted, extemporaneous preparation of concentrated atropine sulfate should be compounded for administration (Table 28-9). If true cholinergic excess exists, the administration of atropine should produce no ill effects. However, excessive amounts of atropine, either from giving too much to a symptomatic patient or from giving atropine to an unexposed person, can produce anticholinergic effects such as dry mouth, blurred vision, dilated pupils, urinary retention, tachycardia, and inability to sweat. These side effects are generally considered minor though they can last for 24–48 hours. Physostigmine should not be administered to counteract the adverse effects of atropine in a nerve gas exposure.

Significant caution should be exercised when hypoxia is present in cases of severe nerve agent poisoning. Intravenous administration of atropine to animals with hypoxia caused by severe respiratory complications of nerve agent poisoning has produced ventricular fibrillation. Therefore, hypoxia should be corrected first, if possible, before atropine administration. However, atropine should not be withheld from a victim of severe nerve poisoning because of a concern about precipitating a life-threatening arrhythmia, especially if the victim is an apparently healthy young person with an otherwise healthy heart.

TABLE 28-9

PROTOCOL FOR EXTEMPORANEOUS PREPARATION OF ATROPINE SULFATE FOR INJECTION

- Reconstitute 30 g of atropine sulfate USP powder in 30 mL of normal saline (1 g/mL)
- Draw up 1 mL into a syringe
- Attach a Millex 0.22 micron filter to the syringe
- Add 1 mL (1 g atropine sulfate) to a 500 mL container of normal saline (2 mg/mL)
- Add 1 mL (1 g atropine sulfate) to a 1 L container of normal saline (1 mg/mL)

Children appear to tolerate large doses of atropine better than some adults. Following the Gulf War, a retrospective national survey was conducted on atropine autoinjector poisonings in Israeli children. Several hundred children received accidental doses of atropine, often in the finger or palm. The doses were up to 17 times higher than the standard, age-appropriate doses. About 50% experienced some systemic effects, but only 8% suffered from severe atropinization. There were no seizures, hyperthermia, or deaths associated with this accidental atropine intoxication.

Pralidoxime (2-PAM)/Other Oximes

Pralidoxime (2-PAM) is an oxime, a chemical that reacts with the nerve agent-inhibited cholinesterase enzymes to remove the nerve agent from the enzyme, allowing the cholinesterases to reactivate and metabolize acetylcholine. The timing of pralidoxime administration is critical because the binding of the nerve agents to cholinesterase can become irreversible with time. This irreversible binding is called "aging." Once aging has occurred, the cholinesterase enzyme will never be able to metabolize acetylcholine. Aging occurs at different rates for different nerve agents (Table 28-6). For VX, the RBC cholinesterase enzyme deactivates at roughly 0.5–1% per hour for the first 48 hours. It takes approximately 5 hours for 50% of the sarin-cholinesterase enzyme complex to age. In contrast, the soman enzyme complex is completely, irreversibly aged within less than 10 minutes with 50% of the enzyme aged after only 2 minutes.

2-PAM is recommended for all cases of moderate to severe nerve agent poisoning. The optimal dosage is dependent on the nerve agent, time since exposure, and the cholinesterase activity of the victim. One human study assessed regeneration of cholinesterase activity when IV 2-PAM was given 1 hour after sarin exposure. A 2-PAM dosage of 10 mg/kg reactivated 28% of RBC cholinesterase activity. A 2-PAM dosage 20 mg/kg reactivated 58% of RBC cholinesterase activity. If therapy was delayed for 3 hours and the dose reduced to 5 mg/kg, only 10% was reactivated, but if the dose was increased to 10 mg/kg, the reactivation was over 50%. After exposure to VX, pralidoxime, given in doses of 2.5–25 mg/kg from 0.5 to 24 hours reactivated more than 50% of the inhibited enzyme.

Normally, 2-PAM is given intravenously in a 1–2-g loading doses (in 250 mL of normal saline or D_5W) after exposure, over 5–10 minutes, for a 70 kg person. The U.S. Armed Forces issue an autoinjector containing 600 mg of pralidoxime with 2 mg of atropine for intramuscular self-administration (Mark I autoinjector, Bethesda, Maryland). A total of three autoinjector syringes are issued to each person. This autoinjector is not recommended for children under 10 years of age. The recommended dose of pralidoxime for nerve agent exposure is variable, depending on the route of exposure and the severity of the poisoning. The current U.S. Surgeon General recommendation for 2-PAM is a maximum single dosage of 30 mg/kg or 2 g. Higher doses, for example, (4 g) may be necessary in severe cases. Sidell has suggested 2-PAM can be given up to a maximum cumulative dose of 2.5 g over 1–1.5 hours with additional doses repeated one or two times, every 60–90 minutes. Data on administration of 2-PAM to children are limited. One suggested routine for pediatric victims is to begin with a dose of 15–20 mg/kg given by slow intravenous infusion. 2-PAM is rapidly excreted unchanged in the urine, with 80–90% of an intramuscular or intravenous dose excreted within 3 hours.

A continuous IV infusion of pralidoxime of 500 mg/h (5–10 mg/kg/h in pediatric patients) has been utilized successfully for organophosphate insecticide poisoning and should be given after the loading dose for at least 24 hours in patients exhibiting moderate to severe nerve agent intoxication. The maximum daily infusion dose is 12 g in adults. Criteria to terminate a continuous pralidoxime infusion include resolution of signs and symptoms of intoxication and stabilization of cholinesterase levels. Once these criteria are met, the pralidoxime continuous infusion can be terminated. However, immediately prior to its termination, obtain cholinesterase levels. If the patient's signs and symptoms of intoxication recur, rebolus with pralidoxime, and restart the continuous IV infusion for 24 hours. If the patient's signs and symptoms do not recur, recheck the cholinesterase levels 6 hours after termination of the continuous pralidoxime infusion. If the patient does not exhibit any reoccurrence of signs and symptoms by 6 hours and the patient's red blood cell or plasma cholinesterase level is within 10% and 20% respectively, of the level obtained 6 hours previously, then the therapeutic endpoint is reached and further pralidoxime is unnecessary. It should be noted that cholinesterase levels display significant intraindividual variability with RBC and plasma cholinesterase levels varying 10% and 20% respectively, from one blood draw to the next in a given individual without any organophosphate toxicity.

In case of true cholinergic crisis, no side effects are expected from 2-PAM administration. When pralidoxime is given to healthy adults without nerve agent toxicity, it can cause brief effects such as dizziness and blurred vision. Hypertension is the side effect of greatest concern. Hypertension can occur with normal doses and recommended infusion rates. At doses of 45 mg/kg, systolic pressures can increase by over 90 mm Hg and diastolic pressures can increase by 30 mm Hg. These elevations can persist for several hours. Increasing the infusion time to 30–40 minutes can minimize this potential side effect. Phentolamine, 5 mg IV in adults, has been used to reduce excessive elevation of blood pressure in adults.

Oximes other than pralidoxime have been utilized. Obidoxime chloride (CAS# 7683-36-5 or 114-90-9) is a quaternary oxime used primarily in Europe for organophosphate poisoning; it appears that it may be useful for sarin or tabun exposure. In addition to its primary antidotal property of reactivating cholinesterase, it also exhibits weak anticholinergic

activity. Its half-life is about 2 hours. The adult dose is 250 mg given by slow intravenous administration. This dose may be repeated up to two times at 2-hour intervals, for a maximum daily dose of 750 mg. A 5-day course can be considered for severe exposure. Autoinjectors of atropine and obidoxime (220 mg) have been developed by the Dutch military. A continuous infusion of about 0.5 mg/kg/h up to a maximum dose of 750 mg daily has also been used. Pediatric dosing is 4–8 mg/kg, not to exceed 250 mg per dose. Side effects include nausea, vomiting, diarrhea, paresthesia, transient elevation of hepatic transaminases, and tachycardia (at doses exceeding 5 mg/kg). HI-6 is an investigational oxime (CAS# 34433-31-3) which is also known as asozime chloride. The usual dosage is 500 mg IM 4 times daily to a total dose of 4–14 g. Intramuscular absorption half-life is 7–8 minutes in humans. HI-6 appears to be particularly effective (in rodent studies) for VX, soman, or GF toxicity while obidoxime appears to be less useful for GF toxicity. Trimedoxime (TMB-4 or dioxime) is an investigational oxime given in doses of 125–250 mg to treat tabun exposure.

Other Therapeutic Modalities

Nebulized ipratropium bromide can be used as adjunctive therapy in treating nerve gas bronchospasm. Benzodiazepines are useful in controlling seizures. Diazepam (10 mg IV in adults or 0.2–0.4 mg/kg in pediatric patients) should be given to individuals with severe exposure to prevent seizures. A diazepam autoinjector containing 10 mg of diazepam in 2 mL of fluid is to be administered after 3 Mark I autoinjectors have been utilized. It should be noted that intramuscular absorption of diazepam may be erratic. Hemodiafiltration (4-hour tenure) followed by hemoperfusion has been used successfully in one patient exposed to sarin after the Tokyo subway attack who was resistant to pharmacologic therapy. Biphasic extrathoracic cuirass ventilation may be an effective tool in providing on-scene noninvasive respiratory support.

It appears that there may be utility in utilizing surfactant, N-acetylcysteine, or dexamethasone when combined with atropine to inhibit mucous secretions due to pulmonary toxicity from VX, although this has not been extensively studied.

Disposition

Delayed sequelae are unlikely to develop in asymptomatic individuals exposed to nerve agents by inhalation. Dermally exposed individuals should be observed for at least 18 hours. Individuals exhibiting only miosis can then be safely discharged.

Pre-Exposure Prophylaxis

Pyridostigmine bromide was used by soldiers during Operation Desert Storm, for pretreatment of anticipated nerve agent exposure. It has been suggested that use of this drug, in combination with atropine and pralidoxime chloride can increase survival following exposure to nerve agents versus atropine and pralidoxime therapy alone. The dosage regimen was 30 mg orally every 8 hours, for up to 7 days. About half of the military personnel noted mild gastrointestinal symptoms (increased flatus, abdominal cramps, and soft stools). Of the 41,650 soldiers taking pyridostigmine bromide, the drug was discontinued in 28 (0.07%) soldiers due to adverse effects (exacerbation of asthma, hypertension, allergic reactions, and intolerable gastrointestinal complaints).

A dermal topical protective agent containing a 50:50 mixture of perfluoroalkylpolyether and polytetrafluoroethylene has been utilized by military personnel wearing mission-oriented protective posture (MOPP) gear, when chemical warfare is deemed possible. Known as "Serpacwa" (skin exposure reduction paste against chemical warfare agents) it is manufactured for the U.S. Army by McKesson Bioservices. It is applied to the skin until a barely visible white film layer is present. Prior to its application, a dry towel should be used to remove perspiration, insect repellants, camouflage paint, or dirt, from the skin. Animal studies have demonstrated decreased toxicity of sulfur mustard, VX, soman, T-2 mycotoxins, and CS (a lacrimator). Serpacwa's duration of action has not been evaluated for more than 6 hours. Its major side effect is an occasional, mild flu-like syndrome. There is no systemic absorption through intact skin, but it has not been studied in pediatric patients. Standard decontamination techniques should still occur after a nerve agent or other chemical agent exposure.

Forensic

Cholinesterase activity in postmortem analysis can be assayed for up to 1 week after death. Bodies contaminated with nerve agents should be washed with an alkaline solution. Prosectors should wear self contained breathing appiratus.

Suggested Reading

Abraham RB, Weinbroun AA. Resuscitative challenges in nerve agent poisoning. *J Emerg Med.* 2003;10:169–175.

Barr JR, Driskell WJ, Aston LS, et al. Quantitation of metabolites of nerve agents sarin, soman, cyclohexyl sarin, VX and russian VX in human urine using isotope-dilation gas chromatography—tandem mass spectrometry. *J Anal Tox.* 2004;28:372–378.

Eyer F, Huberkorn M, Kelgenhauer, et al. Toxicity of parathion, cholinesterase status, and neuromuscular function during antidotal therapy in a fatal case of parathion poisoning. *J Toxicol Clin Tox.* 2001;39(3):318.

Gur I, Bar-Xishay E, Ben-Abraham R. Biphasic extrathoracic cuirass ventilation for resuscitation. *Am J Emerg Med.* 2005;23:488–491.

Jortiani SA, Snyder JW, Valdes R Jr. The role of the clinical laboratory in managing chemical or biological in terrorism. *Clin Chem.* 2000;46:1883–1893.

Kassa J., Kuca K., Bartosova L., Kunesova G. The development of new structural analogues of oximes for the antidotal treatment of poisoning by nerve agents and the comparison of their reactivating and the therapeutic efficacy with currently available oximes *Currr Org Chem* 2007.11:267–283.

Keller JR, Hurst CG, Dunn MA. Pyridostigmine used as a nerve agent pretreatment under wartime conditions. *JAMA.* 1991;266:693–695.

Leikin JB, Thomas RH, Walter FG, et al. A review of nerve agent exposure for the critical care physician. *Crit Care Med.* 2002;30:2346–2354.

Liu DK, Wannemacher RW, Snider TH, et al. Efficacy of the topical skin protectant in advanced development. *J Appl Toxicol.* 1999;19 (suppl):541–545.

Mars TC. The roles of diazepam in the treatment of nerve agent poisoning in a civilian population. *Toxicol Rev.* 2004;23(3):145–157.

Niven AS, Roop SA. Inhalation exposure to nerve agents. *Respir Care Clin N Am.* 2004;10(1):59–74.

Okumura T, Takasu N, Ishimatsu S, et al. Report on 640 victims of the Tokyo subway sarin attack. *Ann Emerg Med.* 1996;28:129–135.

Quail M. T, Shannon MW. Pralidoxime safety and toxicity in children. *Prehosp Emerg Care* 2007:11:36–41.

Thierman H, Worek F, Szinicz L, et al. Principles of oxime treatment and its limitations: assessment of oxime effectiveness. *J Toxicol Clin Tox.* 2001;39:256.

Thomas RG. Chemoterrorism: nerve agents. Walter FB, Klein R, Thomas RG: *Advanced Hazmat Life Support Provider Manual.* 3rd ed, Tucson, AZ: Arizona Board of Regents; 2003:295–314.

Waeckerle JF, Seamans S, Whiteside M, et al. Executive summary: developing objectives, content, and competencies for the training of emergency medical technicians, emergency nurses to care for casualties resulting from nuclear, biological, or chemical (NBC) incidents. *Ann Emerg Med.* 2001;37:587–601.

Worek F, Aurbek N, Koller M et al: Kinetic Analysis of Reactivation and Aging of Human Acetylcholinesterase Inhibited by Different phosphoramidates *Biochem Pharmacol* 2007 June 1; 73(u): 1807–17.

Worek, F, Eyer P., Aurbek, N et al. Recent advances in evaluation of oxime efficacy in nerve agent poisoning by in vitro analysis. *Toxical Appl Pharmacol.* 2007:219:226–234.

29

BLISTER AGENTS

Kimberly A. Barker and Christina Hantsch Bardsley

BLISTER AGENTS

- Mustard exposure produces rapid tissue damage; however, development of actual signs and symptoms, including pain, does not occur until after a latent period.
- There is no antidote for mustard. The focus of treatment after mustard exposure is supportive measures.
- Lewisite exposure produces immediate burning sensation.
- British Anti-Lewisite (BAL) is the antidote for lewisite poisoning.
- None of the blister agents present a significant risk to health-care workers caring for exposed patients.

INTRODUCTION

Blister agents, or vesicants, are chemical agents that produce blisters or vesicles on contact with skin. The three most likely to be encountered in a chemical threat include mustard, lewisite, and phosgene oxime. Each of these agents produces a distinct clinical presentation that is outlined in Table 29-1. Bis-(2-chlorethyl) sulfide is the agent commonly referred to as mustard. Other mustard forms, specifically nitrogen mustards, exist but are not considered chemical agent threats as they have not been found suitable for weaponization. The discussion of mustard in this chapter will focus on sulfur mustard. Originally synthesized in the 1800s, mustard was used in the 1930s during World War I as well as other times including by Iraq in the 1980s during the Iran-Iraq war and later against the Kurds. Lewisite, B-chlorovinyldichloroarsine, was first synthesized during World War I but the history of its use on the battlefield is less clear. Although categorized by the United States military as a vesicant, phosgene oxime or dichloroformoxime is not a true vesicant since

exposure to it does not result in fluid-filled blisters. Rather, typical skin lesions after phosgene oxime are urticarial. There are no verified reports of the use of this agent in military conflicts.

MUSTARD

Pathophysiology

Mustard is an oily liquid with a garlic or mustard-like odor. The military designation for mustard is "H" or "HD." While mustard is recognized as an alkylating agent causing immediate damage to cellular DNA, questions still remain regarding its full mechanism of action. Mustard is recognized to have cholinergic action at both muscarinic and nicotinic receptors. Other possible mechanisms postulated include cellular depletion of glutathione and free radical-induced cellular damage.

Mustard induces separation of the epidermis (upper layer of skin) from the dermis (lower layer of skin). When these two layers separate, the space between becomes a blister. Associated DNA damage prolongs the healing process. Due to biochemical breakdown of the mustard, the fluid-filled blisters do not actually contain mustard.

Cellular level damage also occurs with pulmonary and ocular exposure but blisters do not form in these organ systems. The eye is the most sensitive organ to mustard exposure. Rather than blisters, injury including irritation and redness after minimal exposure to severe corneal destruction and loss of the eye with extensive exposure can occur. Pulmonary exposure produces progressive necrosis of the upper and then lower airway mucosa. Resultant inflammation and pseudomembrane formation may lead to airway obstruction. Mustard exposure may also induce laryngospasm.

BLISTER AGENTS

Agent	Onset of Symptoms	Presentation
Mustard gas	3–6 hours for mild to moderate exposures	Mild exposures may develop erythema, ocular irritation and cough in first 3–12 hours
	Severe ocular exposures may have symptoms within the first 2 hours	Moderate and severe exposures will develop vesications >12 hours after exposure
Lewisite	Seconds to minutes	Erythema and possibly respiratory irritation initially, blisters develop several hours later
Phosgene oxime	Immediate	Extreme pain, dermal necrosis, respiratory irritation, dimmed vision, and corneal lesions

Confirming the Threat

While exposure to mustard produces immediate tissue damage, the onset of clinical effects is delayed for several hours. Because of this delay mustard exposure may not be recognized for several hours. Victims exposed to mustard gas may report a distinctive odor, likened to mustard, garlic, onions, leeks, or horseradish. However, this odor is not always reported due to faintness and/or olfactory accommodation. Mustard is an oily liquid with a low volatility. In cool weather it produces little vapor as its freezing point is 57°F. This property makes it an undesirable chemical for dispersal in wintertime or from airplanes. However, liquid agent dispersed at night in cooler temperatures will vaporize as the day warms. In World War I, mustard attacks were frequently conducted by these means. To more effectively use mustard in colder weather, it may be mixed with another substance and thereby lower its freezing point.

Mustard detection can be done with certain military testing devices. Mustard vapor at ≥ 0.1 mg/m^3 will be identified by a chemical agent monitor (CAM.) Mustard liquid will turn M8 paper ketchup red. Mustard liquid will also change M9 paper to pink, red, or purple. These reactions are not specific to mustard liquid as chemical nerve agents and other vesicants will produce the same effect.

Personal Protective Equipment and Decontamination

Decontamination of skin and eyes following mustard exposure is only fully effective if performed within 1–2 minutes of exposure. However all victims with possible exposure should have decontamination performed as soon as possible even if it is after this time frame. Later decontamination may still prevent ongoing damage or spread of the agent. Mustard quickly penetrates cloth but it also penetrates leather and wood with time. Unless the skin has been occluded, any nonabsorbed mustard quickly evaporates from skin. Decontamination with copious amounts of water is recommended for dermal and ocular exposure. Patients should be quickly removed from the area to decrease respiratory exposure. Personal protective equipment (PPE) for personnel going into an area with possible mustard includes pressure demand self-contained breathing apparatus (SCBA). Charcoal in protective respiratory masks and chemical protective overgarments will absorb mustard. In addition, butyl rubber in chemical protective gloves and boots is impermeable to mustard.

Resources

Access to sources of water for decontamination and biohazard bags for clothing items will be needed. If no biohazard bags are available for clothing, double bagging is recommended. If there are other possible injuries involved from a secondary source, gurneys and backboards should be of a type that can be decontaminated for any possible chemical exposure. A chemical resuscitation device, a bag valve mask equipped with a chemical agent canister, may be used for any patients in immediate respiratory distress.

Clinical Manifestations

As noted previously, the tissue damage from mustard occurs immediately but the clinical effects take several hours to manifest. See Table 29-2 as well for information on the onset of symptoms. Skin, eyes, and airways are most commonly involved due to direct contact with mustard. The early effects on these organ systems have already been discussed. Patients with late developing dermal, ocular, or respiratory manifestations are unlikely to have had a significant exposure. Other potential systems affected include the

TABLE 29-2

MUSTARD GAS EXPOSURE

Time Postexposure	1–2 hours	3–6 hours	4–12 hours	>12 hours
Mild exposure	No symptoms	May develop erythema	• Ocular irritation, lacrimation and burning sensation • Rhinorrhea, sneezing, epistaxis, hoarseness and cough	• Erythema • Worsening hoarseness and cough
Moderate exposure	No symptoms	• Ocular irritation, lacrimation burning sensation, lid edema, and pain • Erythema		Erythema and vesication
Severe exposure	Severe ocular pain and lid edema	• Rhinorrhea, epistaxis, hoarseness, productive cough and mild to severe dyspnea • Erythema		Erythema and vesication

gastrointestinal tract, central nervous system (CNS), and hematologic system. Mild nausea and vomiting, likely due to cholinergic activity of mustard or a nonspecific reaction to the exposure, may develop in the first few hours following exposure but severe gastrointestinal symptoms are uncommon. Late (days after exposure) developing nausea and vomiting are more likely due to generalized cytotoxic effects and damage to the mucosa of the gastrointestinal tract. While CNS effects are usually clinically nonspecific, causalities of mustard gas exposure in military conflicts have reported nonspecific symptoms such as depression, intellectual dullness, and apathy. In animal models, CNS effects occurred following exposure to large amounts of mustard. These effects included hyperexcitability, seizures, and other neurologic manifestations. Lastly, systemic effects of absorbed mustard may include suppression of the hematopoietic system after large exposure.

Patients with moderate to severe exposure may have further effects occur after the first 24 hours. These may include worsening of dermatologic symptoms following severe exposure. While the early erythema may resemble sunburn and be accompanied by pruritus and a burning sensation, small vesicles may develop within this erythematous area. These vesicles will later merge to form larger blisters. These areas may appear similar to second or third-degree thermal burns. The typical blister contains fluid that is initially thin and clear, which then progresses to a yellowish discoloration. This fluid does not contain mustard and is itself not a vesicant or a risk to health-care personnel. Severe lesions have prolonged healing time and take longer to heal than a similar appearing thermal burn. Necrosis and secondary inflammation and infection occur in severe cases. Changes in pigmentation of the skin may also be seen. Vesication is not necessary for these changes

to occur. Initially the skin may have hyperpigmentation with a blanched, or hypopigmentated, area around it. In severe exposures, the respiratory tract may be damaged and bronchitis may occur. This bronchitis is initially noninfectious but bacterial infection may develop 4–6 days postexposure. Most mustard-induced damage to the lungs occurs via inflammation of the airway and tissue immediately surrounding the airway. Death following mustard exposure is most often caused by severe pulmonary damage. In the early postexposure period, likely mechanisms of death are mechanical obstruction or laryngospasm. Deaths in the later postexposure period are caused by pulmonary infection and/or sepsis.

Laboratory Studies

There is no specific laboratory study that can confirm mustard exposure. Patients with significant exposure are at risk for bone marrow suppression. A complete blood count (CBC) should be checked in all patients 3–5 days after exposure. Other laboratory studies needed to assist with supportive care measures should also be obtained.

Referral

All victims exposed to mustard should be decontaminated as soon as possible. Patients with early symptoms of dyspnea or ocular burning and pain are most likely to develop severe manifestations of exposure and should receive priority in transport for further medical care. All other patients should be observed for 6 hours for development of symptoms. Patients who develop mild to moderate symptoms within 6 hours should be observed a minimum of 24 hours postexposure for development of worsening symptoms. While some patients may develop symptoms greater than 6 hours following exposures, these are the patients with mild exposures.

Treatment

There is no antidote for mustard exposure. Treatment involves initial decontamination followed by symptomatic and supportive care. Guidelines similar to those for thermal burn patients including pain control and expectant management for immunosuppression and multiorgan system involvement should be followed. One notable difference from thermal burn patients however, is fluid and electrolyte management. While monitoring and correction of volume and electrolyte status is important, victims of mustard exposure do not have the magnitude of fluid loss that thermal burn patients do.

LEWISITE

Pathophysiology

Lewisite is an oily, colorless liquid reported to smell like geraniums. The military designation for lewisite is "L." The exact mechanism by which lewisite causes cellular damage is unknown. However, since lewisite is an arsenical vesicant, it shares many biochemical mechanisms with other arsenical compounds. Recognized actions of lewisite include loss of protein thiol status, loss of calcium homeostasis, lipid peroxidation, inhibition of pyruvate dehydrogenase complex, loss of ATP, inactivation of carbohydrate metabolism, and cell death. The overall effect of lewisite is increased capillary permeability. In high concentrations, all capillaries of the body are sensitive to damage. Pulmonary capillaries appear to be more readily damaged because of absorption via the respiratory tract and because absorbed lewisite reaches the lungs before the systemic circulation.

Confirming the Threat and What to Expect

As opposed to mustard, lewisite produces immediate symptoms. Dermal exposure produces pain within seconds to minutes. Erythema develops within 15–30 minutes and blisters form over the next few hours. This initial pain and burning allows victims to immediately recognize the exposure. Direct ocular exposure to lewisite liquid produces severe ocular damage and can cause perforation. The ocular effects of lewisite vapor are irritating but less severe than those of mustard exposure. This is in part due to lewisite-induced blepharospasm and immediate irritation, which help to reduce subsequent exposure to the vapor. Lewisite vapors will also produce irritation of other mucous membranes including those of the airway as evidenced by coughing and rhinorrhea.

In addition to the immediate symptoms, victims exposed to lewisite may report a distinctive odor of geraniums.

However, as with mustard exposure, the odor of lewisite is not always reported due to faintness and/or olfactory accommodation.

As with mustard, lewisite detection can be done with certain military testing devices. Lewisite vapor at ≥ 2 mg/m^3 will be identified by a CAM. Lewisite liquid will turn M8 paper ketchup red and M9 paper to pink, red, or purple. As noted previously, these reactions are not specific to lewisite as chemical nerve agents and other vesicants will produce the same effects.

Personal Protective Equipment and Decontamination

All victims with possible lewisite exposure should be decontaminated as soon as possible. Decontamination with copious amounts of water is recommended for dermal and ocular exposure. Patients should be removed from the area as quickly as possible to decrease respiratory exposure. PPE for personnel going into an area with possible lewisite includes pressure demand SCBA. Charcoal in protective respiratory masks and chemical protective overgarments will absorb lewisite. Butyl rubber in chemical protective gloves and boots is broken down by lewisite. The protection level is considered adequate for field concentrations and these PPE items should still be used. Replacement gloves and boots should be obtained after lewisite exposure.

Resources

Immediate availability of water for decontamination and biohazard bags to discard clothing are needed. If biohazard bags are not available, then clothing should be double-bagged for disposal. The chelating agent British Anti-Lewisite (BAL) is a specific antidote developed for treatment of lewisite poisoning. While it is effective if used to decontaminate skin and eyes, currently there are no forms of BAL available for this purpose.

Clinical Manifestations

As opposed to mustard, lewisite produces an immediate, painful burning to exposed skin and mucous membranes. Erythema of the area develops within 30 minutes and blisters start to form within the first few hours following exposure. Initially the blister begins as a small lesion in the center of the erythematous area. Eventually it spreads to include the entire area of erythema. The immediate pain lewisite vapor produces following contact with the eye leads to blepharospasm and prevents exposure to significant amounts of lewisite. However, ocular exposure to even a drop of lewisite can lead to perforation and loss of the eye. The immediate irritant effects are also responsible for limited respiratory exposure as victims will quickly seek protection after exposure. This irritation will lead to rhinorrhea and coughing.

The airway lesions produced are similar to those from mustard. Pulmonary edema and "lewisite shock" may develop following severe exposure. "Lewisite shock" is the result of capillary leak and subsequent hemoconcentration and hypotension. As opposed to mustard, lewisite does not suppress the hematopoietic system.

Laboratory Studies

Urinary arsenic excretion may assist in identifying lewisite exposure. However, the clinical diagnosis of exposure can usually be made without this test and there is no specific laboratory test confirmation. Other laboratory studies needed to assist with supportive care measures should also be obtained.

Referral

All patients who experience initial symptoms of exposure should receive decontamination and be referred for further medical care. Since the optimal treatment of exposure is early use of BAL, health-care facilities should be alerted to incoming patients; so BAL can be administered as soon as possible. Patients in the area of lewisite release that are asymptomatic should be assumed to be nonexposed and no referral is needed.

Treatment

Treatment of lewisite exposure involves initial decontamination followed by symptomatic and supportive care similar to that for mustard exposure. In comparison to similar severity mustard exposure, lewisite-related fluid loss from capillary leak is greater and necessitates closer attention to fluid and electrolyte status. The risk of infectious complications is lower, however, as lewisite does not cause immunosuppression. In addition, a specific antidote, BAL, (dimercaprol), is available for parenteral administration. Although BAL's early use for dermal and ocular exposures has been recommended, there are not topical or ophthalmologic formulations currently available. There is no data on the use of parenteral BAL used directly on the skin or instilled into the eye to either suggest benefit or harm. BAL is in a peanut oil vehicle. Administration to patients with recognized peanut allergies may precipitate an anaphylactoid or anaphylactic response. While no guidelines exist on the treatment of this subpopulation of patients, the pretreatment with H1 and H2 antagonist therapy and epinephrine available at the bedside would be prudent. The recommended dose of BAL is 3 mg/kg administered as a deep intramuscular (IM) injection. Doses should be repeated every 4 hours for 2 days, then every 6 hours on the third day, and every 12 hours for up to 10 days. Due to administration as a deep IM injection, BAL injections are very painful. Other side effects include tachycardia, hypertension, nausea and vomiting, headache, burning sensation

of the lips, and feeling of chest constriction. These are typically dose-related and subside within 30–60 minutes after administration. The use of 2,3-dimercaptosuccinic acid (DMSA) as an effective chelator of arsenic has been demonstrated in animal studies. It has the benefit of being an oral agent and having less potential side effects than BAL. However use of DMSA in lewisite toxicity has not been studied. A compound related to DMSA, 2,3-dimercapto-1-propanesulfonic acid (DMPS) has been shown to protect rabbits exposed to lewisite. It may be administered intravenously or orally. Side effects of DMPS are typically rate related and include hypotension, weakness, dizziness, and nausea following too rapid of an injection. DMPS is not FDA approved, but is available in the United States at some compounding pharmacies.

PHOSGENE OXIME

Pathophysiology

Pure phosgene oxime is a colorless, crystalline solid. The military designation is "CX." The solid material and the vapors produced by it cause symptoms after exposure. Phosgene oxime is not a true vesicant because it does not produce fluid-filled blisters. It is an urticant or nettle agent because its lesions can resemble nettle stings. The mechanism of action is unknown. The lesions produced are similar to those produced by acids; it is considered a corrosive type agent. It is believed to cause injury either by the necrotizing action of the chlorine, the direct effect of the oxime, or the direct effect of the carbonyl group. The direct injury involves enzyme activation, cell death, corrosive injury, and rapid local destruction of tissue.

Confirming the Threat and What to Expect

As with lewisite, there is immediate pain and burning following exposure to phosgene oxime. It causes more severe tissue damage than other vesicants. No other agent produces such immediate profound pain followed by rapid necrosis.

Phosgene oxime may have a pepperish or pungent odor, however, as with other vesicants, faintness of the odor and/or olfactory accommodation makes this an unreliable indicator of exposure. Military detection devices including a CAM as well as M8 and M9 paper are also unreliable for detection of phosgene oxime.

Personal Protective Equipment and Decontamination

Decontamination principles after phosgene oxime exposure are similar to those of other vesicants. The immediate tissue damage caused by this chemical agent makes rapid decontamination essential.

PPE for personnel going into an area with possible phosgene oxime includes pressure demand SCBA. Charcoal in protective respiratory masks and chemical protective overgarments will adsorb phosgene oxime. As with lewisite, the butyl rubber in chemical protective gloves and boots is broken down by phosgene oxime but the protection level is considered adequate for field concentrations and these PPE items should still be used. Replacement gloves and boots should be obtained after phosgene oxime exposure.

Resources

Decontamination materials as discussed with mustard and lewisite are needed for management of phosgene oxime exposure victims. There is no specific antidote to be obtained or prepared in anticipation of a patient with phosgene oxime exposure.

Clinical Manifestations

Limited information is available about the effects of phosgene oxime. It is known to cause extensive tissue damage including injury primarily to the skin, eyes, and lungs. The main characteristic of exposure to phosgene oxime is extreme pain that is rapid onset and prolonged. Skin necrosis occurs shortly after dermal contact. Ocular exposure results in immediate irritation, dimming of vision, and corneal lesions. Respiratory symptoms include irritation and pain in upper airways. Pulmonary edema may occur after significant exposure.

Laboratory Studies

There are no specific laboratory studies to confirm exposure to phosgene oxime. There is no hematologic toxicity associated with phosgene oxime. Laboratory studies needed to assist with supportive care measures should be obtained.

Referral

All patients with symptoms following exposure should be referred to a health-care facility. Patients in the area of chemical release who have no early symptoms do not require referral.

Treatment

There is no antidote for phosgene oxime. As with mustard exposure, treatment includes rapid decontamination followed by symptomatic and supportive care. Necrotic lesions should be kept clean to avoid infection.

SUMMARY

Blister agents, or vesicants, are chemical agents that produce blisters or vesicles on contact with skin. The three most likely to be encountered in a chemical threat include mustard, lewisite, and phosgene oxime. Exposure to any of these vesicants produces rapid onset of tissue damage, particularly of the skin, eyes, and airway. Signs and symptoms develop rapidly after lewisite or phosgene oxime exposure but are associated with a latent period after mustard exposure. Characteristic skin lesions are blisters after mustard or lewisite exposure, and urticaria and necrosis after phosgene oxime exposure.

Mustard and possibly other vesicants have been used previously in military situations. Stockpiles currently maintained by other countries are believed to contain vesicants including in particular mustard and lewisite. Healthcare professionals need to be familiar with vesicants and the management of victims of exposure to these agents as part of their emergency preparedness procedures.

Suggested Reading

Anderson DR, Holmes WW, Lee RB, et al. Sulfur mustard-induced neutropenia: treatment with granulocyte colony-stimulating factor. *Mil Med.* 2006;171(5):448–453.

Beheshti J, Mark EJ, Akbaei HM, et al. Mustard lung secrets: long term clinicopathological study following mustard gas exposure. *Pathol Res Pract.* 2006;202(10):739–744.

Cowan FM, Broomfield CA, Lenz DE, et al. Putative role of proteolysis and inflammatory response in the toxicity of nerve and blister chemical warfare agents: implications for multi-threat medical countermeasures. *J Appl Toxicol.* 2003;23: 177–186.

Jortani SA, Snyder JW, Valdes R. The role of the clinical laboratory in managing chemical or biological terrorism. *Clin Chem.* 2000;46(12):1883–1893.

Le HQ, Knudsen SJ. Exposure to a first world war blistering agent. *Emerg Med.* 2006;J23:296–299.

Rice P. Sulfur mustard injuries of the skin: pathophysiology and management. *Toxicol Rev.* 2003;22(2):111–118.

Sidell FR, Urbanetti JS. Vesicants. In: Sidell, Takafuji ET, Franz DR, eds. Textbook of Military Medicine, Part I, Warfare, Weaponry, and the Casualty. Washington DC, Office of the Surgeon General, Walter Reed Army Medical Center, 1997.

Vilensky JA, Redman K. British Anti-Lewisite (Dimercaprol): an amazing history. *Ann Emerg Med.* 2003;41(3):378–383.

30

CHEMICAL ASPHYXIANTS

Brandon K. Wills and Mark B. Mycyk

S T A T   F A C T S

CHEMICAL ASPHYXIANTS

- Cyanide, hydrogen sulfide, and sodium azide interrupt cellular respiration and can be rapidly fatal.
- Clinical manifestations can include rapid unconsciousness and severe metabolic acidosis.
- Preentry considerations for chemical asphyxiants include removal of patients from exposure, decontamination, and institution of supportive care.
- Hydroxocobalamin or the cyanide antidote kit (amyl nitrite, sodium nitrite, sodium thiosulfate) are essential antidotes and should be administered early in suspected exposures.
- Our health-care system would be unprepared to manage a cyanide mass casualty event due to inadequate hospital supplies of the antidote kit.
- Hydroxocobalamin has been successfully used as a cyanide antidote in France and was recently approved for use in the United States.

INTRODUCTION

The cellular asphyxiants cyanide, hydrogen sulfide, and sodium azide are potential chemical terrorism agents due to their substantial lethality at relatively low doses. Despite their considerable toxicity, cellular asphyxiants are unlikely to be effective if dispersed as a gas due to difficulty achieving a lethal concentration in open environments. They could potentially be employed by dispersal in closed environments, contaminating foodstuffs, or targeting industrial areas, which utilize these agents. Cyanide is well-known for its use in capital punishment, Nazi concentration camps and for mass suicide. Several reported events have raised the level of concern for the utilization of cyanide for the purpose of chemical terrorism. Canisters containing cyanide were discovered in the Chicago subway system and have been confiscated during raids of suspected domestic terrorists. There is some suggestion that the 1993 Trade Center attack utilized explosives containing cyanide. Cyanide was unsuccessfully used in Tokyo subways several weeks after the initial sarin attack. In a recent analysis of 161 suspicious powders submitted during the post-9/11 anthrax scare, four samples contained cyanide. Fortunately, successful use of cellular asphyxiants for the purpose of chemical warfare remains absent.

PATHOPHYSIOLOGY AND PROPERTIES OF EXPOSURE

Pathophysiology

The cellular asphyxiants all share a common mechanism and therefore have similar clinical and pathophysiologic effects. Cyanide has a high affinity for ferric iron (Fe^{3+}) and binds reversibly to cytochrome aa3 in the mitochondrial electron transport chain. Once bound, electron transport is arrested preventing utilization of oxygen and cellular respiration. Adenosine triphosphate (ATP) production becomes dependent on nonoxidative metabolism, resulting in profound lactic acidosis. Organs with large metabolic demands (e.g., central nervous system and myocardium) will manifest early and sustain more significant toxicity.

Properties of Exposure

Cyanide

Hydrogen cyanide (HCN) and cyanide salts are used in many industries including chemical production, metal extraction, and electroplating. HCN may also be liberated with combustion of organic compounds or formed by bioconversion of ingested cyanogenic compounds such as amygdalin (seeds from most *Prunus* species) or nitriles (e.g., acrylonitrile, acetonitrile). Exposure could be from inhalation of gas or ingestion of a solid or liquid. HCN gas does have irritant properties but lacks sufficient warning properties. Concentrations greater than 90 ppm can be fatal. Cyanide salts are solids at room temperature and could be toxic from oral ingestion, large dermal exposures, or liberation of HCN gas when mixed with acidic or aqueous liquids.

Cyanogen Chloride

Cyanogen chloride (ClCN) is a gas that was used by the French during World War I for chemical warfare. Like HCN, cyanogen chloride is also a respiratory irritant but has moderate solubility and can cause delayed pulmonary injury similar to phosgene. Cyanide toxicity can also occur with concentrated exposures.

Hydrogen Sulfide

Hydrogen sulfide (H_2S) can be formed by fermentation of organic material and is associated with a vast number of industrial processes. It is a gas under normal conditions, can oxidize metals, and is flammable. Similar to cyanide, hydrogen sulfide can produce rapid unconsciousness and death due to its effects on cellular respiration.

Sodium Azide

Sodium azide (NaN_3) is a chemical used in many industries and is a propellant in automobile airbags. Azide salts can form hydrazoic gas when exposed to aqueous or acidic solutions. Like the other cellular asphyxiants, sodium azide interrupts cellular respiration; however, there is some suggestion that azides can form cyanide in vivo.

CONFIRMING THE THREAT AND WHAT TO EXPECT

Confirmation of cyanide exposure will likely be made clinically. If a suspicious substance is identified without patient exposure, confirmation of cyanide can be performed with gas chromatography/mass spectroscopy (GCMS) or Fourier transform infrared spectroscopy (FTIR). A history of exposed patients experiencing nonspecific initial symptoms followed by rapid "knockdown" or collapse is highly suggestive of a cellular asphyxiant. The utility of laboratory testing is discussed under laboratory studies.

PERSONAL PROTECTIVE EQUIPMENT/DECONTAMINATION

Personal protective equipment (PPE) for first responders and hospital-based providers will depend on the phase of the cellular asphyxiant (Table 30-1). Patients exposed via ingestion of contaminated foodstuffs will not present a substantial risk to the provider. It would be prudent to refrain from mouth-to-mouth resuscitation and exercise caution when performing endotracheal intubation, which could result in "off-gassing" or emesis and subsequent exposure to providers. The National Institute for Occupational Safety and Health PPE recommendations for on-site responders are listed in

TABLE 30-1

CHEMICAL PROPERTIES AND RECOMMENDED PERSONAL PROTECTIVE EQUIPMENT FOR CELLULAR ASPHYXIANTS

Compound	Chemical Formula	CAS#	Physical State (BP)	Personal Protective Equipment (PPE)
Cyanogen chloride	ClCN	506-77-4	Gas or compressed liquid (13.8°C)	Inhalation: SCBA, CBRN, or APR Skin: Butyl rubber gloves. Teflon, Responder, or Tychem protective clothing Eyes: Eye protection in combination with breathing protection
Cyanide salts	KCN NaCN	151-50-8 143-33-9	Solid (1625°C) Solid (1496°C)	Inhalation: Above, prevent dispersion of dust
Hydrogen cyanide	HCN	74-90-8	Gas or liquid (26°C) *Flammable*	Inhalation: Above or gas mask with HCN canister
Hydrogen sulfide	H_2S	7783-06-4	Gas (−60.6°C) *Flammable*	Above
Sodium azide	NaN_3	26628-22-8	Solid (decomposes)	Above

APR—air-purifying respirator; CBRN—chemical, biological, radiological, nuclear; SCBA—self-contained breathing apparatus
Source: From NIOSH Emergency Response Card. The Centers for Disease Control and Prevention, National Institute for Occupational Safety and Health. Available at: http://www.bt.cdc.gov/agent Accessed January 2006.

Table 30-1. Decontamination for gas exposures generally only requires removal of patients from the source and removing clothing. For dermal exposures to solid or liquid forms, removal of clothing and copious irrigation is necessary. Gastrointestinal decontamination for ingested cyanide compounds is unlikely to prevent toxicity; however, activated charcoal could be considered for those who are minimally symptomatic.

RESOURCES NEEDED BEFORE THE FIRST PATIENT APPEARS, WHEN MASSES APPEAR

Hospitals are inadequately prepared for a successful cyanide terrorist attack. Receiving hospitals would need to be prepared to manage critically ill patients in need on intensive supportive care including mechanical ventilation and vasopressors. It is doubtful that a large number of patients would require antidotal therapy given that many patients would expire at the scene while those who are alert and minimally symptomatic are unlikely to require them. Most centers however, stock limited quantities of the cyanide antidote kit.

CLINICAL MANIFESTATIONS/DIFFERENTIAL DIAGNOSIS

The clinical presentation will vary depending on dose and exposure type. Inhalational exposures from a concentrated (indoor) source will result in rapid unconsciousness and death within minutes of exposure. Symptoms from oral exposures may begin up to 30 minutes after ingestion or several hours for precursors that require metabolic conversion to cyanide (e.g., acetonitrile, amygdalin). Initial symptoms from a mild to moderate exposure are nonspecific and can include dyspnea, dizziness, headache, nausea, anxiety, and altered mental status. Due to its irritant properties, exposures to cyanogen chloride can include lacrimation, rhinorrhea, and bronchorrhea, which could be potentially confused with organophosphate or nerve agent exposure. Vital sign abnormalities can be variable with hypertension and tachycardia seen initially, followed by hypotension and bradycardia or tachycardia, and arrhythmias. More severe exposures may produce seizures, apnea, and cardiovascular collapse. Physical examination findings are generally not helpful to distinguish cyanide from other agents. Abnormally elevated oxygen content of venous blood may manifest as bright red skin or retinal veins on funduscopy. Cyanosis is generally not observed unless due to apnea and cardiovascular collapse. The characteristic smell of bitter almonds may be detected in some cases, but the ability to detect this is a genetically determined trait not possessed by every examiner. Differential diagnosis for industrial or potential chemical terrorism agents causing rapid unconsciousness are listed in Table 30-2.

TABLE 30-2

DIFFERENTIAL DIAGNOSIS FOR AGENTS, WHICH CAN CAUSE RAPID UNCONSCIOUSNESS

Simple asphyxiants*
Carbon dioxide
Methane
Cellular asphyxiants
Carbon monoxide
Cyanide
Hydrogen sulfide
Sodium azide
Other agents
Nerve agents
Inhalational anesthetics
Arsine

*Any gas that displaces atmospheric oxygen could potentially be a simple asphyxiant.

LABORATORY STUDIES

Obtaining whole blood cyanide concentrations is possible but is usually performed at reference laboratories and would not be available for medical decision-making. Plasma thiocyanate levels may confirm exposures but will likely take several hours to obtain. For significant exposures, the hallmark finding is a profound lactic acidosis. Despite having a large differential diagnosis for lactic acidosis, in the right clinical setting (i.e., a large number of individuals with a similar clinical presentation), a plasma lactate level greater than 8 mmol/L may be suggestive of cyanide toxicity.

While oxygen is not being adequately utilized for cellular respiration, a relative increase in central mixed venous oxygen saturation may be observed. A decreased arterial-venous oxygen difference (AO_2-VO_2) is observed when comparing arterial and venous blood gas determinations, resulting in apparent "arteriolization" of venous blood. The upper limits of normal for venous oxygen saturation obtained from the superior vena cava and pulmonary artery are 87% and 84% respectively. With critical illness, saturations can be lower. Obtaining true mixed venous blood from the pulmonary artery is not realistic in most cases however, a peripheral venous saturation above 90% should be considered abnormal. Because of patient variation in cardiac output, arterial oxygen content, and hemoglobin level, venous saturations less than 90% unfortunately cannot "rule out" cyanide toxicity. Cyanide or thiocyanate levels will not be available to guide decision-making and antidote utilization in the event of cyanide poisoning. Obtaining a simultaneous ABG and VBG could potentially provide the most useful data in the acute setting because these tests have a rapid turnaround time and are available in every hospital.

Numerous nonspecific electrocardiographic changes may occur in cyanide toxicity. Sinus bradycardia may be noted early or may be observed as a preterminal event. Later, sinus tachycardia may be seen, as well as atrial fibrillation, atrioventricular block, ventricular ectopy, and ventricular dysrhythmias. A shortened QT segment or T waves originating high on the R wave may be seen.

EARLY INTERVENTIONS

Initial treatment following decontamination should be focused on maintaining airway patency, providing positive-pressure ventilation with 100% oxygen, and establishing intravenous access and circulatory support with crystalloids and vasopressors. Severe metabolic acidosis may be treated with bolus administration of sodium bicarbonate; however, its efficacy in altering clinical outcome in cases of cyanide poisoning is not known. Utilization of antidotes is discussed under treatment.

WHO TO REFER AND WHEN

Asymptomatic patients exposed to a gas may be selectively referred to a health-care facility. Symptomatic individuals require immediate evaluation. Patients who have ingested contaminated food or water supplies should be referred for hospital evaluation.

TOXICOKINETICS

HCN gas is rapidly absorbed in the lungs and may cause profound toxicity within seconds. Ingested cyanide salts, such as sodium or potassium cyanide, are also rapidly absorbed across the gastric mucosa and may result in toxicity within minutes. Ingestion of amygdalin and other cyanogenic glycosides require hydrolysis to release cyanide, so toxicity may be delayed up to several hours after ingestion. Acetonitrile and acrylonitrile release cyanide through oxidative metabolism by the hepatic cytochrome P_{450} system, thus delaying clinical manifestations of toxicity for 2–6 hours from the time of ingestion. [Blood cyanide concentrates in the erythrocytes, with an RBC:plasma ratio of 100:1]. Sixty percent of plasma cyanide is protein-bound.

Cyanide elimination occurs by four separate routes. The widely distributed endogenous enzyme rhodanese (sulfurtransferase), in the presence of thiosulfate, converts cyanide to nontoxic thiocyanate. This accounts for the majority (80%) of elimination with thiosulfate availability being the rate-limiting factor. Some cyanide is converted in the presence of hydroxocobalamin (vitamin B_{12a}) to cyanocobalamin (vitamin B_{12}), which is also nontoxic. Clinically insignificant amounts of cyanide are excreted in expired air and in sweat. The reported elimination half-life in humans is variable, ranging from 20 minutes to 1 hour in nonlethal exposures, to a mean of 3 hours in fire victims who had been treated with antidotes. Thiocyanate elimination half-life in humans with normal renal function is 2.5 days.

TREATMENT

In addition to intensive supportive measures, early administration of a cyanide antidote is essential. The Taylor antidote package contains amyl nitrite for inhalation, sodium nitrite, and sodium thiosulfate (Table 30-3). Since cyanide has an affinity for ferric iron (Fe^{3+}), induction of methemoglobin with nitrites will reduce the amount of cyanide bound to cytochrome aa3. Nitrites appear to have beneficial effects not exclusive to the induction of methemoglobin. Other beneficial mechanisms may be due to augmentation of blood flow to viscera and increasing endothelial detoxification of cyanide. Nitrites may also be effective therapy for hydrogen sulfide but do not appear to be helpful for sodium azide. Adverse effects of nitrites include hypotension and the potential for markedly high methemoglobin levels. Although dose response for nitrites can be erratic, high methemoglobin levels are not common. One series of smoke inhalation patients treated with sodium nitrite demonstrated methemoglobin levels between 8% and 13%. Methylene blue is relatively contraindicated for the treatment of markedly elevated methemoglobin concentrations due to the theoretic risk of liberating free cyanide.

TABLE 30-3

CYANIDE ANTIDOTES

Antidote	Dose
Cyanide antidote package[*] (Taylor pharmaceuticals)	
Amyl nitrite (0.3 mL ampules for inhalation)	Crush and inhale for a 15–30-second and on/off cycle
Sodium nitrite (3% for injection, 10 mL)	10 mL (300 mg) IV over 2–4 minutes
	Pediatric dose: 0.33 mL/Kg for a hemoglobin of 12g/dL[†]
Sodium thiosulfate (25% for injection, 50 mL)	50 mL (12.5 g) IV
	Pediatric dose: 1.65 mL/Kg, up to 12.5 g
Hydroxocobalamin	Cyanokit®
	5 g IV over 15 minutes
	Typically given with 8 g sodium thiosulfate
	Pediatric dose: unknown, 70 mg/kg has been used

[*]May be repeated in 30 minutes at half initial dose
[†]Adjust dose by 0.03 mL/kg for every 1 g/dL higher or lower than 12 g/dL

Cyanide is normally metabolized by the enzyme rhodanese to thiocyanate, a less toxic, renally excreted product. This bioconversion requires endogenous sulfur donors, which are rapidly depleted in large cyanide exposures. Sodium thiosulfate serves as a sulfur donor to accelerate this process. Sodium thiosulfate is synergistic with nitrites but can also be effective as monotherapy. Since it has very few side effects it may be reasonable to use sodium thiosulfate alone for equivocal cases.

The recommended regimen and doses for the Taylor cyanide antidote components are summarized in Table 30-3. It is prepackaged to rapidly administer to adult patients; however, dosing adjustments are necessary for pediatric patients. Amyl nitrite pearls are administered first while establishing an intravenous line and preparing the sodium nitrite solution. The pearls should be crushed in gauze and held near the nose and mouth for 15–30 seconds. Amyl nitrite administration will produce a methemoglobin level of 3–7%. Once an intravenous line is established and sodium nitrite solution prepared, amyl nitrite administration may be discontinued. Sodium nitrite is administered at a rate of 2.5 mL/min. In an unstable or hypotensive patient, or when there is concomitant CO poisoning, the dose may be given more slowly, over 30 minutes. With the slower rate of infusion, the methemoglobin level peaks 35–70 minutes following administration and rises to roughly 10–15%. Methemoglobin levels should be monitored periodically after the infusion.

Hydroxocobalamin is a vitamin B_{12} precursor which effectively complexes with cyanide to form cyanocobalamin (vitamin B_{12}), which is nontoxic and renally excreted. Unlike nitrites, it does not form methemoglobin therefore does not interfere with oxygen delivery. It has been successfully used in France for treatment of cyanide and was recently approved in the United States. Recommended doses for significant exposures is 5 g, given intravenously (or 70 mg/kg in pediatric patients); the initial dose may be repeated as necessary, it is distributed through Dey L.P. as the Cyanokit® and can be obtained by calling 800-755-5560. Sodium thiosulfate may possibly be synergistic and can be given (over a 15-minute time period and in a separate I.V. line) with hydroxocobalamin.

Typically, symptoms and signs of cyanide poisoning begin to respond within several minutes of the administration of antidotes. If symptoms recur following antidote administration, both the sodium nitrite and sodium thiosulfate may be given again at half the original doses. Repeated doses of hydroxocobalamin can also be administered in severe cases.

DISPOSITION, FORENSIC ISSUES

Forensic Issues

Testing of materials at the incident can be performed by the National Guard's Weapons of Mass Destruction Civil Support Team, forensic or private reference laboratories, or many state health laboratories. Identification of the various cellular asphyxiants can usually be performed with GS-MS or FTIR. Patients who have expired due to suspected cyanide toxicity can have confirmatory levels sent from whole blood. The major risk to autopsy personnel is volatilization of cyanide from tissues, especially from gastric contents. It should be noted that the presence of hydroxocobalamin can interfer with the cooximetry measurements of carboxyhemoglobin, methemoglobin and oxyhemoglobin value.

Disposition

Patients who are asymptomatic from mild exposures can be observed for 4–6 hours. Those ingesting nitriles or cyanide precursors should be observed 12–24 hours. Patients requiring antidotal treatment are cared for in an intensive care unit where vital signs, mental status, arterial blood gases, methemoglobin and carboxyhemoglobin levels can be checked frequently. Following recovery, patients are observed for 24–48 hours. Rarely, late neurologic syndromes have been reported following cyanide toxicity, and periodic outpatient follow-up is advised.

Suggested Reading

Abrams J, el-Mallakh RS, Meyer R. Suicidal sodium azide ingestion. *Ann Emerg Med.* Dec 1987;16(12):1378–1380.

Akintonwa A, Tunwashe OL. Fatal cyanide poisoning from cassava-based meal. *Hum Exp Toxicol.* Jan 1992;11(1):47–49.

Barratt-Boyes BG, Wood EH. The oxygen saturation of blood in the venae cavae, right-heart chambers, and pulmonary vessels of healthy subjects. *J Lab Clin Med.* Jul 1957;50(1): 93–106.

Baud FJ, Borron SW, Megarbane B, et al. Value of lactic acidosis in the assessment of the severity of acute cyanide poisoning. *Crit Care Med.* Sep 2002;30(9):2044–2050.

Borron S.W., Baud, F., Bariot P et al: Prospective study of hydroxocobalamin for acute cyanide poisoning in smoke inhalation: *Ann Emerg Med* 2007;49:794–801.

Borron, S.W., Baud, F.J., Megarbane, B., Bismuth, C.: Hydroxocobalamin for severe cyanide poisoning by ingestion or inhalation. *Am. J. Emerg. Med.* 2007;25:551–558.

Brennan RJ, Waeckerle JF, Sharp TW, et al. Chemical warfare agents: emergency medical and emergency public health issues. *Ann Emerg Med.* Aug 1999;34(2):191–204.

Chang S, Lamm SH. Human health effects of sodium azide exposure: a literature review and analysis. *Int J Toxicol.* May–Jun 2003;22(3):175–186.

Cyanide, arsenal stirs domestic terror fear. Available at: *http://www.cnn.com/2004/US/Southwest/01/30/cyanide.probe.ap* Accessed January 13, 2006.

Dart RC. Hydroxocobalamin for acute cyanide poisoning: new data from preclinical and clinical studies, new results from the pre-hospital emergency setting. *Clin Toxicol* (Phila). 2006;44 Suppl 1:1–3.

Dart RC, Stark Y, Fulton B, et al. Insufficient stocking of poisoning antidotes in hospital pharmacies. *JAMA.* Nov 13, 1996;276(18): 1508–1510.

Erdman A.R: Is Hydroxocobalamin safe and effective for smoke inhalation: Searching for guidance in the haze. *Ann Emerg Med* 2007:49:814–816.

Feierman DE, Cederbaum AI. Role of cytochrome P-450 IIE1 and catalase in the oxidation of acetonitrile to cyanide. *Chem Res Toxicol.* Nov–Dec 1989;2(6):359–366.

Forsyth JC, Mueller PD, Becker CE, et al. Hydroxocobalamin as a cyanide antidote: safety, efficacy and pharmacokinetics in heavily smoking normal volunteers. *J Toxicol Clin Toxicol.* 1993;31(2):277–294.

Gill JR, Marker E, Stajic M. Suicide by cyanide: 17 deaths. *J Forensic Sci.* Jul 2004;49(4):826–828.

Hall AH, Linden CH, Kulig KW, et al. Cyanide poisoning from laetrile ingestion: role of nitrite therapy. *Pediatrics.* Aug 1986;78(2):269–272.

Hall AH, Rumack BH. Clinical toxicology of cyanide. *Ann Emerg Med.* Sep 1986;15(9):1067–1074.

Hall, A.H, Dart R., Bogdan G. Sodium thiosulfate or hydroxocobalamin for the empiric treatment of cyanide poisoning? *Ann Emerg Med.* 2007:49:806–813.

Johnson RP, Mellors JW. Arteriolization of venous blood gases: a clue to the diagnosis of cyanide poisoning. *J Emerg Med.* Sep–Oct 1988;6(5):401–404.

Kirk MA, Gerace R, Kulig KW. Cyanide and methemoglobin kinetics in smoke inhalation victims treated with the cyanide antidote kit. *Ann Emerg Med.* Sep 1993;22(9):1413–1418.

Lambert W, Meyer E, De Leenheer A. Cyanide and sodium azide intoxication. *Ann Emerg Med.* Sep 1995;26(3):392.

Lee J. Mukai, D., Krevter K et al: Potential interference by hydroxocobalamin on coaximetry hemoglobin measurements during cyanide and smoke inhalation treatments. *Ann Emerg Med* 2007:49:802–805.

Marquet P, Clement S, Lotfi H, et al. Analytical findings in a suicide involving sodium azide. *J Anal Toxicol.* Mar–Apr 1996;20(2):134–138.

Martin C. Chemical terrorism update: cyanide toxins. *http://www.emedmag.com/html/pre/fea/features/071502.asp*

Mass suicides in recent years. Available at: *http://www.cnn.com/US/9703/27/suicide.list/index.html* Accessed January 13, 2006.

Morocco A. Cyanides. *Crit Care Clin.* 2005;21(4):691–705.

NIOSH Emergency Response Card. The Centers for Disease Control and Prevention, National Institute for Occupational Safety and Health. Available at: *http://www.bt.cdc.gov/agent* Accessed January 2006.

Rotenberg JS. Cyanide as a weapon of terror. *Pediatr Ann.* Apr 2003;32(4):236–240.

Schulz V, Bonn R, Kindler J. Kinetics of elimination of thiocyanate in 7 healthy subjects and in 8 subjects with renal failure. *Klin Wochenschr.* Mar 1, 1979;57(5):243–247.

Suchard JR, Wallace KL, Gerkin RD. Acute cyanide toxicity caused by apricot kernel ingestion. *Ann Emerg Med.* Dec 1998;32(6):742–744.

Sun P, Borowitz JL, Kanthasamy AG, et al. Antagonism of cyanide toxicity by isosorbide dinitrate: possible role of nitric oxide. *Toxicology.* Dec 15, 1995;104(1–3):105–111.

Thier R, Lewalter J, Bolt HM. Species differences in acrylonitrile metabolism and toxicity between experimental animals and humans based on observations in human accidental poisonings. *Arch Toxicol.* Jul 2000;74(4–5):184–189.

van Heijst AN, Douze JM, van Kesteren RG, et al. Therapeutic problems in cyanide poisoning. *J Toxicol Clin Toxicol.* 1987;25(5):383–398.

Wills BK LJ, Rhee J, Weidner K. Analysis of suspicious powders in Northern Illinois following the post 9/11 Anthrax Scare. *J Toxicol Clin Toxicol.* 2005;43(6):696–697 (abstract).

31

FLAMMABLE INDUSTRIAL LIQUIDS AND GASES

Mary Powers and David D. Gummin

INTRODUCTION

Flammable gases and liquids are abundant throughout North America. These substances range from fuels to paint solvents to industrial precursors. A majority are stored or transported in bulk, often in or near major metropolitan areas. All flammable gases and liquids are classified as hazardous materials by the Occupational Safety and Health Administration (OSHA) and by the U.S. Department of Transportation (U.S. DOT). OSHA regulates storage of flammable compounds, and their transport is regulated by the DOT. DOT-regulated transporters must prominently display placards that identify the class of agent being transported. Flammable liquids constitute DOT Class 3, while compressed gases (flammable or nonflammable) are in Class 2. Substances that fall into more than one class may require posting of more than one placard. While toxicity can result from exposures after the release, explosion, or combustion of these agents, primary health concerns resulting from fire or explosion relate to blunt physical trauma and thermal burns.

WHAT TO EXPECT

- The FBI Bomb Data Center (BDC) and other intelligence data indicate that most large-scale terror events involve explosions.
- Since 9/11, planners increasingly include "soft," or lightly guarded targets over "hard," very secure targets.
- A carefully placed explosive or incendiary device in or near a bulk storage facility or refinery could be catastrophic, particularly if in proximity to human traffic.
- A bulk storage or transport vessel ideally satisfies the primary objective of the terrorist—to maximize impact and public fear by employing resources already available.
- An explosion in a school could quickly overwhelm a community's pediatric care and resources.
- Familiarity with specifics of a given locale is prerequisite to determining risk and potential targets. Is there a large chemical plant in the vicinity? Is there

a single thoroughfare into and out of the location? Do tank trucks or rail cars transport chemicals past schools, governmental buildings, stadiums, or other populated public areas?

- The answers to these questions can help communities and providers prepare for potential injuries and exposures.

PERSONAL PROTECTIVE EQUIPMENT/DECONTAMINATION CONSIDERATIONS

- Personal protective equipment (PPE) protects emergency responders, prevents secondary contamination, and reduces morbidity and mortality of rescuers and victims.
- To be beneficial, appropriate size and type of PPE must be appropriately worn.
- Positive pressure self-contained breathing apparatus (SCBA) equipment is most appropriate for rescuers in the immediate vicinity of these substances.

RESOURCES NEEDED BEFORE THE FIRST PATIENT APPEARS

- In each of the fifty states, a State Emergency Response Commission (SERC) designates local emergency planning districts, and appoints Local Emergency Planning Committees (LEPCs) for each district. Each SERC supervises and coordinates the activities of each subordinate LEPC and reviews local emergency response plans.
- Each LEPC maintains a database of the substances available within its district. This information is used to develop regional and local emergency plans, and is available through each municipality's Emergency Management Office and LEPC.
- EMS providers, poison centers, and HCFs are integral to each local plan. Active participation by EMS and health-care providers is essential in developing and implementing these plans, and in conducting drills to test them.
- Hazmat teams, Federal Bureau of Investigation (FBI), local law enforcement, Red Cross, city, county, and regional Emergency Management should all be included in planning.
- Ongoing planning and drills are essential to develop and to maintain local and regional capabilities and networking.
- Field decontamination facilities are essential, as patient decontamination should occur prior to transport to a HCF. Nevertheless, during real mass casualty events, the majority of patients present to

HCFs without accessing EMS. Providers and facilities must recognize this, must develop capabilities for patient decontamination, and must train staff to perform decontamination properly.

RESOURCES NEEDED IN A MASS CASUALTY EVENT

- Internal and external disaster plans must be initiated.
- Municipal disaster plans must identify specific resources available and systems required to manage mass casualties.
- Public Health and Poison Center resources should be mobilized early, to offer guidance and assist in accessing supplemental resources.
- Field triage of patients occurs in a reversed paradigm, with the most severely injured arriving after the less injured. This system is designed to do the greatest good for the greatest possible number of victims. See Chap. 25.

CLINICAL MANIFESTATIONS

Under conditions of sufficient temperature and oxygenation, flammable gases or liquids assume substantial risk of exploding. Explosions inflict multiple levels of injury on victims, including multisystem blast trauma, thermal burns, and inhalational injury. With larger explosions, more victims can be expected. Injury patterns depend on multiple factors, including the composition of the explosive, the surrounding environment, distance between victim and blast, and presence of protective barriers. Explosions involving flammable gases or liquids carry additional risk of toxicity related to the flammable agent itself, as well as to products of combustion. (See Table 31-1.)

Rupture of tympanic membranes is common in blast injury, and may portend serious solid organ injury. Alternatively, significant injury may be present despite intact tympanic membranes. Blunt and penetrating injuries can occur in an explosive blast, including impalement by flying debris. Protruding objects must be evaluated and handled cautiously, and may require surgical management. Significant eye injuries occur in up to 10% of all blast survivors. These include globe penetration, keratoconjunctivitis, foreign bodies, hyphema, and lid lacerations.

Inhalation of hydrocarbon gases or volatilized liquid solvents may lead to central nervous system (CNS) depression due to general anesthetic properties of these agents. High concentration of gas or volatilized liquid in a small space may displace oxygen and lead to asphyxia. Carbon monoxide toxicity may result from inhalation of combustion products or may even result from exposure to certain flammable liquids themselves. Some products may be oxidants that can induce methemoglobinemia.

TABLE 31-1

COMMON EXPLOSIVES INJURIES

System	Injury or Condition
Auditory	TM rupture, ossicular disruption, cochlear damage, foreign body
Eye, orbit, face	Perforated globe, foreign body, air embolism, fractures
Respiratory	Blast lung, hemothorax, pneumothorax, pulmonary contusion and hemorrhage, AV fistulas (source of air embolism), airway epithelial damage, aspiration pneumonitis, sepsis
Digestive	Bowel perforation, hemorrhage, ruptured liver or spleen, sepsis, mesenteric ischemia from air embolism
Circulatory	Cardiac contusion, myocardial infarction from air embolism, shock, vasovagal hypotension, peripheral vascular injury, air embolism-induced injury
CNS injury	Concussion, closed and open brain injury, stroke, spinal cord injury, air embolism-induced injury
Renal injury	Renal contusion, laceration, acute renal failure due to rhabdomyolysis, hypotension, and hypovolemia
Extremity injury	Traumatic amputation, fractures, crush injuries, compartment syndrome, burns, cuts, lacerations, acute arterial occlusion, air embolism-induced injury

Source: Reproduced from CDC: Emergency Preparedness and Response, available at http://www.bt.cdc.gov/masscasualties/explosions.asp

In industry, the term, "solvent" often refers to an organic solvent, and this term typically means hydrocarbon liquid mixtures used to dissolve other substances. While aerosols, fumes, dust, and smoke can cause deleterious health effects, the most flammable and explosive form of hydrocarbon liquids are the vapors of volatilized agents mixed with air or another oxygen source. Fire and explosion have obvious health implications. But vapor clouds (unlike smoke or aerosol plumes) are usually invisible, and may go undetected, particularly if personnel are wearing eye and respiratory protective equipment. Solvent vapors are invariably heavier than air, and tend to pool in low-lying areas. Oxygen is typically displaced by these "vapor pools," resulting in a hypoxic environment. Invisible vapor clouds can travel significant distances before encountering an ignition source. Specific caution is required by firefighting personnel and EMS providers.

Significant exposure to some hydrocarbons, especially those that are chlorinated, can cause liver or kidney damage. Blast injury damages tissues, including muscles, causing rhabdomyolysis. This can result in electrolyte abnormalities and kidney dysfunction. Contact with skin or mucous membranes may lead to chemical burns. Prolonged skin contact may lead to dermatitis by defatting the lipid components of the skin.

INITIAL MEDICAL CARE

The first management priority is to protect rescuers. In terror events, secondary explosions are increasingly common. No medical rescuer should enter a hazardous environment, until that environment is deemed safe by the response incident commander. Personal protection is mandatory at each level of health-care delivery.

Next, remove the exposure from the patient, and the patient from the exposure. External contamination (especially clothing) must be removed prior to the patient's transport to an HCF. Isolate the patient from the environment by wrapping in a blanket or sheet to prevent spread of any residual contamination. Attention to the airway, breathing, and circulation remain top priorities for rescuers, but the usual multivictim triage process must be reversed when handling mass casualty events (see Chaps. 23, 25).

EMS rescuers should obtain and record details about the nature of fire or explosion, potential toxic exposures or other environmental hazards, and casualty location from incident commanders.

STUDIES

- Arterial blood gas (ABG) testing may be helpful to assess oxygenation for those with significant vapor or smoke inhalation. Significant metabolic acidosis with an elevated anion gap suggests inhalation of hydrogen cyanide, commonly produced during combustion of synthetic polymers. In this setting, the arterial lactate concentration provides a reliable screen for cyanide toxicity. An arterial lactate greater than 10 mmol/L, without major trauma or exsanguination, strongly suggests cyanide toxicity.
- ABG testing will often concurrently assess for methemoglobinemia or carboxyhemoglobinemia. Specific testing for these abnormal hemoglobins should be considered if not concomitantly performed on ABG.
- Baseline electrolytes should be obtained, with special attention to potassium abnormalities. Initial renal function and liver enzymes should be assayed in the

setting of inhalational injury, blunt trauma, or smoke inhalation.

- Urinalysis screens for evidence of hemoglobinuria or myoglobinuria.
- Baseline chest x-ray should be obtained for inhalational injuries, as well as for blast injuries. Blast lung occurs rapidly. This is recognized as a "butterfly" pattern on chest x-ray. Prophylactic bilateral thoracostomy tubes are indicated prior to general anesthesia or air transport in these patients.
- Law enforcement and a poison center or toxicologist should be consulted to determine whether additional bioassays or specific levels are required for forensic or diagnostic purposes.

EARLY INTERVENTIONS

- Initial actions should be to limit exposure and to decontaminate the victim.
- Ensure that the airway is open and support respirations if necessary. Aggressive airway management may be necessary especially with inhalation exposure. Many inhaled agents cause inflammation and may compromise the airway.
- Administer oxygen by high-flow non–rebreather mask. Hoarseness, cough, or respiratory stridor suggest inhalation injury and require further evaluation.
- If a burn is present, estimate the body surface area (BSA) of the burn. Cover burned areas with dry sterile dressings. Administer IV fluids. The burn should be treated similarly, whether it is a chemical or a thermal burn. Administer pain medications as needed. Evaluate need for surgical intervention. Consider referral to a specialized burn unit.
- Evaluate for systemic toxicity. If the substance is known, treat for specific agent toxicity.

WHEN TO REFER

These decisions are greatly influenced by local capabilities, local and regional resources, and the scale of the event. Regional capacities determine the ability to perform timely referral. Frontline providers must entertain early and ongoing contact with resources such as the local emergency management office, local public health officials, the regional poison center, and regional burn center. Regional trauma triage protocols may provide access to regional trauma care, and typically address disaster contingencies. When needed, consider patient transfer to regional tertiary care centers with resources to provide mechanical ventilation. Poison centers can assist with referral and follow-up of issues related to chemical toxicity. Providers should consider ophthalmologic referral for those with eye complaints.

COMBUSTION AND FLAMMABILITY

Health-care providers may be unfamiliar with the science of fire and explosions. At minimum, a working knowledge of accepted terminology is helpful. For detailed information, the reader is referred to *The National Fire Protection Association's Flammable and Combustible Liquids Code.*

A *flammable* material can be solid, liquid, or gas (including the vapor phase of a liquid). OSHA defines flammable (pertaining to liquids) as "any liquid having a flash point below 100°F" (or 37.8°C). In contrast, *combustible* liquids are somewhat harder to ignite (flash point ≥100°F). OSHA further divides liquids into Classes I–III, with lettered subclasses. The lower the OSHA class, the higher the combustion or explosion risk at low temperatures. Gasoline's flash point is −40°C, and it is quite flammable (Class Ib). An outdated term, "inflammable," simply means flammable. To avoid confusion, use of the term "flammable" is preferred. Material that does not burn is called *nonflammable*.

The *flash point* is the lowest temperature at which a liquid can form an ignitable mixture in air. This value is determined under test conditions, and actually measures the minimum temperature at which the liquid gives off sufficient vapor concentration to form an ignitable mixture, near the surface of the liquid. The *fire point* is the temperature at which a flame will become self-sustaining, allowing the liquid to continue to burn. The fire point is usually a few degrees above the flash point, and generally indicates susceptibility to ignition.

The physical phase of a material influences its flammability. Vapor (gas phase) mixes readily with air (and therefore with oxygen) to contribute the first two requirements for the fire triad. All that's required is heat (or a spark). Hydrocarbons in the liquid state generally do not support flame, since oxygen cannot dissolve into liquids in quantities sufficient to ignite or to sustain combustion. Only the vapor phase, near the surface of the liquid, will burn or ignite. Liquids with high vapor pressure enter the gaseous phase more readily at a given temperature, so are more likely to be available for ignition.

The flash point serves as the basis for classifying flammable and combustible liquids because it directly relates to a liquid's vapor pressure, that is, its volatility. Since only the vapor of a liquid burns, the vapor pressure is the main property that determines its fire hazard. Liquids with flash points below ambient temperatures demonstrate rapid spread of flame over the surface of the liquid. More heat is available to the fire, since less energy is expended in heating the liquid to generate vapor.

A common misconception is that all halogenated (e.g., chlorine, bromine or iodine-containing) hydrocarbon compounds are not flammable. While some halogenated liquids do not have a "flash point"—considered "nonflammable" by this definition—these liquids can exist in atmospheric mixtures that will still support combustion. Examples include carbon tetrachloride, chloroform, ethylene dibromide, methyl chloroform, methylene chloride, perchloroethylene, and trichloroethylene. Moreover, some halogenated hydrocarbons (notably: ethyl chloride; 1,2 dichloroethane; 1,1-dichloroethylene; 1,2-dichloroethylene; 2-chloropropane; and dichloroacetylene) have low flash points and boiling points, and are OSHA Class I liquids. These are highly flammable and explosive. Trichloroethylene (TCE) decomposes readily at temperatures >60°C to dichloroacetylene. Decomposition can be rather violent at low temperatures. The degradation product has no measurable flash point, but is both combustible and explosive. Similarly, organic peroxides undergo autoaccelerating thermal decomposition. Essentially, these substances can explode without exposure to external air or to oxygen, so are excluded from flash point determination methods.

For anything to catch fire or to explode, there must be just the right mix of heat, fuel, and oxygen (the fire triad, or triangle). There exists a minimum concentration of vapor in air, below which propagation of flame does not occur on contact with an ignition source (mixture too lean). Similarly, there is a maximum concentration of vapor in air above which propagation of flame does not occur (insufficient oxygen—too rich).

The tendency for flammable liquids to burn, when mixed with air in the proper proportion, is delineated by its flammable limits (also called the explosive limits, or the explosive range). In the explosive concentration range, the presence of an ignition source will result in rapid combustion: an explosion. Proportional boundaries of vapor with air are known as the lower and upper flammable or explosive limits (respectively). These are usually expressed in terms of percentage (by volume) of vapor in air. (See Fig. 31-1.)

Flowing liquids (e.g., through a pipe) generate static electricity. This can provide the spark that completes the fire triad. Workers transferring liquids from one container

to another, or managing pipe or other leaks, must follow proper bonding and grounding procedures.

DISPOSITION

Major blunt or penetrating injury requires trained and experienced evaluation and disposition should generally be to an appropriate trauma center. Deep partial thickness or full thickness burns require special evaluation, and transfer or disposition should be coordinated in consultation with a burn center or an experienced burn surgeon. Mild carbon monoxide toxicity should be treated with high-flow oxygen for at least 4–6 hours, and until all symptoms have resolved. More severe or complicated carbon monoxide toxicity may benefit from hyperbaric oxygen therapy. Disposition should be planned in consultation with a toxicologist or a regional poison center.

Significant inhalation of hydrocarbons may result in pulmonary toxicity. Radiographic evidence of pneumonitis may lag behind clinical symptoms. In the setting of fire or explosion, it may be difficult to distinguish pulmonary hydrocarbon injury from injury due to smoke inhalation. Further complicating this distinction is the possibility of "blast lung" from an explosion.

Blast lung is rapidly progressive, involving cough, pain, dyspnea, and tachypnea, with pulmonary capillary leak and/or hemorrhage. The course is rapidly progressive over the first 1–2 hours after the blast. Patients who were not present in the blast zone, who sustain no blunt or penetrating injury, and give no history of smoke exposure are still at risk for hydrocarbon pneumonitis. Hydrocarbon pneumonitis progresses over the first 1–4 hours. Patients with hydrocarbon inhalation who are symptomatic on arrival to the emergency department will likely develop progressive pneumonitis. Conversely, the majority of asymptomatic patients after hydrocarbon inhalation are not likely to manifest delayed toxicity. Those who are asymptomatic, have normal oxygen saturation, and a normal chest x-ray performed 6 hours after exposure, are unlikely to deteriorate. On the other hand, patients with significant smoke inhalation, regardless of the etiology, may progress in delayed fashion. The majority develop increasing symptoms over 18–24 hours after the exposure.

Special caution should be paid to patients who were exposed to hydrocarbons that cause cardiac sensitization. These patients may develop malignant cardiac rhythms, and should be observed on a cardiac monitor for at least 6 hours after exposure. Mental status depression, seizures, or arrhythmias attributed to a known cardiac sensitizer (or to an unknown HC ingestion) warrant at least 6 hours of continuous cardiac monitoring.

Appropriate outpatient disposition can be made by 6 hours after exposure. All patients should be instructed to return immediately, if respiratory symptoms occur, particularly if smoke inhalation is a possibility.

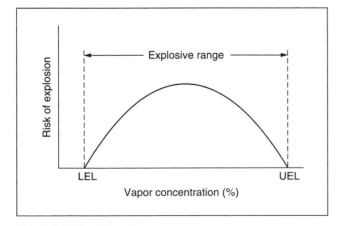

FIGURE 31-1

EXPLOSIVE RISK FOR FLAMMABLE VAPOR IN ATMOSPHERE
LEL—Lower explosive limit; UEL—Upper explosive limit

Patients with depressed mental status or ongoing pulmonary or cardiac toxicity 6 hours after exposure require hospitalization.

FORENSIC ISSUES

Most important is to recall that, in a terrorist event, the incident scene is a crime scene. In fact, your emergency department may be declared a crime scene. Patient care warrants top priority. But in the interest of justice, the clinician will want to cooperate with the needs of law enforcement, and also has a legal obligation to do so. Rescuers should document details about the nature of a fire or explosion, potential toxic exposures or other environmental hazards, and casualty location. Each patient's personal effects and even body specimens may become part of a criminal investigation. When possible, clothing should be bagged and labeled, and chain of custody maintained. Health-care providers need to interface with law enforcement to determine whether additional bioassays or specific specimens should be obtained for forensic purposes. As in any legal evaluation, physical findings should be carefully examined and documented. In the United States and its territories, the FBI has jurisdiction over terror events, regardless of the scope.

Suggested Reading

Barceloux DG. Halogenated Solvents, Trichloroethylene, and Methylene Chloride. In: Sullivan JB, Krieger GR, eds. *Clinical Environmental Health and Toxic Exposures*. Philadelphia, PA: Lippincott, Williams & Wilkins. 2001, 733–50.

CDC (Centers for Disease Control and Prevention): Emergency Preparedness & Response. Available at *http://www.bt.cdc. gov/masscasualties/explosions.asp* Accessed October 29, 2006.

FBI (Federal Bureau of Investigation). 1998. 1997 Bomb Summary. FBI Bomb Data Center, General Information Bulletin 97-1. Washington, D.C.: U.S. Department of Justice. Available at *http://www.depts.ttu.edu/museumttu/disasters/ US%20Response%20Files/SupportDocs/FBI%20reports/1997 bombrep.pdf* Accessed October 13, 2006.

Flammability definitions available at *http://www.chemistry.ohio-state.edu/ehs/handbook/flammabl/oshafire.htm* Accessed October 13, 2006.

International Policy Institute for Counter-Terrorism. *http:// www.ict.org.il/* Accessed April 13, 2006.

LEPC contact information from the US EPA. Available at: *http:// yosemite.epa.gov/oswer/CeppoWeb.nsf/content/epcraOverview. htm?OpenDocument* Accessed October 14, 2006.

Morse, LH, Owen DJ, Fujimoto G, et al. Toxic Hazards of Firefighters and Combustion Toxicology. In: Sullivan JB, Krieger GR, eds. *Clinical Environmental Health and Toxic Exposures*. Philadelphia, PA: Lippincott, Williams & Wilkins. 2001, 630–6.

NFPA 30, Flammable and Combustible Liquids Code. Available at: *http://www.nfpa.org/freecodes/free_access_document.asp* Accessed October 13, 2006.

The OSHA Standard 29 CFR 1910.106, Flammable and Combustible Liquids. Available at *http://www.osha.gov/* Accessed April 13, 2006.

U.S. Department of Transportation. 2004. Emergency Response Guidebook, 2004. ISBN 0-16-072282-9. Available at *http:// hazmat.dot.gov/pubs/erg/erg2004.pdf* Accessed October 13, 2006.

32

CORROSIVE INDUSTRIAL AGENTS

Richard T. Tovar, Ernest Stremski, and Mary Powers

STAT FACTS

CORROSIVE INDUSTRIAL AGENTS

- If a corrosive injury to the skin is suspected, the patient must be immediately evacuated and decontaminated. "Time is tissue."
- Water, preferably warm, to avoid hypothermia, is the decontaminating agent of choice.
- The only corrosive materials in which water decontamination is contraindicated are reactive metals such as sodium, lithium, and potassium.
- Time to decontamination is up to 2 hours for acids and 12 hours for alkalis.
- Identification of the corrosive chemical may not be possible at the scene. Determination of the pH of the chemical at the scene is usually possible.
- Do not delay basic and advanced airway and cardiac care. Consider the simultaneous use of decontamination with airway management.

- Most corrosive chemical weapons of mass destruction will be released as a liquid or gas in a public place.
- Have a high index of suspicion for systemic or protoplasmic corrosive poisons.
- Involve burn center specialists early in the treatment of the victim(s).
- Acidic corrosives cause a coagulation dermal necrosis, via protein denaturation (hence a "dry" appearing coagulum) that causes less dermal layer penetration and is more amenable to decontamination.
- Basic or alkali corrosives cause a liquefaction necrosis, which can penetrate deeper into tissue. Besides causing more injury as compared to acids, the necrosis decreases ability of water to dilute and decontaminate tissue.
- Alkali burns resemble a more "wet" burn due to protein and fat denaturation.

INTRODUCTION

Corrosive materials are ubiquitous in the settings of industry, research, and even in the home. Corrosive materials have been used interchangeably in the literature with other terms such as caustics, acids, bases, and alkalis. Basically, a corrosive is a substance that causes both histological and functional damage after contact with body tissues. The Occupational Safety and Health Administration (OSHA) definition of a corrosive in 29 CFR 1919.1200 App A is as follows.

Corrosive: A chemical that causes visible destruction of, or irreversible alterations in, living tissue by chemical action at the site of contact. For example, a chemical is considered to be corrosive if, when tested on the intact skin of albino rabbits by the method described by the U.S. Department of Transportation in appendix A to 49 CFR part 173, it destroys or changes irreversibly the structure of the tissue at the site of contact following an exposure period of four hours. This term shall not refer to action on inanimate surfaces.

Acids are defined as proton donors, which cause injury below a pH below 3. Alkalis are proton acceptors that

TABLE 32-1

EXAMPLES OF CORROSIVE/CAUSTIC CHEMICALS
AVAILABLE AS WEAPONS OF MASS DESTRUCTION

Chemical	Commercial Use
ACIDS	
Chloroacetic acid	Pigments, drugs
Trichloroacetic acid	Tissue fixation
Acetic acid	Disinfectants, dyes
Formic acid	Cellulose, tanning
Phenol, cresols	Resins, plastics
Sulfuric acid	Toilet cleaners
Nitric acid	Engraving
Hydrofluoric acid	Rust remover
ALKALIS	
Ammonia	Cleaners, detergent
Calcium oxide	Plaster, cement
Sodium carbonate	Detergent
Lithium hydride	Absorb CO
Sodium Silicate	Detergents
Sodium/Calcium hypochlorite	Bleach
Sodium/Potassium hydroxide	Drain/oven cleaners
METALS	
Lithium, sodium, potassium	
OXIDIZERS	
Peroxides	
Bleaches	
Chromates	Tanning, dyes
Permanganates	Disinfectants

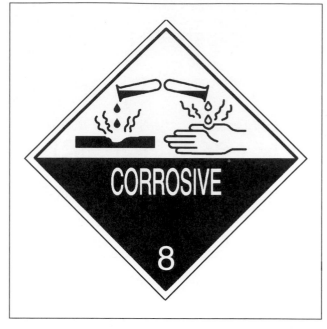

FIGURE 32-1

HAZARDOUS MATERIAL CORROSIVE PLACARD

cause injury at a pH above 11. With acidic or basic substances, injury actually occurs in the tissues as the process of neutralization occurs. A secondary process occurs with release of heat/thermal energy with further tissue damage. Some caustics such as phenol can cause tissue damage and have near neutral pHs. Corrosive or caustic agents can be either synthesized or be readily available by numerous chemical processes that are available and ongoing in our communities. An example of this can be found in Table 32-1.

CONFIRMING THE THREAT

Because of their extremely irritating properties to both the respiratory and dermatological systems, corrosive agents usually exhibit immediate signs and symptoms that can be visualized by innocent bystanders, suspects, and first responders. Identification of the type of corrosive agent can be accomplished by several means. Site-specific identification includes direct visualization of the actual chemical agent or identification labels such as hazardous material placards (Fig. 32-1). Other identifiers include shipping papers, and United Nations chemical identification numbers.

The American Association of Poison Control Centers (AAPCC) in 2003 reported over 100,000 exposures to caustics. Mortality was surprisingly low, with 20 deaths. Morbidity included those with major toxicity at 120 cases, and moderate toxicity at 2322 cases.

According to Department of Transportation (DOT) data, corrosive material ranked second in 2002 for documented hazardous incidents. It is unclear how much chemical injury is to be expected with these types of incidents. Multiple factors enter into these types of incidents, which include weather patterns, chemical type, time of day, population demographics, etc.

PERSONAL PROTECTIVE EQUIPMENT/DECONTAMINATION

Due to the potential for immediate injury to both respiratory and dermatological systems, the maximum amount of personal protective gear is recommended until there is a thorough understanding of the chemical hazards. Decontamination procedures for victims and responders alike include basic principles such as complete clothing removal, rapid evacuation, and washing with copious amounts of water to remove the chemicals.

PREINCIDENT RESOURCES

Depending on the size of the incident, exposure to corrosive acid or bases centers on the treatment of respiratory and dermatological injury. If dilution with water at the scene or at a safe location (cold zone) adjacent to the scene can be accomplished, then the mucous membrane and skin injury can be mitigated. Rapid decontamination can decrease morbidity thereby decreasing the need for in-hospital burn center specialty resources. Obviously, local and regional capability to decontaminate mass casualties is variable throughout each jurisdiction. It cannot be stressed however that first responders should have the ability to perform "dilutional" decontamination to a large amount of victims on a rapid basis.

The incident command (IC) structure (law enforcement, fire, EMS) should have access to available material data and safety sheets (MSDS), eye witness reports, and hazardous material placard signs, in order to perform risk assessment of the incident. IC should also plan for secondary chemical or explosive devices aimed at first responders.

CLINICAL MANIFESTATIONS

Dermatological manifestations of injury have been reviewed in the medical literature along with treatment. The amount of damage by a corrosive/caustic to a tissue is influenced by several factors: volume/concentration of toxin, time of contact/exposure, and pH. For mucosal surfaces, the concept of titratable alkaline/acid reserve (TAR) is used. TAR is the amount of "neutralizing substance" needed to turn the pH of a caustic into the physiologic pH of the surrounding tissue. The larger the TAR, the more damaging the agent. Two chemicals, such as phenol and zinc chloride, have near physiologic pHs, and are very corrosive (high TAR).

Generally, corrosives cause tissue damage via a chemical reaction and less importantly a hyperthermic reaction. The keratin layer of skin is destroyed and then the deeper layers are injured. Visualization of skin burns can range from obvious skin changes to pain without skin lesions. Acids cause direct chemical protein denaturation that results in a tissue coagulum. The coagulum, an acid-protein complex, then results in cellular dehydration and further cell damage. This type of injury, termed coagulation necrosis, is histologically different and may be less penetrating than alkali burns.

Alkalis have been described to cause a liquefaction tissue necrosis, which is deeper and more aggressive with respect to tissue damage than acid injury. The alkali-protein complex, similar to acids, causes cellular dehydration. Alkalis further cause saponification of fatty tissue. Alkali burns cause much more cellular dehydration than acids. Some corrosives, such as phenols, zinc and mercuric chloride, and hydrofluoric acid, may also cause systemic as well as dermal or mucosal toxicity. Some corrosives have a characteristic color of dermal burn (Table 32-2).

Lab Studies

Once the patient has arrived in a medical treatment environment and has been decontaminated, further medical workup can proceed. Most corrosives exhibit only dermal injury and do not usually cause systemic toxicity. Exceptions to this include but are not limited to hydrofluoric acid, phenols, and zinc and mercuric acid. Since the above three corrosive chemical classes can initially present with skin or respiratory signs and symptoms and then proceed to systemic toxicity, all patients should have preliminary baseline laboratories, including serum electrolytes, calcium, liver enzymes, and renal function tests. If possible, documentation of skin pH should also be accomplished before and after the decontamination process.

Patients with respiratory symptoms should have chest x-rays and measurement of pulmonary function parameters such as pulse oximetry and peak flow on an emergent basis. More detailed pulmonary function tests can be performed after the initial stabilization of the patient. Early intervention is crucial. Timely treatment of the dermal and respiratory effects of corrosive exposure is extremely important. As previously stated, the concentration of the corrosive agent and its duration of contact determine the amount of tissue damage. Tissue injury continues to occur until the causative agent is removed or neutralized. Therefore, any witness to a dermal exposure to a corrosive must initiate water decontamination (hydrotherapy) as rapidly as possible. Again, the victim's clothes must be removed first as this will remove any reservoir effect from the clothing. Experimental animal studies have demonstrated that the depth of burn is far greater if decontamination is begun at 3 minutes versus just 1 minute. Furthermore, these studies demonstrate that with acid substances, the tissue pH may return to neutral after 2 hours of continuous water irrigation. Dermal pH may not return to baseline for up to 12 hours with alkali exposure. This delay in return to baseline dermal pH is due to the hydroxyl (OH$^-$) alkali group combining with proteins or fats to form insoluble proteins or soaps. These complexes allow the hydroxyl ions to pass deeper into the tissue layers thereby sequestering them from dilution from water on the dermal surface. Acids do not form these types of tissue complexes, thereby allowing for more skin surface dilution and removal.

TABLE 32-2

EXAMPLES OF CHARACTERISTIC SKIN BURNS

Chemical	Burn/Skin Color
Copper salts	Green skin stain
Arsenic, Arsine	Bronze
Oxalic acid	Blue
Formaldehyde, phenol, Nitric acid, picric acid	Yellow to brown
Osmium tetroxide, silver salts	Black to silver
Phenol	Gray to brown
Sulfuric acid	Black to brown

Specialty Medical Referral

Depending on first responder resources, all victims at a WMD corrosive incident should be referred to medical personnel that can provide definitive monitoring and treatment. An incident medical command system should be established to provide continued treatment and stabilization during a mass casualty incident. This type of treatment facility may be established at a receiving hospital(s) or at a secure secondary site. Literature recommendations for dermal hydrotherapy include 2 hours for strong acids and 12 hours for strong alkali corrosive injury. This may or may not be possible with the first responders and hospital resources. Respiratory exposure requires symptomatic treatments as indicated. These symptomatic treatments include, but are not limited to, nebulized β-agonists, oral or intravenous steroids, and invasive airway management. Further specialty referral to plastic or general surgeons is case-specific. Patients that exhibit systemic toxicity either via direct dermal injury or protoplasmic mechanisms mandate hospital admission and multispecialty care. Other general guidelines for admission are for parenteral pain control and circumferential or large surface area burns. Other indications for specialty referral include chemical burns to the face, genitalia, hands, and feet. Close coordination with a burn center can help expedite these types of cases.

TOXICOKINETICS/PATHOPHYSIOLOGY

The systemic manifestations of caustic burns can be divided into 2 areas: systemic effects from skin surface injury and protoplasmic poisoning. The systemic effects seen by dermal/respiratory mucosal injury are similar to thermal injury patients. These manifestations include but are not limited to fluid third spacing with resultant volume issues, infection, pulmonary complications such as acute respiratory distress syndrome (ARDS), and cosmetic/healing concerns. Protoplasmic poisoning is common in hydrofluoric acid, phenols, formic acid, copper sulfate, and others (see Table 32-3). The pathophysiology of

TABLE 32-3

EXAMPLES OF SYSTEMIC CORROSIVE AGENTS

Agent	Systemic Toxicity
Hydrofluoric acid	Hypocalcemia, hyperkalemia, hypomagnesemia
Phenols	CNS toxicity, hypotension, metabolic acidosis
Formic acid	CNS toxicity
Copper sulfate	Increased copper levels with hemolysis, hepatitis
Chromic acid	Renal toxicity
White phosphorus	Hypokalemia, hyperphosphatemia

dermal corrosive burns has been covered elsewhere in this chapter.

Special chemical agents include white phosphorous, which causes more of a thermal burn in deference to other corrosive agents that cause liquefaction or coagulation necrosis.

PROPHYLAXIS/STAFF PROTECTION

Most hazardous materials teams and specialized law enforcement units approach a chemical release as an unknown. Therefore, the incident is approached with Level A hazardous material personal protective gear. Hospital personnel should also protect themselves with at least Level B or C protective gear, especially if field decontamination has been brief or nonexistent.

Special situations for both field and hospital decontamination include reactive elemental metals such as sodium, lithium, and potassium. If these metals are activated by water, an exothermic reaction occurs with the release of heat and generation of hydrogen gas and hydroxide. The evolved heat is sufficient to ignite the resultant hydrogen gas, which results in even greater heat and causes additional thermal burns. Furthermore, formation of hydroxide compound may cause a liquefaction necrosis injury to the tissue along with the thermal burn. The water-exothermic reaction occurs more rapidly with elemental potassium than with sodium. These deleterious effects of potassium have been attributed to trace amounts of potassium superoxide released on exposure to water and air. Therefore, hydrotherapy is contraindicated in these circumstances.

In the prehospital setting, use only a Class D fire extinguisher (containing sodium chloride, sodium carbonate, or graphite base) or sand to suppress flames. The patient then has the reactive metal swept or vacuumed off the skin. When the fire is extinguished, the metal is covered by oil (e.g., mineral oil, cooking oil) to isolate metal from water. Transport the patient to the ED for further wound debridement and cleansing. Remove small pieces of metal from the skin via brushing or metal forceps. Metal particles removed from the patient may be placed in oil as above. It must be remembered that all foreign bodies removed from patients whether solid or liquid have the potential to become forensic evidence. Therefore, consider the labeling and cataloging of these materials, even though they may still be hazardous.

DISPOSITION

Follow-up of patients with either dermal or respiratory corrosive injury or exposure is case-specific. As previously stated, consultation with a burn center or specialist is advisable for both admission and future follow-up. Systemic or protoplasmic poisoning can be managed by a multispecialty team including but not limited to medical toxicology, primary care, pulmonology, and so on.

FORENSIC ISSUES

Most experts state that a public exposure to a corrosive agent would probably be via a liquid or gaseous route. It is understandable that clothing, decontamination fluid, and other materials may remain hazardous if kept with the patient or with medical providers. Nonetheless, if precautions are taken by medical and hazardous material personnel, this evidence can be preserved for law enforcement personnel. Again, chain of evidence must be preserved, and incorporated into any treatment protocol. Finally, any observations with respect to the incident that are stated to medical providers can be referred to law enforcement, to assist in the investigation.

Both hospitals and first responders should develop a list of chemical "targets of opportunity." Local law enforcement may also assist with such a list. As much as can be known about the chemical composition of each location via MSDS sheets should be organized. The amount of medical and first responder resources to treat a mass casualty incident should be proposed to those administrators and public officials who can allocate assets before an incident occurs.

Interaction with the local poison center can benefit both the first responder and the hospital treatment team. Most U.S. poison centers participate in the toxic exposure surveillance system (TESS). This system can assist all participants in a potential corrosive intentional release by facilitating early warning of covert chemical outbreak events. Real-time and on-scene management information can also be given to medical providers.

Suggested Reading

Andrews K. The treatment of alkaline burns of the skin by neutralization. *Plast Reconstr Surg.* May 2004;111(6):1918–21.

Baker D. Civilian exposure to toxic agents: emergency medical response. *Prehospital Disaster Med.* Apr–Jun 2004;19(2): 174–8.

Baker DJ, Critical care requirements after mass toxic agent release. *Crit Care Med.* Jan 2005;33(1 Suppl):S66–74.

Banin E, Morad Y, Berenshtein E, et al. Injury induced by chemical warfare agents: characterization and treatment issues. *Invest Ophthalmol Vis Sci.* 2003;44: 2966–72.

Berkowitz Z, Haugh GS, Orr MF, et al. Releases of hazardous substances in schools: data from Hazardous Substances Emergency Events Surveillance System, 1993–1998. *J Environ Health.* 2002;65:20–7.

Betts-Symonds. Major disaster management in chemical warfare. *Accid Emerg Nurs.* Jul 1994;2(3):122–9.

Bond, Sheldon J, Gregory C, et al. Cutaneous burns caused by sulfuric acid drain cleaner. *J Trauma.* March 1998;44(3): 523–6.

Burda AM. Pharmacy preparedness for incidents involving weapons of mass destruction. *Am J Health Syst Pharm.* 2001;58: 2274–2284.

Edlich RF, Farinholt HM, Winters KL, et al. Modern concepts in treatment and prevention of chemical injuries. *J Long Term Effect Med Implants.* 2005;15(3);303–18.

Jelenko C. Chemicals that burn. *J Trauma.* 1974;14(1);65–72.

Karayilanoglu T, et al. Evaluations over the medical emergency responding to chemical terrorist attack. *Mil Med.* Aug 2003;168(8):591–4.

Krenzlok EP, et al. The poison center role in biological and chemical terrorism. *Vet Human Toxicol.* 2000;42:297–300.

Belson M, et al. Case definitions for chemical poisoning. *MMWR.* Jan 14, 2005;54(RR01): 1–24.

Moles TM, et al. Toxic trauma. *Prehospital Disaster Med.* Apr–Jun 2001;16(2):78–80.

Salzman M., O'Malley R.N: Updates on the evaluation and management of caustic exposures. *Emerg Med Clin N Am.* 2007:25:459–476.

Schwek M. Chemical warfare agents—still taboo poisons? *Toxicology.* Oct 30, 2005;214(3):165–6.

Schwenk M. Toxicological aspects of preparedness and aftercare for chemical-incidents. *Toxicology.* Oct 2005;214(3):232–48.

Wolkin AF, Patel M, Watson W, et al. Early detection of illness associated with poisonings of public health significance. *Ann Emerg Med.* Feb 2006;47(2):170–6.

Zavotsky KE, Valendo M, Torres P. Developing an emergency department based special operations team: Robert Wood Johnson University Hospital's experience. *Disaster Manag Response.* Apr–Jun, 2004;2(2):35–9.

Zilker T. Medical management of incidents with chemical warfare agents. *Toxicology.* 30;214(3):221–31. Epub 2005 Aug 10.

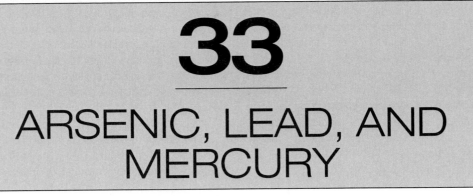

33

ARSENIC, LEAD, AND MERCURY

Gerald Maloney and Rachel Goldstein

STAT FACTS
ARSENIC, LEAD, AND MERCURY

Arsenic

- Arsenic is a naturally occurring element with three oxidation states. The trivalent form (arsenite) is considered the most toxic.
- Arsenic is released via various industrial sources (mining, metal smelting) and can contaminate both groundwater and the food chain. Arsenic is also found in pesticides, herficides, and herbal remedies.
- Toxicity varies by amount and duration of exposure, and acute and chronic variations are present.
- From a terrorism perspective, the most significant routes of exposure would be large-scale contamination of the water supply or release of arsine gas in a confined space.

Lead

- Lead exists in both organic and inorganic states. In Western countries, most lead exposure is to the inorganic state, and is from industrial exposures, paint, or moonshine manufacture. Most organic lead exposure comes from leaded gasoline.
- Inorganic lead has both acute and chronic toxicity, both of which can ultimately result in encephalopathy and neurologic impairment.

- Parenteral chelation with British Anti-Lewisite (BAL) and calcium disodium EDTA is recommended for all encephalopathic patients, or asymptomatic patients with blood levels >70 µg/dL.
- From a terrorism perspective, the most likely scenario is poisoning of the water or food supply with either organic or inorganic lead species.

Mercury

- Mercury is a naturally occurring element in the environment and is contributed by human industrial activity.
- The organic form: methylmercury is the most dangerous in regards to the food chain.
- Most common route of exposure for the general population is via fish from streams and oceans as they feed. Food processing and cooking techniques do not significantly reduce the amount of mercury in fish.
- The greatest concern from a bioterrorism standpoint in regards to mercury would be a large vapor exposure in a closed space. In this case it would be more of an irritant or in severe exposures could lead to respiratory distress.

INTRODUCTION

With the exception of arsenic, the heavy metals have not been weaponized in any large scale previously. However, their use as potential terrorist weapons or agents of opportunity should not be underestimated. Arsenic in particular has a long history of use in individual and mass murders, and lead and mercury have been the culprits behind several large-scale environmental disasters. A detailed review of these metals, and their toxic properties, will follow.

ARSENIC

Arsenic is not widely discussed as a potential terrorist chemical weapon, as its ability to acutely affect large numbers of persons simultaneously is limited. However, it does have a long and vibrant history in both intentional and unintentional poisonings and has been developed as a weapon (though never actually deployed in battle) in the Second World War. In addition to intentional poisonings, chronic toxicity from arsenic contamination in the water supply has led to epidemic arsenic poisonings in nations such as China, Taiwan, and Bangladesh. Use of arsenic in Chinese "herbal balls" and some ayurvedic medications has also been described.

Historically, arsenic's use as a weapon was limited primarily to the development of the blistering agent known as *lewisite*. This agent was developed by an American chemist Winford Lee Lewis in 1918 as an alternative to sulfur mustard as it caused immediate pain upon exposure, as opposed to the often delayed effects of sulfur mustard, thereby providing some warning of its presence on the battlefield. It also persisted in the environment for a shorter period of time than sulfur mustard, so that its use on the battlefield would not preclude U.S. forces from occupying any territory vacated by retreating enemy troops. Though developed in 1918, it was not deployed in the First World War but was instead stockpiled and researched during the antebellum period between the wars. Ultimately, lewisite was found to be not as effective an agent as mustard and although some 20,000 tons were produced it was never deployed to the battlefield. U.S. stockpiles of lewisite were chemically neutralized and disposed of decades ago. However, stockpiles of leftover lewisite from the Second World War have been discovered in Korea and China, where ongoing decontamination efforts are occurring.

The most important development related to lewisite, however, is likely the fact that the British Army developed an antidote for lewisite exposure that has become one of the most widely used chelating agents for acute metal toxicity in the world, dimercaprol, or British Anti-Lewisite (BAL). BAL was first synthesized by British biochemists at Oxford University during the Second World War and has since taken its role as a primary chelating agent for acute and chronic heavy metal toxicity, as well as management of Wilson's disease.

Arsenic has been used in poisonings for centuries. The ancient Greeks described topical arsenic for treatment of a variety of skin conditions. Later, when arsenic trioxide was synthesized, it became widely popular as a homicidal agent during the Middle Ages. Arsenic has been used medicinally more recently, as well; Fowler's solution, which was potassium arsenite, was used to treat a variety of conditions including asthma until the 1900s; arsenicals were used to treat syphilis and other spirochetal and protozoal infections into the 1900s. Much more recently, in 2000, the FDA approved the use of arsenic trioxide as a chemotherapeutic agent for acute myelogenous leukemia. Arsenic was widely used as a herbicide and a pesticide (in its arsenite and arsenate forms). Arsine gas, which has unique toxicity, is used in semiconductor manufacturing. Arsenic continues to be an agent of both intentional and unintentional acute poisonings; two recent high-profile cases in New England in which arsenic was used for a mass homicidal poisoning at a church in New Sweden, ME, and ingestion of an arsenical pesticide resulted in the death of a child in Marblehead, MA, occurred in 2003.

Arsenic exists in three valence states, and as arsine gas. *Elemental arsenic* exists in a zero-valence state and has little to no acute human toxicity. It is also the least commonly encountered form. *Inorganic arsenic* is associated with human toxicity and has two primary valence states: the trivalent form [As^{3+}], *arsenite*, and the pentavalent form [As^{5+}], *arsenate*. The trivalent form is usually more toxic than the pentavalent form; however, after ingestion the pentavalent form is converted to varying degrees into the trivalent form and their clinical patterns of toxicity overlap significantly. Arsenic trioxide [As_2O_3] in addition to its medical uses is frequently a by-product of the copper smelting industry. Sodium arsenite and sodium arsenate are also highly soluble inorganic forms of arsenic that have been associated with human toxicity. *Arsine* [AsH_3], unlike the other arsenicals which primarily exist in solid or liquid form, is a gas, and the only arsenical associated with a primarily inhalational exposure. Arsine is primarily produced by the mixing of metallic compounds (primarily zinc) with an acid. Arsine can be rapidly fatal and produces toxicity different from the other arsenicals. *Lewisite*, as described above, is not produced any more but may still be found in old munitions. Lewisite is primarily a dermal exposure, although inhalational exposures have occurred as well and these can result in significant morbidity and death.

PHARMACOKINETICS/TOXICOKINETICS

There are limited data on the kinetic properties of arsenic. Human volunteer studies using radiolabelled arsenic compounds injected intravenously demonstrated a two-phase Vd—initially Vd was calculated at 0.2 L/kg, but redistribution after initial plasma clearance yielded a delayed Vd of ~6 L/kg. It appears to exhibit low protein binding and is excreted primarily (>95%) via the urine. While half-lives in volunteer studies were relatively short, with a majority of arsenic excreted in 2.1 days, the half-life may be significantly prolonged in acute overdose. Inorganic arsenic is converted to both trivalent and pentavalent compounds, with pentavalent compounds being formed in greater amounts in chronic exposure cases. While toxicokinetic data on arsenic are relatively limited, the median lethal dose in humans appears to be 3–4 mg/kg.

The primary route of exposure for inorganic arsenicals is via ingestion, either directly of the compound itself or through ingestion of contaminated meat or water. Arsine is an inhalational exposure; lewisite can involve either inhalational or cutaneous exposure.

PATHOPHYSIOLOGY

Arsenic has a complex pathophysiology that results from multiple interactions at the cellular level. Arsenite binds to intracellular sulfhydryl groups and also inhibits pyruvate dehydrogenase, resulting in disruption of the tricarboxylic acid cycle. Arsenite and its metabolites also inhibit glutathione reductase, thus enhancing cellular susceptibility to oxidative stress. There is also some suggestion that arsenite will increase oxidative free radical formation. Arsenate can substitute in phosphorylation reactions and can also interfere with heme synthesis. Additionally, a wide variety of cellular toxicity involving alterations in DNA expression and cellular signaling has been attributed to arsenic. Arsenic is considered a carcinogen, although experimental models of carcinogenicity are lacking.

Arsine gas possesses a different mechanism of toxicity than the other forms of arsenic. Arsine causes an increase in intracellular calcium in erythrocytes, presumably through binding to sulfhydryl groups and altering ion transport across the cell membrane. This is an effect seen with arsine, not arsenite, suggesting there may be a unique interaction or metabolite formed by the heme-arsine interaction. Arsine begins to exhibit effects almost immediately in the erythrocyte, with hemolysis generally occurring 60 minutes following exposure. Additionally, some arsine is transported to tissues and may be converted to arsenite, resulting in a multisystem toxicity.

Lewisite is primarily a liquid that is a vesicant agent, rapidly causing burning and blistering of the skin. It also has a significant ocular toxicity. Inhalational toxicity, resulting in airway injury and pulmonary edema from loss of the alveolar/capillary membrane, can be seen as well with significant exposures.

CLINICAL MANIFESTATIONS

Arsenic toxicity will present with differing clinical pictures based on whether the exposure is to inorganic arsenic, arsine, or lewisite. It will affect most body systems and especially in chronic or subacute poisonings can have an insidious course.

Inorganic Arsenic (Arsenate, Arsenite)

Inorganic arsenic produces the typical clinical spectra of symptoms associated with arsenic poisoning. For discussion purposes, acute and chronic toxicity will be discussed under the heading of the different organ systems affected.

Central Nervous System

Inorganic arsenic affects the central nervous system (CNS) in both acute and chronic toxicity. The hallmark of arsenic neurotoxicity, whether acute or chronic, is development of a peripheral neuropathy. This is a mixed motor/sensory neuropathy that occurs typically in a stocking-glove distribution and is ascending in nature. Rarely does this result in inhibition of the respiratory muscles. The neuropathy is often described as a "pins and needles" sensation early in its course that gradually progresses with loss of strength, reflexes, and posterior column signs (loss of vibration and position sense). During the recovery phase, a burning pain with allodynia may be seen. Rarely, symptoms may progress to the point of respiratory muscle paralysis. Guillain-Barre Syndrome may be incorrectly diagnosed in these cases. The other major CNS findings in acute toxicity may be encephalopathy and less commonly seizures. Isolated neuropathies of cranial or phrenic nerves have also been reported.

Cardiovascular

The acute cardiovascular effects of inorganic arsenic poisoning are hypotension, which may be orthostatic and related to vasodilation, or due to direct myocardial suppression, and dysrhythmias. QTc prolongation has been commonly reported in arsenic toxicity from both acute and nonacute exposures, with resultant bradycardia, ventricular dysrhythmias, and death. This same phenomenon is noted with subacute and chronic exposures, even with controlled administration of arsenic. Arsenic trioxide chemotherapy has been noted to cause dysrhythmias as well. The other major cardiovascular toxicity, seen in chronic poisoning primarily, is arteriosclerosis. This can be both peripheral and central in nature, and has been linked to increased rates of myocardial infarction, stroke, and peripheral vascular disease. Blackfoot disease, a progressive obliterative peripheral arteriopathy of the lower extremities seen in Taiwan, is related to chronic arsenic exposure.

Gastrointestinal

The primary gastrointestinal (GI) effects in acute toxicity are vomiting and abdominal pain, which generally occurs rapidly after ingestion. The GI symptoms may be prolonged and nonresponsive to IV fluids, which casts doubt on an incorrect diagnosis of gastroenteritis. Pancreatitis, hepatitis, and GI mucosal ulcerations have all been reported with acute poisoning.

Chronic toxicity can cause vomiting and diarrhea as well, but is more commonly associated with hepatotoxicity. Portal hypertension, noncirrhotic portal venous thrombosis, and hepatic angiosarcoma have been reported with chronic arsenic poisoning.

Renal

Acute renal failure that develops from arsenic exposure is generally due to volume depletion, or a pigment nephropathy from rhabdomyolysis. There may be direct nephrotoxicity as well due to depletion of glutathione. Chronic exposure is associated with a progressive nephropathy. Also, genitourinary (GU) tract malignancies, specifically transitional cell carcinoma of the bladder, have been associated with chronic arsenic poisoning.

Hematologic

Hematologic disorders resulting from acute inorganic arsenic poisoning include hemolysis (though to a lesser degree than that associated with arsine) and anemia. Significant myelosuppression may be seen in acute exposure though hematologic disorders are generally seen in chronic toxicity.

Chronic arsenic poisoning can result in aplastic anemia and agranulocytosis. As pentavalent arsenic can also interfere with heme synthesis, this may be another mechanism for development of anemia. In patients receiving arsenic trioxide chemotherapy, a leukemoid reaction, with WBC counts in excess of 100,000/L have been reported.

Pulmonary

Acute inorganic arsenic toxicity may cause an acute lung injury (ALI) picture indistinguishable from that occurring with SIRS or sepsis. Chronic toxicity has been associated with the development of a restrictive lung disease and lung carcinomas (both small cell and nonsmall cell).

Musculoskeletal

Acute toxicity may cause an acute myopathy with rhabdomyolysis. There have been commonly reported musculoskeletal pathologies with chronic arsenic poisoning.

Dermatologic

Acute and chronic poisonings produce different dermatologic findings. Acute toxicity can result in an exfoliative dermatitis or erythroderma. Less commonly, oral mucosal lesions may be seen. Alopecia takes several weeks to develop and may be seen after an acute exposure, or with repeated acute exposures. Mee's lines are uncommon, reportedly occurring in less than 5% of cases. They do not show until a minimum of 30 days after exposure and represent not arsenic deposition but rather disruption of the nail matrix and hyperkeratinization. They can be seen after a large acute exposure or with chronic exposure.

Chronic poisoning causes several different lesions. Hypopigmentation ("raindrops on a dusty road"), hyperkeratosis of the palms and soles, and dermatologic malignancies (squamous and basal cell carcinomas, and Bowen's disease) are reported with chronic exposure.

Arsine

The clinical presentation of arsine gas is rapid onset of jaundice, myalgias, hypotension, hematuria, and mental status changes. The arsine itself is odorless and not an irritant gas, so initial exposure may go unnoticed. Massive hemolysis with profound anemia and cardiovascular collapse may occur. ALI is also a possibility.

Lewisite

Lewisite generally results in a near-immediate burning sensation of the skin or eyes. Blistering and vesiculation of the skin occurs within a few hours. Pulmonary symptoms may occur rapidly with a large inhalational exposure and include ALI; delayed presentation of ALI in patients exposed to lewisite has not been reported.

DIAGNOSTIC TESTING

Diagnosis of acute arsenic poisoning and chronic poisoning are similar in that urine arsenic collection is a mainstay for both. Due to the previously described rapid clearance of arsenic from the plasma, blood testing is of little value with chronic poisoning and limited value in acute poisoning unless done shortly after exposure. Whole blood levels >5 µg/L are considered elevated. Urine testing can be a spot urinary arsenic level, though variations in urinary excretion of arsenic can cause a false-negative test. 24-hour collection is the preferred method. A 24-hour level >50 µg/L is indicative of an elevated urinary arsenic level. If the patient has been eating fish recently, then speciation of the arsenic to determine organic versus inorganic arsenic is needed. Hair and nail testing can be done as well, though there is a more defined body of literature on hair testing. With large exposures to inorganic arsenic, accumulation in the hair within 30 hours of ingestion has been reported, though in general, hair is used as a secondary test if arsenic toxicity is strongly suspected but urine collection fails to yield results.

Given the wide variety of clinical manifestations, laboratory testing for complete blood count, peripheral smear, measurement of renal function, hepatic enzymes, and electrocardiograph are all prudent in the evaluation of suspected arsenic poisoning. Radiography may be helpful to evaluate for radio-opaque foreign bodies in the GI tract.

MANAGEMENT

Management of arsenic toxicity differs somewhat by acute versus chronic, and form of arsenic poisoning. Acute arsenic poisoning cases should first undergo decontamination, of the skin if use of a liquid or vapor form was identified, then of the GI tract if ingestion occurred. Many acute cases will be vomiting already, so induction of emesis is not recommended. Arsenic does not bind to activated charcoal well. If radio-opaque foreign bodies are present in the GI tract, then attempted decontamination with whole bowel irrigation using 1–2 L/h of polyethylene glycol should be undertaken assuming there are no contraindications.

Standard resuscitation including airway management, volume resuscitation with IV crystalloids and blood, and management of dysrhythmias with continuous ECG monitoring should occur. In cases of significant hemolysis after arsine exposure, exchange transfusion may be attempted.

Specific treatment for arsenic involves chelation therapy, irrespective of whether the poisoning is acute or chronic. This is accomplished using dimercaprol (BAL), given in doses of 3–5 mg/kg deep IM every 4 hours. This can be followed with dimercaptosuccinic acid, or succimer, an oral analog of BAL, which is given as 10 mg/kg/dose every 8 hours for the first 5 days, followed by 10 mg/kg/dose every 12 hours for 14 days. The endpoint for chelation is a urinary arsenic level <50 μg/L. D-Penicillamine is not useful for arsenic poisoning. Hemodialysis does not significantly affect arsenic elimination and is not indicated in cases with normal renal function. Arsine is generally not amenable to chelation and supportive care is the preferred method of treatment.

DISPOSITION

Patients with arsenic poisoning should generally be managed on an inpatient basis. Very few cases with acute toxicity will be well enough to go home, and most patients with acute exposure will have been exposed either via a suicidal ingestion or attempted homicidal poisoning. Likewise, chronic toxicity cases are generally suffering a recurrent environmental exposure and will need to have the source of their exposure investigated. Early acute arsenic toxicity may be difficult to differentiate from any other number of conditions, including sepsis. The occurrence of a peripheral neuropathy and QTc prolongation on the ECG should prompt the practitioner to screen for arsenic.

LEAD

Lead is likely the best known, and most commonly screened-for, heavy metal. Though advances in environmental safety in the past four decades have markedly reduced most human lead exposures, it still remains a problem in children, particularly inner-city residents, in industry, and in certain cultures. While lead has not been described as a likely choice for large-scale weaponization, use of smaller quantities of lead to affect a limited number of patients may be possible. More commonly, the emergency or primary care practitioner will see lead poisoning in acute or chronic toxicity.

Much like arsenic and mercury, lead has a colorful history. As lead has a lower melting point than most metals, it was one of the first metals used to formulate weapons, armor, and cookware. Use of lead-based paints stretches back thousands of years. The recognition of clinical lead toxicity dates back almost that far, with descriptions of lead encephalopathy dating back to the ancient Greeks and Romans. The term plumbism was coined in reference to the chemical symbol for lead, Pb. Lead has more recently become an occupational exposure, as well as an exposure for those in environments where lead is still plentiful.

Current lead exposure comes from a multitude of sources. Childhood lead exposure is still a major problem, particularly in urban areas where older (pre-1978) homes may still have lead paint. Children eating paint chips are one of the most common sources of exposure. Also, lead dust on the carpets and in the yards of homes with lead paint, aerosolized lead from sandblasting of leaded paint from homes, lead from older plumbing, lead from clay or pottery glaze, and lead from moonshine production in old radiators are all current common sources of exposure. Other sources include ingestion of lead weights or buckshot. Glass makers, lead smelters, and firing range instructors make up many of the current occupational exposures.

Like arsenic and mercury, lead exists in both inorganic and organic forms, which have markedly different characteristics. Inorganic lead, which accounts for the overwhelming majority of lead exposures, is found in most of the solid lead preparations. Organic lead, or alkyl lead, is more commonly liquid and is found mostly in leaded fuels. Organic lead exposure is uncommon in the United States.

PHARMACOKINETICS/TOXICOKINETICS

Inorganic lead can be absorbed primarily by ingestion and inhalation, with ingestion being the more efficient route. Oral absorption rates of lead with adults and children differ; adults will absorb 10–15% of an ingested dose on average, with children absorbing 30–40%. Cutaneous absorption of inorganic lead is minimal. After absorption, 99% of lead is initially bound to erythrocytes, from which it undergoes a complex redistribution into the CNS, soft tissue, and bone. Half-lives of lead vary by compartment, with bone stores of lead lasting 10–20 years. Organic leads have different absorption and kinetics. Tetraethyl lead is readily absorbed across the skin and is lipophilic, resulting in a rapid distribution to the CNS. Some organic lead may also be converted back into inorganic lead, so in a patient with organic lead exposure they may manifest kinetics and features of both types of poisoning.

PATHOPHYSIOLOGY

Lead has a complex pathophysiology that affects multiple organ systems. It has an affinity for sulfhydryl groups, which allows it to bind to affect several enzymatic structural proteins. It is structurally similar to calcium and can interfere in calcium-mediated processes. It also has mutagenic and cytotoxic effects. One example is lead's well-known ability to interfere with heme synthesis, resulting in accumulation of erythrocyte protoporphyrin (which often binds to zinc, elevating the levels of zinc protoporphyrin).

CLINICAL EFFECTS

Lead has a multitude of acute and chronic effects across several organ systems. The most worrisome involve both acute and chronic effects in the CNS.

Central Nervous System

Lead has a multitude of acute and chronic CNS effects. These are primarily due to lead's interference with neurotransmitter function and cellular function, with resultant encephalopathy, seizures, and cerebral edema. Acute lead encephalopathy is the most dramatic presentation and more commonly described in children though it has also been described in adults. Acute encephalopathy presents with headache, mental status changes, vomiting (often severe), papilledema, seizures, and coma. Cerebral edema may be noted on CT. Encephalopathy may also follow a slower, more insidious course with progressive mental status changes. More subtle chronic findings may include hyperactivity, difficulty concentrating, and developmental delay. Peripheral neurotoxicity of lead is rare now, though the classic description is the motor neuropathy of the radial nerve that resulted in wrist drop. This is more commonly seen in adults who have experienced acute lead encephalopathy.

Cardiovascular

In both adults and children, cardiovascular effects of lead poisoning are rare. ECG abnormalities or myocardial dysfunction have been only infrequently reported.

Gastrointestinal

GI complaints are common in patients of all ages with chronic lead poisoning. Colicky abdominal pain, constipation, and ileus are most commonly reported. Hepatitis, pancreatitis, or surgical illness is rare. Perforation of the stomach or bowel by ingested lead pellets has been reported but is extremely uncommon.

Renal

Lead nephrotoxicity is more commonly reported in adults with lead exposure and has been reported to progress to the point of needing renal replacement therapy. More commonly, a progressive decline in renal function with resulting hypertension has been reported. Significant renal impairment may exacerbate the chronic anemia seen in most cases of lead toxicity (Table 33-1).

Hematologic

The primary hematologic effect of lead is anemia caused by interference with heme synthesis. This is most often a normocytic or microcytic hypochromic anemia with the classically described finding of basophilic stippling.

Pulmonary

Lead rarely causes acute pulmonary toxicity but significant inhalational exposures can present with a SIRS-like picture. ALI and bronchospasm are rare in both acute and chronic lead exposure.

Musculoskeletal

Lead deposits to a large degree in bone and soft tissue. While this rarely causes any direct effects beyond occasional myalgias or arthralgias, the potentially large bone burden of lead can be a reservoir from which lead can gradually equilibrate into the central compartment and result in a recrudescence of blood lead levels (BLL) after chelation treatment.

Dermatologic

As opposed to arsenic and mercury, there are no significant pathognomonic skin lesions for lead toxicity. A bluish-purple

TABLE 33-1

OVERVIEW OF LEAD TOXICITY

Mild	Moderate	Severe
BLL <45 µg/dL	BLL 45–69 µg/dL	BLL 70 µg/dL and higher
Clinical findings: Asymptomatic, mild CNS symptoms (confusion, cognitive impairment); may see mild anemia or elevated EPP/ZPP levels	Clinical findings: may be asymptomatic; GI: vomiting, abdominal pain CNS: headache, confusion; anemia, elevated EPP/ZPP level	Clinical findings: rarely asymptomatic; headache, encephalopathy, seizures, vomiting, abdominal pain
Treatment: controversial; currently routine chelation not recommended	Treatment: if no vomiting or significant CNS symptoms, dimercaptosuccinic acid (Succimer)	Treatment: IV calcium disodium edetate and intramuscular dimercaprol

line across the gingiva, related to lead deposition, is called the Burton Line.

Reproductive

Lead exposure is associated with fertility issues, with direct toxicity to the gametes in chronic lead exposure. The effects after a single acute exposure are unclear.

Organic Lead

The clinical presentation of organic lead toxicity differs somewhat from inorganic, with CNS symptoms including mental status changes, delirium, seizures, coma and death reported, as well as tremors and increased DTRs. Hepatitis and acute renal failure have been reported. However, hematologic disorders are rare.

DIAGNOSTIC TESTING

The whole BLL is the standard measurement used to clinically correlate lead exposure. This is most commonly reported in μg/dL and is often used to guide therapy. The erythrocyte protoporphyrin (EPP), or zinc protoporphyrin (ZPP) level can gauge chronicity of exposure but is in itself not sensitive enough to guide therapy. Urine and hair screening is not routinely employed in either screening or diagnosis of lead toxicity. In addition to the BLL, a complete blood count (evaluate for anemia), chemistry (for electrolytes and renal function), and urinalysis (for proteinuria) are recommended screening tests.

Radiographic imaging of the patient with lead exposure can be done to detect the presence of ingested lead (such as paint chips) in the GI tract, or as a marker of total body lead burden in children (skeletal survey for lead lines). Lead lines represent regions of grow arrest in the diaphyseal regions, not actual lead deposition, though their presence suggests significant lead skeletal burden. In patients with encephalopathy, cranial CT imaging evaluating specifically for cerebral edema is recommended.

MANAGEMENT

Management of lead poisoning differs based on age, symptoms, and BLLs. The general breakdown is acute versus chronic toxicity and adult versus pediatric. The common thread in both groups is removal from the source of lead exposure first and foremost.

General supportive care for seizures, as well as treatment for elevated ICP, is the initial mainstay for encephalopathic patients. For nonencephalopathic patients, appropriate symptomatic care while waiting for BLLs is indicated.

The encephalopathic patient, regardless of age, needs immediate chelation therapy. This is accomplished with use of BAL 3–5 mg/kg IM every 4 hours for 5 days, with initiation of calcium disodium EDTA therapy after the first

dose of BAL at 1500 mg/m^2 as either a continuous drip or bid-qid in separate IV doses. The EDTA therapy is continued based on BLLs and symptoms (resolution of encephalopathy). The combination of BAL and EDTA is considered superior to either alone.

In patients who are not encephalopathic, a BLL >100 in adults or >70 in children is considered an indication for combined BAL/EDTA therapy. In adults with levels between 70 and 100, oral chelation with succimer for 14–19 days should be initiated. Adults who are asymptomatic with a level <70 do not routinely require chelation and will benefit primarily from removal from the environment.

Children are managed differently, largely due to the effects of lead of cognitive development. Children at levels >70 will require BAL and EDTA chelation regardless of symptoms. Children with levels between 45 and 70 can be managed with succimer or a combination of succimer and EDTA. Children at levels <45 are controversial; while routine chelation is not recommended, there are some experts who will chelate at levels as low as 20.

Organic lead compounds represent a special case. The BLL does not correlate to neurotoxicity and the benefits of chelation therapy are unclear. Supportive care is still recommended, and chelation may be attempted, but firm evidence of its efficacy is lacking.

DISPOSITION

All acutely symptomatic or encephalopathic patients need to be admitted, as do any patients requiring parenteral chelation. Importantly, even in patients not requiring parenteral chelation, if a return to a lead-free environment cannot be secured then admission for social reasons may be required. This is especially true for pediatric patients. Patients with mild symptoms not requiring parenteral chelation, who can be guaranteed a safe environment and close outpatient follow-up, can be discharged. BLLs should be monitored until the completion of chelation therapy with target BLLs reached.

MERCURY

Although mercury toxicity is not a commonly encountered clinical diagnosis, fear of mercury effects is substantiated. Clinicians are unlikely to see a true case of mercury poisoning in a decade; however, they are very likely to be questioned weekly regarding mercury exposure from a variety of sources, including dietary, medicinal, and environmental.

Mercury is an element that has a long history of use in industry, medicine, and dentistry. It is present in all soil and water, and is mined from ore in locations throughout the world. Its release into the air and accumulation in water has been greatly enhanced over the last century by industrial activity, but has always occurred from volcanoes, erosion, and fires. Once extracted from ore, it is a liquid in its elemental form. It is heavy, having a density approximately 14 times that of water. It has several valence states (0, +1, +2) meaning that it can exist in its elemental form or bound to other compounds.

The toxic effects depend both on the form of mercury present and the route of exposure to the patient. Mercury is biopersistent; in other words, once incorporated by an organism, its elimination is slow or incomplete. Mercury can be bioconcentrated, bioaccumulated, and biomagnified.

PROPERTIES

The most common forms of mercury are metallic, cinnabar ore, mercuric chloride, and methylmercury. These different forms are differentiated below:

Metallic Mercury

Metallic mercury (i.e., elemental, inorganic, and organic) is the most familiar form to most people; this is a silvery, shiny metal that is liquid at room temperature. Mercury vapor is colorless and odorless. Its most common use has been in thermometers, barometers, batteries, fluorescent lights, and electrical switches. Liquid metallic mercury is also used in producing chlorine gas and caustic soda, and in extracting gold from ore. Dental amalgams (contain tin, silver, and sometimes gold dissolved in mercury) contain up to 50% metallic mercury. Controversy exists around replacing silver fillings to decrease mercury exposure. It has been found to be more dangerous to remove multiple fillings than to leave them in place. The danger occurs when heating the filling material to remove it thereby releasing high levels of mercury vapor.

Inorganic Mercury

Inorganic mercury compounds occur when mercury combines with oxygen, sulfur (aka cinnabar red powder, which turns black with ultraviolet [UV] exposure), or chlorine. This forms a mercury salt, which is identified as a white powder or crystalline material. Mercury is mined as cinnabar ore, which contains mercuric sulfide. Mercuric sulfide is then heated to vaporize the mercury, which is then captured and cooled to form liquid metallic mercury.

Inorganic mercury was a common ingredient in disinfectants and topical preparations. Mercurous chloride was regularly used as a laxative, teething powder, and deworming medication. Thimerosal is a common ingredient in vaccines as a preservative agent. Some reports have linked exposure to thimerosal in childhood vaccines as a cause for autism, but this has not been proven to date.

Organic Mercury

Organic mercury is formed when mercury combines with oxygen forming many different compounds. The one of most concern to human exposure (and that which will be discussed in this text) is methylmercury (MM). Bacteria and fungi bioconvert to produce different forms of mercury, with MM being the most common. Bioconcentration and bioaccumulation are characteristics of all persistent contaminants that are incorporated into organisms low on the food chain, which are then consumed by higher predators. In the case of mercury, aquatic anaerobic bacteria convert elemental mercury into organic MM. This form of mercury is a potent neurotoxin; thus the effect of mercury has been magnified by these organisms. These features have raised concern regarding the effects of environmental mercury on human health.

MM used to be found in antifungal agents in seed grains and interior/exterior paints. This use has been banned as mercury vapor was released during painting.

TOXICOKINETICS/ROUTES OF EXPOSURE

Metallic Mercury

The American Association of Poison Control Centers received calls for more then 21,000 mercury exposures in 2001. More than 80% of these were the result of broken thermometers. Of all these calls, there was one reported death. This resulted from inhalation of a large volume of mercury fumes released in a small space. Vacuuming metallic mercury increases the temperature of mercury therefore increasing one's vapor exposure.

Inorganic Mercury

Historically, pediatric mercury toxicity was most commonly seen with inorganic mercury salts. The use of calomel (mercurous chloride) as a teething agent resulted in large numbers of children receiving small, repeated doses of mercury salts. Although most clinicians today will encounter questions regarding exposures to elemental mercury, such as from broken thermometers, the driving force behind expressed concerns are fears related to possible effects of organic mercury.

Organic Mercury (MM)

Despite the rarity of significant acute effects from casual exposure to elemental mercury, a very emotionally charged debate continues because of the possibility of neurologic effects from chronic exposure, predominantly to organic mercury compounds. The high-profile neurologic disasters of Minamata Bay and the Iraqi grain episodes serve as a reminder of the possible neurotoxic effects of large amounts of mercury. In Minamata, Japan, 23 infants with cerebral palsy and retardation were born to mothers who ingested contaminated seafood. The mothers had some numbness of fingers and fatigue as the only symptoms of exposure. The Iraqi grain episode consisted of ingestion of grain tainted with organic mercury as a fungicide. This also resulted in cerebral palsy and mental retardation. These two large population exposures demonstrated the transplacental fetal exposure to mercury.

MM crosses the placenta and binds with higher concentration to fetal RBCs than to maternal RBCs (This indicates that MM binds more strongly to fetal hemoglobin than maternal hemoglobin). This is the source of debate on the role of exposure to much smaller amounts of mercury that are applicable to the general population, and to higher risk groups such as pregnant women and neonates.

PATHOPHYSIOLOGY

Once absorbed systemically, mercury has a predilection for the kidneys, liver, spleen, and CNS. Short-chain alkylmercurials (methyl- and ethylmercury) penetrate RBCs and bind to hemoglobin. MM crosses the blood-brain barrier (BBB), with mercury being sequestered in the lysosomal dense bodies of neurons. Mercurials are attracted to sulfhydryl groups and bind to enzymes and metalloproteins. As one example, mercury combines with the sulfhydryl group of S-adenosylmethionine, which is a cofactor for catecholamine-O-methyltransferase (COMT). The inhibition of COMT allows accumulation of norepinephrine, epinephrine, and dopamine; this may account for some of the symptoms seen in acrodynia and erethism.

Metallic Mercury

Swallowing elemental mercury is considered nontoxic and may pass relatively unchanged. Although, the presence of anatomic defects such as a fistula, abdominal perforation, or slow GI transit may be associated with increased absorption.

Mercury vapor is rapidly absorbed through the respiratory tract. Once absorbed through the alveolar membrane, mercury has a predilection for the kidneys, liver, spleen, and nervous system. The CNS peak concentrations may be delayed for a few days following an intense vapor exposure. The elimination of elemental mercury has a biphasic pattern with an initial rapid decline followed by a slower phase resulting in a biological half-life of approximately 60 days. Both the fecal and urinary routes eliminate mercury.

Inorganic Mercury

Contrary to metallic mercury, inorganic mercury is primarily absorbed through the GI tract, although only 10% of a given dose will be absorbed. The most common salt is mercuric chloride (divalent), which requires dissociation before it can be absorbed. Calomel (mercurous chloride) a monovalent salt requires transformation to a divalent compound to be absorbed. Tegumental absorption of inorganic salts is well-documented by various cases of toxicity following dermal application of ointments or powders containing calomel.

Once absorbed, inorganic mercury concentrations drop rapidly. Inorganic mercury concentrates within the kidneys primarily affecting the renal tubules. In the blood, the inorganic mercury is equally distributed within the RBCs and protein plasma bound. Due to its poor liposolubility, inorganic mercury poorly penetrates the CNS but once it crosses the BBB it will concentrate in the cerebral and cerebellar cortices. Excretion of inorganic mercury is primarily fecal however urinary excretion is observed following chronic exposure.

Organic Mercury (Methylmercury)

Organic mercury (like inorganic mercury) is primarily absorbed through the GI tract although dermal and inhalational absorption may be a concern. MM is approximately 90% absorbed through the GI tract. This percentage decreases with longer alkyl chains. Given their lipid solubility, once absorbed, organic mercurial compounds readily cross the BBB as well as the placenta and adhere to RBCs. The half-life of methylmercury in the child is uncertain. Adult data reveal a half-life of approximately 40–50 days. In a study of metabolism of thimerosal in infants following vaccinations found that the elimination half-life of mercury was approximately 7 days and that the GI tract is a possible mode of elimination of parenterally administered thimerosal. When ingested, MM is primarily (90%) eliminated through feces.

Although CNS damage is diffuse, MM's neurotoxicity is characterized by damage within the cerebellum, calcarine fissure, and precentral gyrus. The classic triad of MM toxicity includes dysarthria, ataxia, and constricted visual fields. Perinatal exposure to MM has resulted in mental retardation and cerebral palsy type syndrome as previously mentioned. The fetus is most sensitive to the effects of mercury during the third and fourth months of pregnancy. The effects of toxicity may not be noticed until developmental milestones are delayed (i.e., walking, talking, memory, language, and attention span). Once the baby is born, the health threat from maternal mercury exposure is not of concern. This includes exposure to breast milk.

CLINICAL MANIFESTATIONS

Clinical manifestations for mercury compounds affect mostly the respiratory, nervous, skin, GI, and GU systems.

RESPIRATORY SYSTEM

Metallic Mercury

Inhalation of mercury vapor results in acute respiratory distress and noncardiac pulmonary edema.

NERVOUS SYSTEM

Metallic Mercury

Vapor exposure can produce a variety of symptoms. These include personality changes, tremors, visual changes (narrowing of visual field), deafness, muscle incoordination, loss of sensation, and memory difficulties.

Organic Mercury

Symptoms following acute exposures to organic mercurials are delayed by several days. Progressive neurologic deterioration with personality changes, visual field constriction, cerebellar dysfunction, and coma may ensue. Acrodynia (aka Pink disease) is the usual presentation of mercury poisoning in children. Clinical features include an erythematous rash involving the extremities that later desquamates, insomnia, personality changes, irritability, profuse sweating, hypertension, and tachycardia. Although rarely seen now following the removal of mercury salt containing teething powders (calomel), individual cases still occur following inhalation exposure to elemental mercury, and previously to phenylmercuric fungicide containing house paint. A case presentation in 2001 describes an 11-year-old boy presenting with all of the aforementioned symptoms. There was a delay in his diagnosis, highlighting the other conditions in the differential. Presumably because mercury causes accumulation of norepinephrine, epinephrine, and dopamine, the symptoms can easily be confused with pheochromocytoma, minus the rash. Also of similarity in presentation is Kawasaki's disease (fever, rash, adenopathy, eye changes, mucous membrane involvement, and extremity involvement), especially atypical Kawasaki's disease.

SKIN AND MUCOUS MEMBRANES

Metallic Mercury

Short-term exposure (in hours) to metallic mercury can damage the lining of the mouth and irritate lungs and airways.

This results in chest tightness, burning sensation in lungs, and coughing. Direct skin contact can cause rashes. A larger inhalation exposure following the recovery from the inhalation effects of mercury vapor leads to an erosive dermatitis and a neurologic syndrome called erethism. Patients with erethism commonly have mood swings and shyness or social withdrawal.

GASTROINTESTINAL

Metallic Mercury

The GI absorption of metallic mercury from ingestion is negligible and is considered nontoxic.

Inorganic Mercury

The ingestion of mercury salts is very rare, although may be seen with accidental or suicidal ingestion of pesticides containing mercuric chloride. Vomiting, abdominal cramps, diarrhea, and resulting cardiovascular collapse are secondary to volume loss.

GENITOURINARY

All forms of mercury can affect the kidneys secondary to accumulation of mercury. If the damage to the kidneys is not too great, the kidneys can recover once the mercury load has been cleared from body tissues.

Inorganic Mercury

Acute tubular necrosis may result after oral ingestion as well as immune-mediated glomerulonephritis. (See Table 33-2.)

LABORATORY ANALYSIS

The diagnosis of mercury poisoning is done via a combination of clinical and laboratory features. Tests involve

TABLE 33-2

MERCURY SIGNS AND SYMPTOMS SUMMARIZED

Form(HG)	Route of Exposure	Target Organ	Symptoms	Biomonitoring	Treatment
Metallic	Inhaled vapors	Pulmonary CNS	Occur within hours: dyspnea, which may progress to ARDS; delayed neurologic symptoms	Urinary excretion (Timed)	Chelation
Inorganic	Ingestion	GI and renal	Vomiting, bloody diarrhea, ATN	Urinary excretion (Timed)	IVF/Volume
Organic	Ingestion	CNS	Paresthesias, ataxia, visual field constriction, behavioral changes, coma	Whole blood	Chelation

urine, blood, and hair samples. Nursing mothers may have their breast milk tested for mercury levels if any of the aforementioned sources do not contain significant levels of mercury. Although it must be noted that none of these will give perfect results.

Of critical importance is modification of dietary intake (no seafood or seaweed-based dietary supplements for several days prior to collection) and avoiding potential external contaminants (collection container and transport media). Fish that is known to contain larger levels of mercury are the predatory species: shark, ray, swordfish, orange roughy, and bluefin tuna. In general, a timed urine collection is the most reliable method for determining body burden of mercury. This will generally reflect exposures over the previous month or two. Although hair analysis at a reputable laboratory may be useful for documenting long-term excessive exposure, this is generally more of a research, rather than clinical, tool. Hair will also reflect exogenous environmental contaminants that may not contribute to mercury body burden or toxicity. Blood mercury determinations are greatly effected by recent dietary intake and quickly decline following acute exposures. For chronic exposures, concentration of mercury in hair is 300 times that of blood. Spot urine measurements of urinary mercury may be inconsistent secondary to diurnal variations in excretion. Nonetheless, they may be useful as screening tests or at the initiation of therapy in a clinically poisoned patient. Twenty-four-hour urine mercury measurements yield the best estimate of mercury excretion. A practical compromise would be a measurement of mercury concentration in a first void or early AM collection (e.g., bagged overnight), as this would reflect an approximately 8-hour collection. Urinary excretion under normal conditions should generally not exceed 50 μg in 24 hours.

It is important to note that levels are only used to reflect any adverse health effects that may be likely to occur. Mercury in urine is for exposure to metallic mercury vapor and inorganic forms. Whole blood and hair is used for MM exposure. None of these measurements can tell the exact quantity of exposure. The exception is MM due to its predicted decrease in blood by one-half every 3 days once exposure is ceased. This is most useful after short-term exposures, not long-term. Hair samples for MM can give a snapshot of exposure for up to 1 year (depending on length of hair). Short-term exposure to metallic mercury vapor can be measured in the breath (some people will report a metallic taste after exposure). This method only works for acute exposures and can be inaccurate.

DECONTAMINATION/TREATMENT

Decontamination always begins with removing oneself from the source. With regard to metallic mercury immediate ventilation and moving to fresh air immediately is critical, containing any spill of metallic mercury in an airtight container and not vacuuming up mercury beads. Wash with soap and water and remove all contaminated clothing and place in a plastic bag. Always contact local or state health department. In the event of ingestion of inorganic mercury or metallic mercury, an x-ray is a good choice to follow foreign body. The use of chelating agents has not been proven and is controversial. This applies to MM as well.

Elemental Mercury Exposure

Ingestion: GI absorption of elemental mercury may become a clinical concern when the mercury is trapped in the appendix and bacterial action creates organic mercurials that are readily absorbed. There is ongoing controversy over the proper management of retained mercury in the appendix. It is reasonable to obtain an abdominal radiograph after a large ingestion (e.g., a ruptured Miller-Abbott tube) and follow urinary excretion if there is residual retained mercury.

Inhalation: Significant symptoms require exposure to amounts of mercury in vapor form greatly in excess of those found immediately after a household or office mercury spill. The importance of minimizing vaporization after a spill should therefore be emphasized. Protocols for spill management include visualizing mercury droplets with a bright light, scraping together all visible mercury using an adsorbent product if possible, and avoiding dispersion or vaporization by such methods as sweeping or vacuuming. A special mercury vacuum with restricted exhaust is available for larger spills. Assistance should be sought from the state Department of Environmental Protection and the regional poison control center for spills larger than a household clinical thermometer. Efforts to reduce the reliance on mercury measuring devices (such as sphygmomanometers and thermometers) are worthwhile, given the cost and environmental concern with spills from these items.

Inorganic Mercury

Treatment is focused on volume resuscitation and prevention of acute tubular necrosis and resultant renal failure.

Organic or Methylmercury

The progression of neurologic dysfunction following organic mercurial exposure is poorly amenable to treatment. A radiograph to document the source of any ongoing absorption is reasonable. As the central nervous system uptake is very rapid, chelation therapy with such agents as dimethylsuccinic acid or other chelators is ineffective. Nonetheless, it is often offered, with monitoring of urinary excretion during and after treatment.

DISPOSITION

Current recommendations from the federal government to protect public health include levels that are acceptable in drinking water, workplace, and dietary levels in regards to fish and shellfish. Both the EPA (Environmental Protection Agency) and FDA have set a limit of 2 parts inorganic mercury per billion parts water in drinking water. EPA recommends 144 parts per trillion inorganic mercury in lakes, streams, and rivers.

FDA limit on seafood products is 1 ppm MM. If levels exceed 1 ppm MM, fish and shellfish may be seized as well as grains.

Current recommendations for pregnant women or women to become pregnant in the next 6 months are to avoid predatory fish all together (shark, ray, swordfish, barramundi, gemfish, orange roughy, ling, or bluefin tuna). Limit tuna steaks to one portion per week and canned tuna to two (140 g) cans per week. Currently there is no restriction on salmon (fresh or canned). Levels of mercury in breast milk are generally not high enough to be of concern. Once the baby is out of the womb, the risk of mercury toxicity from maternal consumption is not of issue. It is best to avoid feeding young children any of the aforementioned predatory fish. For the most part unless one is eating large quantities of fish containing mercury regularly, the concern for mercury toxicity following the above guidelines is low as the body does clear mercury over time. The greatest concern from a bioterrorism standpoint in regards to mercury would be a large vapor exposure in a closed space. In this case it would be more of an irritant or in severe exposures could lead to respiratory distress.

Suggested Reading

ATSDR Public Health Statement for Mercury 1999. Toxicological Profile for mercury. Atlanta, GA: U.S. Department of Health and Human Services, Public Health Service.
American Academy of Pediatrics Committee on Environmental Health. Lead exposure in children: prevention, detection, and management. *Pediatrics.* 2005 Oct;116(4):1036–46.
Azziz-Baumgartner, E., Luber, G., Schurz-Rogers H, et al. Exposure assessment of a mercury spill in a Nevada school–2004. *Clin Toxicol* 2007.
Brodkin E, Copes R, Mattman A, et al. Lead and mercury exposures: interpretation and action. *CMAJ.* 2007 Jan 2;176(1):59–63.
Bush A, DuRoss F. Mercury monitoring. Vermont Monitoring Cooperative. May 19, 1995. Available at *http//www.uvm.edu/~snrdept/hg.html*
Canfield RL, Henderson CR, Cory-Slechta DA, et al. Intellectual impairment in children with blood lead concentrations below 10 microg per deciliter. *N Engl J Med.* 2003 Apr 17;348(16):1517–1526.
CDC: Elemental Mercury Releases Attributed to Antiques—New York, 2000-2006. *MMWR,* June 15,2007:56(23):576–579.
Clarkston TW. Mercury: an element of mystery. *N Engl J Med.* 1990;323(16):1137–1139.
Duenas-Laita A, Perez-Miranda M, Gonzalez-Lopez MA, et al. Acute arsenic poisoning. *Lancet.* 2005 Jun 4–10;365(9475):1982.
Drasch G., Bosese-O' Reilly S., Illig S., Increase of renal excretion of organo-mercury compounds like methylmercury by DMPS. (2,3-Dimercapto-1-propane-sulfonic acid, Dimaval® *Clin Toxicol* 2007:45:266–269.
Erickson T, Ahrens W, Aks S, et al. *Pediatric Toxicology: Diagnosis and Management of the Poisoned Child.* New York: McGraw-Hill. 2004, pp. 468–475.
Graeme KA, Pollack CV Jr. Heavy metal toxicity, Part I: arsenic and mercury. *J Emerg Med.* 1998 Jan–Feb;16(1):45–56.
Ibrahim D, Froberg B, Wolf A, et al. Heavy metal poisoning: clinical presentations and pathophysiology. *Clin Lab Med.* 2006 Mar;26(1):67–97.
Katz SA, Katz RB. Use of hair analysis for evaluating mercury intoxication for evaluating mercury intoxication of the human body: a review. *J Appl Toxicol.* 1992;12:79–84.
Kosnett MJ, Wedeen RP, Rothenberg SJ et al, Recommendations for medical management of adult lead exposure. *Environ Health Perspective.* 2007:115:463–471.
Mahaffey KR. Recent advances in recognition of low-level methylmercury poisoning: a review. *Curr Opin Neurol.* 2000 Dec;13(6):699–707.
Morgan BW, Todd KH, Moore B. Elevated blood lead levels in urban moonshine drinkers. *Ann Emerg Med.* 2001 Jan;37(1):51–4.
Phleps RW, Clarkston TW, Kershaw TG, et al. Interrelationship of blood and hair mercury concentrations in North American population exposed to methyl mercury. *Arch Environ Health.* 1980;35:161–8.
Shih H, Gartner JC Jr. Weight loss, hypertension, and limb pain in an 11 yr old boy. *J Pediatr.* 2001 Apr;138(4):566–9.
Sixteenth report of the joint FAO/WHO expert committee in food additives, 1972, No. 505.

34

PULMONARY AGENTS

James W. Rhee

INTRODUCTION

Any gas can cause toxicity in humans—even inert gases can cause toxicity by displacing oxygen. However, gases with irritant properties are the ones that are typically used as warfare or mass casualty agents. Pulmonary irritant gases have been used since World War I to cause mass casualties. The prototypical agents when used for warfare are chlorine and phosgene gases.

On April 22, 1915, the German army released over 150 tons of chlorine gas against the Allied Forces resulting in injuries or death to more than half of Allied soldiers present. This was the first time a pulmonary agent was used effectively in modern warfare. Later that same year, the German army used phosgene gas with more lethal results. These events marked the introduction of pulmonary agents as weapons of mass destruction. Given the devastating effects of the chemical agents—including the pulmonary agents—the League of Nations instituted a ban on chemical weapons in 1918.

However, pulmonary agents are still widely available as they are used in many industries worldwide. Industrial and transportation accidents—not war or acts of terrorism—account for most of the injuries and deaths from these agents.

EPIDEMIOLOGIC OVERVIEW

During World War I, there were reportedly 100,000 deaths and 1.2 million casualties. While this accounts for less than 3% of the deaths during the war, these gases had a profound psychological impact on the soldiers. These toxic gases created immense fear as they were viewed as a silent and unseen killer.

In day-to-day life, many individuals are exposed to irritant gases. People are exposed to chlorine gas at very low levels when around swimming pools without any significant clinical effects. Some more significant exposures result when an unwary individual mixes ammonia and chlorine bleach together in an attempt to create a cleaning solution—this combination results in the formation of chloramine gas. Most individuals will remove themselves from the exposure before significant injury can occur given the highly irritating property of this gas.

Industrial accidents have resulted in mass casualties. One of the most significant disasters occurred in Bhopal, India, when a Union Carbide plant involved in the manufacture of pesticides accidentally released methyl isocyanate gas. This incident killed at least 3800 people and led to significant morbidity and premature death of many thousands more.

PATHOGENESIS

Irritant gases dissolve in the mucosal water to form an acid or alkali. Some irritant gases may also generate reactive oxygen species and other free radicals. Once these damaging mediators are formed, direct injury to the surrounding tissue ensues.

Precipitation of the irritant gas in the eyes and oropharynx leads to pain, erythema, injection, and induration. In the lungs, injury to the bronchopulmonary tree can lead to acute lung injury with subsequent impaired gas exchange and resulting hypoxemia.

In general, irritant gases fall into one of three categories (see Table 34-1). These differ based on the solubility of the chemical in water. Agents that are highly water-soluble are highly irritating in low concentration—these include ammonia, chloramine, hydrogen fluoride, hydrogen chloride, and sulfur dioxide.

Since these highly water-soluble agents are highly irritating, they are said to have good warning properties, since they produce burning in the eyes, nose, and throat immediately on exposure. More intense exposures may lead to more significant sequelae such as corneal injury, dyspnea, stridor, bronchospasm, or upper airway obstruction. Prolonged exposures may allow these gases to travel further down the respiratory tract resulting in injury to the lower respiratory tract.

Agents that are only slightly water-soluble are often nonirritating in moderate to high concentrations—some agents, in fact, may even be pleasant leading an unwary individual to breathe in even deeper. Phosgene, the agent used so effectively during World War I, is the prototype of these slightly water-soluble agents. It has an odor described as "freshly mown hay," and was more effective than chlorine during World War I because it lacked the adverse qualities even at toxic doses. Because of this property, exposed individuals do not feel the need to remove themselves from the exposure and subsequently tend to remain in the toxic environment. The resulting prolonged exposure allows the gas to reach the lower respiratory tract and alveoli. The ensuing dissolution of the gas in this area leads to direct injury and inflammation with resulting acute lung injury.

Ozone and oxides of nitrogen such as nitrogen dioxide are examples of some other slightly water-soluble gases. Although initially asymptomatic, patients exposed to significant concentrations of these slightly water-soluble agents may not have any marked initial symptoms—however, they can develop pulmonary edema several hours after exposure.

The agents that are moderately water-soluble fall in between the other two classes of irritant gasses. They are irritating in high concentrations but may be quite tolerable at low levels. Chlorine, the first effective pulmonary agent used by the German army in World War I, is the prototypical agent of this class.

CLINICAL PRESENTATION

Patients exposed to irritant gases will present differently based on the water solubility of the gas (see Fig. 34-1). Gases that are highly water-soluble will produce symptoms predominantly around the eyes and the mucous membranes of the oropharynx and upper respiratory tract. Symptoms may include conjunctival irritation, lacrimation, pharyngitis, nasal irritation, rhinorrhea, hoarseness, stridor, and coughing. If the exposure is significant or prolonged, then symptoms may become more severe and can lead to airway obstruction, pulmonary edema, and/or acute lung injury.

Pulmonary irritants that are less water-soluble produce a much more insidious picture as the ocular, upper airway, and oropharyngeal effects may not be pronounced after an exposure. These agents typically diffuse down into the lower respiratory tract and alveoli subsequently causing injury at these sites. Symptoms from these exposures may be delayed up to a day after the initial exposure.

TABLE   34-1

SOME COMMON IRRITANT GASES AND RELATIVE WATER SOLUBILITY

Highly Water-Soluble	Moderately Water-Soluble	Slightly Water-Soluble
Ammonia (NH_3)	Chlorine (Cl_2)	Nitrogen dioxide (NO_2)
Chloramine (NH_2Cl)	Hydrogen sulfide (H_2S)*	Ozone (O_3)
Formaldehyde (HCHO)		Phosgene ($COCl_2$)
Hydrogen chloride (HCl)		
Hydrogen fluoride (HF)*		
Methyl isocyanate (C_2H_3NO)		
Sulfur dioxide (SO_2)		

*Hydrogen fluoride and hydrogen sulfide have associated systemic toxicity not addressed in this chapter.

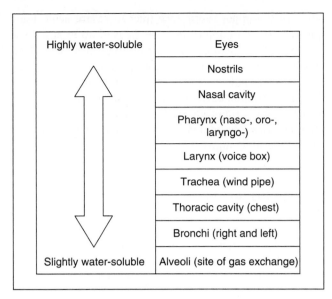

Highly water-soluble	Eyes
	Nostrils
	Nasal cavity
	Pharynx (naso-, oro-, laryngo-)
	Larynx (voice box)
	Trachea (wind pipe)
	Thoracic cavity (chest)
	Bronchi (right and left)
Slightly water-soluble	Alveoli (site of gas exchange)

FIGURE 34-1

Highly water-soluble gases have greater effects on the upper respiratory tract while the slightly water-soluble gases have greater effects on the lower respiratory tract.

DIAGNOSIS

Diagnosis is based primarily on the history. There is no definitive test that can confirm a diagnosis of toxicity from a pulmonary agent. A clinician, however, should be wary if multiple patients present for respiratory symptoms (Table 34-2). The constellation of symptoms may vary based on the properties of the offending agent as well as the dose of exposure. Patients may present early after exposure to a pulmonary agent with upper airway symptoms—the severity may range from mild irritation to life-threatening airway obstruction. However, given that a lot of the early symptoms can be fairly mild and self-limited, some patients may not seek medical care early after an exposure. For those who have had more intense or prolonged exposure to an irritant gas, they may present later with dyspnea, productive cough, rales, hypoxemia, and decreased breath sounds—evidence of acute lung injury.

Chest radiographs can help with the diagnosis of injury to the lungs. However, radiographic findings often lag behind clinical findings—a normal chest radiograph early

TABLE 34-2

DIFFERNTIAL DIAGNOSIS OF PULMONARY AGENT EXPOSURE

- Riot control agents (Pulmonary edema is rare)
- Nerve agents (Rhinorrhea and bronchial secretions occur)
- Vesicant inhalation (Pulmonary hemorrhage occurs rather than pulmonary edema)
- Arsine (Dyspnea is due to hemolysis)

after exposure is the rule rather than the exception. Classically, acute lung injury manifests as bilateral pulmonary infiltrates on chest radiographs.

Arterial blood gases and pulse oximetry can help detect hypoxemia that results from pulmonary agent-induced acute lung injury. However, initial normal oxygenation is not a reliable marker of good prognosis as the lung injury may be delayed after exposure.

Corneal fluorescein staining and examination with a cobalt-blue slit lamp or a Wood's lamp can reveal evidence of corneal damage.

MEDICAL MANAGEMENT

Removal from exposure and decontamination is paramount. Continued exposure to a pulmonary irritant gas will only lead to more injury. However, appropriate protection should be provided to the first responders. The patient's clothes should be removed as well and appropriately bagged. Dermal decontamination with copious amounts of water may be necessary if there is any concern about the presence of residual liquids or other toxic products on the skin.

Because upper airway swelling may be profound and lead to stridor and upper airway occlusion, aggressive airway management is critical. Visualization of the vocal cords and supraglottic area is indicated in these severely symptomatic patients. Although, when establishing an airway, orotracheal or nasotracheal intubation is preferred—cricothyrotomy may become necessary in the setting of profound airway edema.

Supplemental oxygen should be used as needed to treat hypoxemia. Bronchospasm should be treated with inhaled β-adrenergic agonists.

The role of corticosteroids in the setting of irritant gas exposures is not clear. However, the administration of corticosteroids is probably warranted in cases where severe symptoms are present—such as, severe upper airway edema, severe bronchospasm, or severe acute lung injury.

Sodium bicarbonate solution administered by inhalation has been shown to provide symptomatic relief and improve pulmonary function in patients exposed to chlorine—inhaled sodium bicarbonate is probably useful with all irritant gases that liberate acid.

A 3.75% sodium bicarbonate solution for nebulization can be prepared by diluting 2 mL of a standard 7.5% sodium bicarbonate solution with 2 mL of normal saline—this can then be administered through a standard nebulizer.

Patients with Phosgene exposure should be given supplemental oxygen. The use of intravenous prednisolone (250 mg IV) or aerosolized dexamethasone or beclomethasone has been recommended to prevent pulmonary edema although it has not been well studied. N-acetylcysteine administered by nebulizer (20 mL of a 20% solution) has been efficacious in an animal model.

Patients who require mechanical ventilation should be placed on low tidal volumes (5–7 mL/kg) to minimize further lung injury. Positive end-expiratory pressure can be used to help optimize oxygenation.

Irritated eyes should be irrigated with copious amounts of normal saline until a neutral pH is obtained. Ophthalmologic consultation or follow-up is recommended if symptom resolution is not rapid or there is evidence of significant corneal injury.

Patients should be observed after exposure to irritant gases. Those who only had a brief exposure to a highly water-soluble irritant gas may be medically cleared if they are asymptomatic after a couple of hours—delayed symptoms would not be expected in these patients.

Hospital admission is required for all persistently symptomatic patients and those who were exposed to intermediate or poorly soluble gases because the extent of toxicity is unpredictable—24 hours of hospital observation with continuous pulse oximetry is warranted.

ADMISSION CRITERIA/TRIAGE

Individuals with bronchospasm, signs of pneumonitis or abnormal chest radiograph signs should be admitted. Significant phosgene exposures over 150 ppm per minute will probably require admission. Hydrogen Fluoride exposures over 30 ppm will also probably require admission.

SUMMARY

Pulmonary agents act as direct irritants to the respiratory tract. The water-solubility of the gas largely dictates the location of their action. The clinical effects range from irritation of the upper respiratory tract to severe acute lung injury. Acute lung injury may be delayed up to at least a day after initial exposure. After removal from exposure and dermal decontamination, treatment centers on supportive care and maintenance of oxygenation and ventilation. Sodium bicarbonate nebulization treatment may help with acid-forming irritant gases. If mechanical ventilation is required, then low-tidal volumes should be the rule to prevent further lung injury.

Suggested Reading

Aslan S, Kandis H, Akgun M, et al. The effect of nebulized NaHCO$_3$ treatment on "RADS" due to chlorine gas inhalation. *Inhal Toxicol.* 2006;18:895–900.

Borak J., Diller W. F., Phosgene Exposure: Mechanisms of Injury and Treatment Strategies. *J. Occup Environ Med* 2001:43:110–119.

Bosse GM. Nebulized sodium bicarbonate in the treatment of chlorine gas inhalation. *J Toxicol Clin Toxicol.* 1994;32:233–241.

Broughton E. The Bhopal disaster and its aftermath: a review. *Environ Health.* 2005;4:6.

Duffy M. Weapons of War: Poison Gas. Available at: *http://www. firstworldwar.com/weaponry/gas.htm* Accessed Oct 16, 2006.

Eckert WG. Mass deaths by gas or chemical poisoning: a historical perspective. *Am J Forensic Med Pathol.* 1991;12:119–125.

Meduri GU, Headley AS, Golden E, et al. Effect of prolonged methylprednisolone therapy in unresolving acute respiratory distress syndrome: a randomized controlled trial. *JAMA.* 1998;280:159–165.

Tanen DA, Graeme KA, Raschke R. Severe lung injury after exposure to chloramine gas from household cleaners. *N Engl J Med.* 1999;341:848–849.

Vinsel PJ. Treatment of acute chlorine gas inhalation with nebulized sodium bicarbonate. *J Emerg Med.* 1990;8:327–329.

35

PESTICIDES

Christian A. Herrera and Randall Myers

S T A T   F A C T S

PESTICIDES

- Organophosphate and carbamates inhibit the enzymatic function of acetylcholinesterase (AChE).
- Organophosphate binding to the enzyme AChE is permanent; carbonate binding is transient.
- Organochlorine agents cause neuronal irritability while pyrethrin compounds block neuronal sodium and γ–aminobutyric acid (GABA) chloride channels.
- Various herbicide and rodenticide exposures can result in coagulation, neurologic, metabolic, and pulmonary complications.

INTRODUCTION

On March 30, 1995, the Tokyo subway system experienced a bioterrorist attack. Sarin gas was placed in five subway cars during the busy morning rush hour. That day about 5000 people were exposed to sarin and 11 commuters died. Many hospitals participated in the care of these patients.

In this chapter pesticides will be discussed. An attack similar to the Tokyo attack can occur with any of the pesticides that will be discussed. Clinical presentation of toxicity, pathophysiology, and treatment will be reviewed.

CONFIRMING THE THREAT

On the day of the Tokyo attack, it took about 3 hours for the authorities to identify and announce the biochemical agent as being sarin. With a biochemical terrorist attack, it is difficult to determine the causative agent quickly with an accurate laboratory analysis. Thus, health-care providers will have a window of treating exposed victims before the authorities confirm an attack and the agent used. The diagnosis must be

made on the clinical picture. In Tokyo, health-care providers recognized that the victims were showing signs of organophosphate poisoning and treated them as such before the authorities confirmed the agent as being sarin.

HOSPITAL RESPONSE

Personal Protective Equipment

During the Tokyo attack, 23% of the hospital staff at St. Luke's International Hospital experienced secondary exposure because of a lack of personal protective equipment (PPE) and on-site decontamination facilities. PPE consists of respiratory protection and skin protection. PPE has a classification system from level A to D used by the Environmental Protection Agency (EPA). Level A equipment uses a protective suit and pressure-demand breathing apparatus (air cylinder) contained within the suit. Level B is similar but has the breathing apparatus outside of the protective suit. When the causative agent is known, level C equipment is used. This protective suit uses a cartridge for breathing that is preselected to absorb a specific causative agent. Another option for respiratory protection is a contained breathing apparatus called the powered air-purifying respirator (PARF).

The biochemical agent used in a chemical terrorist attack may not be identified for hours. Level C equipment requires identification of the agent so the proper air cartridge may be used. As such, level B or PARF are better suited for medical facilities because they offer a broader protection from chemical agents.

Decontamination

A designated area for decontamination must be preselected to limit contamination of the hospital facilities and secondary exposures of the staff. Hospitals will also need high ventilation in the emergency room and any other locations where patients may be located prior to decontamination. Tokyo hospitals did not have on-site decontamination and this is why a significant portion of the staff had secondary exposure.

INSECTICIDES

Organophosphate and Carbamates Insecticides

Organophosphates were created during the Second World War as chemical agents to be used in battle as nerve gases (soman, sarin, tabun, VX). After the war, these agents found a new use as a key ingredient in pesticides. At the end of the past century, carbamates have become much more common in pesticides than organophosphates. Carbamates are similar to organophosphates in mechanism and in toxicity profile.

Organophosphate pesticides include malathion, parathion, chlorpyrifos, diazinon, pirimiphos methyl, and coumaphos.

Organophosphate compounds are composed of carbon and phosphorous acid derivatives and are highly lipid-soluble. With low-level exposures, accumulation can occur in adipose tissue. Toxicity can occur by dermal, inhalation, and gastrointestinal (GI) exposure. Carbamate compounds are composed of carbamic acid. Carbamates are also absorbed by dermal, inhalation, and GI exposure.

With organophosphate exposure, oral and respiratory exposures generally result in signs and symptoms of toxicity within 3 hours. With dermal exposure, toxicity may be apparent by 12 hours. Agents that are highly lipophilic may show delayed toxicity and toxicity of longer duration due to adipose accumulation.

Organophosphates bind to neural or red blood cell (RBC) acetylcholinesterase (AChE) and deactivate its enzyme activity. AChE is an enzyme that causes the hydrolysis of acetylcholine into choline and acetic acid. Inhibition of AChE by organophosphates causes an accumulation of acetylcholine at specific neural synapse sites that include autonomic nicotinic and muscarinic synapses, skeletal muscle nicotinic synapses, and central nervous system (CNS) sites.

Each different organophosphate has a specific period of time at which its action on AChE is permanent. After it binds and forms the AChE-organophosphate complex, it goes through a conformational change called "aging." At this point of "aging" the function of AChE cannot be salvaged with antidotal treatment.

Carbamates are similar to organophosphates. They too inhibit the enzymatic function of AChE but their binding of AChE is transient. Carbamates are associated to AChE for less than 48 hours. Once they dissociate from AChE, it regains its function of hydrolyzing acetylcholine. Thus with carbamates there is no "aging" and the duration of carbamate toxicity is shorter than organophosphates.

With either exposure it is important to remember that children have a greater risk of toxicity due to their size and lower baseline levels of AChE. Also, chemical warfare agents (soman, sarin, tabun, VX) are rapid acting and "age" within minutes of inhalation or dermal exposure, causing a rapid death.

Organophosphate Toxicity

Acute Toxicity The signs and symptoms of cholinergic crisis will be the initial presentation of acute organophosphate poisoning. Acetylcholine plays a strong role in the parasympathetic system through nicotinic and muscarinic cholinergic receptors. It is also involved at neuromuscular junctions and the CNS. Clinical signs include bradycardia, miosis, lacrimation, salivation, bronchorrhea, bronchospasm, urination, emesis, and diarrhea. Diaphoresis can occur from stimulation of postganglionic muscarinic receptors from the autonomic nervous system. Tachycardia can occur from nicotinic stimulation of the sympathetic nervous system. The combination of these muscarinic, nicotinic, and CNS effects on the respiratory system may result in fatality.

There are two mnemonics used for muscarinic signs:

SLUDGE/BBB—salivation, lacrimation, urination, defecation, gastric emesis, bronchorrhea, bronchospasm, bradycardia
DUMBELS—defecation, urination, miosis, bronchorrhea/bronchospasm/bradycardia, emesis, lacrimation, salivation

Not included in these mnemonics are the effects of nicotinic and CNS stimulation. At neuromuscular junctions the nicotinic effects of fasciculations and muscle weakness may occur, similar to the effect of depolarizing agents. CNS effects include lethargy, coma, and seizures.

Intermediate Toxicity A significant number of patients with organophosphate poisoning develop "intermediate syndrome" 24–96 hours after exposure. Symptoms include neck flexion weakness, cranial nerve abnormalities, proximal nerve weakness, decreased deep tendon reflexes, and respiratory depression. Most patients recover within 2–3 weeks. RBC AChE turnover correlates with this recovery. Early antidote therapy may prevent this syndrome.

Delayed Toxicity Organophosphorus agent-induced delayed neuropathy (OPIDN) may occur 1–3 weeks after ingestion of certain organophosphorus agents. It is thought that the inhibition of neuropathy target esterase (NTE), not AChE, causes this delayed neurotoxicity. This enzyme metabolizes ester compounds. The locations of this enzyme include the brain and peripheral nerves.

The symptoms for OPIDN include transient, painful paresthesias followed by symmetrical flaccid weakness of the lower extremities with ascension into the upper extremities. Sensory disturbances can also occur. Most cases will resolve with time.

Carbamate Toxicity

Symptoms of toxicity are similar to organophosphorus agents. Both cause cholinergic crisis but with carbamates the duration of the toxicity is shorter. The CNS is not penetrated well by carbamates. Thus, central toxicity is less common and seizures do not occur.

The degree of organophosphate toxicity and effectiveness of therapy can be followed by direct and serial measurements of RBC AChE activity. This is not a routine lab and needs to be sent out at most institutions, making it less helpful in acute management. Measuring plasma AChE does not correlate well with toxicity or therapy.

With carbamate poisoning RBC AChE levels may return to normal spontaneously within 10 hours after exposure. Thus, spontaneous decarbamylation makes the RBC AChE assay unhelpful in treatment of carbamate toxicity.

Clinical

The diagnosis of organophosphate or carbamate poisoning is based on history and toxidrome. In the case of the comatose patient with an unknown history, the clinical picture of cholinergic excess suggests the toxicity. An odor of petroleum or garlic-like smell may be present with organophosphate poisoning. If doubt exists, a trial of 1 mg of atropine (0.02 mg/kg in children) may be given. The absence of anticholinergic effects with the atropine is suggestive of organophosphate or carbamate poisoning.

Decontamination is a priority. In topical exposure, the patient must be disrobed of their clothes and the patient needs to be washed with water and a mild soap. The patient's belongings should be considered as contaminated items and discarded with hazardous materials. For GI exposure, activated charcoal should be given to all and gastric lavage should be considered if the patient is intubated.

Patients who are mildly poisoned can quickly develop respiratory failure from CNS respiratory depression, diaphragmatic weakness, bronchospasm, and bronchorrhea. These patients should be placed on 100% oxygen and intubated early if needed. When paralyzing the patient for intubation, a nondepolarizing agent should be used for neuromuscular blockade. Succinylcholine should not be used because it is metabolized by plasma cholinesterase and prolonged paralysis will occur.

Volume resuscitation should be given to all patients with organophosphate poisoning. With moderate poisoning, bradycardia and hypotension may be present. Also, transient tachycardia may occur from nicotinic stimulation of the sympathetic nervous system.

With moderate to severe cholinergic poisoning, atropine is given at a dose of 2–5 mg IV for adults and 0.05 mg/kg IV for children. Atropine competes with acetylcholine and binds to muscarinic receptors preventing cholinergic activation. Every 3–5 minutes the dose is doubled and titrated to the endpoint of clearing respiratory secretions and relief in pulmonary bronchoconstriction. Tachycardia should not be used as a measure of titration since it may represent hypoxia or hypovolemia. Hundreds of milligrams of atropine may be needed over many days in a patient with severe poisoning.

Atropine does not bind nicotinic receptors. Thus, it is ineffective in alleviating neuromuscular dysfunction. Pralidoxime (2-PAM) and other oximes (HI-6 and obidoxime) have an effect on muscarinic and nicotinic symptoms. These antidotes are cholinesterase reactivating agents. They displace organophosphates from cholinesterases if given before "aging."

Any patient showing cholinergic toxicity, neuromuscular dysfunction, or with known exposure to organophosphorus agents known to cause delayed neurotoxicity should be started on oxime treatment. It is not given to asymptomatic patients. The World Health Organization recommends treatment with an IV bolus of pralidoxime of 30 mg/kg for adults and 25–50 mg/kg for children. Early treatment with oximes reduces the risk of intermediate toxicity and organophosphorus induced delayed neuropathy. Rapid infusion of pralidoxime has been associated with cardiac arrest. It should be administered slowly over 30 minutes.

Benzodiazepines are used to treat seizures associated with organophosphate cholinergic toxicity. Diazepam is the benzodiazepine of choice. It has been shown to decrease neurocognitive dysfunction with organophosphorus toxicity.

With acute carbamate poisoning the treatment is similar to that of organophosphate poisoning. Atropine is used for muscarinic symptoms and is usually given for 6–12 hours while decarbamylation from AChE occurs spontaneously. Since carbamate is transiently bound, pralidoxime is not needed. However, with a patient in cholinergic crisis and unknown agent exposure or a known mixed poisoning pralidoxime should be used. With isolated carbamate poisoning pralidoxime should be avoided.

All caring for patients exposed to carbamates or organophosphates should wear PPE.

Asymptomatic patients with minimal exposure require decontamination and 6–8-hour observation. Patients with moderate to severe toxicity require admission to the intensive care unit. Within 48 hours, most patients on 2-PAM therapy will show an increase in RBC AChE level. Toxicity may be more prolonged with fat-soluble toxins. For these patients, respiratory and supportive care may be needed for weeks until new enzymes are synthesized. For those with fatal exposure, death usually occurs due to respiratory failure from respiratory muscle weakness, CNS depression, and bronchorrhea. After recovery, patients may have lifelong nonspecific neurologic symptoms after acute exposure.

Carbamates are less toxic than organophosphates. Most patients with moderate carbamate poisoning recover completely within 24 hours and as such, only need an observation period.

Organochlorine Insecticides

Organochlorine pesticides include dichlorodiphenyltrichloroethane (DDT), chlordane, heptachlor, dieldrin, hexachlorocyclohexane, and adrin. These pesticides are chlorinated hydrocarbons. Hexachlorocyclohexane (lindane) is a scabicide that was banned in 2000 for human use because of its toxicity and is now used as a garden insecticide. In the United States, most organochlorines have been restricted because of their persistence in the environment and long metabolic life. However, other countries continue to use them.

Organochlorines are lipid-soluble compounds. They accumulate in fatty tissues and produce toxicity by dermal, inhalation, and GI exposure.

Organochlorines affect neuronal membranes. The toxicity is caused by neuronal irritability. The neuron membrane repetitively discharges as a result of its decrease in sodium channel permeability. Also, the hepatic microsomal enzyme system may be activated by many of these agents. Thus medications that function through this system will have diminished activity when used in presence of organochlorine toxicity.

There are also cardiac affects from organochlorines. The myocardium may show increased sensitivity to catecholamines in the presence of organochlorines causing ventricular dysrhythmias.

Toxicity

Organochlorine intoxication presents with neurotoxicity. Mild poisoning can present with symptoms of neurological stimulation such as confusion, apprehension, combativeness, irritability, tremulousness, myoclonus, and facial paresthesias. Fever and hyperthermia can also occur. Seizures are sometimes seen with severe toxicity. Ventricular dysrhythmias can arise from sensitization of the myocardium to endogenous catecholamines. Organochlorines often are contained in hydrocarbon solvents. With ingestion, these solvents may cause sedation and a state of coma.

Diagnosis may be difficult from patient examination alone. Prehospital information concerning scene, the exposure, the pesticide, and package label if available will be helpful.

No specific routine laboratory will confirm the diagnosis. Some specialty laboratories may have special assays to detect organochlorines in the serum and urine.

Clinical

Skin decontamination should be initiated with water and soap to decrease acute dermal exposure. GI decontamination

is indicated for ingestion. Short-acting benzodiazepines or barbiturates are used for seizure control. If a patient is in status, high-dose barbiturates and paralyzing agents should be used. Exposed patients should be placed on the monitor because of the risk of ventricular dysrhythmias, which may occur during seizures secondary to circulating catecholamines. Patients should not be given atropine or epinephrine because of the sensitization of the myocardium to catecholamines. β-Adrenergic antagonists should be given to reduce the catecholamine effect.

Decontamination of the patient and protective gear is important to prevent exposure of staff providing care.

With organochlorine toxicity, hospitalization is required until seizures are controlled and neurological symptoms resolve. This may take 24–48 hours.

Pyrethrin Insecticides

Pyrethrins are natural occurring compounds found in chrysanthemum flowers. Pyrethroid pesticides are synthetic derivatives from pyrethrin analogs. These insecticides are used in a wide variety of settings from agricultural fields to homes. These agents are considered relatively safe and are used in many over-the-counter insecticides.

Pyrethroid pesticides occur mostly as aerosols. Thus exposures usually occur through inhalation.

The sodium channel of neuronal membrane is blocked by pyrethroids, resulting in repetitive neuronal discharges. Chloride channel is also inhibited in GABA receptors with these compounds. Nonsynthesized pyrethroids or natural occurring forms may cause hypersensitivity dermal reactions. Pyrethroid compounds are rapidly degraded in the liver making systemic toxicity uncommon.

Toxicity

Allergic reactions can occur through inhalation or dermal exposure. Symptoms may include allergic dermatitis, rhinitis, rhinorrhea, cough, shortness of breath, wheezing, and anaphylaxis. Also, pyrethrin antigens have cross-reactivity with ragweed pollen antigens.

Blocking of sodium channels and GABA chloride channels may lead to neurological symptoms. They may be nonspecific, such as headache, fatigue, and dizziness or neurological such as confusion, tremors, incoordination, and seizures.

No routine laboratory study will confirm the diagnosis of pyrethroid toxicity.

Clinical

Like other pesticides, decontamination is a priority. Treatment is mainly supportive and focuses on allergic and respiratory symptoms.

With pyrethroid pesticide exposure, the intensity of the symptoms will determine the disposition. Patients often are discharged from the ED.

N,N-Diethyl-3-methylbenzamide (DEET) Insecticides

DEET or N,N-diethyl-m-toluamide is an insect repellent. It is found in most over-the-counter insect repellents, formulations ranging from 5% to 100%. Children should not have greater than 10% formulations applied.

DEET is a lipid-soluble compound. Toxicity can occur by dermal or GI exposure.

Toxicity affects the CNS. DEET is a neurotoxin, however, its mechanism of action is unknown.

Toxicity

Contact dermatitis may occur with prolonged skin exposure. With ingestion or repeated dermal applications of DEET, neurological symptoms can occur. Symptoms include restlessness, confusion, CNS depression, muscle cramps or tremors, and seizures.

Routine labs will not confirm the diagnosis of DEET toxicity.

Clinical

Skin decontamination should be initiated with water and soap. For GI exposure, activated charcoal should be given for ingestion. Otherwise, general care is supportive for DEET exposure. Benzodiazepines should be used if seizures occur.

DEET exposures that manifest neurological symptoms require admission for observation. Ingestions that are symptomatic can be observed for a couple of hours.

HERBICIDES

Chlorophenoxy Herbicides

2,4-Dichlorophenoxyacetic acid (2,4-D) and 4-chloro-2-methylphenoxyacetic acid (MCPA) are commonly used chlorophenoxy herbicides. The herbicide Agent Orange used in the Vietnam War had 2,4-D as a component. Chlorophenoxy compounds affect broadleaf plants and are used as weed killers.

The mechanism of toxicity is unknown. Toxicity can occur by dermal exposure, inhalation, and ingestion.

Toxicity

Nausea, vomiting, and diarrhea can occur with ingestion. Pulmonary edema can occur with inhalation. Exposure can also lead to muscle toxicity, presenting with fasciculations and rhabdomyolysis, and cardiovascular findings of dysrhythmias and hypotension.

Routine laboratories will not confirm exposure. A metabolic acidosis and renal dysfunction may be found. Elevated CPK and myoglobinuria suggests rhabdomyolysis.

Clinical

Skin decontamination should be initiated. Otherwise, treatment is supportive. Patient should be monitored for rhabdomyolysis and treated appropriately.

Mild symptoms can be observed and discharged after 4–6 hours. Patients with significant toxicity, which is rare, should be admitted.

Biphyridyl Herbicides

Paraquat and diquat make up this class of nonselective contact herbicides.

Death from paraquat toxicity has occurred from dermal exposure, ingestion, and inhalation. Most manufactured paraquat herbicides contain a blue dye, a stenchant, and an emetic. Diquat is much less toxic. Diquat formulations do not include blue dye, a stenchant, or emetic.

Paraquat is minimally absorbed through skin if dermis is intact. However, it will cause local irritation. Through ingestion, paraquat is rapidly absorbed and is distributed to most organs, with kidneys and lungs acquiring the largest amount.

Toxicity

Paraquat accumulates in the lungs and here becomes a superoxide radical in alveolar cells. This radical formation from paraquat is augmented by oxygen. As a radical, it causes lipid peroxidation disrupting the cell membrane and causing cell death. This causes inflammation and reversible damage of alveolar type 1 and type 2 cells. Within weeks, permanent interstitial fibrosis can form. In other places, it is just damaging. It causes renal tubular necrosis, myocarditis, liver necrosis, adrenal necrosis, and ulcerations of the GI tract.

Paraquat is a strong caustic agent. With dermal exposure, it will cause local corrosive irritation and ulceration. With inhalation a patient may experience dyspnea, chest pain, pulmonary edema, epistaxis, and hemoptysis. Ingestion causes mucosal irritation and ulceration. Patients' lips, oral cavity, and GI tract can develop caustic ulcerations, producing abdominal pain and vomiting. Fluid losses occur from the lesions and with decreased oral intake the patient may be in a state of hypovolemia. Ingestion of greater than 30 mg/kg will result in multisystem effects, including pulmonary edema and fibrosis (with refractory hypoxemia occurring days later), GI perforation and hemorrhage, acute tubular necrosis and renal failure, and congestive heart failure from cardiovascular collapse. With massive ingestion, death from multiorgan failure may occur in days.

Lethal dose of diquat is similar but death is less common. Diquat has less of an affinity for pulmonary tissue, causing less extensive pulmonary injury.

Some specialty laboratories such as assays for paraquat in the urine and blood assist in the diagnosis. Nomograms have been created that predict survival based on plasma paraquat concentration and time of ingestion. A chemistry panel may show lactic acidosis from hypoxemia and multi-organ failure. Chest radiographs diffuse parenchymal injury and pneumomediastinum or pneumothorax from corrosive rupture of the esophagus.

Clinical

Like other exposures, decontamination is a priority. Clothing should be removed and the skin washed with soap and water. Any exposure requires hospitalization because of the potential for delayed pulmonary toxicity. To prevent superoxide radical formation low inspired oxygen (FIo_2 <21%) should be used unless severe respiratory failure occurs. Fluids and electrolytes should be given aggressively to replace losses from GI tract damage and vomiting and to prevent volume depletion and prerenal failure. Gut decontamination with activated charcoal (1–2 g/kg) is indicated and should be repeated every 4 hours. Gastric lavage is also recommended. Other supportive care includes airway protection, fluid resuscitation, and pain relief.

The amount ingested correlates with outcome. Large or concentrated ingestions result in development of GI ulceration, renal failure, extensive pulmonary injury, and fibrosis, causing death in most patients. These large ingestions cause death from multiorgan failure and cardiogenic shock. Death from smaller ingestions occurs from pulmonary fibrosis and respiratory failure. With smaller ingestions, death may not occur for 2–3 weeks.

Urea-Substituted Herbicides

This group of compounds includes chlorimuron, diuron, fluometron, and isopturon. Urea-substituted herbicides act on plant life by inhibiting photosynthesis. With ingestion methemoglobinuria may occur. A patient with GI exposure requires decontamination, supportive care, and methylene blue if methemoglobinuria is present.

RODENTICIDES

Rodenticides are a heterogeneous group of compounds that exhibit different toxicity in humans and rodents. These are among some of the most toxic substances found in the homes of the general public.

Arsenic

Arsenic is a semimetallic, naturally occurring substance found in food, water, and household items. It was commonly used as a rodenticide until about two decades ago. It may still be found in liquid form in old barns and storage sites. Arsenic is a notorious poison because it has no odor or taste. Throughout history, there have been many incidents of

murder by arsenic poisoning. Arsenic became a favorite murder weapon of the Middle Ages. Arsenic poisoning often went undetected because the symptoms were similar to those of cholera, which was common at that time. Over the past century, several notorious American serial killers used arsenic as their poison of choice. In 2003 in Maine, homicide investigators said arsenic-laced coffee served at the church reception killed a 78-year-old man and made several others sick.

Arsenic affects nearly all organ systems. Arsenic's toxicity functions by two mechanisms. Arsenic hydrolyzes high-energy bonds of ATP effectively uncoupling oxidative phosphorylation and disrupts sulfhydryl containing enzymes.

Toxicity

Acute ingestion of a toxic amount of arsenic typically causes severe GI signs and symptoms including severe abdominal pain, nausea and vomiting, and bloody or rice-water diarrhea. Cardiovascular effects include hypotension, shock; ventricular arrhythmias, congestive heart failure, and pulmonary edema. Neurologic symptoms include light-headedness, weakness, lethargy, delirium, convulsions, and coma. Other complications include rhabdomyolysis and DIC. Patients may also exhibit a garlic odor on their breath.

Early clinical diagnosis of arsenic toxicity is often difficult. The key diagnostic laboratory test for recent exposure is urinary arsenic measurement, with a 24-hour urine collection. A spot urine testing may also be performed in many emergency departments.

Clinical

Hemodynamic stabilization and gut decontamination are key factors in the initial management of acute arsenic intoxication. Fluid replacement and transfusion of blood products as required are the mainstays of initial treatment and should begin as soon as possible, even in the absence of hypotension. Chelation therapy administered within hours of arsenic exposure may prevent the full effects of arsenic toxicity by curtailing the distribution of arsenic in the body. The agent most frequently recommended is dimercaprol. It is administered intramuscularly at 3–5 mg/kg of body weight every 4–12 hours until symptoms resolve. Contraindications to dimercaprol include pregnancy, pre-existing renal disease, concurrent use of medicinal iron, and glucose-6-phosphate deficiency. Oral agents such as 2,3-dimercaptocuccinic acid (DMSA) or D-penicillamine are alternatives to dimercaprol.

Barium

Barium is a silvery white metal that exists abundantly in nature in ores. No commercially available rodenticides containing barium are currently available in the United States. Barium metaborate is a microbiocide/microbiostat used as an industrial preservative in the manufacturing of paints, bricks, ceramics, glass, and rubber.

Barium has been found to cause GI disturbances and muscular weakness when people are exposed to it at elevated levels. Barium drives potassium intracellularly. Consuming very large amounts of soluble barium compounds can cause arrhythmias, hypotonia or paralysis, and possibly death. Potassium infusion is used clinically to reverse the toxic effects of barium. There is no routine medical test to determine whether patients have been exposed to barium.

Yellow Phosphorous

This compound causes chemical burns. Clinical presentation in humans includes a garlic odor breath, oral burns, vomiting, and phosphorescent smoking feces.

PNU (N-3-pyridylmethyl-Np-nitrophenyl urea)

This compound destroys the pancreatic β-cell.

Sodium Monofluoroacetate (Compound 1080)

Sodium monofluoroacetate ($CH_2FCOONa$), also known as Compound 1080 belongs to a class of chemicals known as fluoroacetates. It is a tasteless and odorless, water-soluble rodenticide of high potency that has been used widely to control gophers, squirrels, prairie dogs, coyotes, and other rodents. The widespread use of 1080 in pest control has led to accidental deaths of livestock, pets, and humans and several suicides from drinking 1080 rat poison solutions.

When consumed fluoroacetate is converted to fluorocitrate, a compound that inhibits the enzymes aconitase and succinate dehydrogenase, causing an accumulation of citrate, which interferes with energy production and cellular function.

Clinical effects usually develop within 30 minutes to 2.5 hours of exposure but might be delayed as long as 20 hours. The predominant manifestations of Compound 1080 are metabolic, cardiovascular, and neurologic signs and symptoms. Effects of acute exposure include metabolic acidosis, hypotension, dysrhythmias, seizures, coma, and respiratory depression. There is no laboratory test to detect Compound 1080. There is no effective antidote.

Strychnine

Strychnine is a white, odorless, bitter crystalline powder that is used primarily as a rodenticide to kill rats. Strychnine is a powerful poison and only a small amount is needed to produce severe effects in humans including death (LD_{50} 1 mg/kg). Ingestion is the primary route of exposure. Strychnine exposure is known to occur through contaminated drinking water, food, or exposure to contaminated street drugs. Strychnine exposure can also occur through absorption of membranes of the nostrils, eyes, or mouth if released in aerosolized form.

Strychnine acts as an antagonist at the strychnine-sensitive Glycine receptor (GlyR), a ligand-gated chloride channel in the spinal cord and the brain. Inhibition results in severe painful spasms throughout the body. Symptoms of poisoning occur within 15 to 60 minutes after exposure. Signs and symptoms of low to moderate poisonings of strychnine include agitation, tachycardia, hypertension, muscle pain and soreness, uncontrolled arching of the neck and back, difficulty breathing, and convulsions. Initially strychnine has no effect on consciousness and thus victims are aware of their symptoms. An individual exposed to high levels typically will exhibit respiratory failure, coma, and rapid death, 15–30 minutes after exposure.

Treatment consists of activated charcoal to decontaminate the GI tract and supportive medical care. For convulsions and spasms diazepam is given. Cooling measures should be taken for high temperatures. If a person survives the initial toxic effects of strychnine poisoning, long-term health effects are unlikely.

Thallium

Thallium sulfate is an odorless and tasteless compound widely used in the past as a rat poison and ant killer. Thallium-containing rodenticides were banned in the United States during the 1960s. These compounds are still used in some tropical countries and accidental poisonings are common. Contaminated food with thallium is the major source of human exposure.

Toxicity stems from its ability to replace important alkali metal compounds such as sodium and potassium in the body. It disrupts many cellular processes. Immediate effects of thallium exposure include nonspecific GI symptoms, including abdominal pain and nausea. Subacute symptoms of thallium poisoning are loss of hair and damage to peripheral nerves, exhibited as neuropathy, ataxia, and seizures. The presence and levels of thallium can be tested for in the urine and hair.

Zinc Phosphide

Zinc phosphide is a gray-black powder with a decaying fish odor that is used as a rodenticide. Zinc phosphide is a popular rodenticide because it is fairly specific for rodents and there is no true secondary poisoning. Although there are documented cases of adults dying from massive doses of the pesticide (4000–5000 mg), the LD_{50} is 45.7 mg/kg.

Poisoning occurs when the zinc phosphide comes into contact with the dilute acids in the stomach and phosphine gas is liberated and rapidly absorbed into the bloodstream. This results in damage to blood vessels and irritation of the alimentary tract. Symptoms of acute zinc phosphide poisoning include nausea, vomiting, diarrhea, agitation, hypotension, and loss of consciousness. Symptoms are usually evident within 15 minutes to 4 hours of ingestion of a toxic dose. In fatal cases there is liver, kidney, heart, and brain damage. Death is usually due to anoxia. There have been no observed symptoms of chronic poisoning due to zinc phosphide exposure in humans.

There is no specific antidote for zinc phosphide but several treatments can be given to offset the effects of the chemical. Sodium bicarbonate can be given orally to neutralize the stomach acidity; calcium gluconate and sodium lactate can be given intravenously to combat systemic acidosis.

Cholecalciferol

Cholecalciferol-containing rodenticides cause hypercalcemia. However, overdoses are not likely to occur with this type of rodenticide because these products are not commonly available, and they require extremely large doses to create toxicity in humans.

Bromethalin

This compound uncouples oxidative phosphorylation.

Norbormide

This compound leads to vasoconstriction with ischemia.

Red Squill

The botanical preparation of red squill was used as a rodenticide for many years. It contains a cardiac glycoside as an active ingredient. Rodents ingest the product, and because they are incapable of vomiting, develop glycoside intoxication and pulmonary edema. Humans instead are capable of vomiting, and as such red squill was considered harmless. This product is not used much today because of its limited effectiveness as a rodenticide.

Anticoagulants

The vast majority of rodenticide exposures to humans are due to anticoagulants. Warfarin was the first anticoagulant rodenticide used in the United States. It is used for controlling rats and house mice at the public and agricultural level. It is odorless and tasteless and effective in very low dosages. A dose of 200 mg/m^3 is considered highly toxic and immediately dangerous to life. Warfarin is an established human teratogen during any trimester of pregnancy.

Brodifacoum

Brodifacoum is a rodenticide found in many common mice and rat traps. This compound prevents the production of essential blood-clotting factors. Both intentional and unintentional poisoning incidents in humans have been reported. Also, known as superwarfarin, it was developed as a second-generation anticoagulant after resistance of warfarin was noted in some rodent species. It is absorbed through the gut and inhibits the vitamin K-dependent steps in the synthesis of multiple clotting factors. Death usually occurs through gastric hemorrhage. It is highly effective at small doses—usually a rodent ingests a fatal dose after a single feeding and will die within 4 to 5 days.

Symptoms of acute intoxication by brodifacoums in humans vary from an excessive bruising, nose and gum bleeding, and blood in urine in less severe poisonings to massive hemorrhage in more severe cases. The signs of poisoning develop with a delay of one to several days after ingestion. The average fatal dose for adult man is estimated to be approximately 15 mg brodifacoum or 300 g of 0.005% bait.

Treatment has to be tailored to individual circumstances. It is thought that if only a small amount has been ingested, no action is required other than to measure the prothrombin time at about 36–48 hours. Vitamin K (5–10 mg IV) should be given as a prophylactic measure to replete depleted coagulation factors. If bleeding is already evident, fresh frozen plasma will be necessary for immediate control since vitamin K will not be effective for about 24 hours. Repeated doses of vitamin K may be required depending on the amount and specific nature of the compound involved. Prothrombin time is a satisfactory guide to the severity of acute intoxication and also for the effectiveness and duration of therapy.

Suggested Reading

Bradberry SM et al: Mechanisms of toxicity, clinical features, and management of acute chlorophenoxy herbicide poisoning: a review, *Clin Toxicol.* 38:111–122, 2000.

Centers for Disease Control and Prevention. Third National Report on Human Exposure to Environmental Chemicals. Atlanta (GA): CDC, 2005.

Dorman DC, Beasley VR: Neurotoxicology of pyrethrin and the pyrethroid insecticides, *Vet Hum Toxicol.* 33:238, 1991.

Eddleston M, Roberts D, Buckley N. Management of severe organophosphorous pesticide poisoning. *Crit Care.* 2002;6:259.

Eddleston M, Szinicz L, Eyer P, et al. Oximes in acute organophosphorous pesticide poisoning: a systematic review of clinical trials. *QJM.* 2002;95:275.

Eyer P. The role of oximes in the management of organophosphorous pesticide poisoning. *Toxicol Rev.* 2003;22:165.

Fradin MS: Mosquitoes and mosquito repellents: a clinician's guide, *Ann Intern Med.* 128:931–940, 1998.

Glynn P. Neuropathy target esterase. *Biochem J.* 1999;344 Pt 3:625.

Hayes WJ: Pesticides studied in man, Baltimore, 1982, Williams and Wilkins.

Hart TB, Nevitt A, Whitehead A. A new statistical approach to the prognostic significance of plasma paraquat concentrations. *Lancet.* 1984;2:1222.

Holstege CP, Baer AB. Insecticides. *Curr Treat Options Neurol.* 2004;6:17.

Holstege CP, Bechtal LK, Reilly TH, et al: Unusual but potential agents of terrorism. *Emerg Med Clin N Am.* 2007:25:549–566.

Jones GM, Vale JA: Mechanisms of toxicity, clinical features, and management of diquat poisoning: a review, *Clin Toxicol.* 38:123–128, 2000.

Khurana D, Prabhakar S. Organophosphorous intoxication. *Arch Neurol.* 2000;57:600.

Kumura T, Hisaoka T, Yamada A, et al. The Tokyo subway sarin attack—lessons learned. *Toxicol Appl Pharmacol.* 2005;207: s471–s476.

Kumura T, Suzuki K, Fukuda A, et al. The Tokyo subway sarin attack: disaster management, Part 2: hospital response. *Acad Emerg Med.* 1998;5:618–624.

Kumura T, Suzuki K, Fukuda A, et al. The Tokyo subway sarin attack: disaster management, Part 1. community emergency response. *Acad Emerg Med.* 1998;5:613–617.

Scherrmann JM, Houze P, Bismuth C, et al. Prognostic value of plasma and urine paraquat concentrations. *Human Toxicol.* 1987;6:91.

Senanayake N, Karalliedde L. Neurotoxic effects of organophosphorous insecticides: an intermediate syndrome. *N Engl J Med.* 1987;316:761.

Tuovinen K. Organophosphate-induced convulsions and prevention of neuropathological damages. *Toxicology.* 2004;196:31.

World Health Organization. Environmental Health Criteria No 63. Organophosphorous Pesticides: A General Introduction. World Health Organization, Geneva 1986.

36

NONLETHAL WEAPONS OR INCAPACITATING AGENTS

Katherine A. Martens, Christina Hantsch Bardsley, and
Brian L. Bardsley, Jr.

STAT FACTS

NONLETHAL WEAPONS OR INCAPACITATING AGENTS

- The goal of incapacitating agents is to temporarily impair performance of victims rather than seriously injure or kill.
- Riot control agents cause temporary inability to fight due to pain or discomfort during the exposure period and shortly after it.
- The anticholinergic compound 3-quinuclidinyl benzylate (BZ) is an incapacitating agent whose effects generally last for 48–72 hours.
- Physostigmine can reverse the effects of BZ.

INTRODUCTION

Incapacitating agents are designed as nonlethal, less-than-lethal or, perhaps more accurately, less-lethal weapons. The goal of their use is to impair the performance rather than seriously injure or kill the victims. This goal is distinctly different than that of the chemical warfare agents categorized as lethal agents, including pulmonary agents, "blood" agents, blister agents, and nerve agents, which are discussed in other chapters in this book.

Another group of nonlethal compounds is riot control agents. However, riot control agents are not recognized by the United States as official chemical warfare agents (*United States Army Field Manual* 8-285). Also called irritants, harassing agents, lacrimators, and sternutators (which cause sneezing), riot control agents are utilized for purposes similar to incapacitating agents. Rather than seriously injure or kill the victims, riot control agents are intended to deter or render temporary inability to fight or resist due to pain or discomfort. The duration of riot control agent effects is shorter than incapacitating agents with symptoms often ending after cessation of exposure and decontamination. Riot control agents are discussed in Appendix K.

Nonlethal weapons or incapacitating agents encompass a wide variety of armaments. The National Institute of Justice has categorized these weapons into acoustics, chemical, electric shock, impact projectiles, light, and physical restraints. Even olfactory assault with noxious odors has been investigated as a possible approach to incapacitation.

Calmative agents are non lethal methods to control crowds and hostage situations offer an advantage of being administered without the need for direct contact. Such calmatives—sleeping agents if you will, have spurred increased interest by several governments including the US and Russia as the likelihood of terrorist threats and potential for hostage situations grows. Although early efforts focused on fentanyl and single agents, multiagent regimens are now being investigated.

This chapter will focus on chemical incapacitating agents as defined by the Chemical Casualty Care Division of the U.S. Army Medical Research Institute of Chemical Defense. Objectives of the chapter include obtaining an understanding of the pharmacology, clinical effects, differential diagnosis, and treatment of chemical incapacitating agents. In addition, a brief review of their historical use and discussion of their future prospects will be presented.

BACKGROUND

Chemical warfare agents include lethal agents, designed to cause serious injury and death, and incapacitating agents. The U.S. Department of Defense defines an incapacitating agent as "an agent that produces temporary physiological or mental effects, or both, which will render individuals incapable of concerted effort in the performance of their assigned duties." Theoretically, an individual or crowd is thus unable to function in combat or resistance on a temporary basis, without mortal or permanent consequences, as a result of exposure to these agents. In the military context, this impairment is based primarily on the central nervous system (CNS) or psychobehavioral effects as opposed to physical symptoms.

HISTORY

The use of chemical agents to incapacitate opposing forces dates back to ancient times. In 1961, Goodman systematically reviewed 100 years of 4 major American and British journals as well as several German medical journals and reported an "astonishing" number of reports of pharmacological induction of "behavioral toxicity," particularly utilizing atropine and related drugs, which produce anticholinergic effects. It was felt that many of these incidents could be considered as historical precedent in the use of drugs as "weapons of mass destruction." Table 36-1 lists historical incidents that support the view that incapacitating chemical weapons are not a modern concept.

Incapacitating agent use has continued in more recent times. In 1995, 3-quinuclidinyl benzylate (BZ) was alleged to have been used by the Serbians on civilians fleeing Srebrenica in the Bosnia and Herzegovina war. Use of an incapacitating agent in Moscow in October 2002 generated much discussion regarding these agents. On October 23, over 700 people attended a musical in a Moscow theatre. During the performance, 40 Chechen terrorists demanding the withdrawal of Russia from Chechnya captured the building and took performers and customers hostage. Explosives were planted throughout the theatre, supporting the claim of the terrorists that they preferred death to surrender. The hostages, which included many children, were deprived of food and water while conditions deteriorated. On October 26, Russian Special Forces piped in an anesthetic gas reported to be fentanyl or a fentanyl derivative in order to incapacitate the terrorists prior to storming the theatre. All of the Chechens were killed; a reported 128 of the hostages also died, presumably from a combination of fentanyl and dehydration.

WEAPONIZATION

Research into chemical incapacitating agents was initiated by the U.S. military following World War II. The criteria for selection of a suitable incapacitating agent include military, medical, and budgetary considerations:

1. Effectiveness—the enemy must be rendered unable to fight
2. Relative lack of toxicity—compound must result in few deaths or permanent injuries
3. Persistence—effects must be temporary, lasting a maximum of a few days
4. Logistical feasibility—compound must be potent, chemically stable, and capable of being incorporated into practical munitions

TABLE 36-1

HISTORICAL INCIDENTS EXCERPTED FROM THE MEDICAL MANAGEMENT OF CHEMICAL CASUALTIES AND GOODMAN'S HISTORICAL REVIEW

Date	Historical Incident
600 BC	Hellebore roots were thrown into the streams supplying enemy troops to cause diarrhea by Solon's soldiers. [Ketchum JS, et al.]
200 BC	"According to Sextus Julius Frontinus, Maharbal, an officer in Hannibal's army... sent by the Carthaginians against the rebellious Africans, knowing that the tribe was passionately fond of wine, mixed a large quantity of wine with mandragora, which in potency is somewhere between a wine and a soporific. Then, after an insignificant skirmish, he deliberately withdrew. At the dead of night, leaving in the camp some of his baggage and all of the drugged wine, he feigned flight. When the barbarians captured the camp and in a frenzy of delight greedily drank the drugged wine, Maharbal returned, and either took them prisoners or slaughtered them while they lay stretched out as if dead." [USAMRICD]
AD 1672	"During his assault on the city of Groningen, the Bishop of Muenster tried to use grenades and projectiles containing belladonna against the defender. Unfortunately, capricious winds often blew the smoke back, creating effects opposite to those intended. As a result of this and other incidents in which chemicals were used in battle, a treaty was signed in 1675 between the French and the Germans, outlawing further use of chemical warfare." [USAMRICD]
1881	*Hyoscyamus falezlez* was used to contaminate dates eaten by members of a railway survey expedition by tribesmen of the Tuareg territory in North Africa. [Ketchum JS, et al.]
1908	Poisoning with a plant related to *H. falezlez* caused delirium in 200 French soldiers in Hanoi. [Ketchum JS, et al.]
1988	An intelligence report from the British Ministry of Defense accused Iraq of stockpiling Agent 15, a glycolate anticholinergic incapacitating agent. [Ketchum JS, et al.]

Source: As reported in the Textbook of Military Medicine, Medical Aspects of Chemical and Biological Warfare.

5. Treatability—effects should be reversible by medical treatment
6. Predictability—behaviors produced must be relatively predictable and unlikely to result in serious secondary consequences to civilians or noncombatants
7. Manageability of casualties—incapacitated individuals must be controllable
8. Expense—production must be affordable

Other considerations include manufacture, storage, and transport of the compound as well as training of both troops and medical personnel.

In the United States, significant resources were devoted to the development of incapacitating agents. In addition to anticholinergic compounds, other substances such as indoles (D-lysergic acid diethylamide, LSD, and cogeners), cannabinoids (marijuana and cogeners), and antipsychotic tranquilizers were investigated. After extensive consideration, only a single agent, BZ, was selected for standardization by the U.S. Army Chemical Corps. BZ became the primary agent in the United States inventory, was weaponized in the 1960s and stockpiled through the 1970s for possible use in military combat. Originally developed to enhance gastrointestinal radiographic imaging due to its ability to decrease gastrointestinal motility, BZ was discovered to cause mental status changes and therefore eliminated for use as a pharmaceutical agent. However, this capacity to induce confusion led to the selection of BZ for manufacturing as an incapacitating agent. Other desirable properties of BZ as an incapacitating agent include a prolonged duration of action, predictable effects, rapid transit through the blood-brain barrier, and high safety margin. The dose sufficient to cause incapacitation in 50% of the population exposed, known as the ID_{50}, is 112 mg·min/m^3; the lethal concentration in 50%, LD_{50}, is 200,000 mg·min/m^3.

The use of BZ was portrayed in the 1990 movie *Jacob's Ladder* in which BZ was the agent causing hallucinations and violent deaths in a fictitious American battalion in Vietnam. In actuality, BZ was never used in a military operation. The destruction of BZ supplies began in 1988 and although the U.S. military no longer maintains a supply of BZ, other countries or entities may possess this agent. In addition to use by the military in other countries, BZ may be encountered in civilian settings in terrorist actions or in conflict with sequestered groups in scenarios such as prison riots, hijackings, or hostage situations. BZ is also used by neuropharmacologists as a research standard for measuring central antimuscarinic activity.

The Chemical Casualty Care Division of the U.S. Army Research Institute of Chemical Defense currently addresses two agents in their training for medical management of incapacitating chemical casualties: BZ and Agent 15. Agent 15 is an incapacitating agent alleged to be contained in the Iraqi arsenal. It is believed to be similar, if not identical, to BZ. Therefore, for the purpose of this chapter, the details of the pharmacology and therapeutics of incapacitating agents will focus on BZ, an anticholinergic compound. General characteristics of other classes of drugs, which may be encountered as incapacitating agents, will also be discussed.

CHARACTERISTICS

Incapacitating agents, by military definition, are those agents that produce temporary and nonlethal impairment of military performance due to psychobehavioral or CNS effects. Anticholinergic compounds produce these desired effects. Table 36-2 lists anticholinergic compounds. These may be encountered outside of the military context as there is wide use of pharmaceutical agents and many naturally occurring plants with anticholinergic properties. The Toxic Exposure Surveillance System of the American Association of Poison Control Centers reported over 2.4 million cases of human poisoning in 2005, including 7,013 anticholinergic drug presentations and 75,762 antihistamine presentations. The highest morbidity was experienced in the patients with CNS manifestations. Due to unpleasant side effects, there is very little market for the illicit use of these substances.

3-QUINUCLIDINYL BENZYLATE (BZ)

General

BZ is the NATO code for 3-quinuclidinyl benzylate, designated QNB in the scientific community. BZ is a glycolate related to other anticholinergic compounds such as atropine and scopolamine, in addition to plant alkaloids such as hyoscine. It is an odorless substance, which is in a solid state at ambient temperatures. BZ has a high melting point and can be made into a fine powder; it is therefore ideal for release by explosive munitions. It can be dissolved in most solvents, including DMSO, which enhances percutaneous absorption, and dispersed as an aerosol. There is no mechanism for the detection of BZ in the environment where it can persist for long periods; the half-life is 3–4 weeks in moist air.

Pharmacodynamics

Mechanism of Action

Anticholinergic glycolates such as BZ are competitive inhibitors of the neurotransmitter acetylcholine. Sites of action are at the postsynaptic receptor in neurons and postjunctional muscarinic receptors in cardiac and smooth muscle and exocrine glands. BZ has minimal, if any, agonist activity. Nicotinic receptors are not effected.

TABLE 36-2

ANTICHOLINERGIC COMPOUNDS

Anticholinergics	• Clomipramine
• Atropine, scopolamine	• Desipramine
• Glycopyrrolate	• Doxepin
• Benztropine, trihexyphenidyl	• Imipramine
Antihistamines	• Nortriptyline
• Chlorpheniramine	• Protriptyline
• Cyproheptadine	**Mydriatics**
• Doxylamine	• Cyclopentolate
• Hydroxyzine	• Homatropine
• Dimenhydrinate	• Tropicamide
• Meclizine	**Miscellaneous drugs**
• Promethazine	• Carbamazepine
Antipsychotics	• Cyclobenzaprine
• Chlorpromazine	• Orphenadrine
• Clozapine	**Plants**
• Mesoridazine	• *Amanita muscaria* (fly agaric)
• Olanzapine	• *A. pantherina* (panther mushroom)
• Quetiapine	• *Arstium lappa* (burdock root)
• Thioridazine	• *Atropa belladonna* (deadly nightshade)
Antispasmodics	• *Cestrum nocturnum* (night blooming jessamine)
• Clidinium	• *Datura suaveolens* (angel's trumpet)
• Dicyclomine	• *D. stramonium* (jimson weed)
• Hyoscyamine	• *Hyoscyamus niger* (black henbane)
• Oxybutynin	• *Lantana camara* (red sage)
• Propantheline	• *Solanum carolinensis* (wild tomato)
Cyclic antidepressants	• *S. dulcamara* (bittersweet)
• Amitriptyline	• *S. psuedocapsicum* (Jerusalem cherry)
• Amoxapine	• *S. tuberosum* (potato)

Absorption, Distribution, and Elimination

Exposure to BZ can occur through inhalation or oral consumption; it is absorbed through the mucous membranes. BZ can also be absorbed through damp skin; when contact occurs through skin, the onset of effect is delayed about 24 hours. After mucous membrane exposure, the onset of action of BZ varies from 30 minutes to 20 hours and generally occurs between one-half to four hours; the duration of action is 3–5 days. There is very little difference in pharmacokinetics after intravenous or intramuscular administration. Relative to parenteral administration, the effectiveness of BZ is approximately 80 percent by oral administration, 40–50% by inhalation of optimal particle size (1 micron diameter) and 5–10% when applied to the skin. BZ is distributed throughout the organs and tissues of the body resulting in the peripheral nervous system effects; BZ crosses the blood-brain barrier and causes CNS effects. It is unknown whether BZ crosses the placenta or is excreted in breast milk. It is metabolized in the liver and both active compound and metabolites are excreted primarily in the urine.

CLINICAL MANIFESTATIONS

The effects of anticholinergic agents in humans are well-known; BZ causes similar clinical manifestations, which are summarized in Table 36-3. Note these effects are generally the opposite to symptoms resulting from exposure to nerve agents.

The CNS effects of BZ are of primary interest from a military perspective; patients may develop drowsiness and progress to coma. However, the peripheral nervous system effects are easily recognizable and useful in diagnosis. The cutaneous effects, in particular, are also important from a management perspective as decreased stimulation of sweat glands results in an inability to dissipate heat through evaporative cooling and may cause an elevation in core temperature. Hyperthermia is both an important differential in the diagnosis as well as an effect from the exposure. Although, like other anticholinergic compounds, BZ does not interfere with neurotransmission at the postjunctional nicotinic receptors of the skeletal muscle, these patients still manifest weakness along with increased deep tendon reflexes.

TABLE 36-3

CLINICAL EFFECTS OF BZ

	Peripheral Nervous System	
Organ	Effect	Mnemonic
Eyes	Mydriasis	
	Paralysis of accommodation	"blind as a bat"
Mouth	Xerostomia	"dry as a bone"
	Thirst	
Skin	Decreased sweating	"dry as a bone"
	Cutaneous vasodilatation ("atropine flush")	"red as a beet"
	Heat retention, increase core temperature	"hot as a hare"
Heart	Heart rate labile	not useful diagnostically
	Inconsistent effect	
Gastrointestinal Tract	Motility decreased	
	Secretions decreased	
Genitourinary Tract	Bladder tone decreased	
	Bladder distention	

	Central Nervous System	
Effect on Brain	Description	Mnemonic
Poor judgment	Lack of social restraint	
	Disrobing	
Altered level of consciousness	Drowsiness	
	May progress to coma	
Ataxia	Uncoordinated movements	
Slurred speech		
Illusions	Misperceptions of objects actually seen	"mad as a hatter"
Visual hallucinations	Observing an object that does not exist	
	Hallucinations may be shared	
Paranoia	Labile affect	
Perseveration	Repetitive actions	
	Automatic behaviors—climbing and crawling motions referred to as "progresso obstinato"	

Source: Army, U.S. [Computer Based Learning Program] 2004 [cited 2006 10/5/2006]; Available from: https://ccc.apgea.army.mil/sarea/courses/ imi/WebExport/Incaps_2004/incaps_1/index.html

CLINICAL COURSE

Following a latent period prior to onset of action, symptoms may develop in as little as 30 minutes or as long as 20 hours after exposure. The usual period prior to development of symptoms is one-half to four hours. Initial symptoms reflect parasympathetic blockade in addition to mild CNS effects. In general, decline in performance reaches a peak at approximately eight hours. In the period between 4 and 20 hours after exposure, patients may manifest stupor, ataxia, and hyperthermia. From 20 to 96 hours, patients may demonstrate fluctuating mental status with delirium. During the recovery period, the patient may vacillate between periods of paranoia when awake and in deep sleep. Climbing and crawling automatisms may appear.

The effects of BZ, generally 48 to 72 hours in duration, can persist for up to 6 days. At the IC_{50} level of exposure, the duration of incapacitation is 24 hours. If the exposure dose is doubled, recovery period extends to 48 hours.

CDC case definition criteria for laboratory diagnosis is

- Biologic—a case in which BZ is detected in the urine.
- Environmental—no method available for detecting BZ in environmental samples.

TRIAGE

With respect to BZ intoxication, military triage categories are defined as follows:

Immediate casualty—cardiorespiratory compromise or severe hyperthermia

Delayed casualty—severe or worsening anticholinergic CNS signs

Minimal casualty—mild peripheral or central anticholinergic effects

Expectant casualties—severe cardiorespiratory compromise in a situation where resources are inadequate to provide treatment or evacuation

TREATMENT

Decontamination

Since BZ is a solid at ambient temperature, chemical decontamination measures must be instituted for cases of possible exposure by BZ dissemination as either a solid or liquid. Protection of health-care workers is a primary consideration in care of these patients and appropriate personal protective equipment should be donned. For military purposes, the HEPA filter in the C2A1 canister of the chemical protective mask prevents inhalation exposure to aerosolized BZ. The battledress overgarment (BDO) and the Joint Service Lightweight Integrated Suit Technology (JSLIST) equipment will protect the skin against contact with BZ whether dispersed as fine particles or in solution. Decontamination follows standard recommendations; patients should remove all clothing, which should then be sealed in plastic bags for disposal or decontamination. The patients must be completely disrobed and their skin and hair washed thoroughly with soap and water.

Isolation and decontamination measures may be compromised by the nature of the compound, which is odorless and nonirritating and has a latent period before clinical symptoms are exhibited. In addition, there is no means of identifying BZ in the field and environmental samples must undergo laboratory analysis for diagnostic confirmation. These circumstances may result in a delay in recognition of exposure and thus failure to assume appropriate precautions. Persistence of this compound in the environment is another characteristic to bear in mind in considering potential for further exposure.

Supportive Measures

Again, primary consideration must be given to safety of health-care personnel. Therefore any weapons or potential weapons must be confiscated immediately. Patients may also require restraint for their own protection. Although BZ is intended as a nonlethal, incapacitating agent, there is some risk. In BZ poisoning, the life-threatening risks to patients include (1) injury from their erratic behavior or the behavior of other patients with BZ intoxication and (2) hyperthermia. Hyperthermia is a particular risk in hot, humid environments or when complicated by dehydration.

In addition to cooling measures, electrolytes and cardiac rhythms monitoring should be done. In battlefield scenarios, the need for evacuation to a higher level of care should be considered in view of the prolonged duration of action.

Antidote Therapy

Therapy in BZ poisoning is directed to increasing the concentration of acetylcholine at the synapses and junctions and reversing the clinical anticholinergic effects. Any compound which can accomplish this can potentially reverse BZ intoxication, including administration of the nerve agent VX when administered under controlled conditions. However, the specific antidote available for the treatment of anticholinergic poisoning is the carbamate anticholinesterase physostigmine (eserine; Antilirium). The natural source of physostigmine is the calabar bean, which is the fruit of Physistigma veneosum found in West Africa.

The mechanism of action of physostigmine is to bind with acetylcholinesterase, thereby inhibiting its action and allowing increased quantities of acetylcholine to compete more effectively with BZ at the muscarinic nerve receptor sites. Physostigmine acts in both the peripheral and central nervous systems. However, in the case of BZ intoxication, physostigmine is primarily indicated for behavioral management. BZ is a nonpolar compound and therefore it is capable of crossing the blood-brain barrier. As significant CNS manifestations do not occur until after 4 hours, physostigmine is not useful in the early period of exposure. The duration of action of physostigmine is 45–60 minutes. While physostigmine is effective in treating the CNS symptoms, it does not shorten the clinical course. Relapse will occur unless physostigmine is dosed repeatedly with dose and interval based on serial mental status examination. Due to the prolonged duration of action of BZ, physostigmine dosing may have to be continued for up to 5 days and requiring up to 70 doses.

Physostigmine may be administered intramuscularly, by mouth or intravenously.

Physostigmine dosages:

IM   45 mcg/kg (adult)   20 mcg/kg (child)
PO   60 mcg/kg
IV   30 mcg/kg not to exceed 1 mg/min

Oral administration of physostigmine requires a cooperative patient because of its bitter taste; it is better tolerated if mixed in juice. One and one-half times the parenteral dose is usually required. The onset of action between intravenous and intramuscular injections varies by only minutes, so the difference is unlikely to be clinically important. Because of the repeated dosing required, it appears logical to consider an intravenous infusion. However, this is generally advised against unless the setting is conducive to the provision of careful monitoring for cholinergic symptoms. Administration of intravenous physostigmine should not exceed 1 mg/min to minimize the complications of seizures or arrhythmias. Physostigmine should be avoided in patients with QRS prolongation. It is contraindicated in a patient with cardiorespiratory compromise, hypoxia, or acid-base imbalance with a history of seizures or arrhythmias. Other side effects of physostigmine include cholinergic symptoms such as sweating, abdominal cramps, nausea, vomiting, muscle fasciculations, tremors, weakness, and bradycardia.

Whatever route of administration is used for physostigmine, the dose should be titrated to the patient's mental status examination using simple tests such as serial sevens. A mental status examination should be recorded every hour with modification of the dose and interval based on improvement in the patient's condition.

If the diagnosis of anticholinergic poisoning is in doubt, a test dose of 1–2 mg intramuscularly can be considered. This can be repeated once after 20 minutes if no improvement with the initial dose is noted.

Interestingly, the antagonism between physostigmine and atropine was first reported in 1864 when a physician treated a prisoner who became delirious after drinking tincture of belladonna. Use of physostigmine was again ignored by the medical community when its use in treating psychiatric patients who had been administered up to 50 mg of atropine was reported in the 1950s. It was not until 1967 that a controlled study reported the reversal of anticholinergic intoxication by physostigmine.

DIFFERENTIAL DIAGNOSIS

Heat stroke is a disease entity difficult to distinguish from BZ intoxication. The diagnosis would rely primarily on the lack of response to resuscitation measures for hyperthermia. Other anticholinergic agents must be considered in the differential and would cause similar symptoms to BZ. In particular, atropine poisoning from a MARK I autoinjector may cause some confusion in the patient, but this would not be likely to appear until six injections had been received. Exposure to indoles such as LSD would also present with hallucinations, but of a different nature. LSD-related hallucinations are not based on reality and are more panoramic. Cannabinoids may cause lethargy but are not associated with the peripheral anticholinergic symptoms discussed. Anxiety and other intoxicants would also be included in the differential. Lead, barbiturates, and bromides poisoning can lead to confusion and erratic behavior. The peripheral nervous system effects of BZ when associated with CNS findings provide the main clues to the diagnosis.

OTHER INCAPACITATING AGENTS

Also grouped with agents of chemical warfare are a variety of chemicals, which produce incapacitation through physiological as opposed to psychological or behavioral effects. Blister agents, such as mustard and Lewisite, and chlorine incapacitate but cause extremely painful injuries as well as death. Irritants, including chlorobenzylidene malonitrile (CS) and chloroacetophenone (CN), are safe and effective but their duration is only about 30 minutes after exposure and tolerance can develop. These factors make irritants including CS and CN undesirable as incapacitating agents. However, irritants have a role in riot control and are discussed in Appendix K. The safety margin of 10-chloro-5,10-dihydrophenarsazine (DM), a nausea-producing agent, was unacceptable. There also exist several noninfectious biological agents, such as the staphylococcal enterotoxins, which could be used to cause symptoms resulting in inability to fight. In addition, sublethal levels of nerve agents were considered. These systemic agents were also deemed unacceptable as incapacitating agents due to low safety margins.

The psychochemical agents can be classified into four general categories of stimulants, depressants, psychedelics, and deliriants; all of these agents result in CNS effects and disrupt higher brain function by virtue of their ability to cross the blood-brain barrier. Stimulants include amphetamines, cocaine, caffeine, nicotine, and eliptogenic substances, strychnine, and metrazole. These agents lacked sufficient potency for aerosolized dispersal. Depressants have not proved useful for a variety of reasons, their dosage requirements or safety margins being too high or too low. Agents studied in the category include barbiturates, opioids, antipsychotics, and minor tranquilizers. No reports describe the use of aerosolized opioids or benzodiazepines as incapacitating agents in the American population; a report of the international use of an aerosolized opioid in Moscow in 2002 was previously discussed. The mortality and morbidity associated with the use of aerosolized benzodiazepines or opioids as incapacitating agents is unknown, but many deaths resulted from the Moscow event. The class of psychedelics, including LSD, was given serious consideration by the military with systematic testing conducted from 1950 to 1965. LSD proved too unpredictable while its analogs lacked potency. Other synthetic psychedelic compounds including 3,4-methylenedioxymethylamphetamine (MDMA or ecstasy) also proved unpredictable. After briefly observing the effects of phencyclidine (PCP), the military also was deemed it unsuitable for use. Finally, large doses of delta-9-tetrahydrocannabinol (THC) may cause confusion, amnesia, delusions, hallucinations, anxiety, and agitation; however, the effects generally resolve rapidly without intervention. Deliriants proved to be the most logical candidates for chemical incapacitating agents, and the anticholinergic category was intensely investigated for this purpose. The chosen agent, BZ, met necessary criteria and production was pursued as discussed. However, these other compounds may still be encountered in small-scale covert operations with simpler logistics. In likely scenarios, their use must be considered in the differential diagnosis of altered mental status.

DISCUSSION AND FUTURE PROSPECTS

General public indignation occurred as a result of the chemical weapons such as chlorine, mustard, and phosgene used in World War I. As a consequence, an international ban on chemical weapons was adopted by the Geneva Convention in 1925. Although the United States did not sign until 1975, the concept in theory was supported. In World War II, chemical weapons were not used, although stockpiles of several lethal anticholinesterase nerve agents were found in Germany. "Debate about the legality of this new kind of weapon has revolved around whether their development and use are permitted for law enforcement (as opposed to armed combat), which is not prohibited by the 1993 Chemical Weapons Convention." A report from the National Academy of Sciences concluded there was sufficient ambiguity in the Chemical Weapons Convention to permit the use of some nonlethal weapons. At present no incapacitating agents exist in the U.S. military armamentarium. Wartime use of riot control agents is limited to defensive measures by presidential order. In addition, there are accepted peacetime uses of riot control agents. The significance of less lethal weapons is demonstrated by the fact that on June 22, 2006, in Boeblingen, Germany, the United States European Command focused this year's Summit and Capability Exercise on current and emerging nonlethal weapon systems and techniques.

While any weapon can be misused, most weapons have a legitimate use. Changing technology does not alter human intent, which is the source of abuse of any weapons system. While less lethal weapons do not resolve all issues with the abuse of force, they do offer hope of minimizing casualties while protecting public or national interests. Either denying legitimate use or permitting uncontrolled use of less lethal technology may result in unnecessary suffering and death. In defense of the use and development of less lethal weapons, a case can be made for their having a legitimate place on the "use of force" continuum; these are the cases where they provide an alternative to lethal force.

Others caution about the development of these weapons even for use by law enforcement due to the risk to noncombatants in a domestic situation, as well as the risk of terrorists equipping themselves with an equivalent arsenal. Some argue that the promise attached to the development of less lethal weapons has not lived up to expectations. A minimum framework proposed for the assessment of nonlethal weapons contends: alternatives to new force options should be pursued first, weapons should be subject to rigorous and transparent testing procedures, the approval of weaponry should be a transparent and accountable process, postapproval monitoring and feedback is essential. Some experts contend that "the introduction of nonlethal options has not functioned as a substitute for lethal or other force options, but increased the range of situations in which force is used."

It has also been proposed that a medical perspective should be brought to this debate to discuss the inevitable role of physicians with respect to aspects such as development, training, and treatment. The development of emerging nonlethal technologies will produce new challenges for medical personnel not only in the management of physical and psychological effects, but in maintaining an awareness of the symptoms of human rights abuse. The development of nonlethal weapons raises ethical dilemmas about how and when they should be used and how they can be tested on people. It has been suggested that an independent entity such as the Institute of Medicine study these emerging ethical dilemmas related to less lethal weapons in the context of terrorism and national security.

Suggested Reading

Alexander JB. An overview of the future of non-lethal weapons. *Med Confl Surviv.* 2001;17(3):180.

Army, U.S. [Computer Based Learning Program] 2004 [cited 10/5/2006]; Available from: *https://ccc.apgea.army.mil/sarea/courses/imi/WebExport/Incaps_2004/incaps_1/index.html*

Bruns JJ. Toxicity, Anticholinergic. *eMedicine J.* [serial online] 2006; Available at: *www.emedicine.com/emerg/topic36.htm*

Center for Disease Control, 2005 [cited 4/13/2006]; Available from: *www.bt.cdc.gov/chemical*

Chemical Incapacitating Weapons Are not Non-lethal—Position Paper. 2006 [cited 4/13/2006]; Available from: *www.armscontrolcenter.org/cbw/wg/pp/pp_chemical_incapacitants.pdf*

Coupland RM. Incapacitating chemical weapons: a year after the Moscow theatre siege. *Lancet.* 2003;362(9393):1346.

Department of Defense, 2006 [cited 10/1/2006]; Available from: *www.defenselink.mil/transformation/*

Dobrowolski A, Moore S. Less than lethal weapons and their impact on patient care. *Top Emerg Med.* 2005;27(1):44.

Holstege CP, Baer A. CBRNE—Incapacitating Agents, Opioids/Benzodiazepines. *eMedicine J.* [serial online] 2004; Available at: *www.emedicine.com/emerg/topic944.htm*

Jussilla J. Future police operations and nonlethal weapons. *Med Confl Surviv.* 2001;17(3):248.

Ketchum JSaS, Frederick R. Incapacitating agents. In: Zajtchuk R, ed. *Medical Aspects of Chemical and Biological Warfare.* Washington, DC, Office of the Surgeon General, Department of the Army, United States of America, 1997; p 287.

Lewer N. Non-lethal weapons: operational and policy developments. *Lancet.* 2003;362S:s20.

Moreno JD. Medical ethics and non-lethal weapons. *Am J Bioeth.* 2004;4:W1.

Pasternak D. A softer touch. The U.S. is developing weapons that would subdue, but not kill. *US News World Rep.* 2002;133 (18):32.

United States Army Medical Research Institute of Chemical Defense. *Medical Management of Chemical Casualties Handbook.* 3rd ed. Aberdeen Proving Ground: 2000.

Rappert B. A framework for the assessment of non-lethal weapons. *Med Confl Surviv.* 2004;20(1):35.

37

OTHER CHEMICAL AGENTS

Christopher P. Holstege, Tracey H. Reilly, and Laura K. Bechtel

STAT FACTS

OTHER AGENTS

- There are a multitude of potential chemical agents capable of causing mass toxicity following a terrorist attack.
- Chemical agents utilized by terrorists may come from commercial (i.e., sodium monofluoroacetate), natural (i.e., trichothecene mycotoxins), military (i.e., vomiting agents), or industrial (i.e., dioxin) sources.
- Rapid detection systems for these agents are lacking; confirmatory tests may take days to weeks for final results.
- The majority of potential chemical agents that could be utilized by terrorists have no associated antidote and symptomatic and supportive care will be the primary focus of the medical teams.

INTRODUCTION

There are numerous chemical agents that could be utilized by terrorists to cause injury to a single individual or to a large gathering of people. There is not a unified consensus of what these potential agents might be, and part of each community's local plan should focus on the potential chemical agents available in their region that could be utilized by terrorists. For example, the Virginia Department of Health released a list of potential agents that could be utilized against its citizens (Table 37-1) by terrorist groups. The Center for Disease Control (CDC) did likewise in 2005 (*MMWR.* 2005;54:1–24). The challenge for first responders and local hospitals is to prepare for an event that might utilize one or multiple of these agents.

The CDC has created a multilevel laboratory response network (LRN) to provide surge capacity testing for

exposure to chemical or biological terrorist agents. The LRN links 126 clinical laboratories to public health agencies in all states by providing state-of-the-art facilities that can analyze potential biological and chemical terrorist agents. At the onset of an event, state laboratories are capable of performing some initial testing. More specialized analyses from one of the seven CDC-funded Level 1 facilities may be required. Furthermore, the CDC directly may employ a Rapid Toxic Screen to analyze human blood and urine samples for a large number of potential terrorist agents. If medical personnel suspect patient exposure to a chemical or biological terrorist agent, the health-care team should immediately contact their respective state or local health department. The majority of detection methods require collection and shipping of human specimens as specified by the CDC Laboratory Information for Chemical Emergencies Web page *(http://www.bt.cdc.gov/ chemical/lab.asp).*

It is beyond this chapter's scope to describe all the potential chemical agents that might be utilized by terrorists. Rather, it will focus on unique representatives from the four groups of toxin sources, namely the commercial (i.e., sodium monofluoroacetate), industrial (i.e., dioxin), natural (i.e., trichothecene mycotoxins), and military (i.e., vomiting agents) sources.

SODIUM MONOFLUOROACETATE (COMPOUND 1080)

Sodium monofluoroacetate (also known as SMFA, ratbane 1080, and compound 1080) is a potent rodenticide initially derived from plants that is used commercially against vertebrate species in a number of countries, including the United States, Australia, New Zealand, Israel, and Mexico. Although banned from use by the general public in the

TABLE 37-1

A PARTIAL LISTING OF POTENTIAL CHEMICAL AGENTS THAT COULD BE UTILIZED BY TERRORIST GROUPS AS PROVIDED BY THE VIRGINIA DEPARTMENT OF HEALTH

Abrin	Acids	Adamsite
Ammonia	Arsenic	Arsine
Barium	Benzene	Brevetoxin
Bromine	Bromobenzylcyanide	BZ
Carbon monoxide	Caustics	Chlorine
Chloroacetophenone	Chlorobenzylidenemalononitrile	Chloropicrin
Colchicine	Cyanide	Cyanogen chloride
Dibenzoxazepine	Digitalis	Diphosgene
Ethylene glycol	Hydrogen fluoride	Lewisite
Long-acting anticoagulants	Mercury	Methyl bromide
Methyl isocyanate	Mustard	Nerve agents
Nicotine	Opioids	Organic solvents
Osmium tetroxide	Paraquat	Phosgene
Phosphine	Phosphorous	Saxitoxin
Sodium azide	Sodium monofluoroacetate	Stibine
Strychnine	Sulfuryl fluoride	Tear gas
Tetrodotoxin	Thallium	Trichothecene

United States in 1972, it is currently restricted for use solely in livestock protection collars to protect sheep and cattle from coyotes. There is currently concern for the potential use of SMFA by terrorist groups through the contamination of potable water or food.

Properties

The synthetic form of the SMFA (CAS # 62-74-8) exists as a white powder (similar in appearance to flour or powdered sugar) that remains stable for long periods of time. It is odorless, tasteless, and readily dissolves in water. It is relatively insoluble in organic solvents such as ethanol or vegetable oils. The only reported distinguishing characteristic is that it has a weak vinegar taste when mixed with water. It is heat-stable; it does not decompose until temperatures approach 200°C. SMFA is highly toxic to vertebrates, although the sensitivity of different species varies dramatically. In man, the estimated lethal poisoning dose ranges from 2 to 10 mg/kg body weight.

Routes of Exposure

Compound 1080 is well-absorbed from the gastrointestinal tract, the respiratory tract, open wounds, mucus membranes, and the eye. The majority of human exposures reported in the medical literature have been through ingestion. Toxicity has been reported to be the same whether it is administered orally, subcutaneously, intramuscularly, or intravenously. Dusts containing SMFA are effectively toxic by inhalation.

Pathophysiology

The toxicologic mechanism of SMFA involves disruption of cellular energy production resulting in multisystem organ failure (Fig. 37-1). The parent compound, fluoroacetate, has very low cellular toxicity. However, once ingested and absorbed, enzymatic reactions within cells convert fluoroacetate to fluoroacetyl-CoA. Fluoroacetyl-CoA, in the presence of oxaloacetate, is converted by citrate synthase to

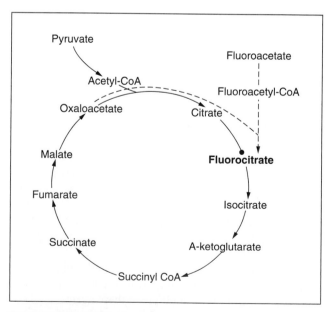

FIGURE 37-1

KREBS CYCLE DEMONSTRATING THE REGION OF INHIBITION BY FLUOROACETATE

fluorocitrate, a potent inhibitor of the enzyme aconitase. Aconitase catalyzes the reversible Krebs cycle reaction converting citrate to isocitrate. The inhibition of aconitase results in the interruption of the energy producing Krebs cycle and the buildup of citrate. Fluorocitrate also inhibits transport of citrate into and out of mitochondria, contributing to the buildup of citrate. Elevated citrate levels disrupt energy production via glycolysis, by inhibiting the enzyme phosphofructokinase. Elevated citrate levels may also cause life-threatening hypocalcemia. Because it takes time for the metabolic conversion of fluoroacetate to fluorocitrate, there is a delay from the time that the poison is ingested to the initial onset of signs and symptoms.

Clinical Manifestations

Clinical signs and symptoms associated with SMFA poisoning are nonspecific. SMFA poisoning is characterized by a latent period of 30 minutes to 3 hours following the administration of the compound by any route. Even massive doses do not elicit immediate responses, although the latent period may be reduced. In animal studies, the early stages of poisoning are typically reported as displaying a range of signs including lethargy, vomiting, trembling, excessive salivation, incontinence, muscular weakness, incoordination, hypersensitivity to nervous stimuli, and respiratory distress. Early neurological signs include muscular twitches often affecting the face, such as nystagmus and blepharospasm. These then progress to generalized seizures, initially tonic and then becoming cyclically tonic-clonic with periods of lucidity in between. Partial paralysis may be seen that lasts for prolonged time periods. Death typically results from depression of the respiratory center and/or ventricular fibrillation.

Numerous human reports exist in the literature. Trabes et al, for example, described a 15-year-old who attempted suicide by ingesting SMFA. She developed nausea, vomiting, and abdominal pain within 30 minutes of ingestion followed by a grand mal seizure 1 hour later with associated tachycardia (150 beats/min) and profuse diaphoresis. She was described as disorientated, demonstrated signs of psychomotor agitation, and over the ensuing 4 hours developed three additional grand mal seizures and then became comatose. She recovered, but developed a chronic cerebellar ataxia and computerized tomography findings of moderate diffuse brain atrophy. Reigart et al. described an 8-month-old who developed two episodes of nausea and vomiting after ingesting SMFA, but was otherwise asymptomatic until seizures developed 20 hours postingestion. In a retrospective study of 38 human cases of SMFA poisoning, Chi et al. noted the most frequent symptom to be nausea and/or vomiting (74%). Electrocardiograph changes were quite variable, ranging from mild nonspecific ST- and T-wave abnormalities (72%), to ventricular tachycardias and asystole. The most common electrolyte abnormalities included hypocalcemia (42%) and hypokalemia (65%). Seven of the thirty-eight patients died in this series. Discriminate analysis identified hypotension, increased serum creatinine, and decreased pH as the most important predictors of mortality, with sensitivity of 86% and specificity of 96%.

Laboratory Testing

Chemical detection methods are currently utilized to detect SMFA in human blood specimens. Derivatized extracts are analyzed using gas chromatography mass spectroscopy (GC/MS) or gas chromatography with electron-capture detection. Since the exact mechanism for SMFA metabolism has not been elucidated, rapid collection of blood specimens should be done and the blood immediately stored at 4°C. The limits of detection are approximately 0.1 mg/kg (ppm), providing highly sensitive methods for detecting toxic levels (LD_{50} 2–10 ppm) in human biological samples.

Treatment

There is no specific antidote for SMFA toxicity and therapy is primarily focused on supportive care. A number of different treatments have been explored for SMFA toxicity. Because SMFA induces hypocalcemia, calcium supplementation through administration of either calcium gluconate or calcium chloride has been shown to be of benefit. In animal models, sodium succinate has also been shown to be of benefit as a potential antidote to revive the Krebs cycle, especially when utilized with calcium. All patients with known oral exposure to SMFA should be observed for a minimum of 24 hours following exposure.

DIOXIN

Dioxin is a term applied to a family of compounds known as the chlorinated dibenzo-*p*-dioxins. The basic structure of a dioxin consists of two benzene rings joined via two oxygen bridges at adjacent carbons on each of the benzene rings (Fig. 37-2). The family of dioxins contains 75 distinct types: 2 monochlorodibenzo-*p*-dioxins; 10 dichlorodibenzo-*p*-dioxins; 14 trichlorodibenzo-*p*-dioxins; 22 tetrachloro-dibenzo-*p*-dioxins; 14 pentachlorodibenzo-*p*-dioxins;

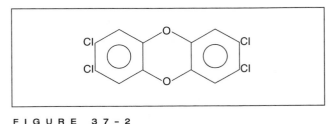

FIGURE 37-2

DIOXIN BASIC STRUCTURE

10 hexachlorodibenzo-*p*-dioxins; 2 heptachlorodibenzo-*p*-dioxins; and 1 octachlorodibenzo-*p*-dioxin. The most thoroughly studied dioxin is 2,3,7,8-tetrachloro-dibenzo-*p*-dioxin (TCDD). Dioxins are within a larger grouping of compounds called the polyhalogenated aromatic hydrocarbons (PAH), consisting of polyhalogentated naphthalenes, polyhalogenated biphenyls, polyhalogenated dibenzofurans, polychlorodibenzofurans, tetrachloroazobenzene, and tetrachloroazo-oxybenzene. All these compounds are capable of causing similar health effects, though TCDD is reportedly the most toxic of the group.

PAHs have been associated with numerous adverse human health effects. Historically, there have been massive environmental exposures that lead to the toxicity of thousands of people. These historical events include the BASF accident in Ludwigshafen, Germany (1953); Philips-Duphar Facility explosion in Amsterdam, Netherlands (1963); *Yusho disease* (rice oil), Japan (1968); Coalite explosion, England (1973), Seveso disaster, Italy (1976); and *Yu-Cheng disease* (rice oil), Taiwan (1979). Dioxin has recently been reported to have been utilized in a number of criminal poisoning cases (i.e., Austria and Ukraine) and has been a focus of various terrorism preparedness programs (i.e., The American College of Medical Toxicology Chemical Agents of Opportunity for Terrorism Course).

Properties

TCDD has no odor or warning characteristics and is soluble in oils. TCDD has been shown to form a stable complex with α-fetoprotein (AFP). The apparent solubility of TCDD in water increases 10^5-fold after TCDD:AFP complex formation.

Routes of Exposure

Dioxins are well-absorbed by inhalation, ingestion, and dermal contact. TCDD bioaccumulates in the highest concentrations within the fat, pancreas, liver, and skin; the lowest concentrations are found within the nervous tissue, lung, and kidney. Elimination occurs via the feces through biliary secretion. Enterohepatic recirculation occurs. The elimination half-life is approximately 7 years. There is a tremendous interspecies variation of clinical toxicity. The LD_{50} is reportedly 70 μg/kg (ppb) in the monkey and 0.6 μg/kg in the guinea pig. The reported mean toxic dose is 0.1 μg/kg in humans. It is the marked toxicity of the pure form and the long elimination half-life that make TCDD a potent terrorist weapon.

Pathophysiology

Dermatologically, TCDD alters the pattern of keratinocyte terminal differentiation; keratinocytes become hyperplastic. Comedones form, consisting of numerous accumulated layers of keratinized cells and sebum. Hyperproduction of melanin occurs by a normal number of melanocytes.

Triglycerides may elevate. This is thought secondary to a number of processes. First, there is increased triglyceride synthesis in the liver. Second, there is decreased lipoprotein lipase activity. Third, triglyceride storage is decreased in adipose tissue thereby causing increased serum triglycerides and a wasting syndrome. Fourth, TCDD also stimulates the aryl hydrocarbon receptor which depresses adipogenesis. Finally, TCDD enhances lipolysis, resulting in hyperlipidemia and steatosis.

TCDD causes an inhibition of uroporphyrinogen decarboxylase, which leads to a rise in porphyrins. There has been a documented genetic predisposition to this effect, resulting in porphyria cutanea tarda in 14% of exposed patients.

Clinical Manifestations

Reports describing TCDD's clinical effects vary widely in the literature. The clinical effects associated with dioxin exposure depend on a number of factors, including the route of the exposure, the presence of other chemicals, the total dioxin body burden, the duration of dioxin exposure, the age of the person exposed, and the preexisting health of the exposed person. Initial clinical signs and symptoms associated with TCDD poisoning are nonspecific. TCDD poisoning is characterized by a latent period of hours to days following the administration of the compound by any route. Anorexia, irritability, weight loss, fatigue, headache, and insomnia have all been associated with dioxin toxicity. Gastrointestinal symptoms including nausea, vomiting, abdominal pain, and gastritis may occur. Hepatitis and pancreatitis have been reported. TCDD causes peripheral neuropathies. Sensory neuropathies tend to be delayed in onset, persistent, and most commonly affect the legs. Polyneuropathic electromyogram abnormalities are frequently observed. The neuritis may cause limb pain of disabling severity. The motor nerves are rarely affected. Severe myalgias of the extremities, shoulders, and thorax have been reported. Hormonal alterations, including elevated luteinizing hormone and follicle stimulating hormone with lowered testosterone, have been noted in association with elevated TCDD levels. Sexual impotence has been reported as well as loss of libido.

The dermatologic effects following TCDD exposure may be pronounced and have been well described, lasting for decades from severe exposure. Chloracne (also known as halogen acne) is one of the most common findings in humans exposed to dioxin. Chloracne is a symmetrical dermatologic condition involving the change of undifferentiated sebaceous gland cells to keratinocytes resulting in a disappearance of sebaceous glands and the substitution of closed comedones and keratin cysts. The malar crescent of the face and retroauricular folds are the areas of the skin that are most commonly involved. The cheeks, forehead, neck, forearms, trunk, back, legs, and genitalia are also commonly afflicted. The nose, eyelids, and the auricular region are often less severely affected, except in patients with markedly elevated levels. The hands, forearms, feet, and legs are involved less. Cystic lesions containing straw-colored fluid develop, especially on the face in the "crow's feet" area, giving a "plucked chicken skin" appearance. Lesions in the axilla may mimic hidradenitis suppurativa. Xerosis, alopecia, and granuloma annulare have also been reported. Hypertrichosis, primarily involving the temporal area of the face and the eyebrows, occurs primarily in association with dioxin-induced porphyria cutanea tarda. Punctate keratoderma, primarily involving the palms and soles, has been described and is histologically characterized by cone-shaped hyperkeratosis invaginating, but not penetrating, into the dermis. Palpebral edema and meibomian gland cysts have been reported. Hyperhidrosis of the palms and the soles may occur. Increased nail growth and nail plate thickening also have been reported.

Numerous abnormalities in laboratory values have been reported including anemia, leukocytosis, thrombocytopenia, and decreased numbers of natural killer cells. Reports also demonstrate elevated erythrocyte sedimentation rate, C-reactive protein, fibrinogen, uroporphyrins, alkaline phosphatase, lipase, amylase, and liver transaminases (GGT, GPT, GOT). Prolonged elevation of γ-glutamyltransferase (GGT) has been documented in numerous reports. Dioxin-induced alternations in serum lipid levels have been shown, with elevated triglycerides best characterized in the medical literature. Elevated total cholesterol and lowered high-density lipoprotein (HDL) may also occur.

TCDD is classified to be carcinogenic to humans (Group 1) by the International Agency for Research on Cancer (IARC). TCDD has been associated with soft-tissue sarcoma, Hodgkin's disease, non-Hodgkin's lymphoma, gastric cancer, nasal cancer, and liver cancer in various reports.

Laboratory Testing

Since dioxin levels in biological specimens are extremely low, testing requires very sensitive and specific methods for analysis. Two types of testing procedures are available for measuring dioxins in human blood and urine specimens—bioanalytical and chemical detection methods. The preferred method for identifying the TCDD congener in blood and urine specimens is chemical detection using gas chromatography coupled to ^{13}C-labelled isotope dilution sector high-resolution mass spectrometry (GC-ID-HRMS). The sensitivity for this method (20 pg/g serum, 0.020 ppb) is within the estimated TCDD levels (1–1000 ppt) found in the general population of the United States, Canada, Germany, and France. The long half-life for TCDD permits a large collection window when analyzing human specimens and results can be available in several hours.

Unfortunately, the long half-life for TCDD and poor bioaccumulation and exposure data available in human studies make the "toxic exposure" assessment particularly difficult. Therefore, interpretation of quantitative TCDD values obtained from the analysis of human samples requires expert and knowledgeable personnel.

The high cost for screening human samples for TCDD using GC-ID-HRMS is due to the requirement of expensive equipment, highly qualified operators, and qualified personnel to interpret the data. Two less costly chemical detection methods have been developed: quadruple ion storage mass spectrometry (QUIST-MS) and two-dimensional gas chromatography time-of-flight mass spectrometry (GCxGC-TOF-MS). Although these alternative methodologies have lower resolution, the level of sensitivity for a particular congener is within an acceptable range for detection.

Due to the limited data available for assessing elevated TCDD levels in the general public, bioanalytical tools are an alternative method for assessment of human exposure levels in human samples. These methods may be used to screen a large number of samples if a TCDD-related terrorist event is suspected. For example, the enzyme immunoassay (EPA method 4025) and CALUX (EPA method 4425) are currently approved for determining a scientific basis for the quantitative assessment of environmental health risks. Numerous other bioassays are currently available that are based on the ability of biological molecules to recognize a unique structural property of the dioxin compound, or have a unique response to dioxin compounds.

Treatment

The treatment options for dioxin toxicity are limited, primarily due to its prolonged elimination half-life. Due to its enterohepatic recirculation, a number of treatments have been suggested to enhance the elimination of TCDD. These have included cholestyramine with dietary fiber, colestimidine, and olestra. High-dose vitamin A and E have also been advocated to potentially decrease the incidence of cancer formation. The treatment of chloracne is especially problematic, and numerous therapies have been attempted without success, including isotretinoin, topical retinoic, ultraviolet light, prednisone, and tetracycline. Dermabrasion and light cautery under EMLA topical anesthesia have been utilized with some success.

TRICHOTHECENE MYCOTOXINS

The trichothecene mycotoxins constitute a family of more than 60 compounds produced by a number of fungi, including *Fusarium, Myrothecium, Phomopsis, Stachybotrys, Trichoderma, and Trichothecium.* All trichothecenes contain a common 12,13-epoxytrichothene skeleton and are subdivided into four chemical groups (type A, B, C, D).

T-2 toxin is one of the most extensively studied of the trichothecenes.

The trichothecene mycotoxins have a long and sordid history. In the Ukraine in the early 1930s, a disease unique to horses was recognized, that was characterized by lip edema, stomatitis, oral necrosis, rhinitis, and conjunctivitis. The clinical effects often progressed through well-defined stages including pancytopenia, coagulopathy, neurologic compromise, superinfections, and death. When autopsies were performed on the afflicted animals, the entire alimentary tract was found to have diffuse hemorrhage and necrosis, giving rise to the name *alimentary toxic aleukia*. During World War II, a large population within Orenburg, Russia, became ill following the ingestion of overwintered grain colonized by mold, giving a similar disease pattern as noted in previous animal outbreaks. These outbreaks subsequently lead to the discovery of the trichothecene mycotoxins, with T-2 toxin isolated in 1968. The trichothecenes were reported to have been used in the "yellow rain" incidents in the mid to late 1970s and early 1980s, killing thousands in Southeast Asia and Afghanistan.

Properties

The trichothecene mycotoxins are extremely stable proteins, resistant to heat, autoclaving, hypochlorite, and ultraviolet light. However, when exposed to sodium hydroxide, the toxins are rendered inactive. Of the naturally occurring trichothecenes, T-2 is one of the most potent toxins in animal studies and the most extensively studied. These toxins can be delivered as dusts, droplets, aerosols, or smoke from a variety of dispersal systems and exploding munitions. They are highly soluble in a number of organic solvents, such as ethanol, and only slightly soluble in water. T-2 toxin is distributed rapidly to tissues, with the hepatobiliary system being the major route for the metabolism and elimination. The median lethal dose is mammalian species dependent, between 0.5 and 50 mg/kg.

Routes of Exposure

The trichothecene mycotoxins are well absorbed by topical, oral, or inhalational routes.

Pathophysiology

The trichothecene mycotoxins are markedly cytotoxic. These toxins bind to the 60S ribosomal subunit and inactivate its peptidyl transferase activity at the transcription site, thereby inhibiting protein synthesis. Actively proliferating cells are particularly sensitive. As a result, these toxins have both cytotoxic effects and immunosuppressive effects.

Clinical Manifestations

The various trichothecenes cause a wide range of clinical effects. The trichothecene mycotoxins can cause mucosal

and skin irritation if exposed topically. Cutaneous signs and symptoms include erythema, edema, pain, pruritus, and blisters. Ultimately, necrosis and sloughing of large areas of skin may occur. Severe ocular irritation and corneal ulceration may also be seen. Airway and intestinal necrosis may occur, depending upon the route and dose of exposure. A late effect of systemic absorption is pancytopenia, predisposing to bleeding and sepsis.

Laboratory Testing

The parental compound T-2 is rapidly metabolized to HT-2, T2-triol, and T-2 tetraol within hours after consumption. Therefore, detection methods have been developed that measure T-2 metabolites with intrinsically longer half-lives found in human specimen. Current methods rely on inexpensive and rapid enzyme-linked immunosorbent assay (ELISA) for T-2 metabolite detection in urine samples within a week after exposure. The sensitivity for T-2 and its metabolites using the ELISA method (ppb) is well below the estimated LD_{50} (3.7 ppm) for T-2 toxin. Results from the ELISA assay can be available within hours.

T-2 metabolites can be detected in blood samples for as long as a month using a highly sensitive modified liquid chromatography tandem mass spectroscopy analysis (LC-MS/MS). Results may take hours to days using the LC-MS/MS method. Due to the high equipment cost, requirement of highly trained personnel, and lack of quality standard controls, LC-MS/MS is not the preferred analytical method. Unfortunately, until other methods are available for analyzing T-2 and T-2 metabolites outside the 1-week collection window, LC-MS/MS will continue to be utilized. With this in mind, development of bioassays for cytotoxic screening of T-2 metabolites is currently being investigated. These assays may be used to analyze acute and chronic exposure to T-2 toxins and help assess toxic exposures subsequent to extensive metabolism.

Treatment/Disposition

Adsorbents such as activate charcoal may be useful in treatment if utilized early following oral exposure. Washing the exposed skin with water and detergent may have benefit. No specific antidote is currently available and care is focused on symptomatic and supportive treatment. Steroids, such as methyl prednisolone and dexamethasone, may be of benefit following skin exposure.

VOMITING AGENTS

The chemical warfare agents diphenylchlorarsine (DA), diphenylcyanoarsine (DC), and diphenylaminearsine (DM, adamsite) belong to a group of chemicals classified as the "vomiting agents." The synthesis of these agents dates back to the early twentieth century. In 1915, Heinrich Wieland, a German chemist, synthesized the agent DM. Three years later, an American chemist, Robert Adams, independently developed this same compound and named it adamsite. Since that time, these agents have been produced for two purposes, as riot control agents and as emesis-inducing agents to promote removal of personal protective gear during chemical warfare.

The use of vomiting agents has been reported during international conflicts. DA was first used by German troops in 1917. DA was not well-filtered by the standard issue gas masks at that time. It resulted in nausea and vomiting, causing enemy troops to remove their masks. This rendered those personnel vulnerable to the toxic effects of other agents such as phosgene and chlorine gas. The Germans also produced DC and DM, but limited documentation exists for use of these agents during World War I. Questionable reports exist of vomiting agents used in other countries as riot control agents.

Properties

DA appears as colorless crystals, DC as a white solid, and DM as light yellow-to-green crystals. DA and DM are odorless; DC reportedly has an odor similar to garlic or bitter almonds. All three agents are insoluble in water.

DM is the most toxic agent of this group, with an estimated LCt_{50} of 11,000 mg·min/m^3 (i.e., an estimated 50% lethality for a group of patients breathing air with a concentration of 11,000 mg/m^3 for 1 minute). Other factors also are important, such as the exposed patient's preexisting health status and the time from exposure to medical care. The dose at which vomiting reportedly begins for DM is estimated as 370 mg·min/m^3.

Routes of Exposure

Vomiting agents typically are disseminated as aerosols. The primary route of absorption is through the respiratory system. Exposure also can occur by ingestion, dermal absorption, or eye contact.

Clinical Manifestations

The effects of the vomiting agents by any route of exposure are slower in onset and longer in duration than typical riot control agents (e.g., CS). On initial exposure, vomiting agents are irritants. This irritation is delayed for several minutes after contact. As a result of this delay, less early warning properties are present for those exposed. By the time symptoms of irritation occur and personnel consider donning their protective equipment, significant contamination already may have occurred. Systemic signs and symptoms follow the initial irritation and consist of headache, nausea, vomiting, diarrhea, abdominal cramps, and mental status changes. Symptoms typically persist for several

hours after exposure. Death has been reported with excessive exposure.

Laboratory Testing

These agents are enzyme inhibitors that have high affinity for sulfhydryl groups. Following absorption, DA and DC are rapidly hydrolyzed to diphenylarsinic acid (DPAA), then conjugated to glutathione (DPAA-GS) and excreted. Therefore, blood and urine samples should be collected within 24 hours. Current methods can quantitate DPAA and DPAA-GS levels within hours using gas chromatography and mass spectroscopy analysis (GC-MS/MS). Inadequate data is available regarding DM metabolic products thereby limiting GC-MS/MS methods to the parental DM molecule and creating a shorter collection window predominantly from blood samples. The collection window can be opened significantly when measuring organic arsenic levels as opposed to specific metabolites in blood or tissue samples using gas chromatography mass spectroscopy (GC-MS). Arsenic levels in combination with a patient's cytogenetic profile and clinical presentation may help pinpoint exposure to specific organoarsenic agents.

Treatment/Disposition

The initial care of patients exposed to vomiting agents primarily is supportive. No specific antidotes are available. Care is focused on relieving irritant and systemic effects.

CONCLUSION

It will be a challenge to diagnosis and direct appropriate therapy for victims who develop an unexpected illness resulting from an intentional release of a chemical substance. There are numerous potential chemical agents that could be utilized by terrorists. Using an organ system approach to identifying the agent and focusing initial management is critical. While chemicals can have multisystem manifestations, never the less, many will have primary organ targets which should be treated agressively and can also be used to identify the class of agent. It behooves those in clinical practice to have a general understanding of these agents and to be able to recognize a sentinel case that may present itself.

Suggested Reading

Bennett JW, Klich M. Mycotoxins. *Clin Microbiol Rev.* 2003;16:497–516.

Bigalke H, Rummel A. Medical aspects of toxin weapons. *Toxicology.* 2005;214:210–220.

Chi CH, Chen KW, Chan SH, et al. Clinical presentation and prognostic factors in sodium monofluoroacetate intoxication. *J Toxicol Clin Toxicol.* 1996;34:707–712.

Eason C. Sodium monofluoroacetate (1080) risk assessment and risk communication. *Toxicology.* 2002;181–182:523–530.

Geusau A, Abraham K, Geissler K, et al. Severe 2,3,7,8-tetrachlorodibenzo-p-dioxin (TCDD) intoxication: clinical and laboratory effects. *Environ Health Perspect.* Aug 2001; 109(8): 865–869.

Goh CS, Hodgson DR, Fearnside SM, et al. Sodium monofluoroacetate (Compound 1080) poisoning in dogs. *Aust Vet J.* 2005;83:474–479.

Henriksson J, Johannisson A, Bergqvist PA, et al. The toxicity of organoarsenic-based warfare agents: in vitro and in vivo studies. *Arch Environ Contam Toxicol.* Feb 1996;30(2):213–9.

Koch P. State of the art of trichothecenes analysis. *Toxicol Lett.* 2004;153:109–112.

Madsen JM. Toxins as weapons of mass destruction: a comparison and contrast with biological-warfare and chemical-warfare agents. *Clin Lab Med.* 2001;21:593–605.

Michalek JE, Akhtar FZ, Arezzo JC, et al. Serum dioxin and peripheral neuropathy in veterans of Operation Ranch Hand. *Neurotoxicology.* Aug 2001;22(4):479–490.

O'Hagan BJ. Fluoroacetate poisoning in seven domestic dogs. *Aust Vet J.* 2004;82:756–758.

Pelclova D, Fenclova Z, Preiss J, et al. Lipid metabolism and neuropsychological follow-up study of workers exposed to 2,3,7,8-tetrachlordibenzo-p-dioxin. *Int Arch Occup Environ Health.* Oct 2002;75 Suppl:S60–66.

Reigart JR, Brueggeman JL, Keil JE. Sodium fluoroacetate poisoning. *Am J Dis Child.* 1975;129:1224–1226.

Rosenbloom M, Leikin JB, Vogel SN, et al. Biological and chemical agents: a brief synopsis. *Am J Ther.* 2002;9:5–14.

Sherley M. The traditional categories of fluoroacetate poisoning signs and symptoms belie substantial underlying similarities. *Toxicol Lett.* 2004;151:399–406.

Sudakin DL. Trichothecenes in the environment: relevance to human health. *Toxicol Lett.* 2003;143:97–107.

Sweeney MH, Mocarelli P. Human health effects after exposure to 2,3,7,8-TCDD. *Food Addit Contam.* Apr 2000;17(4):303–316.

Tornes JA, Opstad AM, Johnsen BA. Determination of organoarsenic warfare agents in sediment samples from Skagerrak by gas chromatography-mass spectrometry. *Sci Total Environ.* Mar 1, 2006;356(1–3):235–46.

Trabes J, Rason N, Avrahami E. Computed tomography demonstration of brain damage due to acute sodium monofluoroacetate poisoning. *J Toxicol Clin Toxicol.* 1983;20:85–92.

V

BIOLOGICALS

INTRODUCTION

If the anthrax events of 2001 taught us anything it was that an astute physician could save lives. Conversely, physicians who do not know the common signs of deadly, albeit uncommon illnesses, will lose lives. In October 2001 a private practice infectious disease specialist in concert with an alert laboratorian diagnosed the sentinel case of inhalation anthrax – the first known intentional release in the United States. While the sentinel patient ultimately lost his life, the alarm was raised in time to prevent other deaths. Another patient in a different region of the country also with symptoms consistent with inhalation anthrax subsequently presented to a health-care facility; was misdiagnosed and died. Does training pay off? Absolutely!

Emerging infectious diseases can pose as deadly a threat as the intentional dissemination of deadly toxins. We are all too aware of the influenza pandemic of 1918 resulting in millions of deaths. Avian flu (H5N1) related deaths and the rapid spread of this highly pathogenic strain of influenza have raised public concern about another pandemic. In the last few years we have seen the appearance of monkey pox, severe acute respiratory syndrome (SARS), and avian flu affecting humans. As recent as February 2004, the toxin ricin was found in the U.S. Capitol. Not long after, two cases of bubonic plague occurred in New York City - contracted naturally from the victims' home in the Southwest. It could just as easily have been the result of biowarfare.

The question we need to ask ourselves: would we have been able to make a rapid diagnosis based upon our current skill levels?

This new reality of biological weapons led the United States to embark upon a smallpox vaccination program. Many physicians were unfamiliar with vaccinia and inexperienced in the use of bifurcated needles; a reminder that diseases considered long since eradicated or quiescent may re-emerge. At the same time, the number of experienced physicians who have seen or treated such long forgotten illnesses continues to dwindle. Medical management of biological weapons or bioterrorism remains inadequately taught in spite of current events. Often referred to as the poor mans nuclear weapon, biological weapons offer terrorists important advantages. The former Soviet Union employed over 60,000 scientists at their bioweapon institute Biopreparat. Many of these scientists are now working for other countries.

Estimates suggest that more than 20 countries have some form of bioweapons program. The Centers for Disease Control and Prevention (CDC) has categorized biologicals into three levels—A, B, and C— based upon pathogenicity, and likelihood of use.

As practicing physicians we will also face a variety of emerging health threats. Because we live in a global world, our Atlantic and Pacific shores no longer protect us from diseases that are rare on this continent but endemic or epidemic in many other parts of the world. The increase in international travel, cruise ships and immigration from other countries, makes it likely that we will see a variety of unusual illnesses. We also face a global biological threat. Our adversaries know our vulnerabilities, and there is a black market on pathogens—especially deadly ones.

With a covert bioterrorism or bioweapon attack, the most likely indicator of the event would be patients presenting to health care facilities, often with a cascade of similar symptoms. Biodrome recognition is an important tool for early diagnosis. 'Patients with symptoms unusual for a given region, transmission vector, season or area, or a single case of a highly virulent, rare disease such as Ebola should alert the clinician. Whether considering a bioweapon or virulent emerging threat, remaining alert to clinical clues is essential. The following chapters will address the CDC Category Agents, emerging pathogens, and the tools necessary to increase preparedness as well as the likelihood of diagnosing such illnesses.

38

CDC CATEGORY EXPLANATION (A, B, C) OVERVIEW

John D. Charette

STAT FACTS

CDC CATEGORY EXPLANATION (A, B, C) OVERVIEW

- CDC has developed a categorization system for biological exposures based primarily on dissemination, mortality rates, and other clinical criteria.
- Category A agents exhibit high dissemination and high mortality rates with smallpox being the ultimate Category A agent.
- Examples of Category B agents include Brucellosis, Q fever, and glanders.
- Nipa virus is an example of a Category C agent.

INTRODUCTION

The Center for Disease Control (CDC) has classified biological agents into three classes: Types A, B, and C. This classification scheme is based on their ease of dissemination, mortality rates, potential to induce public panic, and special procedures required for identification and management. This chapter will review these categories and the agents that are included in them. The reader is referred to the organism-specific chapters for detailed information about their pathology and treatment. This chapter will address the essentials necessary to justify their place in the CDC classification scheme.

CENTER FOR DISEASE CONTROL CATEGORY A AGENTS

CDC Category A agents are easily disseminated from person to person or have high mortality rates with profoundly negative public health implications. They also have potential to create public panic and social disruption and require special public health planning. Anthrax is caused by *Bacillus anthracis,* a gram-positive spore-forming organism that causes cutaneus, inhalational, and gastrointestinal presentations. Fatality rates for cutaneus anthrax have been reported as less than 1% with antibiotic therapy and 20% without intervention. Case fatality rates for inhalational anthrax have been reported as high as 75% even with appropriate therapy. Gastrointestinal anthrax has a fatality rate of 25–50%. During the 2001 mail attack in the United States the fatality rate for inhalational anthrax was 45%. Unlike some other Category A agents, anthrax does not have significant person-to-person transmission. Although cutaneous lesions are potentially infectious, person-to-person spread of the cutaneous disease is rare. Person-to-person spread of inhalational anthrax has not been reported. Special actions specific to anthrax exposure include environmental sampling to identify the organism, cultures on exposed individuals, and postexposure prophylaxis.

Botulism is caused by a toxin produced by *Clostridium botulinum.* This toxin is the most lethal toxin in the world. One gram of this toxin, if appropriately delivered, could theoretically kill more than a million people. This toxin is of major concern because in addition to its lethality, it is easy to produce and its victims require prolonged intensive care. Public health surveillance is critical. Clinicians suspecting clinical botulism should notify public health authorities immediately. Clinical features include asymmetric, descending flaccid paralysis with prominent bulbar palsies in an afebrile patient with a clear sensorium. The prominent bulbar palsies can be summarized in part as "4 Ds": diplopia, dysarthria, dysphonia, and dysphagia. There are four potential sources of infection: cutaneous, inhalational, intestinal, and wound botulism. The common pathway is absorption of the toxin from a mucosal surface of damaged skin, gut, or lung. The cornerstone of therapy is the administration of antitoxin.

Surveillance of a potential outbreak is critical. Features suggesting a botulism attack include unusual botulinum type (type C, D, F, or G, or type E toxin not acquired from an aquatic food), common geographic factor among cases without a common dietary exposure, and simultaneous outbreaks with no common source. Person-to-person spread of botulism would not be expected unless the organism was genetically modified.

Naturally occurring plague occurs as the result of a bite from a flea infected with *Yersinia pestis*. The organism invades and destroys regional lymph nodes and causes bacteremia and sepsis. In some cases, secondary spread to the lungs occurs. This organism is a Class A agent because of its potential mortality and documented lethality. There have been three plague pandemics, one of which killed one-third of the European population. Plague has been engineered and deployed by military forces. Four of seven patients with primary pneumonic plague in the United States over the last 50 years died. The primary bioterrorist threat would be aerosolized *Y. pestis*, which would directly infect the respiratory tract causing pneumonic plague. Infection would be manifested by fever, cough, dyspnea, and bloody, watery, or purulent sputum, which may be accompanied by nausea, vomiting, abdominal pain, and diarrhea. The subsequent clinical course is consistent with a rapidly progressive pneumonia. Bioterrorist-induced pneumonic plague or anthrax should be suspected in the setting of many cases of fulminant fever, cough, shortness of breath, chest pain, and death. The presence of hemoptysis in this setting would strongly suggest plague. Because there are no effective methods of detecting aerosolized *Y. pestis*, diligence in reporting unusual numbers of cases of fulminant progressive pneumonia is the primary means of identifying and defending an outbreak. Unlike anthrax and botulism, the high mortality of pneumonic plague is accompanied by significant risk of person-to-person transmission.

Smallpox is the ultimate Category A agent due to its significant mortality and potential for high person-to-person infectivity. Smallpox is caused by the *Variola* virus, and is spread via aerosol. It causes four types of disease. Variola major has a 30% mortality rate. Variola minor has a 1% mortality rate. Hemorrhagic and malignant smallpox are 90% fatal. Adding to its potential as a Class A agent is the absence of effective therapy and its high infectivity. In addition to transmission via direct contact and aerosol, smallpox can be transferred via contact with contaminated clothing or bed linens. Studies of past outbreaks have demonstrated the generation of as many as ten secondary infections for each primary case. The absence of routine vaccinations, our high trans and intercontinental mobility, the nonspecific nature of early disease and high infectivity

of smallpox give this disease the potential to create an international health disaster of unprecedented proportions. Vaccinating at risk populations within 7 days of exposure is the best strategy for containing the disease.

Tularemia is caused by *Francisella tularensis*, a gram-negative coccobacillus that is one of the most infectious pathogenic bacteria known. As few as ten microorganisms can cause significant disease. Although there is no person-to-person transmission, *F. tularensis* is considered to be dangerous because of its ease of dissemination, high infectivity, and capacity to cause serious illness and death. A study by the World Health Organization estimated 250,000 casualties and 19,000 deaths from an attack utilizing 50 kg of virulent *F. tularensis* against a metropolitan area of 5 million people. Furthermore, illness would be expected to last several months, relapses would occur and immunized people would only be partially protected. The CDC has estimated that the economic impact of an attack would be $5.4 billion for every 100,000 exposures. The ability to weaponize *F. tularensis* has been clearly demonstrated by multiple countries, including the United States and the Soviet Union, over the last century. The most likely bioterror scenario is the use of an aerosol, which would result in life-threatening pneumonitis.

The viral hemorrhagic fevers are caused by *Filo*, *Arena*, *Bunya*, and *Flavi* viruses. Of greatest concern from the bioterrorism standpoint are Ebola and Marburg (*Filoviridae*), Lassa fever and New World arena viruses (*Arenaviridae*), Rift Valley fever (*Bunyaviridae*) and Yellow fever, Omsk hemorrhagic fever, and Kyasanur Forest disease (*Flaviviridae*). There are multiple factors, which earn these agents a Category A rating. They are highly available and environmentally stable organisms with high morbidity and mortality at low infective dose. Animal studies have demonstrated successful transmission via aerosol. There is significant risk of person-to-person transmission, creating potential for large sustained outbreaks and public panic. These agents have been weaponized by the United States and the Soviet Union.

The nonspecific nature of early viral hemorrhagic fevers (VHF) disease makes early diagnosis of a potential bioterrorist attack difficult. After an incubation period of 2–21 days, prodromal symptoms of fever, headache, malaise, arthralgias, myalgias, nausea, abdominal pain, and nonbloody diarrhea develop. Hypotension, relative bradycardia, tachypnea, conjunctivitis, pharyngitis, and a variable rash follow. The petechiae, mucous membrane and conjunctival hemorrhage, hematuria, hematemesis, melena, DIC, neurologic symptoms, and shock that distinguish these infections from more common diseases are late developments. A significant percentage of victims of a VHF outbreak may require intensive supportive care including vasopressors, mechanical ventilation, and renal dialysis. Although ribavirin has shown effectiveness against Arena and Bunyaviridae, it is ineffective against the other two categories of VHF.

CENTER FOR DISEASE CONTROL
CATEGORY B AGENTS

Q fever is a zoonotic disease caused by *Coxiella burnetti*, an organism, which normally uses cattle sheep and goats as its natural reservoir. *C. burnetti* organisms are shed in milk feces, amniotic fluids, and placentas of infected animals. Humans usually acquire the infection by inhaling air contaminated by barnyard dust containing animal feces, urine, and placental and amniotic fluids from infected animals. Clinical illness is manifested by fever, headache, malaise, myalgias, sore throat, chills, sweats, nonproductive cough, nausea, vomiting, diarrhea, abdominal and chest pain. Up to half of infected patients will develop pneumonia and many will get hepatitis. Only 1% of patients who acquire naturally occurring Q fever die. Chronic Q fever may develop 1–20 years after initial infection. Up to 65% of patients acquiring Q fever may die. Endocarditis is a particularly serious complication. One organism can cause clinical infection. It is resistant to heat and drying, and can be aerosolized and delivered as an airborne agent.

Brucellosis is a zoonotic disease caused by several *Brucella* organisms that have cattle, goats, pigs, and dogs as their natural reservoir. Natural infections of humans usually occur through contact with infected animals. Acute infections (less than 8 days) are manifested by nonspecific symptoms such as fever, sweats, malaise anorexia, headache, and back pain. Undulant brucellosis is manifested by arthritis, undulant fevers, and epididymo-orchitis. Chronic fatigue syndrome, depression, and arthritis are chronic complications. This organism is considered a bioterrorism threat because of its high infectivity via aerosol.

Glanders is caused by *Burkholderia mallei*, an organism that normally infects horses but has also been found in mules, donkeys, cats, goats, and dogs. Natural human infection is rare and normally occurs as a result of prolonged contact with infected animals or inhalation. Clinical syndromes include localized cutaneous infections, pneumonia, bacteremia, and chronic infections with abscess formation in the arms, legs, spleen, or liver. Human-to-human transmission has been reported. Its potential as a weapon lies in the low number of organisms required to cause infection, potential for aerosolization, and its endemic availability in Africa, Asia, the Middle East, and Central and South America.

Melioidosis or Whitmore's disease is caused by *B. pseudomallei*. The clinical presentation of melioidosis is similar to glanders and like glanders can be spread from person to person. Melioidosis is endemic in Southeast Asia where it is a common contaminant of laboratory cultures and is often isolated from soldiers serving in endemic areas.

Psittacosis is caused by *Chlamydia psittaci*, an organism that normally infects birds. Naturally occurring human disease occurs after close contact with infected birds or their droppings. Short exposures can produce infection and the organism can infect humans via the respiratory route. It can cause severe pneumonia, pericarditis, myocarditis, mental status changes, and delirium. Typhus fever is caused by Rickettsia prowazeki, the rickettsial agent that has inflicted the most misery on humanity. It infects humans through the body louse. This organism is secreted into the feces of the louse and is autoinoculated into the bloodstream when the victim scratches their infected skin. Epidemic typhus has a long history of decimating military and civilian populations, particularly when there are marginal living conditions.

Ricin is a highly potent toxin derived from waste material from the castor plant (*Ricis communis*) during production of castor oil. Multiple factors favor it as a potential biological warfare agent. As little as 500 µg of ricin can kill a human adult. It remains stable at extremes of temperature, is colorless, tasteless, and water soluble. It can be dispersed as an aerosol, used to contaminate water supplies, or injected, and has no known antidote. Respiratory exposures may result in rapid onset of pulmonary edema, hypotension, and respiratory failure. Gastrointestinal exposures cause severe bloody diarrhea, vomiting, shock, and hepatic and renal failure. Death can occur within 36 to 72 hours of exposure.

Bioterrorism-related contamination of food and water supplies could result in widespread outbreaks of cholera (*Vibrio cholerae*), shigellosis (*Shigella spp*), salmonellosis (*Salmonella spp*), typhoid fever (*Salmonella typhi*), and *Escherichia coli O157:H7*. All can result in significant dehydration. Untreated cholera can result in death within hours. *E. coli O157:H7* has been associated with hemolytic uremic syndrome. Staphylococcal enterotoxin B (SEB) can be aerosolized or used to sabotage food supplies. Incapacitating and lethal doses via inhalation are only 30 ng and 1.7 µg. The incubation period is less than 6 hours. This toxin can cause pulmonary edema, acute respiratory distress syndrome (ARDS), severe nausea and vomiting, septic shock, and death. *Clostridium perfringens* is an organism that has heat labile spores, which germinate in the human intestinal tract. The organisms produce an enterotoxin, which causes potentially severe enteritis. These organisms are attractive to potential terrorists because they offer the potential to utilize public water and food supplies to deliver potentially incapacitating or lethal toxins to large numbers of people. In addition to causing potential illness, such delivery methods have the potential to instill panic within the affected populations, and strain public health resources that will be faced with the logistical challenges of testing, purifying, and protecting local water and food supplies. These threats carry the additional bonus of the negative economic impact of removing potentially contaminated food and water resources from commercial markets. The safety of food and water supplies is assumed by most developed nations. The mere threat of contamination of food and water supplies would strike at the core of public confidence and could achieve the panic desired by potential terrorists.

Viral encephalitis can be caused by a variety of agents that cause inflammation of the brain. These agents are of concern for potential bioterrorism use because of their rapid onset and progression of potentially debilitating symptoms and frequency of long-term sequelae. Eastern Equine encephalitis, Western Equine encephalitis causes rapidly progressive potentially debilitating symptoms and have the potential for long-term sequelae.

CENTER FOR DISEASE CONTROL CATEGORY C AGENTS

Nipa virus emerged as new cause of human encephalitis in the late 1990s as the result of molecular evolution in the paramyxovirus family. This organism naturally infects swine and naturally occurring human cases have occurred after close contact with infected animals. This organism produces multiorgan vasculitis. The rapidly progressive febrile encephalitis produced by this virus occurs within 2 weeks of exposure, carries a 30–40% mortality rate, and has no known cure. Hantaviruses cause hemorrhagic fever with renal syndrome (HFRS) or Hantavirus pulmonary syndrome (HPS). Mortality rates are 50–60% for HPS and 1–10% for HFRS. Mortality rates vary based on the specific Hantavirus species. Naturally occurring infections occur as a result of close contact with or bites by infected rodents, or airborne exposure to urine or feces. The potential of Hantaviruses as bioterrorism agents lies in their worldwide distribution, ease of production, and feasibility of aerosol dispersal.

39

ANTHRAX

Larry M. Bush and Maria T. Perez

S T A T   F A C T S

SUSPECTED ANTHRAX INFECTION

Category	Action/Comment
EPIDEMIOLOGY:	
• Diagnosing inhalational anthrax infection implies a link to a bioterrorist event until proven otherwise	• Follow institution's preparedness plans
• Anthrax infection may follow an overt or covert bioterrorist attack	• Notify the health department and criminal authorities
• Proven or suspected anthrax cutaneous lesions should raise the suspicion of widespread exposure	• Designate a clear voice of communication (usually the chairperson of the institution's infection control)
	• Syndromic surveillance data
	• Report to national bioterrorism agencies
CLINICAL EVALUATION:	
• The initial phase of illness is nonspecific and may be indistinguishable from common flu-like conditions	• Review and have at hand a list of signs and symptoms of anthrax infection
• Fulminant disease rapidly ensues in systemic anthrax infection in the form of septic shock	• High index of suspicion is based on concurrent epidemiologic circumstances
	• Employ a multidisciplinary approach to treat a septic patient
DIAGNOSTIC TESTS:	
• Laboratory Studies	• Prior to administration of antibiotics
• Obtain blood cultures	• Gram's stain of blood Buffy coat and smears may disclose the bacilli
• Complete blood cell count and differential	
• Comprehensive chemistry profile	• Notify the hospital laboratory of suspicions of anthrax to ensure biosafety level 2 conditions
• CSF analysis and cultures if meningitis is clinically suspected	• Expedite specimen evaluations
	• Refer samples to a laboratory response network (LRN) facility
	• Initiate empiric antibiotics if delay in obtaining a CSF sample
	• Immunohistochemistry and/or PCR may be necessary to detect the organism in the hemorrhagic pleural fluid
	• Unlikely to be diagnostic
• Pleural fluid analysis if imaging studies demonstrate a significant quantity	• Immunohistochemical and PCR studies
• Sputum culture and Gram's stain	• Not useful in acutely ill patients
• Gram's stain and culture of vesicular fluid if skin lesions present	• Predictive value unknown; should not be used as a clinical diagnostic test. Most useful if obtained during the initial 24 hours
• Punch biopsy of cutaneous lesions	

Category	Action/Comment
• Serologic studies for anthrax anti-PA IgG antibodies	
• Nasal swabs of exposed patients	
• Imaging Studies	
• Chest Radiograph	• Look for widened mediastinum and/or pleural effusions
• Chest computerized tomography scan	• Air space disease is uncommon
	• Mediastinal hilar lymphadenopathy, parenchymal infiltrates (pulmonary edema), and pleural effusions
TREATMENT	
• Proven or suspected inhalational anthrax	• See Table 39-2
• Proven cutaneous anthrax	• See Table 39-3
PROPHYLAXIS	
• Proven or suspected inhalational anthrax	• Identify those at risk
• Valid information of an anthrax bioterrorist attack	• See Table 39-4
PATIENT DISPOSITION/TRIAGE	
• Known exposure	
• Symptomatic	• Admission to ICU and prompt treatment initiation
• Asymptomatic	• Start prophylactic therapy with close clinical follow up
• Possible exposure	
• Symptomatic	• Admission; begin empiric treatment pending evaluation
• Asymptomatic	• Start prophylaxis pending evaluation
• No known exposure	• Routine emergency room evaluation and triage
INFECTION CONTROL	
• Patient	
• Inhalational infection	• Standard barrier precautions
• Cutaneous infection	• Contact isolation; biohazardous waste disposal of dressings
• Environment	• Standard hospital practice; cleanse with hypochlorite solution

CSF: Cerebrospinal Fluid, PCR: Polymerase Chain Reaction, ICU: Intensive Care Unit

INTRODUCTION

"Whenever you have eliminated the impossible, whatever remains, however improbable, must be the truth".

—Sir Arthur Conan Doyle

Anthrax has long been considered a serious biologic agent to be potentially used as a biological weapon for purposes of bioterrorism or biowarfare. Its relatively easy availability, stability in aerosolized form, high illness-to-infection ratio, and unique virulence factors, together with a large case fatality rate if acquired via inhalation, are special characteristics warranting the placement of anthrax on the Centers for Disease Control and Prevention (CDC) Category A list of putative biological threats. Included with anthrax on this list are smallpox, plague, tularemia, botulism toxin, and certain viral hemorrhagic fevers, all of which have in common the greatest potential of achieving the goal of bioterrorism: not as much to do mortal harm, as it is to disrupt our way of life and make us clearly aware of our vulnerability.

The anthrax attacks of October 2001, which utilized the United States Postal Service to deliver the intended biological weapon, resulted in 22 confirmed or suspected cases of anthrax infection. Eleven were inhalational cases (five of whom died) and eleven were cutaneous. More than 33,000 people required postexposure prophylaxis in the 5 geographic areas directly affected.

Two branches of the federal government as well as postal operations around the nation were shut down, with costs directly attributable to these attacks exceeding $3 billion. The consequences of these attacks substantiated many findings and recommendations in the Working Group on Civilian Biodefense Consensus Statement published in 1999; however, the events of 2001 changed much of what was known about anthrax and hopefully served to make us both intellectually and emotionally better prepared.

Early suspicion, detection, and confirmation of a bioterrorist event are also the essential initial steps for triggering an effective emergency response. Various experimental approaches have been formulated and studied in an attempt to ascertain if it might be possible to detect an act of bioterrorism at an earlier moment in time. Syndromic surveillance is one such approach designed to monitor the number of cases with various general types of symptoms by surveying emergency rooms, clinics, and 911 calls. The index case of fatal inhalational anthrax due to bioterrorism in the United States was detected by a practicing clinician.

Thus, through a variety of educational venues and training programs, emphasis can be placed on assuring that emergency room staff, along with other primary care providers, are knowledgeable of aspects including clinical signs and symptoms, diagnosis, treatment, prophylaxis, infection control measures, and public health reporting of anthrax and other infectious agents categorized as potential biological weapons.

HISTORY

Anthrax infection, caused by the bacterium *Bacillus anthracis*, acquired its name from the Greek word *"anthrakis"* meaning "coal," descriptive of the typical black escar associated with cutaneous disease. Anthrax is presumed to have been the fifth plague that killed the cattle of the Egyptians referred to in the Book of Exodus in the Bible. Robert Koch's detailed microbiologic studies of *B. anthracis* in 1876 served as the proof that a single bacterium caused a specific disease, thus formulating his famous postulates. Louis Pasteur capitalized on this information and, in 1882, developed a heat-inactivated anthrax vaccine, which protected animals from infection with live *B. anthracis*.

The theoretical use of anthrax as an agent of bioterrorism or biowarfare has been the subject of much research and speculation. In 1970, the World Health Organization estimated that 50 kg of *B. anthracis* spores released over an urban population of 5 million would cause illness in 250,000 and kill 100,000 persons. The former Soviet Union along with other countries is known to have had significant *B. anthracis* production as part of its offensive weapons program. Prior to the U.S. bioterrorism attacks of 2001, an unintentional release of aerosolized anthrax spores from a military facility in Sverdlovsk, Russia, resulted in the only documented case of inhalation anthrax from weaponized *B. anthracis* spores. As a result of this accident, cases of anthrax in humans occurred as far as 4 km from the site and cases in animals as far as 50 km away. At Sverdlovsk, 68 of the 79 patients with diagnosed inhalational anthrax died. Attempts by the Aum Shinrikyo cult in 1995 to aerosolize anthrax and use it against civilians in Japan were unsuccessful, owing to the fact that the anthrax used was likely a strain employed in animal vaccination and not a significant risk to humans.

EPIDEMIOLOGY

Human infection with anthrax is typically linked to infection of herbivores including cattle, horses, goats, sheep, and pigs, and from the soil where they graze. Spores of *B. anthracis* are prevalent in soil throughout the world and, depending on local conditions, they may survive from months to even decades. Animal vaccination efforts have proven to be very successful in greatly reducing the number of infected animals, but have not altogether eliminated the endemicity of this infection. These animals may become infected with anthrax via ingestion of spores lying dormant in the soil. Animal products that can transmit anthrax infection to humans include wool, hair, hides, meat, bones, and bone meal, or by contaminated foodstuffs, hence the term "wool-sorter's disease."

Human anthrax infection occurs by three major routes: inhalational, cutaneous, and gastrointestinal. Although infection results almost in all instances from exposure to anthrax spores, clinical disease may also develop as a consequence of ingesting the vegetative form of the organism when present in insufficiently cooked contaminated meat. Acquisition of the disease due to direct contamination of food or water with *B. anthracis* spores has not been proven in experimental animal models.

The cutaneous is the most common of the forms of anthrax infections worldwide, yet just two cases were reported in the United States between 1992 and 2000. Eighteen cases of inhalational anthrax were reported in the United States between 1900 and 1976, but none were documented thereafter until the eleven cases associated with the 2001 anthrax attacks. Most reported cases of inhalational anthrax have resulted from occupational exposure to contaminated animal products. Oddly, the index case of inhalational anthrax due to bioterrorism was also caused by occupational exposure to anthrax, although not by a naturally occurring source. In urban areas, the rare occurrence of naturally acquired human anthrax infection should lead to the consideration of bioterrorism as the putative causation.

MICROBIOLOGY AND PATHOPHYSIOLOGY

The Agent

B. anthracis, the etiologic agent of anthrax, is a gram-positive, aerobic, nonmotile bacillus found in soil worldwide, predominantly in agricultural areas. When the environmental conditions are not favorable or nutrients are exhausted, this bacterium transforms into 1–5-μm-sized spores able to remain viable for several decades (Fig. 39-1). The spores germinate when they encounter a nutrient-rich environment such as human or animal tissues and blood, converting to their vegetative (or proliferative) form, a large bacillus, 1–8 μm long and 1–1.5 μm wide (Fig. 39-2), that grows within few (6–24) hours forming nonhemolytic colonies with a peculiar "curly hair" appearance on laboratory culture media. The bacillus has a polypeptide capsule that becomes visible with India ink staining. Its susceptibility to penicillin is one of the characteristics used, along with the Gram's stain and colony morphology, for the preliminary identification of *B. anthracis* in the laboratory.

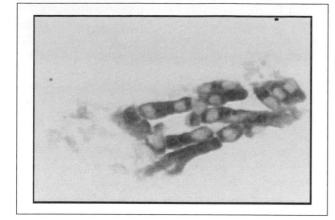

F I G U R E   3 9 - 1

Gram's stain of the colony growth on agar plate, demonstrating subterminal spores within the bacilli.
Source: Courtesy of Dr Larry Bush, Atlantis, Florida.

Virulence Factors and Pathogenesis

The virulence of *B. anthracis* depends on its antiphagocytic (polypeptide) capsule (AC), three toxin components or factors (protective antigen [PA], lethal factor [LF], and edema factor [EF]) and its capability for rapid replication resulting in a large bacterial burden. The pathophysiologic mechanisms of anthrax toxin–induced cell damage and death are not completely elucidated yet. The AC inhibits phagocytosis of the organism by host macrophages. Phagocytosis is also prevented by one of the toxin components, the protective antigen. The PA binds to a specific receptor on the host cell membrane (anthrax toxin receptor),

promoting the transport of the other two toxin factors across the membrane, altering its permeability and resulting in intracellular edema. The binding of PA and EF produces edema toxin, which inhibits neutrophilic function and contributes to the genesis of edema. Similarly, the binding of PA and LF produces lethal toxin, responsible for cell lysis with subsequent release of mediators of cell injury and death such as tumor necrosis factor-α, interleukin-1, oxygen radicals, and lysosomal enzymes.

Genetics

Molecular analysis of the *B. anthracis* species has revealed a highly conserved genetic sequence among the approximately 1200 strains isolated using amplification of restriction fragment length polymorphisms techniques (only 1% of the genetic material is variable from strain to strain). About half of the strains have been fingerprinted by multilocus variable number tandem repeat sequence analysis, providing a reference genomic library for forensic investigation of bioterrorist events involving anthrax.

Mechanisms of Transmission

There are three routes of infection, each corresponding to a particular clinical manifestation:

- Direct contact of skin with spores: cutaneous anthrax
- Ingestion of vegetative bacterial organisms: gastrointestinal anthrax
- Inhalation of spores: inhalational anthrax

CLINICAL MANIFESTATIONS

Generally considered a disease of grazing animals because of its reservoir in soil, anthrax is occasionally reported in humans who had direct contact with animal products contaminated by *B. anthracis* spores. Anthrax may produce several clinical presentations depending on the route of infection, but on occasion, localized forms may gain access to the circulation causing systemic disease. The four distinct clinical presentations of anthrax include cutaneous, gastrointestinal, inhalational, and meningitis or meningo-encephalitis forms.

Cutaneous Anthrax

Also known as "malignant pustule," it is the most common form of anthrax infection, estimated in 20,000–100,000 cases per year worldwide. Reported cases in the United States have fallen from about 200 cases per year in the early 1900s to approximately 200 cases during the period 1955–1992. The lesion develops in exposed areas of the body after contact with infective spores; abrasions, cuts, or wounds increase susceptibility to infection, but infection

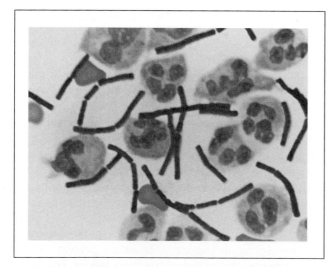

F I G U R E   3 9 - 2

Gram's stain of a cerebrospinal fluid in meningoencephalitis secondary to fatal inhalational anthrax. Note the high burden of large gram- positive bacilli.
Source: Courtesy of Dr Larry Bush, Atlantis, Florida.

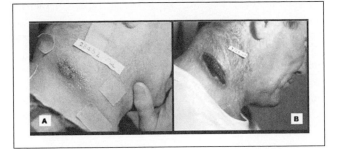

FIGURE 39-3

CUTANEOUS ANTHRAX
(A). Vesiculo-pustular-edematous phase. (B). Black eschar phase.
Source: Courtesy of the Centers for Disease Control and Prevention.

may occur with intact skin. The incubation period ranges from 1 to 10 days after exposure. Once the spores germinate, the organism releases toxins responsible for tissue edema and pruritus, resulting in the formation of a macule, which evolves to a papule, and then to an ulcer, all of which occurs within a period of 48 hours. The ulcer is often surrounded by fluid-filled vesicles that contain the bacillus, therefore useful for diagnostic purposes (Fig. 39-3A). The ulcer evolves into a flat black eschar (Fig. 39-3B) that falls off in 1–2 weeks. It is not uncommon to observe associated regional lymphadenitis. The mortality rate is estimated to be approximately 20% if untreated, but it rarely occurs if antimicrobials are given. Antibiotic therapy, even when initiated early, does not change the usual clinical progression of the skin manifestations. Secondary infection, particularly with streptococci or staphylococci, is uncommon, but it is suggested when there is purulent drainage and fever. Other diseases to be considered in the differential diagnosis would include brown recluse spider bites, community-acquired methicillin-resistant *Staphylococcus aureus* furuncles, erysipelas, cellulitis, cat scratch disease, scrub typhus, rickettsial spotted fevers, rat bite fever, plague, tularemia, and ecthyma gangrenosum.

Gastrointestinal Anthrax

It has rarely been reported in humans. The few documented cases have been linked to ingestion of poorly cooked animal meat contaminated with spores of *B. anthracis*. Animal models of infection using direct instillation of large numbers of spores into the gastrointestinal tract have been unsuccessful, meaning that the infection most likely occurs by ingesting the organism in its vegetative state.

Two clinical subtypes have been described:

- Oropharyngeal: characterized by ulcerations in the mouth, pharynx, and esophagus leading to sepsis
- Intestinal: involves predominantly ileum and cecum, causing acute abdomen presentation, bloody diarrhea, and/or ascites, and progressing to septicemia

The fatality rate is high (approximately 25–60%), probably owed to late diagnosis. Postmortem examinations in Sverdlovsk cases showed submucosal lesions in many of the victims, however, all of them had pathologic evidence of inhalational source of infection.

Inhalational Anthrax

Inhalation of *B. anthracis* spores is the most effective route in contracting lethal infection. Some published data have suggested that as few as three spores are sufficient to cause infection, and that the dose needed to kill 50% of individuals exposed to it (LD_{50}) is in the range of 2500–55,000 spores. However, the recent experience with the anthrax attacks of 2001 would suggest that inhalation of a much smaller quantity of spores can effectively lead to clinical disease. Due to the very small size of the spores (1–5 μm), they are able to reach the respiratory alveoli in the lung parenchyma where they are phagocytized by pulmonary macrophages. Some of the spores are digested within these scavenger cells, whereas others will be transported to the regional lymph nodes in the pulmonary hilum and the mediastinum where they may remain dormant for hours, days, or weeks. The stimuli and/or conditions that trigger the germination of the spores remain unknown. Once in their vegetative state, the bacteria rapidly multiply and produce toxins that are ultimately responsible for tissue damage.

Following an incubation period, which may range from a few days to a few months, the initial symptoms of inhalational anthrax are vague and nonspecific, resembling a flu-like illness syndrome, and therefore precluding early diagnosis and subsequent treatment nonaccessible. The signs and symptoms that were found in all victims of inhalational anthrax following the September 11 attacks included nausea, vomiting, pallor and/or cyanosis, diaphoresis, altered mental status, tachycardia (>110 beats/min), fever (>100.9°F), and increased hematocrit (Table 39-1 lists the most common signs, symptoms, and laboratory findings reported in the inhalational anthrax cases during the 2001 attacks). The rapid onset of a septic syndrome and the development of multisystem organ failure generally follow if appropriate treatment is not initiated in a timely manner. The single most valuable finding is the presence of mediastinal widening by chest radiograph (Fig. 39-4) or computerized tomography (CT) scan films. Such widening is caused by enlarged lymph nodes, most commonly due to hemorrhagic lymphadenitis, which has been described in the majority of the most recent cases of confirmed inhalational anthrax. However, similar changes may be observed with tuberculosis, tularemia, histoplasmosis, sarcoidosis, as well as lymphomatous and other neoplastic processes. In few cases, there is no identifiable mediastinal adenopathy, but hemorrhagic pleural effusions and/or pneumonic infiltrates instead. Blood samples are positive for *B. anthracis* in nearly all patients if obtained prior to the initiation of antibiotics.

TABLE 39-1

INHALATIONAL ANTHRAX INFECTION: REPORTED CLINICAL PRESENTATION AND DIAGNOSTIC TEST FINDINGS

Clinical Features	Physical Findings	Laboratory Abnormalities	Imaging Studies
Fever, chills, sweats*	Fever >37.8°C*	WBC (cells/mm³)*:	Abnormal chest radiograph
Cough, nonproductive*	Tachycardia >100 beats/min*	• Median at admission: 9800	• Widened mediastinum*
Nausea and vomiting*	Hypotension <110 mm Hg	• Median peak: 26,400	• Pleural effusions*
Dyspnea or coryza*	Skin lesions	Elevated liver function tests	• Parenchymal infiltrates
Chest discomfort*		(ALT and AST)*	Abnormal computerized
Confusion		Increased serum creatinine	chest scan (as above)
Headache		Hypoxemia	
Myalgias		Positive blood cultures*	
Meningitis			

*Most common documented findings. WBC—White blood cell count; ALT—Alanine aminotransferase; AST—Aspartate aminotransferase

Source: Data compiled from Inglesby TV, O'Toole T, Henderson DA, et al. Anthrax as a biological weapon, 2002. Updated recommendations for management. JAMA. 2002 207:2236–2252, Bartlett JG, Inglesby TV, Borio L. Management of anthrax. Clin Inf Dis. 2002;35:851–858, and Jernigan JA, Stephers DS, Asford DA, et al. Bioterrorism-related inhalational anthrax: the first 10 cases reported in the United States. Emerg Infect Dis. 2001;7:933–944.

Hemorrhagic Meningitis or Meningoencephalitis

Any route of infection by *B. anthracis* (cutaneous, gastrointestinal, or inhalational) may result in meningitis or meningoencephalitis. Recognition of this clinical syndrome in the context of anthrax is of extreme importance for medical, public health, and national security reasons. It is a medical emergency that requires the earliest of the possible interventions because of its high fatality rate (>95%).

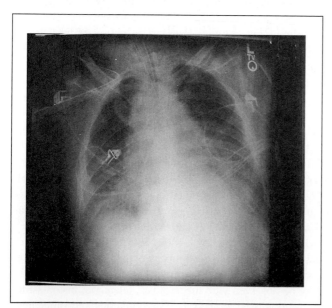

FIGURE 39-4

CHEST RADIOGRAPH OF THE PATIENT IN FIGS. 39-1 AND 39-2, DEMONSTRATING TYPICAL MEDIASTINAL WIDENING IN THE CONTEXT OF INHALATIONAL ANTHRAX INFECTION

Source: Courtesy of Dr Larry Bush, Atlantis, Florida.

The index case of anthrax in the wake of the September 11 attacks was diagnosed in Florida in a man who presented with this syndrome. Making the diagnosis of anthrax implies an immediate response by the local and state public health departments, law enforcement, forensic investigation teams, and governmental resources.

The symptoms of anthrax-related meningitis and meningoencephalitis do not differ from those caused by other organisms. The diagnosis relies in the identification of *B. anthracis* bacteria in the spinal fluid.

DIAGNOSIS

The diagnosis of anthrax relies on the identification of the causative organism in blood, tissue, or fluid samples. It is imperative to obtain samples for culture prior to the administration of antimicrobials, since the bacillus is unlikely to be recovered after a few doses of antibiotic therapy. Preliminary identification of *B. anthracis* is made based on its Gram's stain and encapsulation qualities, rapid growth on blood agar with absence of hemolysis, colony morphology ("curly hair"- or "medusa head"-like), identification of spores from culture plates, sensitivity to penicillin and biochemical testing. Once preliminary identification is accomplished, the samples should be sent for confirmatory testing, to one of the public facilities belonging to the laboratory response network (LRN) for bioterrorism (currently a total of 81 in the country). These tests include enzyme-linked immunosorbent assay (ELISA) for detection of IgG antibodies to the bacterium protective antigen, γ-phage lysis test, the newly Food and Drug Administration (FDA)-approved rapid real-time polymerase chain reaction (RT-PCR) assay and/or immunohistochemical staining. The latter is used on tissue biopsies (i.e., skin punch biopsy of cutaneous anthrax lesions) or necropsy samples (postmortem confirmation). Other rapid assays are being developed, including PCR analysis for amplification of the specific virulence plasmids of *B. anthracis*.

TREATMENT AND POSTEXPOSURE PROPHYLAXIS

Treatment of Inhalational Anthrax

The case mortality rate of the 11 diagnosed inhalational anthrax victims in the 2001 bioterrorism attacks was 45% (5 deaths out of 11 cases). This was significantly less than rates of over 85% in previously reported cases, including those associated with the 1979 Sverdlosk, Russia, event. Early diagnoses together with specific antibiotic therapy are the factors that have contributed most to this improvement in fatality rate. Therefore, given the rapid clinical course of symptomatic inhalational anthrax infection, early effective antibiotic administration is essential. Patients should begin receiving treatment for anthrax infection in the appropriate clinical circumstances while awaiting the results of laboratory studies.

Specific recommendations for antibiotic use in the context of a bioterrorist attack with aerosolized *B. anthracis* spores derive from consensus opinion based on best available evidence, and not on government-sanctioned controlled clinical trials. Most naturally occurring *B. anthracis* strains are highly sensitive to penicillin, which historically has been the preferred anthrax therapy.

The excellent in vitro antimicrobial activity of ciprofloxacin and doxycycline against *B. anthracis*, coupled with proven efficacy in animal models, led to the approval by the FDA of these two antibiotic agents, along with penicillin, for treatment of inhalational anthrax infection. After the demonstration that the strain of *B. anthracis* isolated in the 2001 attacks possessed an inducible β-lactamase, which could possibly lead to penicillin resistance, the CDC recommended that patients with suspected or proven inhalational anthrax be initially treated with ciprofloxacin or doxycycline along with one or two other antibiotics (Table 39-2). The chance of survival was observed to be greater in patients treated in this fashion during the 2001 events. Other suggested antibiotics to be used include rifampin, vancomycin, chloramphenicol, imipenem, penicillin, ampicillin, clindamycin, and clarithromycin.

TABLE 39-2

RECOMMENDED INHALATIONAL ANTHRAX INFECTION TREATMENT

Category	Initial IV Treatment	Prolonged Oral Treatment	Duration
Adults	• Ciprofloxacin 400 mg every 12 h or • Doxycycline 100 mg every 12 h plus • 1 or 2 additional antibiotics*	• Ciprofloxacin 500 mg twice daily or • Doxycycline 100 mg twice daily	• May switch to oral therapy when clinically appropriate • Total duration: 60 days

Children	• Ciprofloxacin 10–15 mg/kg every 12 h
	or
	• Doxycycline:
	  • >8 y/o & weight >45 kg: 100 mg every 12 h
	  • >8 y/o & weight ≤45 kg: 2.2 mg/kg every 12 h
	  • ≤8 y/o: 2.2 mg/kg every 12 h
	plus
	• 1 or 2 additional antibiotics*
		• Ciprofloxacin 10–15 mg/kg twice daily
		or
		• Doxycycline:
		  • >8 y/o & weight >45 kg: 100 mg twice daily
		  • >8 y/o & weight ≤45 kg: 2.2 mg/kg twice daily
		  • ≤8 y/o: 2.2 mg/kg twice daily
			• May switch to oral therapy when clinically appropriate
			• Total duration: 60 days

Pregnant women	• Same as for nonpregnant adults	• Same as for nonpregnant adults	• Same as for nonpregnant adults
* Other therapies	• Corticosteroids (for meningitis and severe mediastinal edema) • Angiotensin-converting enzyme inhibitors • Calcium channel blockers • Specific *Bacillus anthracis* hyperimmune globulin		

*Other antibiotics may include penicillin, ampicillin, imipenem, meropenem, clindamycin, rifampin, vancomycin, and clarithromycin.

Source: Data compiled from Inglesby TV, O'Toole T, Henderson DA, et al. Anthrax as a biological weapon, 2002. Updated recommendations for management. JAMA. 2002;207:2236–2252 and Lucey D. Bacillus anthracis (Anthrax). In: Mandell GL, Bennett JE, Dolin R, eds: Principles and Practice of Infectious Disease. 6th ed. Philadelphia, PA: Elsevier, 2005; p. 2485–2491.

The intravenous route of antibiotic administration is recommended with a switch to oral dosing when clinically appropriate, particularly in the setting of a contained casualty (limited number of patients requiring therapy). However, if the number of individuals requiring antibiotic treatment is substantially high, or in the context of mass casualty, oral administration alone may be the only feasible option. Antibiotic therapy should be continued for at least 60 days. This lengthy treatment course is based on knowledge that antibiotic therapy during anthrax infection may delay or prevent the development of protective antibodies, therefore creating the risk of recurrent disease for an extended period of time, due to the possibility of delayed germination of harbored inhaled anthrax spores.

Treatment of Cutaneous Anthrax

Oral penicillin given for 7–10 days was the standard treatment recommended for cutaneous anthrax infection prior to the 2001 attacks. Currently, for severe cutaneous disease (lesions in the head and neck, extensive edema, and/or signs of systemic involvement), clinical management should employ the same treatment recommendations as summarized above for inhalational anthrax (Table 39-3). Patients presenting with less serious cutaneous disease can be treated with oral ciprofloxacin or doxycycline. Topical antibiotic therapy has not been proven useful. Antibiotic treatment for cutaneous anthrax should be taken for 60 days based on the assumption that inhalational exposure was likely associated with the development of the skin lesions.

Although fluoroquinolone antibiotics are not recommended for use in children younger than 16–18 years old due to the possible development of arthropathy, the significant risks surrounding an inhalational anthrax exposure outweigh these concerns. In similar fashion, though doxycycline use in children less than 9 years of age has been associated with retardation in skeletal growth and discolored teeth, it should be prescribed for anthrax infection in children when ciprofloxacin cannot be given (i.e., adverse reactions, unfavorable antimicrobial susceptibility data, and limited drug supply).

Other Treatment Considerations

Fears of teratogenic effects in the unborn with the use of ciprofloxacin and doxycycline in pregnant women must be balanced with the high death rate associated with anthrax infection. Therefore, the recommendations for treatment during pregnancy are the same as those for nonpregnant adults. Amoxicillin may be substituted for prolonged course of therapy in children, pregnant and lactating women only after 14–21 days of ciprofloxacin or doxycycline administration and with knowledge of antimicrobial susceptibility data pertaining to the isolated strain of *B. anthracis*.

Though limited data are known to exist, other adjuvant treatment modalities to be considered for anthrax infections are systemic corticosteroids (for meningitis or significant mediastinal edema), calcium channel blockers, angiotensin-converting enzyme inhibitors, tumor necrosis

TABLE 39-3

RECOMMENDED CUTANEOUS ANTHRAX INFECTION TREATMENT

Category	Initial Oral Treatment	Alternative Treatment	Duration
Adults*	• Ciprofloxacin 500 mg twice daily or • Doxycycline 100 mg twice daily	• Amoxicillin 500 mg three times daily†	• Total duration: 60 days

Children	• Ciprofloxacin 10–15 mg/kg twice daily (not to exceed 1 g/day)
	or
	• Doxycycline:
	  • >8 y/o & weight >45kg: 100 mg twice daily
	  • >8 y/o & weight ≤45 kg: 2.2 mg/kg twice daily
	  • ≤8 y/o: 2.2 mg/kg twice daily
		• Amoxicillin 80 mg/kg/day, three times daily†	• Total duration: 60 days

Pregnant women	• Same as for nonpregnant adults	• Same as for nonpregnant adults	• Total duration: 60 days

*Cutaneous anthrax with signs of systemic involvement, extensive edema or lesions in the head and neck require the same intravenous and combination therapy as with inhalational anthrax (Table 39-2).

†Amoxicillin may be substituted for prolonged therapy course in patients with a contraindication to ciprofloxacin or doxycycline after 14–21 days of the initial treatment in children, pregnant, and breast-feeding women.

Source: Data compiled from Inglesby TV, O'Toole T, Henderson DA, et al. Anthrax as a biological weapon, 2002. Updated recommendations for management. JAMA. 2002;207:2236–2252 and Lucey D. Bacillus anthracis (Anthrax), In: Mandell GL, Bennett JE, Dolin R, eds. Principles and Practice of Infectious Disease. 6th ed. Philadelphia, PA: Elsevier, 2005; p. 2485–2491.

factor inhibitors, and specific hyperimmune globulin for *B. anthracis*.

Postexposure Prophylaxis

Ciprofloxacin has been approved by the FDA for inhalational anthrax for postexposure chemoprophylaxis (PEP) since August 2000. Following the 2001 attacks, the CDC provided new guidelines for PEP in the event that inhalational anthrax is felt to have occurred (Table 39-4). In addition to ciprofloxacin, doxycycline has been recommended as an equivalent initial PEP option. Amoxicillin has also been offered as an alternative antibiotic for prophylaxis in children, pregnant women, and mothers who are breast-feeding. The duration of PEP recommended is 60 days.

It is imperative that the PEP antibiotics against anthrax be initiated as soon as possible following actual or suspected inhalation of *B. anthracis* spores. Mathematical models have indicated that for each day PEP is delayed after aerosolized anthrax exposure, the case fatality rate can increase by 5–10%. Assessment for possible inhalation exposure to spores must take into consideration the credibility of a perceived or known bioterrorism threat, environmental cultures, tests of potentially contaminated source materials, and cultures of nasal secretions.

The reported adverse event rate associated with PEP following the 2001 attacks of approximately 19% was greater than expected when compared with data from published ciprofloxacin clinical trials. Explanations, which may account for this high rate of adverse events, could include psychological fear surrounding the anthrax attacks as well as the long duration of ciprofloxacin administration. No reported adverse drug reaction was considered serious in terms of hospitalization or death.

There were no reported cases of anthrax infection among those exposed in the 2001 attacks who took PEP antibiotics, including those persons not completing the 60-day treatment course.

VACCINATION

Biothrax, formerly called Anthrax Vaccine Absorbed (AVA), manufactured by Bioport in Lansing, MI, and licensed in 1970, is presently the only available anthrax vaccine in the United States. Made from a cell-free filtrate of a nonencapsulated attenuated strain of *B. anthracis*, the antigen responsible for inducing immunity is almost exclusively the protective antigen (PA). Studies in animals have demonstrated an almost 100% protective efficacy against an aerosolized challenge with *B. anthracis* spores. Preexposure vaccination consists of a series of 6 inoculations over a period of 18 months and is indicated for persons at increased risk of acquiring the disease occupationally, such as laboratory workers, veterinarians, as well as wooden mill workers. A compulsory anthrax vaccine immunization program for military personnel was initiated in 1977 by the U.S. Department of Defense.

Although the anthrax vaccine has not been approved by the FDA for postexposure prophylaxis, the U.S. Institute of Medicine report issued in 2002 concluded that the anthrax vaccine is effective against inhalational anthrax and, when used in conjunction with PEP antibiotics, may

TABLE 39-4

ANTHRAX POSTEXPOSURE PROPHYLAXIS

Category	Oral Treatment	Alternative Treatment	Duration
Adults	• Ciprofloxacin 500 mg twice daily or • Doxycycline 100 mg twice daily	• Amoxicillin 500 mg three times daily*	• Total duration: 60 days[†]
Children	• Ciprofloxacin 10–15 mg/kg twice daily (not to exceed 1 g/day) or • Doxycycline: • >8 y/o & weight >45 kg: 100 mg twice daily • >8 y/o & weight ≤ 45 kg: 2.2 mg/kg twice daily • ≤8 y/o: 2.2 mg/kg twice daily	• Amoxicillin 80 mg/kg/day, three times daily*	• Total duration: 60 days[†]
Pregnant women	• Same as for nonpregnant adults	• Same as for nonpregnant adults	• Total duration: 60 days[†]

*Amoxicillin may be substituted for children, pregnant, and breast-feeding women, if no knowledge of a β-lactamase producing strain of *Bacillus anthracis* has been identified in the attack.

[†]Extended to 100 days if postexposure anthrax vaccination, given on days 0, 14, and 28, is used in conjunction with antibiotics.

help to prevent the development of anthrax disease following exposures. As such, postexposure vaccination consists of a three-dose vaccination series given subcutaneously on days 0, 14, and 28 together with the aforementioned postexposure recommended antibiotics for 60 days. The vaccine must be given under investigational new drug protocols and procedures and requires informed consent. In one large open-label safety study, adverse reactions were reported to have occurred in up to 20% locally at the vaccination site and less than 1% systemically (headache, malaise, myalgias, arthralgias, fever, nausea, diarrhea, dizziness, and anorexia).

Future generation anthrax vaccines under development will contain recombinant protective antigen, and will involve shorter vaccination schedules, fewer doses, and an intramuscular route of administration.

INFECTION CONTROL

Person-to-person transmission of anthrax is not known to occur. Therefore, even in the setting of inhalational anthrax infection, standard barrier isolation precautions are recommended for hospitalized patients diagnosed with, or suspected to have any form of anthrax. Airborne protective measures are not indicated but contact precautions should be used for patients with draining cutaneous lesions. Dressings removed from such lesions need to be disposed as biohazardous waste. Health-care workers, household contacts, friends, and coworkers associated with the patient do not need postexposure prophylaxis or immunization unless it is determined that they, like the patient, were exposed to aerosol or surface contamination with B. anthracis spores. Skin and clothing exposed to spores should be thoroughly washed with water and soap. Disinfectants routinely used for hospital infection control, such as hypochlorite, are effective for cleaning contaminated environmental surfaces. Notification of the hospital epidemiologist, microbiology laboratory, and local as well as state health departments should take place immediately at the earliest indication of an anthrax case. This assures appropriate handling of specimens under biosafety level 2 conditions and referral to the nearest facility in the LRN for bioterrorism. Communication of timely and accurate information must also be a priority.

In the event of death due to anthrax infection, proper burial, and preferably cremation, is important in preventing the further spread of the disease. Embalming infected bodies possesses special risks. Instruments and materials used for autopsies should be autoclaved or incinerated.

DECONTAMINATION

The greatest risk to humans from aerosolized anthrax spores comes at the time when B. anthracis spores are first made airborne, a phenomenon known as "primary aerosolization." Factors such as size of the dispersed particles and hydrostatic properties help to determine for how long the spores will remain in the air. The exposure of large numbers of persons over relatively large geographic areas has previously been estimated assuming the release of large quantities of spores from an aircraft carrier. More recently, less technologically sophisticated systems such as the opening of envelopes containing weaponized anthrax spores in an indoor environment have been proven capable of delivering high concentrations of spores to those in the vicinity to the individual handling the putative envelop. Subsequent transport of those spores to other parts of the building may also occur, increasing the number of individuals susceptible to exposure. The diagnosis of anthrax infection in postal workers who had handled or processed unopened letters in Washington, DC, and New Jersey during the 2001 attacks, provided new evidence that "weapon-grade" spores of B. anthracis could leak from the edges or the pores of the envelop paper.

Resuspension of spores into the air or "secondary aerosolization" following their settlement on surfaces after primary release, is of uncertain risk and would seem to be dependant on the quantity and the quality of the powdered spores, the type of surface where they first settled, as well as the specific activities occurring in the contaminated area. Tests conducted by the Environmental Protection Agency in the U.S. Senate Hart Building, Washington, DC, confirmed that secondary aerosolization related to routine activities in the area contaminated with anthrax spores does occur, but did not assess the specific risk of anthrax infection in persons working in such setting. Although assays for rapid identification of B. anthracis spores are available, they are nonspecific screening tools and should only serve as indications for confirmatory testing.

A consensus has been reached that decontamination of a known contaminated building would be useful in decreasing the probability of acquiring anthrax infection via secondary aerosolization. However, this is a technically difficult task and involves a great monetary expense. The buildings involved in the 2001 anthrax attacks were decontaminated using γ-radiation. Workers involved in decontaminating buildings containing anthrax spores must make use of personal protective equipment and are recommended to follow medical measures such as vaccination and intake of prophylactic antibiotics.

ANTHRAX THREAT PREPAREDNESS IN THE HOSPITAL SETTING

The success of an institution's preparedness for a bioterrorist attack will depend on the coordinated and cohesive efforts of many individuals. In light of the 2001 anthrax attacks along with today's geopolitical and ideological unrest, bioterrorism must now be considered in the differential diagnosis of vague and common conditions, especially if associated with unusual epidemiologic features.

Remembering that diagnostic criteria, management strategies, and epidemiologic principles are common to all infectious diseases regardless of the source, a prepared team of health-care workers can effectively minimize the potentially high morbidity and mortality associated with a bioterrorist event. Emergency room health-care providers are likely to be "first responders" in the event that another bioterrorist attack with anthrax or other biologic agent takes place. The STAT FACTS table at the beginning of this chapter provides a summarized list of considerations for evaluating and diagnosing suspected cases of inhalational anthrax. The response to a bioterrorism attack is a local function, with support from both state and federal agencies. Although emergency room personnel and primary health-care providers are positioned to be among the earliest to detect those possibly sickened by exposure to a biological weapon, a coordinated effort with predefined duties for various clinicians of multiple specialties along with nonclinicians from several hospital departments is essential to effect a rapid and successful response.

The anthrax attacks of 2001 provided us with invaluable lessons. Among those aspects considered to have gone well are medical community's ability to recognize a bioterrorist-related disease, laboratory's identification of the pathogen and collaboration with the LRN, deployment of the National Pharmaceutical Stockpile, and the willingness of volunteers to accept risk and responsibility. However, certain aspects related to the 2001 attacks did not go as well. Specifically, preparedness varied greatly between communities (who is in charge here?); communication, especially from the top, was fragmented, scientific knowledge was old, outdated, and at times incorrect and the legal authority was often unclear (quarantine, jurisdiction, indemnification). With continued vigilance, education, and coordination, until the peoples of the world resolve their differences in an amicable fashion, we will be better prepared for bioterrorism.

Suggested Reading

Altman L. New tests confirm potency of anthrax in Senate Office Building. *New York Times*, December 11, 2001:B6.

Bartlett JG, Inglesby TV, Borio L. Management of anthrax. *Clin Inf Dis*. 2002;35:851–858.

Bush LM, Abrams BH, Beall A, et al. Index case of fatal inhalational anthrax due to bioterrorism in the United States. *NEJM*. 2001;345:1607–1610.

Cole, LA. *The Anthrax Letters. A Medical Detective Story*. Washington, DC: Joseph Henry Press, 2003.

Frist WH. *When Every Moment Counts: What You Need to Know About Bioterrorism from the Senate's Only Doctor*. Lanham, MD: Rowman & Littlefield Publishers, 2002.

Health Aspects of Chemical and Biological Weapons. Geneva, Switzerland: World Health Organization, 1970.

Hepburn MJ, Purcell BK, Paragas J. Pathogenesis and sepsis caused by organisms potentially utilized as biologic weapons: opportunities for targeted intervention. *Curr Drug Targets*. 2007 Apr;8(4):519–32.

Holty JE, Kim RY, Bravata DM, Anthrax: A systematic Review of Atypical Presentations. Ann Emerg Med 2006 Aug; 48(2):200-11 ER62006 Feb 21.

Inglesby TV, Henderson DA, Bartlett JG, et al. Anthrax as a biologic weapon. *JAMA*. 1999;281:1735–1745.

Inglesby TV, O'Toole T, Henderson DA, et al. Anthrax as a biological weapon, 2002. Updated recommendations for management. *JAMA*. 2002;207:2236–2252.

Jernigan JA, Stephers DS, Asford DA, et al. Bioterrorism-related inhalational anthrax: the first 10 cases reported in the United States. *Emerg Infect Dis*. 2001;7:933–944.

Kyriacou DN, Adamski A, Khardori N. Anthrax: from antiquity and obscurity to a front runner in bioterrorism. *Infect Dis Clin N Am*. 2006;20:227–251.

Kyriacou DN, Yarnold PR, Stein AC et al. discriminating inhalational anthrax from community-acquired pneumonia using chest radiograph findings and a clinical algorithm, *Chest* 2007 Feb; 136(2):489–96.

Kyriacou, D. N., Stein, A. C., Yarnold, P. R., Clinical predictors of bioterrorism-related inhalational anthrax. *Lancet* 2004; Jul 31-Aug 6; 449–52.

Lucey D. Bacillus anthracis (Anthrax). In: Mandell GL, Bennett JE, Dolin R, eds. *Principles and Practice of Infectious Disease*. 6th ed. Philadelphia, PA: Elsevier, 2005; p 2485–2491.

Meselson M, Guillemin J, Hughes-Jones M, et al. The Sverdlosk anthrax outbreak of 1979. *Science*. 1994;226:1202–1208.

Place RC, HanFling, Howell JM Mayer TA Bioterrorism-related inhalational anthrax: can extrapolated adult guidelines be applied to a pediatric population? *Biosecur Bioterror*. 2007 Mar;5(1):35–42.

Swartz MN. Recognition and management of anthrax: an update. *NEJM*. 2001;345:1621–1626.

Center for Biologic Counter-Terrorism and Emerging Diseases. *www.bepast.org*

Centers for Disease Control and Prevention. *www.bt.cdc.gov/ anthrax/index.asp*

National Institutes of Health. *www.nlm.nih.gov/medlineplus/ anthrax.htm*

40

YERSINIA PESTIS—PLAGUE

Robin B. McFee

STAT FACTS

YERSINIA PESTIS—PLAGUE

What you should know

- Bubonic plague occurs in the United States (Fig. 40-2—bubonic plague)
  - Most common "natural" presentation of *Yersinia pestis* (plague)
  - Name derived from the development within 1–6 days after a flea bite of an enlarged, painful lymph node ("bubo")
  - Usually bubo found on lower extremity (groin) can occur elsewhere
  - Look alikes are usually *not*
    - As exquisitely painful as plague
    - Associated with rapid development of systemic symptoms
      - Fever
      - Irritability

Pneumonic plague (Fig. 40-2) is

- Most likely bioweapon presentation
- Not the predominant "natural form" but occurs worldwide nevertheless
- Contagious
- Fatal if treatment is delayed
- Associated with these key symptoms
  - Fever
  - Shortness of breath
  - Rapidly progressive respiratory distress
  - 3 Hs
    - Hemoptysis
    - Hematemesis
    - Hemorrhagic diarrhea

NB: Plague in bioterrorism would differ epidemiologically from natural plague as the former would most likely result from an aerosol release, causing numerous patients with severe and

rapidly progressive respiratory distress. The magnitude of the outbreak would be predicated upon the amount and location of the biological release. The occurrence of plague in nonendemic areas, affecting individuals with little preexisting risk for *Y. pestis* exposure and the absence of infected animals would also be important clues. Effective communications among health-care facilities and professionals, sharing information about unusual pulmonary cases, especially increased and nonseasonal, is critical to managing a potential intentional outbreak.

What you should have in advance

- Health-care facility preparedness
  - Professional training with regular updates
  - Medication and other resources
  - Patient triage
  - Early, presumptive diagnosis
  - Patient placement
  - Quarantine capabilities
- Ample supply of personal protective equipment (PPE)
- Ample supply of antimicrobials
  - First and second-line therapy
    - Aminoglycosides
      - First-line streptomycin
      - Gentamicin suitable alternative
    - Tetracyclines (doxycycline)
    - Fluoroquinolones (ciprofloxacin)
    - Chloramphenicol
- Countermeasures for special populations
  - Women who are pregnant
  - Children
  - Elderly
- Contact information for (prominently displayed) familiarity with the response capabilities of appropriate response stakeholders and interactive exercises with the following agencies (bare minimum)

- Local health department
- State health department
- Laboratory response network/State health lab
- Centers for Disease Control and Prevention (CDC) emergency operations office
- Fire-rescue/Emergency medical services
- Law enforcement (local, state, and federal)
- Policymakers/political authorities
- Media liaison
- Coroner's office/Medical examiner

What you should do if presumptive plague patient
- Contact hospital laboratory conveying risk and presumptive diagnosis
  - Antibiotic sensitivity testing of microbe(s)
  - Obtain appropriate samples—transport rapidly per hospital/CDC protocol
- Contact lead infectious disease consultant and hospital epidemiologist
- Contact local health department and/or state health officer and/or CDC
- Contact directly or via health department the state laboratory
- Initiate plague appropriate antimicrobial chemotherapy (*most likely survival advantage conferred if appropriate antibiotics initiated within 24 hours of initial symptoms). Treatment should continue for a minimum of 10 days. Do not use β-lactam antibiotics as they are not generally effective against plague.*
  - First-line antibiotics for **adults** include:
    - Doxycycline
    - Streptomycin
    - Gentamicin
  - First-line antibiotics for **adults with CNS involvement** include:
    - Chloramphenicol
  - For immunosuppressed—current recommendations parallel treatment options for nonimmunosuppressed adults
  - First-line antibiotics for **women who are pregnant** (risk: benefit) include (severe clinical case):
    - Gentamicin or
    - Doxycycline

- First-line antibiotics for **children** include:
  - Streptomycin
  - Gentamicin
- Safe alternatives-
  - If age >2 years old
    - Chloramphenicol
  - If age >8 years old
    - Tetracycline (doxycycline)

Lab specimens and testing
NB: Manipulation of positive cultures may result in aerosol release; BSL 3 practices should be observed in the lab
- Appropriate specimens for analysis include
  - Blood cultures (take three samples each separated by 10–30 minutes)
    - Transport at room temperature
      - Bubo fine needle aspirates (*not* incision and drainage)
      - Cerebral spinal fluid
      - Sputum

Diagnosis
- Based upon history, exposures, symptoms = presumptive
- Laboratory confirmation (CDC Table 40-1)

Isolate patient(s)
- Bubonic plague—minimum 48 hours after administration of plague appropriate antibiotics
- Pneumonic plague—minimum of 96 hours after administration of plague appropriate antibiotics

Initiate Postexposure Prophylaxis (PEP) for contacts (minimum of 7 days)
- Doxycycline
- Ciprofloxacin

NB: All persons developing a temperature of 38.5°C or higher or with symptoms of a new-onset cough/respiratory symptoms should receive antibiotic treatment.
- For infants, new-onset tachypnea is a sufficient indication to start antibiotic treatment.

Initiate hospital response plan to plague
- Mobilize appropriate resources
- Enhance security

BACKGROUND

Yersinia pestis (Plague)

"The plague," also known as the Black Death because of blackened appearance of gangrene of the fingers, toes, and nose associated with septicemic plague, caused the death of millions of Europeans during the Middle Ages. The oldest account of plague is likely found in the First Book of Samuel from the Bible. Stories abound concerning the use of plague as a bioweapon during the siege of Kafka and

throughout history, most recently the infamous Japanese bioweapons program referred to as Unit 731, which, during World War II, was responsible for numerous deaths in Manchuria. Moreover, it is believed the Japanese were working on an effective deployment system to release plague in the western United States. Several terrorist groups have revealed an interest in or access to *Yersinia pestis*.

Plague is a rapidly progressive infectious disease. The causative agent *Y. pestis*, a gram-negative bacillus, was discovered in 1894. It is a member of the Enterobacteriaceae family, and typically transmitted to the human host by a flea bite from a natural reservoir, which includes several different rodent species, resulting in a painful swelling of a lymph node, referred to as a bubo, for example, bubonic plague, which is the most common natural form. The location of the flea bite determines where the bubo or infected lymph node will occur; most commonly the femoral/inguinal lymph nodes are involved given the original flea bite usually occurs on the lower extremity. However other lymph nodes such as the axillary nodes may be affected. Two fleas play a role in plague transmission: *Xenopsylla cheopis* and *Synopsyllas fonquerniei*. *Plague* is still encountered worldwide in areas of enzootic prevalence in local rodent populations (Fig. 40-1). Several countries continue to report human cases of plague illness, including the United States. Recently two tourists in New York City presented to the hospital with a rapidly progressive febrile illness; subsequently they were diagnosed with plague. They lived in New Mexico where studies isolated infected animals near their home. In the United States, approximately a dozen cases of plague occurs—it is a zoonotic disease, appearing mostly in the Southwest and usually affecting Native Americans. So far in 2006, a total of 13 human cases from 4 states, mostly the Southwest—New Mexico, Colorado, California, and Texas—have been reported, as plague remains one of several infections that is reportable to health authorities.

In the event of a bioweapon attack, physicians will be first responders and the front line of defense. Results from a recent study evaluating physician knowledge about the six Centers for Disease Control and Prevention (CDC) Category A agents (anthrax, botulinum toxin, plague, smallpox, tularemia, and viral hemorrhagic fevers) were not overly encouraging; physicians demonstrated the least knowledge about plague. Clearly containing the threat of deadly infections, physicians will need to appropriately diagnose and treat patients infected with biological weapons as well as emerging pathogens. Given the increase in international travel, the prudent physician should consider in the differential diagnosis, global illness, especially if endemic to regions the patient recently visited, or had interaction with persons who may be infected by or exposed to emerging or persistent pathogens such as plague, tuberculosis, measles, and other persistent threats to health that remain a burden to numerous countries.

In the aftermath of 9/11, and the anthrax events of 2001, there are growing concerns among government preparedness agencies about terrorist attacks using biological weapons. Plague has been identified as a leading candidate biological agent, and the CDC has designated it as a Category A organism, based upon ease of access, potential lethality, lack of preventive measures, and rapidity of clinical progression. As *Y. pestis* can be easily obtained and cultured and is highly pathogenic for humans, it poses a serious threat of being used for bioterrorism purposes. Artificially created aerosol containing plague bacilli could cause numerous and almost simultaneous cases of primary pulmonic plague in an exposed population. Persons exposed would most likely develop severe pneumonia with rapidly progressing respiratory and circulatory failure. Infection by flea bite can result in a bubonic or septicemic plague, possibly complicated by secondary pneumonia. The person with pneumonic symptoms may be a source of a droplet-borne infection for other people who consequently develop primary pneumonic plague. Regardless of form, plague is a severe infection characterized by a short incubation period, rapid onset, and quick progress with mortality exceeding 60% if not treated properly. The pneumonic plague is associated with a particularly rapid progression and the mortality rate of almost 100% if not treated properly. Interest in plague as a bioweapon remains strong, with several nations attributed with weaponizing an aerosol version. Unlike anthrax and tularemia, pneumonic plague is highly contagious,

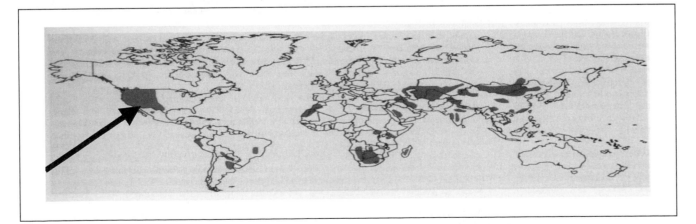

FIGURE 40-1

WORLDWIDE SOURCES OF PLAGUE (Y. PESTIS)
Note the United States (arrow).
(Source: World Health Organization)

making it an especially worrisome potential bioweapon. Intelligence experts suggest bioweapon research conducted in the former Soviet Union (FSU) included the developing strains of *Y. pestis* resistant to antibiotics that would be considered frontline treatment.

Pathogenesis

Y. pestis has a strong ability to overcome the host defense mechanisms. Rapid and overwhelming multiplication of the organism occurs primarily extracellularly. The high mortality rates of this organism are the result of several virulence factors resulting in rapid replication and acclimation to the host environment. *Y. pestis* induces an inflammatory response at the site of inoculation and spreads via the lymphatic system to regional lymph nodes, especially ones closest to the flea bite. Plasmids assist *Y. pestis* to survive the mammalian host. Specific *Y. pestis* proteins such as Yersinia outer proteins (Yops) H have antiphagocytic activity, Yop E is cytotoxic and Yop M binds human thrombin. The F1 capsule, expressed at 37°C has antiphagocytic activity against neutrophils and monocytes and is responsible for eliciting a humoral immune response. While *Y. pestis* can survive in macrophages, neutrophils can kill the bacteria, thus the important role of F1 in *Y. pestis* survival. *Y. pestis* promotes an inflammatory response as well as direct endothelial toxicity of Yersinia toxins. Plasminogen activator is a protease that allows for the degradation of fibrin resulting in fibrinolysis. The V and W antigens enable *Y. pestis* to resist phagocytosis. The V antigen also allows the organism to exist in macrophages. Lipopolysaccharide endotoxin causes endotoxic shock, not unlike the picture of shock associated with other gram-negative bacteria; however, plague is a rapidly progressive and deadly infection that can cause multisystem organ failure in a relatively short period of time. In the later stage of infection, these toxins can cause vascular destruction, local hemorrhages. Plague results in local destruction of tissue and systemic effects of endotoxins, some of which cause peripheral vascular collapse and disseminated intravascular coagulation.

Clinical

Human plague illness appears in three forms—bubonic, septicemic, and pneumonic. The causative agent—*Y. pestis*—is a rod-shaped, gram-negative, nonmotile, nonsporulating bacterium.

Bubonic

Worldwide this is the most common form, representing 85% of all cases and is endemic in the southwest United States. Usually a flea bite will introduce the bacterium into the patient, with the nearest lymph node being affected resulting in lymphadenitis, ultimately enlarging into a "bubo." These can measure routinely from 1 to 10 cm. The overlying skin is often tender to exquisitely painful, warm, erythematous, and often accompanied by extensive edema. The pain and inflammation can be quite severe; guarding and loss of movement may result. Most commonly the inguinal nodes are affected since most flea bites occur on the lower extremity (Fig. 40-2). Cervical and axillary nodes are not uncommon regions, again depending upon where the flea bite occurs. Bubonic plague has an incubation period of 2–10 days. High fever, myalgias, headache, and malaise will accompany the beginning of a swollen, tender bubo. The bubo is exquisitely painful as it is quite enlarged and represents significant infection. These lymph nodes *should not be incised and drained*. However, a sterile aspiration can be both therapeutic and diagnostic. Bubo aspirates can be obtained by using a 20-guage needle on a 10 mL syringe filled with 1 or 2 mL of sterile saline that is infused into the node, withdrawn and then the fluid can be sent off to the laboratory for evaluation. Of note, removal of the fluid provides significant relief to the patient. Fifty percent of patients may have abdominal pain. Sometimes nausea and

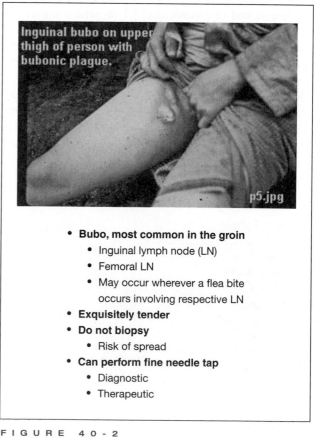

Inguinal bubo on upper thigh of person with bubonic plague.

- **Bubo, most common in the groin**
  - Inguinal lymph node (LN)
  - Femoral LN
  - May occur wherever a flea bite occurs involving respective LN
- **Exquisitely tender**
- **Do not biopsy**
  - Risk of spread
- **Can perform fine needle tap**
  - Diagnostic
  - Therapeutic

FIGURE 40-2

BUBONIC PLAGUE
(Source: CDC)

vomiting occur. The liver and spleen may become enlarged, palpable, and tender. Secondary septicemia can occur. While the list of differential diagnosis can be lengthy of enlarged lymph nodes, when the biodrome or key features of the presenting illness are taken in total, the diagnosis is limited to significant illness, all warranting close evaluation and aggressive intervention. For example, cat scratch fever may cause local discomfort, but patients with bubonic plague suffer a level of pain seemingly disproportionate to the lesion. This is a very telling sign, especially in the context of fever, overall systemic effects. Other diagnoses to consider include streptococcal or staphylococcal lymphadenitis, infectious mononucleosis, lymphatic filariasis, tick-borne typhus, and tularemia. Involvement of intra-abdominal lymph nodes may mimic appendicitis, cholecystitis, or enterocolitis. A thorough travel, occupational, and social (residential) history is critical. Universal precautions should be observed.

It should be noted that the buboes may remain enlarged and somewhat tender for weeks even after appropriate therapy and overall clinical recovery.

Septicemic

A progressive bacteremia in the absence of primary lymphadenopathy is referred to as the primary septicemic form of plague and represents 10–15% of naturally occurring Yersinia pestis illness. Secondary septicemia may occur in association with bubonic plague. While all age groups may be affected, the elderly appear to be at great risk for developing septicemia. Plague septicemia presents much like other gram-negative septicemia. The bacilli rapidly replicate and disseminate causing a profound and deleterious immunological cascade associated with bacterial endotoxin.

Of concern disseminated intravascular coagulopathy (DIC) as well as thrombosis of the acral vessels can occur, resulting in necrosis or gangrene with blackening especially of the nose and digits/extremities, referred to as acral cyanosis (Fig. 40-3). Endotoxemia can cause purpuric lesions. Hematogenous spread to the central nervous system and lungs is possible as well as hepatic and splenic abscesses, with generalized lymphadenopathy. Host response includes multisystem organ failure, DIC, and adult respiratory distress syndrome (ARDS). High fever, chills, vomiting, and hypotension are common symptoms. Plague meningitis occurs in approximately 6% of septicemic and pneumonic cases. Other complications of septicemic plague include plague pneumonia, endophthalmitis, and generalized lymphadenopathy.

Although the clinician may be faced with a nonspecific picture of sepsis syndrome or gram-negative sepsis, fortunately several of the medications common to treat this working diagnosis will work on *Y. pestis*. Nevertheless, plague sepsis is a rapidly progressive illness with a high case fatality rate.

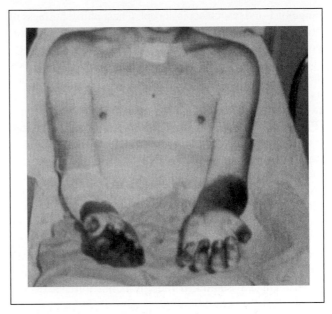

FIGURE 40-3

ACRAL CYANOSIS
Source: McGovern TW, Friedlander AM. Plague. In: Zajtchuk R, Bellamy R, eds. Textbook of Military Medicine: Medical Aspects of Chemical and Biological Warfare. Washington, DC: Office of the Surgeon General, Borden Institute, Walter Reed Army Medical Center; 1997.

Pneumonic

Pneumonic plague is the most fulminant and lethal form of the disease virtually 100% mortality if untreated, with a high case fatality rate if treatment is not administered within 24 hours.

Pneumonic plagues can occur in two forms—primary and secondary. Either should be treated as highly contagious. Primary pneumonic plague, results from inhaling infected respiratory droplets, and initially presents as an infectious pneumonitis with onset of symptoms within 24 to 48 hours of exposures. Sudden disease onset and rapid progression of pulmonary symptoms in an otherwise healthy individual is a typical presentation of primary pneumonic plague. Secondary pneumonic plague occurs in the patient who has been ill for several days prior to lung invasion and the subsequent development of pulmonary symptoms.

The clinical presentation is characterized by fever, chills, headache, generalized body pain, chest pain, dyspnea and resulting in hypoxia, and respiratory distress. Only 1% of naturally occurring plague is pneumonic plague. However, as a biological weapon, this will be the most likely form. Pneumonic plague can result from inhalation of organisms as spread by the weaponized aerosol (primary) or from hematogenous spread from septicemic plague (secondary). The average incubation period is 2–4 days with a range of 1–6 days. Onset is abrupt. Chest pain, shortness of breath, and hypoxia may occur. Concomitant septicemia is possible. The patient may exhibit the three Hs—hemoptysis, hematemesis, and hemorrhagic diarrhea. Bloody sputum is characteristic. Gastrointestinal symptoms such as nausea, diarrhea, and vomiting can occur. The chest x-ray (CXR) most commonly reveals bilateral infiltrates (Fig. 40-4). However, the findings can be varied. Localized areas of necrosis and cavitation or effusion or a picture of noncardiogenic pulmonary edema or ARDS are also possible findings. Pneumonic plague is rapidly progressive and like inhalational anthrax results in shortness of breath, respiratory failure, and death. Heightened concern should arise if a rapidly progressive febrile illness similar to the syndrome of a gram-negative sepsis appears in a young, previously healthy individual. If increasing cases with similar symptoms occur, rapid consult with local health department is essential. If therapy is not initiated within 24 hours, the risk of mortality is high.

Pneumonic plague can initially appear similar to severe community-acquired pneumonias including pneumococcal pneumonia, streptococcal pneumonia, Legionella pneumophila, viral pneumonias, especially in the elderly, *Haemophilus influenza,* Hantavirus pulmonary syndrome, albeit rare, and other bioweapons such as inhalation anthrax and pulmonary tularemia.

PLAGUE DIAGNOSIS

Like other bioweapon illness, the diagnosis of plague must be made quickly and based upon clinical presentation—symptoms and history are key. Context, such as recent travel, occupation, or other exposures and/or the presence of other similarly ill patients, should alert the clinician to the threat of plague (or other emerging pathogen, depending upon the clinical picture and exposures, risks). Unless presumptive diagnosis and early treatment are initiated early, death is likely, especially with pneumonic plague. Untreated bubonic plague has a case fatality rate of 60%, while untreated pneumonic plague is virtually always fatal. Table 40-1 indicates CDC criteria of *Y. pestis* in Level A laboratories.

Any isolate from the respiratory tract, blood, or lymph node containing the major characteristics below should be suspected as *Y. pestis,* including bipolar (closed safety pin appearance) staining rod on Wright, Wayson, or Giemsa stain on direct smear (not typically seen on Gram stain), pinpoint colonies at 24 hours on sheep blood agar (SBA). *Y. pestis* is a nonlactose fermenter that may not be visible on MAC (MacConkey agar) or EMB at 24 hours. It is also oxidase and urease negative, catalase positive. Growth occurs better at 28°C (Tables 40-1 and 40-2). A characteristic "safety pin" appearance of *Y. pestis,* the causative agent of the plague, can be seen on Wayson stain in Fig. 40-5.

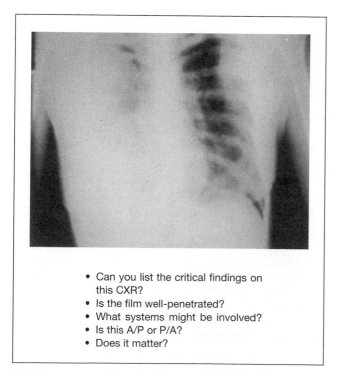

- Can you list the critical findings on this CXR?
- Is the film well-penetrated?
- What systems might be involved?
- Is this A/P or P/A?
- Does it matter?

FIGURE 40-4

CHEST X-RAY (CXR)—PNEUMONIC PLAGUE (Y. PESTIS)
Source: McGovern TW, Friedlander AM. Plague. In: Zajtchuk R, Bellamy R, eds. Cextbook of Military Medicine: Medical Aspects of Chemical and Biological Warfare. Washington, DC: Office of the Surgeon General, Borden Institute, Walter Reed Army Medical Center; 1997.

TABLE 40-1

CDC GUIDELINES LEVEL A LAB PROCEDURES FOR IDENTIFICATION OF YERSINIA PESTIS

Any isolate from the respiratory tract, blood, or lymph node containing the major characteristics below should be suspected as *Y. pestis* if

- Bipolar staining rod on Wright or Giemsa stain on direct smear
- Pinpoint colonies at 24 hours on sheep blood agar (SBA)
- Nonlactose fermenter, may not be visible on MAC or EMB at 24 hours
- Oxidase and urease negative
- Catalase positive
- Growth better at 28°C

Limitation

1. *Y. pestis* will grow on nutrient agar but is slow-growing and more rapidly growing organisms may mask its presence
2. Bipolar staining is not a unique characteristic to *Y. pestis*
3. Some automated systems do not identify *Y. pestis* adequately, resulting in false identification

(www.cdc.gov)

LABORATORY IDENTIFICATION OF PLAGUE (YERSINIA PESTIS)

Essential specimen selection

- Bubonic

    Bubo—lymph node aspirate

- Septicemic

    Blood—organisms may be intermittent. Take three samples 10–30 minutes apart

- Pneumonic

    - *Sputum*
    - *Throat swab*
    - *Bronchial washings*

Testing procedures

- Gram stain

    Small, gram-negative bipolar coccobacilli

- Wayson, Wright, or Giemsa stain

    Pink-blue cells with closed safety pin look

- Growth in Brain Heart

    Infusion Broth *Stalactites on side and bottom of tube—suspended clumps*

- MacConkey agar or sheep broth agar (SBA)
- Optimal growth at 28°C
- NB colonies are much smaller than other Enterobacteriaceae and can be overlooked. Alert the lab you are considering *Y. pestis.*

    24 hours—Tiny, almost invisible, shiny gray translucent

    48 hours—1–2 mm irregular colonies—Fried egg appearance

- Biochemical

    Lactose nonfermenter

    Oxidase negative

    Catalase positive

    Urease negative

    Indol negative

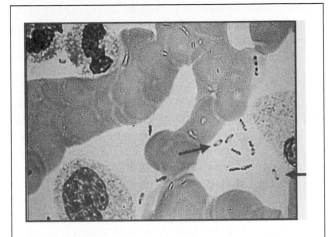

FIGURE 40-5

Note characteristic "safety pin" appearance (see arrows) of *Yersinia pestis*, the causative agent of the plague as seen on this Wayson stain of blood.
Source: McGovern TW, Friedlander AM. Plague. In: Zajtchuk R, Bellamy R, eds. Textbook of Military Medicine: Medical Aspects of Chemical and Biological Warfare. Washington, DC: Office of the Surgeon General, Borden Institute, Walter Reed Army Medical Center; 1997.

Misinterpretation of the bipolar appearance as a gram-positive diplococcus can occur; the acute laboratorian should be aware of potential "look-alikes" or confounding by temperature, transportation, or media used.

The heat-stable F1 capsule antigen is secreted by *Y. pestis* at 37°C universally and found at high concentration in human samples. ELISA (enzyme-linked immunosorbent assay) and dipstick (immunochromatographic) tests to detect F1 antigen are highly sensitive and specific. The F1 antigen monoclonal antibody dipstick assay is a rapid and valuable test especially given reliable results may be obtained in 15 minutes. Since 1999, the World Health Organization (WHO) considers the detection of the F1 antigen in appropriate samples, in addition to symptoms and history consistent with *Y. pestis* to be a presumptive criterion for diagnosing plague. According to the National Plague Control Programme of Madagascar, a nation that continues to have significant *Y. pestis* infections, a patient with suspected plague by symptoms and history would be considered a confirmed case if F1 antigen is detected.

In addition to the laboratory tests recommended, a CXR should be obtained. Laboratory testing may reveal a leukocytosis: total white blood cell (WBC) count of 20,000 with more than 80% PMN. Fibrin split products may indicate DIC. Increased liver enzymes and BUN/creatinine accompany multiple organ involvement. Definitive diagnosis is based upon culturing the organism from aspirates, cerebral spinal fluid, blood, or sputum (Table 40-2). The gold standard technique for diagnosis remains a positive culture.

MEDICAL MANAGEMENT

Plague in bioterrorism would differ epidemiologically from natural plague as the former would most likely result from an aerosol release, causing numerous patients with severe and rapidly progressive respiratory distress. The magnitude of the outbreak would be predicated upon the amount and location of the biological release. The occurrence of plague in nonendemic areas, affecting individuals with little preexisting risk for *Y. pestis* exposure and the absence of infected animals would also be important clues. Effective communication among health-care facilities and professionals, sharing information about unusual pulmonary cases, especially increased and nonseasonal, is critical to managing a potential intentional outbreak.

Antimicrobial therapy as well as appropriate symptomatic and supportive care must be initiated rapidly, and based upon a presumptive diagnosis.

Aspirating the bubo is both therapeutic and assists in diagnosis by providing the organism. As the bubo is exquisitely painful, removing the fluid will relieve much of the discomfort. Although incision and draining pose a risk to health-care workers and should be avoided, needle aspiration is a safe intervention when using universal precautions.

Patients should remain isolated for the first 48 hours of antibiotic therapy and until clinical improvement occurs. In the event of large outbreaks, patients can be cohorted in isolation while undergoing antibiotic treatment. Patients should wear appropriate masks if they are transported. Aerosol generation procedures should be postponed wherever possible.

Chemotherapy

Use symptomatic and supportive care to address hypotension, DIC, and other systemic effects. Streptomycin, was approved by the Food and Drug Administration (FDA) for the treatment of *Y. pestis*. Streptomycin 30 mg/kg/day intramuscular twice a day for 10–14 days. Unfortunately supplies of streptomycin are limited. Nevertheless, streptomycin can be obtained by calling X-Gen Pharmaceuticals in 300 Danial Venker R. Horseheader's NY 148451.866.390.4416 M-F after business hours contact The CDC 24 hour emergency operations center at 1.770.488.7100. Experts suggest other aminoglycosides, such as gentamicin may be suitable alternatives. Gentamicin is a readily available antimicrobial; it is suitable for adults, children, and women, who are pregnant given the risk of plague illness. A limitation of aminoglycosides in the mass casualty setting is the need to administer parenterally. Tetracyclines, specifically doxycycline, can be administered orally. Doxycycline and chloramphenicol are effective. Animal data suggest fluoroquinolones such as ciprofloxacin and ofloxacin may be effective in human treatment. Doxycycline 200 mg IV loading dose followed by 100 mg q 12 hours IV for 10–14 days is a suitable alternative. Ciprofloxacin can be given 400 mg IV BID for 10–14 days. For the treatment of plague meningitis, select an antimicrobial with good blood-brain barrier penetration as well as effective against *Y. pestis*, such as chloramphenicol given as 25 mg/kg IV loading dose followed by 15 mg/kg QID for 10–14 days. (See Table 40-3.)

Special populations should be considered as potential victims. This includes the elderly, who may have underlying health problems or take medications that may confound the clinical picture. In addition, special concerns about adverse reactions from antimicrobials must be taken into account and the decision made based upon the risk-benefit of the situation. Countermeasures for immunosuppressed patients parallel treatment options for nonimmunosuppressed adults. First-line antibiotics for women who are pregnant (consider risk: benefit) include (severe clinical case) gentamicin or doxycycline.

TABLE 40-3

ANTIMICROBIAL TREATMENT OPTIONS

- **Aminoglycosides**
  - **Streptomycin** (avoid for pregnant women)
    - Adults = 1 g intramuscularly (IM) q 12 h
    - Children = 15 mg/kg/dose up to 1 gm maximum dose q 12 h for children
  - **Gentamicin** (preferred for pregnant women)
    - Adults = 5 mg/kg IM or IV q day [or 2 mg/kg load then 1.7 mg/kg q 8 h]
    - Children = 2.5 mg/kg q 8 h
- **Tetracyclines**
  - **Doxycycline**
    - Adults, including pregnant women = 100 mg IV q 12 h
    - Children = 2.2 mg/kg/dose q 12 h up to maximum dose of 200 mg/d for children
- **Fluoroquinolones**
  - **Ciprofloxacin**
    - Adults including pregnant women = 400 mg IV q 12 h
    - Children = 15 mg/kg/dose every 12 h
- *Other fluoroquinolones probably effective
- **Chloramphenicol**
  - Adults and children = 25 mg/kg IV q 6 h

First-line antibiotics for children include streptomycin or gentamicin. Safe alternatives based upon age include chloramphenicol for children aged 2 years or older, and if the child is 8 years of age or older tetracyclines, specifically doxycycline.

Natural resistance to antibiotics has been rare. However in 1995 an isolate from plague in Madagascar demonstrated multidrug-resistant transferable plasmid, which demonstrated resistance capability to streptomycin, chloramphenicol, and *B* lactamase. *Y. pestis* as well as *Escherichia coli* as members of the Enterobacteriaceae family should be able to exchange genetic material including plasmids (1) reports that the FSU engineered multidrug resistant and fluoroquinolone-resistant strains of *Y. pestis* (2) thus it is critical to obtain from the laboratory antimicrobial sensitivities as well as regularly review revised clinical guidelines for the management of plague—natural and potential biological weapons.

Postexposure prophylaxis

Regarding postexposure prophylaxis (PEP), antibiotics should be administered for at least 7 days postexposure with a face-to-face contact of a pneumonic plague patient or aerosolized form of plague. Doxycycline 100 mg PO BID or Ciprofloxacin 500 mg PO BID are appropriate. Tetracycline 500 mg PO QID or chloramphenicol 25 mg/kg PO QID are alternatives. Newer antimicrobial medications continue to be under development. It is important for the clinician to frequently review updates on the medical management of emerging threats as well as to select the most appropriate countermeasures taking into account the impact of antimicrobials as well as the virulence of the pathogen and overall pathophysiological effects, which include the impact of the medications as well as bacteria on immune and organ function.

Vaccine

A formalin-killed whole-cell vaccine was available to the U.S. military and research personnel until 1999, when it was discontinued owing to studies, which revealed it was only protective for bubonic plague. Vaccine prototypes are under investigation, including genetic based. Research is ongoing to develop effective plague vaccines in the United States, United Kingdom, and Israel, especially to protect against primary pneumonic plague with emphasis on developing immunity to the F1 capsular protein and the V antigen. However none are currently available.

Personal Protection, Decontamination

Suspected cases of pneumonic plague require respiratory droplet precautions and should be placed in strict isolation, preferably negative pressure rooms for a minimum of 48 hours of antimicrobial therapy, or for confirmed cases when sputum cultures are negative. Gowns, gloves, and eye protection, as well as N95 or greater mask should be utilized. Negative pressure rooms should be available. Vector tracing and control is required. Soap and water is adequate for decontamination, while a 1:10 mixture of bleach to water is sufficient for surfaces.

AUTOPSY

Handling the dead after a bioweapon event requires advanced planning. An autopsy can subject laboratorians, prosectors and pathologists to blood borne and aerosolized pathogens. While the risk of infectious disease transmission has long been recognized with autopsy, this is especially true of highly pathogenic agents such as Yersinia pestis. In the event of a plague outbreak it is likely it will be considered a public health and security emergency. Law enforcement and federal agents, professionals typically unaccustomed to biosafety and PPE will become involved in all aspects of the event, especially given concerns over evidence, of which the body is, and chain of custody. Adequate resources–PPE, cold storage, transportation and other personnel and materials should be addressed along with preparedness planning that involves experts in handling mass casualties such as DMORT and other agencies.

CONCLUSION

Historically plague has been a deadly pathogen, causing some of the most lethal outbreaks, including the infamous "Black Death." While it remains endemic in several countries worldwide, the annual number of plague deaths remains at about 2000, significantly less than the millions which occurred during the Middle Ages. Of concern, the WHO has designated plague as a reemerging infectious disease. Plague remains a rodent-spread disease and therein lies the challenge in eradicating it as an endemic pathogen. It can survive in animal carcasses for several years. Bioterrorism remains a high consequence threat since numerous nations have studied plague as a potential biological weapon and terrorist groups have expressed interest in this deadly pathogen. Early recognition of a terrorism attack with biological agents, including plague, will rely upon physician diagnosis. Plague, a naturally occurring infection, is a worldwide pathogen and remains a likely bioweapon agent that has already been utilized to cause intentional harm. The health-care community as well as the public at large should remain vigilant against emerging pathogens in general as well as the symptoms associated with the threat of potential biological weapons. While it could be argued that such pathogens can be engineered to be multidrug resistant, nevertheless, it is important to have adequate supplies of numerous antimicrobials. Just as emerging data suggest an antibiotic cocktail may be more effective in the management of anthrax, the same may become true for the management of Y. pestis. Clearly preparedness planning must include such an exigency. Most importantly all critical response stakeholders including the community need to be engaged and interactive if a coordinated and effective response is to occur. The best benefit of all when preparing for biological weapons is the enhanced preparedness of the health-care community in identifying emerging pathogens and providing more rapid care of potentially aggressive pathogens. Optimizing and coordinating the capabilities of public health and community medicine is critical to preparing for plague or other emerging pathogens.

Suggested Reading

American Hospital Formulary Service. *AHFS Drug Information.* Bethesda, MD: American Society of Health System Pharmacists, 2000.

Bockemuhl J, Wong JD. Yersinia. In: Murray PR, ed. *Manual of Clinical Microbiology.* Washington, DC: American Society for Microbiology, 2003: pp. 672–683.

Boyce JM, Butler T. Yersinia species (including plague). In: Mandell GL, Bennett JE, eds. *Principles and Practices of Infectious Diseases.* 4th Ed. New York, NY: Churchill Livingston, 1995: pp. 2070–2078.

Byrne WR, Welkos SL, Pitt ML, et al. Antibiotic treatment of experimental pneumonic plague in mice. *Antimicrob Agents Chemother.* 1998;42:675–681.

Carroll K, Held M, Stombler RE, et al. Laboratory preparedness for bioterrorism: from the phlebotomist to the pathologist. *Lab Med.* 2003;3(34):169–180.

Carus WS. *Bioterrorism and Biocrimes: The Illicit Use of Biological Agents in the 20th Century.* Washington, DC: Center for Counterproliferation Research, National Defense University, 1998.

CDC Plague homepage. *http://www.cdc.gov/ncidod/dvbid/plague/index.htm*

Centers for Disease Control and Prevention. *www.cdc.gov*

Chanteau S, Rahalison I, Ratsitorahina M. Rapid and early diagnosis of bubonic plague using F1 antigen capture ELISA assay and repaid immunogold dipstick. *Int J Med Microbiol.* 2000;290:279–283.

Chanteau S, Ratsitorahina M, Rahalison I, et al. Current epidemiology of human plague in Madagascar. *Microbes and Infection.* 2000;2:25–31.

Cornelis GR. Molecular and cell biology aspects of plague. *Proc Natl Acad Sci USA.* 2000;97:8778–8783.

Cosgrove SE, Perl TM, Song K, et al. Ability of physicians to diagnose and manage illness due to category A bioterrorism agents. *Arch Intern Med.* 2005;Vol 165 Sep:2002–2006.

Dennis D, Chu M. A major new test for plague. *Lancet.* 2003;353:361:191–192.

Duplantier JM, Duchemin JB, Chanteau S, et al. From the recent lessons of the Malagasy foci towards a global understanding of the factors involved in plague reemergence. *Vet Rese.* 2005;6:437–453.

Eitzen EM Jr, Takafuji ET. Historical overview of biological warfare. In: Sidell FR, Takafuji ET, Franz DR, eds. *Medical Aspects of Chemical and Biological Warfare.* Washington, DC: Office of the Surgeon General, Borden Institute, Walter Reed Army Medical Center, 1997: pp. 415–423.

Galimand M, Guiyoule A, Gerbaud G, et al. Multidrug resistance in Yersinia pestis mediated by a transferable plasmid. *N Engl J Med.* 1997;337:677–680.

Human Plague–Four States, 2006–MMWR Dispatch 8/25/06. Last accessed September 28, 2006. *http://www.cdc.gov/mmwr*

Inglesby TV, Dennis DT, Henderson DA, et al. Working Group on Civilian Biodefense. Plague as a biological weapon: medical and public health management. *JAMA.* 2000;283(17): 2281–2290.

Josko D. Yersinia pestis: still a plague in the 21st century. *Clinical Laboratory Science.* 2004;Vol 17(1):1–5.

Koirala J. Plague: Disease, management and recognition of act of terrorism. *Infect Dis Clin North Am.* 2006 Jun; 20(2): 273–87, viii.

Laboratory response network level a laboratory procedures for identification of Y. pestis. *http://www.bt.cdc.gov/agent/plague/ype_la_cp_121301.pdf*

Lutwick LI, Nierengarten MB. Vaccines for category A bioterrorism diseases *Expert opin Biol Ther* 2002 Dec; 2(8): 883–93.

McGovern TW, Friedlander AM. Plague. In: Zajtchuk R, Bellamy R, eds. *Textbook of Military Medicine: Medical Aspects of Chemical and Biological Warfare.* Washington, DC: Office of the Surgeon General, Borden Institute, Walter Reed Army Medical Center, 1997.

Migliani R, Changeau S, Rahalison L, et al. Epidemiological trends for human plague in Madagascar during the second half of the 20th century: a survey of 20,900 notified cases. *Trop Med and Intl Health.* 2006;Vol 11(8):1228–1237.

Nierengarten MB, Lutwick LI. Vaccine development for plague. *Medscape Infectious Diseases.* 2002;4(2). http://www.meoscope.com/ 441260 last accesses 6/4/07.

Norkina OV, Kulichenko AN, Gintsburg Al, et al. Development of a diagnostic test for Yersinia pestis by the polymerase chain reaction. *J Appl Bacteriol.* 1994;76(3):240–245.

Nolte KB, Taylor DG, Richmond JY. Biosafety considerations for autopsy. *Am J Forens Med and Path* 2002;23(2):107–122.

Perry RD, Fetherston JD. Yersinia pestis–etiologic agent of plague. *Clin Microbiol Rev.* 1997;10:35–36.

Plague. In: *WHO Report on Global Surveillance of Epidemic Prone Infectious Disease,* 2000. *http://www.wo.int/emc-documents/surveillances/docs/whocdcsrisr2001.html/plague/plague.html#history*

Prentice MB, Rahalison L. Plague. *Lancet.* 2007 ARR 7: 369(9568): 1196–1207.

Reidel S. Biological warfare and bioterrorism: a historical review. *BUMC Proceedings.* 2004;17:400–406.

Riedel S. Plague: From natural disease to bioterrorism. *BUMC Proceedings.* 2005;18:116–124.

Shih CL, Shih FY. Plague in bioterrorism. *Ann Disaster Med.* 2002;Vol 1 Suppl 1: 526–535.

Smith MD, Vinh DX, Nguyen TT, et al. In vitro antimicrobial susceptibilities of strains of Yersinia pestis. *Antimicrob Agents Chemother.* 1995;39:2153–2154.

Stephenson J. Plague rapid diagnostic test. *JAMA.* 2003; 289(6):691.

Williamson ED. Plague vaccine research and development. *J Appl Microbiol.* 2001;91:606–608.

World Health Organization (WHO) 1999 Plague Manual: epidemiology distribution, surveillance and control (WHO/CDS/CSR/EDC/99.2), 9–4.

41

BOTULISM

Britney B. Anderson, Mark B. Mycyk, and Robin B. McFee

INTRODUCTION

Botulinum toxin is the most lethal biological substance known. Botulinum toxin has a known median lethal dose (LD_{50}) of 1 ng/kg of toxin body mass, thus doses as small as 0.05–0.1 μg can cause death in humans. Even though botulinum toxin has been feared for its deadly effect on humans, this toxin (among other neurotoxins) has recently been identified as a useful treatment modality for many medical conditions in fields such as ophthalmology, neurology, and dermatology. Botulinum toxin has become so popular now that it is universally recognized by the general public as a cosmetic enhancement tool better known as Botox in North America or Dysport in the United Kingdom.

The development and use of botulinum toxin as a bioweapon began about six decades ago. In the 1930s in Manchuria, the head of the Japanese biological warfare group (Unit 731) fed cultures of *Clostridium botulinum* to prisoners resulting in fatalities. The United States bioweapon program first produced botulinum toxin during World War II. The toxin was also investigated as a biologic agent by the British, Canadian, Japanese, and Soviet military. Some terrorist groups have been successful in obtaining the toxin. During World War II, Paul Fildes, a high-ranking British specialist in bacterial weapons, alluded to the fact that by utilizing the toxin, he contributed to assassination of Reinhard Heydrick, the head of the Gestapo. After concerns that the Germans had weaponized botulinum toxin, doses of botulinum toxoid vaccine were made for Allied troops fighting Germany.

Botulinum toxin was one of several agents tested on Vozrozhdeniye Island by Soviets at their Aralsk-7 site. In the early 1990s, before the Sarin gas attack on the Tokyo subway system, the Japanese cult Aum Shinrikyo had released a *C. botulinum* preparation in Japan targeted at a U.S. military installation, but the toxin was ineffectively produced. After the 1991 Persian Gulf War, Iraq told the United Nations inspection team that they had produced 19,000 L of botulinum toxin, and 10,000 L of this was loaded into military weapons. This was three times the amount needed to kill the entire human population by inhalation. Iraq has chosen to weaponize more botulinum toxin than any other of its known biological agents.

PATHOPHYSIOLOGY

C. botulinum is a heterogeneous group of anaerobic, gram-positive, rod-shaped organisms that forms subterminal spores, which elaborate the most potent bacterial toxin known. In addition to *C. botulinum*, *Clostridium baratii* and *Clostridium butyricum* also have the capacity to produce botulinum toxin.

There are eight known serotypes of botulism designated A–G (A, B, C1, C2, D, E, F, and G). Almost all human cases of botulism have been caused by serotypes A, B, and E. There are six forms of botulism that have been reported:

food-borne, wound, infant-intestinal, adult-intestinal, inadvertent injection-related, and inhalational botulism.

Upon entering the body, botulinum toxin finds its way to systemic circulation and is transported to sites of acetylcholine-mediated neurotransmission such as neuromuscular junctions, postganglionic parasympathetic nerve endings, and peripheral ganglia (Fig. 41-1). The active neurotoxin is a

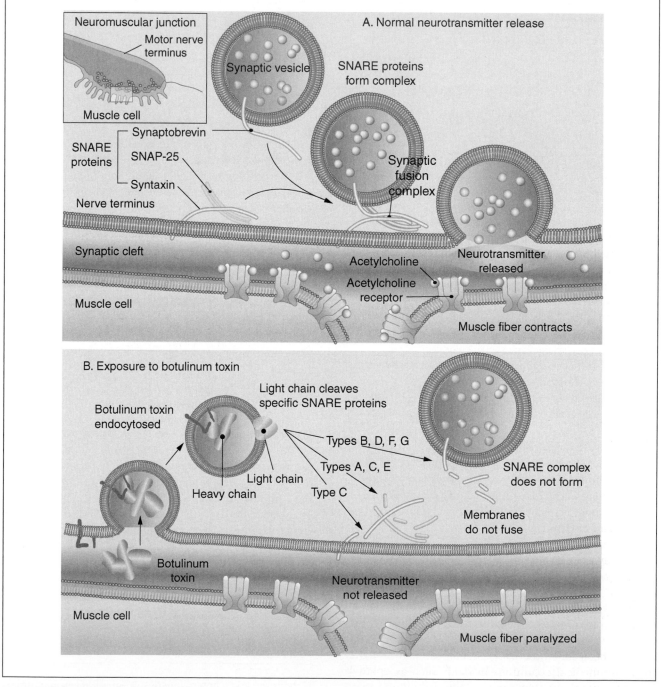

FIGURE 41-1

MOLECULAR BASIS OF BOTULINUM TOXICITY

Source: With permission from St. Louis ME, Peck SH, Bowering P. etal. Botulism from chopped garlic; delayed recognition of a major outbreak. Ann Int Med 1988;108:363–368.

large 150 kDa molecular mass, which is incapable of crossing the blood-brain barrier, therefore, the central nervous system is not involved. The toxin consists of a heavy chain (100 kDa fragment responsible for neurospecific binding and translocation in the nerve cell) and a light chain (50 kDa fragment responsible for intracellular catalytic activity). The toxin binds to the neuronal cell membrane on the nerve, and is taken up by endocytosis into the presynaptic nerve ending. Once inside the neuron, after reduction of a single disulfide bond, the light chain is cleaved free and acts as a zinc-dependent protease, which can attack SNARE proteins (soluble *N*-ethylmaleimide sensitive fusion protein attachment receptor). It is the SNARE protein complex, which is the key process that allows vesicles in the nerve terminus, which contain acetylcholine, to fuse with the neural cell wall and be released into the synaptic cleft. By preventing the release of acetylcholine, muscular contraction cannot occur and flaccid paralysis results. This process renders this neural tissue nonfunctional and recovery occurs only as new neural tissue end plates are regenerated.

FORMS OF BOTULISM ILLNESS

Food-Borne Botulism

In the United States, food-borne botulism results from the ingestion of preformed toxin (types A and B being most common). It usually occurs from exposure to home-canned foods, most commonly vegetables, fruits, and condiments that are improperly preserved or undercooked. Type E outbreaks are frequently associated with fish products. Most cases are initially misdiagnosed, because the early gastrointestinal (GI) symptom complex of nausea, vomiting, and diarrhea is similar to that of other food-borne illnesses.

Infant Botulism

Infant botulism (sometimes referred to as infant-intestinal) is the most commonly reported form of the illness. Most cases occur from 1 week to 1 year of age and are caused by ingestion of spores. The immature GI tract of infants allows the spores to germinate leading to in vivo production of toxin. Honey ingestion, and to a lesser extent, corn syrup and environmental exposures such as living in a rural area, or having a parent who works with soil, have been identified as important risk factors for infant botulism.

Wound Botulism

Wound botulism occurs when a wound is contaminated with spores, which then germinate and produce toxin. Wound botulism has been documented after traumatic injury involving contamination with soil, and after cesarean delivery. Wound botulism from type A and B toxins have also recently become a frequent complication in injection drug users, particularly in those injecting black tar heroin. In 1997, California reported 99 wound botulism cases seen in IV drug users.

Adult-Intestinal Botulism

Adult-intestinal botulism (also classified as undefined or adult-type infant botulism) is a delayed-onset neurologic syndrome. It mainly occurs in adults with abnormal GI pathology in GI disease such as Crohn's disease, peptic ulcer disease, or GI surgery such as Billroth surgery.

Inadvertent Botulism

Inadvertent (injection-related) botulism is an iatrogenic form associated with patients who have been treated with injections of pharmaceutical botulinum toxin. In Florida, a few individuals were the result of unlicensed persons running a cosmetic clinic. They did not use medical grade, appropriately prepared botulinum toxin. Because of the increased prevalence of botulinum use in the medical and cosmetic settings, it is likely that other iatrogenic cases will occur.

Inhalational Botulism

Inhalational botulism can occur through the deliberate release of the botulinum toxin as a biologic weapon.

CONFIRMING THE THREAT AND WHAT TO EXPECT

The early recognition of a botulism outbreak is based upon rapid diagnosis, and is essential to mobilizing vital resources and obtaining appropriate treatment in bioterrorist attacks. The history and motor examination are sufficient to make a presumptive diagnosis and will justify the release of botulism antitoxin from the CDC. There are confirmatory laboratory tests for botulism, but the treatment must be started before the tests are resulted, as they can take 1–2 days for preliminary results. Any case of botulism should raise red flags about the possibility of bioterrorism. A consensus statement published by the *Journal of the American Medical Society* in 2001 listed specific features of an outbreak that would suggest the deliberate release of botulinum toxin. These included (1) the outbreak of a large number of cases of acute flaccid paralysis with prominent bulbar palsies, (2) an outbreak of an unusual botulinum toxin type (i.e., type C, D, F, or G, or type E toxin not acquired from an aquatic food), (3) an outbreak with a common geographic factor among cases but without a common dietary exposure, and (4) multiple simultaneous outbreaks with no common source.

Bioterrorism

Aerosol Dissemination

Aerosol dissemination and food-borne botulism would be the most likely forms of botulism seen in a bioterrorist attack. Cases of botulism acquired by aerosol dissemination would not be difficult to recognize because a large number of the cases would share a common geographical and temporal exposure. Given the ease of travel and mobility in this day and age, a careful history about recent travel, locations, as well as activities and occupation would be important. Not much is known about the rapidity of onset of aerosolized botulism, because so few cases have been reported. Some studies on primates showed the onset of signs and symptoms of inhaled botulism from 12 to 80 hours after the exposure depending on the dose. The only human cases of inhaled botulism known were in laboratory workers handling a deceased animal that had died of botulism. The onset of symptoms in this case was approximately 72 hours after exposure to an unknown amount of reaerosolized toxin. If a deliberate dispersal of botulinum toxin were to occur, there would likely be an upper airway prodrome such as a cold (without a fever) followed by a variable onset of differing degrees of paralysis in the exposed.

Food-Borne Botulism

Food-borne botulism outbreaks would be slightly more difficult in that there would be a need to discern between naturally occurring food-borne disease, and deliberate food-borne disease unless numerous patients with similar symptoms presented. The onset of symptoms of food-borne botulism typically present within 10 to 72 hour range after the meal. The severity of the disease, and rapidity of its onset depend on the amount of toxin ingested. Botulinum toxin is colorless, tasteless, and odorless, and is readily inactivated by heat. Therefore, food-borne botulism is always transmitted by foods that are not heated (or improperly heated) before eating. On the other hand, spores can be dormant, resistant to heat, and germinate in low-acidity, low-salinity environments. Commonly implicated foods include canned vegetables, particularly beans, corn, peppers, and other low acidic vegetables. Items preserved in garlic oil and soups have often been implicated as well. Restaurant outbreaks in the past have been from salads and dips, condiments such as garlic in oil, sautéed onions, and other commercial foods like yogurt. Food is a convenient, ubiquitous, and relatively unnoticed vehicle in which to hide the lethal botulism agent.

Water-Borne Botulism

There have been no reports of cases of water-borne botulism in the past, and water-borne botulism is speculated to be an unlikely scenario. The standard treatment of potable water using chemicals like chlorine and aeration are thought to inactivate the toxin. However, untreated beverages may ensure stability of botulism for days, and should be suspected as a source of contamination if no other source can be identified.

PERSONAL PROTECTIVE EQUIPMENT/DECONTAMINATION

There are no specific guidelines for detoxification of patients exposed to botulism except that clothing and skin should be washed with soap and water. Botulism degrades easily and decays at 1% per minute, therefore substantial inactivation of toxin occurs by 2 days after the aerosolization. All contaminated surfaces should be cleaned with bleach solution if they cannot be avoided for the hours to days required for natural degradation. Victims of botulinum toxin are not contagious, and upon admission to the hospital patients do not need to be placed in any type of isolation environment.

Although symptomatic patients will likely arrive long after their initial exposure to botulinum toxin, activated charcoal should be considered for decontamination of any food-borne or intestinal exposure. Activated charcoal has been shown to adsorb botulinum toxin A in vitro. Wound debridement should be considered for patients with wound exposure.

CLINICAL MANIFESTATIONS

Despite different routes of infection, all adult forms of botulism present similarly. Onset of symptoms after exposure is variable, but with food-borne botulism symptoms usually occur within 1 to 5 days after ingestion of the contaminated food but may be longer after inhalation exposure depending upon the dose and type of toxin. Botulism can be recognized by its classic triad (1) symmetric, descending flaccid paralysis with prominent bulbar palsies in (2) an afebrile patient with (3) a clear sensorium.

The paralysis seen in botulism is an acute, symmetric, descending flaccid paralysis that begins in the bulbar musculature. Usually the bulbar palsies present first as paralysis of the motor functions of the cranial nerves. Initially botulism affects the oculomotor muscles, progressing to facial muscle paralysis and to the muscles of mastication, and swallowing. Prominent neurologic findings in all forms of botulism include ptosis, dry mouth, and the "4Ds": diplopia, dysarthria, dysphonia, and dysphagia. Unlike nerve agent exposure, which usually results in miosis, botulinum can cause mydriasis in approximately 50% of cases. The mucous membranes of the mouth, tongue, and pharynx often appear erythematous and dry due to peripheral parasympathetic cholinergic blockade. The gag reflex is often depressed or absent. As paralysis extends beyond the bulbar musculature, patients experience symmetric descending muscular weakness. Neck muscles, respiratory muscles, and those in the upper and lower extremities are affected. Upper extremities are usually more affected than lower extremities, and proximal muscles weaker than distal. The abdomen may appear distended with hypoactive or absent bowel sounds; ileus may develop. Bladder distension may indicate urinary retention. Eventually the muscles of respiration, including accessory muscles and the diaphragm, are affected. Respirations may become rapid and shallow. Once paralysis progresses to respiratory failure, the patient will need ventilator-assisted support until the motor end plate recovers, often for several months.

A hallmark of the disease is the absence of sensory symptoms and the absence of fever. Sensory examination is normal throughout the disease. The only sensory changes observed are infrequent circumoral and peripheral paresthesias from hyperventilation.

Differential Diagnosis

There is a vast list of metabolic and neurologic causes of motor neuropathies, and the differential diagnosis of botulism includes a wide variety of illnesses (Table 41-1). Two diagnoses in particular seem to be difficult in differentiating from botulism. Myasthenia gravis (MG) often presents with ptosis and is a disease involving bulbar palsies without sensory findings. Due to the subjectivity of the edrophonium test, it is often determined positive in cases thought to be MG, but which turn out to be botulism. However MG is also associated with recurrent paralysis, has different electromyographic (EMG) findings, and has a sustained response to anticholinesterase therapy unlike botulism.

Another clinical mimic of botulism is the Miller-Fisher variant of the Guillain-Barre syndrome (GB). This disease also has been known to present with diplopia, ophthalmoplegia, ptosis, facial and extremity weakness. However this condition is usually associated with a history of antecedent infection, *ascending paralysis,* paresthesias, and early areflexia. On cerebrospinal fluid (CSF) examination, an increase in protein content of the fluid exists, which is characteristic of GB.

Other toxins must also be considered as possibilities. Anticholinergics (atropine, jimson weed, belladonna) cause papillary dilation and erythematous, dry mucous membranes. Aminoglycosides have been known to cause

T A B L E   4 1 - 1

SELECTED MIMICS AND MISDIAGNOSES OF BOTULISM

Conditions	Features That Distinguish Condition from Botulism
Common Misdiagnoses	
Guillain-Barre syndrome[†] and its variants, especially Miller-Fisher syndrome	History of antecedent infection; paresthesias, often ascending paralysis; early aretlexia; eventual CSF protein increase; EMG findings
Myasthenia gravist[†]	Recurrent paralysis; EMG findings; sustained response to anticholinesterase
Stroke[†]	Paralysis often asymmetnc; abnormal CNS image
Intoxication with depressants (e.g., acute ethanol intoxication), organophosphates, carbon monoxide or nerve gas	History of exposure; excessive drug levels detected in body fluids
Lambert-Eaton syndrome	Increased strength with sustained contraction; evidence of lung carcinoma; EMG findings similar to botulism
Tick paralysis	Paresthesias; ascending paralysis; tick attached to skin
Other Misdiagnoses	
Poliomyelitis	Antecedent febrile illness; asymmetric paralysis. CSF pleocytosis
CNS infections, especially of the brainstem	Mental status changes; CSF and EEG abnormalities
CNS tumor	Paralysis often asymmetric; abnormal CNS image
Streptococcal pharyngitis (pharyngeal erythema can occur in botulism)	Absence of bulbar palsies; positive rapid antigen test result or throat
Psychiatric illness[†]	Normal EMG in conversion paralysis
Viral syndrome[†]	Absence of bulbar palsies and flaccid paralysis
Inflammatory myopathy[†]	Elevated creatine kinase levels
Diabetic complications[†]	Sensory neuropathy; few cranial nerve palsies
Hyperemesis gravidarum[†]	Absence of bulbar palsies and acute flaccid paralysis
Hypothyroidism[†]	Abnormal thyroid function test results
Laryngeal trauma[†]	Absence of flaccid paralysis; dysphonia without bulbar palsies
Overexertion[†]	Absence of bulbar palsies and acute flaccid paralysis

CSF indicates cerebrospinal fluid; EMG, electromyogram; CNS, central nervous system; and EEG, electroencephalogram.

[†]Misdiagnoses made in a large outbreak of botulism. (*Source: St. Louis ME, Peck SH, Bowering D, et al. Botulism from chopped garlic: delayed recognition of a major outbreak. Ann Intern Med 1988;108:363–368.*)

neuromuscular blockade. Curare toxin, which contains alkaloids that affect neuromuscular transmission, can cause paralysis without change in mental status. Tick paralysis and hypokalemic periodic paralysis can also cause symmetric myopathies, but tend to have less of an affect on the cranial nerves, and predominantly affect proximal large muscles.

LABORATORY STUDIES

Laboratory testing is confirmatory. Presumptive diagnosis is based upon clinical presentation. The diagnostic laboratory tests for botulism are only available at the CDC (the CDC Director's Emergency Operation Center at (770) 488-7100) and some state and municipal public health laboratories. Samples must be collected and sent to one of these specific locations. Samples include serum, stool, gastric aspirate, and suspect foods. The standard laboratory diagnostic test is the mouse bioassay. Mice which have been pretreated with type-specific antitoxin are subjected to the sample and the toxins therein. The bioassay can detect as little as 0.03 ng of botulinum toxin. Fecal and gastric specimens can also be cultured anaerobically and results of these cultures usually take 7–10 days to become available. Although serum samples must be obtained before therapy with antitoxin, because the antitoxin can negatively affect the mouse bioassay, this is not a reason to delay treatment. Sterile water should be used for enemas to obtain stool samples, as other solutions can confound the mouse bioassay.

Adjunct Studies

Botulism has characteristic findings on EMG studies. An EMG with repetitive nerve stimulation at 20–50 Hz can show normal nerve conduction velocity, normal sensory nerve function, and a pattern of short, small amplitude motor potentials. The most distinctive pattern is an incremental response to repetitive stimulation often seen only at 50 Hz.

Additionally other studies can be utilized to help rule out other diseases on the differential. Cerebral spinal fluid is unchanged in botulism but is abnormal in many central nervous system (CNS) diseases. Other intracranial or spinal pathology such as hemorrhage or neoplasm can be ruled out with neuroimaging techniques such as computed tomography (CT) scans and magnetic resonance imaging (MRI). Simple laboratory tests can rapidly rule out metabolic causes such as hypoglycemia, hypothyroidism, and hypokalemia.

EARLY INTERVENTIONS

Supportive Care

The morbidity of the disease can be severe and usually results from respiratory paralysis. Therefore, treatment should begin as early as possible once botulism is suspected based on history and physical examination. The respiratory status must be closely monitored. Adequacy of gag and cough reflexes should be routinely assessed and close control of oral secretions is beneficial. Monitoring parameters such as oxygen saturation, vital capacity, and negative inspiratory force (NIF) are helpful. Reverse trendelenburg at 20° to 25° with cervical support may improve ventilation by reducing oral secretions, which can pass into the airway, and suspending some of the weight of the abdominal viscera from the diaphragm. Controlled, early anticipatory intubation is indicated when respiratory function deteriorates. The proportion of patients who require mechanical ventilation varies depending on the outbreak. In a large outbreak of botulism, the need for mechanical ventilators and critical care beds could easily exceed the capacity of local resources and would require outside resource allocation.

Antibiotics may be necessary in treating complications from the therapies recommended above, such as nosocomial infections. It should be noted that aminoglycosides and clindamycin can exacerbate neuromuscular blockade and should be avoided unless the clinical benefit outweighs the risk. Maintaining adequate hydration, nasogastric suctioning for ileus, bowel, and bladder care in addition to prevention of decubitus ulcers and deep venous thrombosis.

Botulism Antitoxin

Therapy includes passive immunization with equine antitoxin and supportive care. The antitoxin is available in the United States through the CDC via state and local health departments. Often a direct call to the CDC assistance line will expedite the release of antitoxin. These numbers should be prominently displayed and regularly checked in case they are changed. Early administration of this passive neutralizing antibody is important, as the antitoxin can only neutralize circulating toxin; it cannot reverse the existing paralysis, but does minimize further damage to the nerves.

The antitoxin is a trivalent form, which is active against serotypes A, B, and E. It contains 7500 International Units (IU) of type A, 5500 IU of type B, and 8500 IU of type E antitoxin. Monovalent type E antitoxin is available in Alaska and Canada. Current dosing recommendations for the trivalent antitoxin are 1 vial (10 mL) diluted 1:10 in normal saline intravenously over 30–60 minutes. The package insert should be reviewed with public health authorities before using the product, as dosing recommendations can change. The amount of neutralizing antibody in the antitoxins far exceeds the serum toxin levels seen in food-borne botulism patients. In an instance where a patient could have been exposed to high levels of toxin, such as a bioterrorist attack, the adequacy of neutralization can be confirmed by retesting serum for toxin after treatment. The antitoxin is a horse-derived immunoglobulin and has potential to cause hypersensitivity reactions. There are few published data on the safety of the antitoxin, but a review from 1967 to 1977 done on 268 patients cites the relative risk of hypersensitivity reaction to be 9%. Anaphylaxis occurred in 7 patients in this study (2.6%), and a delayed onset serum sickness occurred in 10 (3.7%). Notably 228 patients (85%) received more than one vial of antitoxin as was the common treatment regimen at that time. To screen for hypersensitivity reactions, a skin test is recommended before receiving a full dose of the antitoxin. Patients who have a reaction to the skin test may be desensitized over 3–4 hours before full infusion occurs. Any decision to give the skin test must weigh the risk and benefits of delayed versus safe treatment. Neither a positive nor a negative skin test can predict or exclude an acute allergic reaction. Diphenhydramine and epinephrine should always be readily available during administration and the clinician should regularly monitor the patient for an adverse reaction. A despeciated heptavalent (A, B, C, D, E, F, and G) antitoxin is available and held by the U.S. military. However 4% of horse antigens remain so there is still a risk for hypersensitivity.

Special Considerations

There is limited information regarding the treatment of botulism in pregnancy, immunocompromised patients, and in children. There are case reports of both children and pregnant women receiving the antitoxin, and the risk to the fetus is unknown.

In a biological warfare event, the prophylactic immunization of designated individuals may be necessary. A pentavalent vaccine exists, and is currently used as pretreatment in laboratory workers and military personnel who are at risk for botulism exposure. The vaccine is active against serotypes A, B, C, D, and E.

DISPOSITION

All patients with significant botulism exposure need to be admitted to the hospital for observation. The proportion of patients who require mechanical ventilation varies depending on the outbreak. In a large outbreak of botulism, the need for mechanical ventilators and critical care beds could easily exceed the capacity of local resources and would require outside resource allocation. Unfortunately, patients who develop respiratory compromise and require ventilatory support may require hospitalization for months. Emotional support and behavioral health care will be a necessary part of therapy.

FORENSIC ISSUES

Whenever botulism is suspected, immediate contact with the CDC and the local health department will speed access to diagnostic and laboratory services and enhance surveillance in the early stages of a mass outbreak. If terrorism is suspected, law enforcement will become involved. Attention to the chain of evidence is a consideration.

Autopsy

Individuals who die of botulism are not generally considered to pose an enhanced risk to autopsy personnel. However aerosolized clostridium botulinum toxins is considered to be dangerous. During necropsy at least a theoretical risk of aerosolization exists. Therefore respiratory precautions are suggested.

Suggested Reading

Arnon SS, Schechter R, Inglesby TV. Botulism toxin as a biological weapon: medical and public health management. *JAMA.* 2001;285:1059–1070.

Bakheit AMO, Ward CD, McLellan DL. Generalized botulism-like syndrome after intramuscular injections of botulism type A: a report of two cases. *J Neurol Neurosurg Psych.* 1997;62:198.

Black RE, Gunn RA. Hypersensitivity reactions associated with botulinal antitoxin. *Am J Med.* 1980;69:567–570.

Cai S, Singh BR Strategies to Design Inhibitors of Clostridium Botulinum Neurotoxins *Infect Disord Drug Targets* 2007 MAR; 7(1):47–57.

Fox CK, Keet CA, Strober JB. Recent advances in infant botulism. *Pediatr Neurol.* 2005;32,3:149–154.

Horowitz BZ. Botulinum toxin. *Crit Care Clin.* 2005;21:825–839.

Hibbs RG, Weber JT, Corwin A, et al. Experience with the use of an investigational F(ab')2 heptavalent botulism immune globulin of equine origin during an outbreak of type E botulism in Egypt. *Clin Infec Dis.* 1996;23:337–340.

Kortepeter M. (Lead Editor). *USAMRIID's Medical Management of Biological Casualties Handbook.* 4th ed. 2001. Fort Detrick, MD: U.S. Army Medical Research Institute of Infectious Diseases; 2001: pp. 118–127.

Kongsaengdao S, Samintarapanya K, Rusmechan S et al. An outbreak of botulism in Thailand: Clinical manifestations and management of severe respiratory failure. *Clin Infect Dis* 2006 Nov; 43 (10): 1247-56 EPub 2006 Oct 16.

MacDonald KL, Spengler RF, Hatheway CL, et al. Type A botulism from sautéed onions: clinical and epidemiological observations. *JAMA.* 1985;253:1275–1278.

Metzger JR, Lewis LE. Human-derived immune globulins for the treatment of botulism. *Rev Infect Dis.* 1979;1:689–692.

Nolte KB, Taylor DG, Richmond JY. Biosafety considerations for autopsy. *Am J Forens Med and Path* 2002;23(2):107–122.

O'Mahony M, Mitchell E, Gilbert RJ, et al. An outbreak of foodborne botulism associated with contaminated hazelnut yoghurt. *Epidemiol Infect.* 1990;104:389–395.

Santos JI, Swensen P, Glasgow LA. Potentiation of Clostridium botulinum toxin by aminoglycoside antibiotics: clinical and laboratory observations. *Pediatrics.* 1981;68:50–54.

Siegel LS. Destruction of botulinum toxin in food and water. In: Hauschild AH, Dodds DL, eds. *Clostridium Botulinum: Ecology and Control in Foods.* New York, NY: Marcel Dekker Inc; 1993: pp. 323–341.

Shapiro RL, Hatheway C, Swerdlow DL. Botulism in the United States: a clinical and epidemiologic review. *Ann Intern Med.* 1998;129:221–228.

Tacket CO, Shandera WX, Mann JM. Equine antitoxin use and other factors that predict outcome in type A food borne botulism. *Am J Med.* 1984;76:794–798.

Townes JM, Cieslak PR, Hatheway CL, et al. An outbreak of type A botulism associated with a commercial cheese sauce. *Ann Intern Med.* 1996;125:558–563.

Werner SB, Passaro D, McGee F, et al. Wound botulism in California, 1951–1998: recent epidemic in heroin injectors. *Clin Inf Dis.* 2000;31:1018–1024.

42

SMALLPOX (VARIOLA) AND POXVIRUSES

Robin B. McFee

VARIOLA AND POXVIRUSES

If your first patient(s) arrives with skin lesions and a clinical picture consistent with smallpox, you must keep the following critical issues in mind as well as have the following personnel and equipment in place to achieve the following:

Diagnosis

History

- Clinical manifestations occur acutely with fever, rigors, vomiting, headache, and backache. By the third day later dermatological lesions will appear and quickly progress from macules to papules to pustular vesicles; distribution extremities/face, synchronous pattern

Clinical

- What does the patient look like? Sick or well?
  - **Smallpox patients generally look sick.**
- Does the patient have a fever? Is it >101°F or <101°F?
  - **Smallpox patients have a fever.**
- Is there a dermatological component? A rash? Where are the lesions? Palms of the hands? Soles of the feet? Trunk?
  - **Palms, soles, extremities, face before trunk suggest smallpox.**
  - Palms, soles with previous genital infection suggest syphilis.
- How do the lesions look? All alike or are they in different stages of development?
  - **All lesions looking alike suggest smallpox.**
  - Lesions looking differently on the same part of the body suggest chickenpox.

- Are there others in the waiting room with similar illness?
- Have any members of the family been sick previous to this patient presenting?
  - Chickenpox often occurs in family/friend clusters.
- Has the patient received a chickenpox vaccine or had natural chickenpox?
- Is there a mental status change?
  - Smallpox may cause encephalitis or delirium.
  - Note that children with high fevers may also experience what may be considered mental status changes.
- Has there been any foreign travel or unusual exposures (animal, occupational)?
  - Monkeypox can present similar to smallpox; exposure in endemic areas or to exotic animals may be a risk.

Preparedness Issues

1. Smallpox plan—
   a. Updated
   b. Involves your department, facility, regional responders
   c. Tested
   d. Readily available to response team
2. Diagnostic chart from CDC or WHO displaying lesions with associated clinical information (Fig. 42-5)
3. Information to contact local public health and CDC if smallpox is suspected
   a. Public health/CDC provide access to advanced lab capabilities
   b. Public health/CDC provide access to newer countermeasures that may only be available as IND products

4. Ability to isolate patient immediately
5. Ability to identify who was in contact with patient
   a. Must be able to access these individuals for follow-up, vaccinations and other contact tracing that the health department will conduct
   b. Your team already should have started working with public health
6. Readily available personal protective equipment (PPE)
7. Trained team to utilize PPE
8. Backup team to assist primary team
9. Additional ventilators available
   a. Sources of ventilators identified
   b. Arrangements/mutual aid agreements/distributor agreements in place
   c. Transportation and other logistics in place
10. Logistics
    a. Cidofovir antiviral medication
    b. Location to triage patients
    c. Location to treat patients
    d. Quarantine sites
    e. Morgue
11. Resources dedicated to health-care teams and their families to ensure attendance and avoid absenteeism
    a. Daycare
    b. Food
    c. Sleeping accommodations
    d. Communications capabilities
    e. Medications/health care
12. Health-care facility team ready to coordinate activities with other response agencies (HICS)
13. On speed dial—
    a. Director of ED
    b. Director of local health department
    c. CDC office of emergency management
    d. Regional LRN lab
    e. Infectious disease consult

Smallpox is contagious. So are chickenpox and monkeypox—the two closest look alikes!

Management Considerations

One case of smallpox is a global emergency—an act of bioterrorism—a public health threat

- Rapid/accurate diagnosis
  - History
  - Physical examination
  - Laboratory studies
    - Notify laboratory; may be variola
    - Only tests that are approved in facility under such circumstances
- Limit contagion—even presumptive concern over potential contagion
- Isolate patient
- Droplet/airborne precautions for a minimum of 17 days following exposure of all contacts. Patients are infectious until all scabs separate.
- Contacts with fever >38°C or 101°F should be considered infected and treated accordingly with home or hospital isolation and appropriate management.
- Initiate preparedness plan
  - Public health notification
  - Protect self and staff
  - Isolate patient
  - Obtain appropriate guidance from experts including CDC
  - Obtain access to laboratory—warn of potential variola samples
  - Obtain countermeasures
    - Vaccine
    - Immunoglobulin
    - Antivirals (Cidofovir). Newer ones may be available as IND.
    - Mental health counselors for staff and ultimately for patient

Handling the Sick

- Negative pressure room
- N95 respirator
- Universal precautions/respiratory-droplet precautions

"The single greatest threat to man's continued existence on earth is the virus."

—Joshua Ledeberg, Nobel Scientist

POXVIRUSES

The poxvirus family is a diverse group of viruses that affect humans and animals. Their nucleosome contains double-stranded DNA; they are among the largest of all animal viruses (200–320 nm) and can be visualized with light microscopes. They preferentially infect skin epithelial cells, replicate in cell cytoplasm and may produce eosinophilic cytoplasmic inclusion bodies, and ultimately cause toxic effects on cells. Among the poxviruses known to affect humans are from the genera Orthopoxvirus, Parapoxvirus, Molluscipoxvirus, and Yatapoxvirus, of which the Orthopoxvirus variola (smallpox) is the most deadly to humans. Different poxviruses are capable of producing a localized, self-limited infection by inoculation to skin such as orf (contagious pustular dermatitis), or systemic disease such as variola (smallpox). Other poxviruses cause localized cell proliferation, that is, molluscum contagiosum. Most cases of poxvirus infection are occupational, and lead to few cutaneous lesions. However smallpox and monkeypox can cause serious illness and death. Therefore from a bioweapon perspective, orthopoxviruses are of greatest interest because they include smallpox, monkeypox, and vaccinia cowpox viruses; the former two are capable of significant illness while the later has been utilized as the basis for vaccination against smallpox. Some preparedness experts express concern that the Orthopoxvirus camelpox poses a risk because being genetically similar to smallpox, not uncommon and owing to its size may be amenable to bioweapon engineering. Infection with one Orthopoxvirus confers protection against other members of the genera.

Vaccinia

Vaccinia is an Orthopoxvirus affecting a wide variety of vertebrate hosts, is among the most widely studied virus, and in 1796 was the first countermeasure developed against smallpox. As a laboratory isolate, this virus does not cause serious disease in immunocompetent humans. Generalized vaccinia viremia can occur 6–9 days after vaccination with full recovery expected. Other vaccine adverse events can occur; the most common is autoinoculation whereby the patient touches the vaccine site, then rubs the eyes without washing hands first (Fig. 42-1). Genetically engineered and attenuated recombinant viruses are being studied as safer alternatives to vaccinia especially for immunecompromised individuals but have not been Food and Drug Administration (FDA) approved as of this writing.

If adverse events occur, especially potentially life-threatening disseminated vaccinia, cardiac sequela associated with vaccinia vaccine, vaccinia immune globulin (VIG) can be administered. (See Smallpox—Vaccination.)

Monkeypox

In 2003, monkeypox appeared for the first time in the Western Hemisphere when several individuals in midwestern United States became ill after contact with prairie dogs and the Gambian giant rat. Importation of exotic animals remains a potential source of human infection with diseases not common to North America. Monkeypox is an Orthopoxvirus that usually affects primates but has infected humans, squirrels, and other animals. According to the World Health Organization (WHO), humans usually contract monkeypox through contact with an infected animal's blood, body fluids, or lesions, or by being bitten. Secondary transmission—human-to-human transmission after close contact with an infected human who was infected by an animal exposure—is approximately 9% based upon cases in the Congo. WHO cautions that outbreaks in one part of the world may not behave similarly to other regions. According to WHO experts, smallpox is clinically indistinguishable from monkeypox, which generally causes less serious illness. Monkeypox does produce lymphadenopathy and skin lesions, which occur in crops (Figs. 42-2 and 42-3). Vaccinia vaccination confers protection. The smallpox vaccine was about 85% effective in preventing human monkeypox during an African outbreak. Vaccination is recommended for those caring for monkeypox patients; vaccination can be given up to 14 days after exposure.

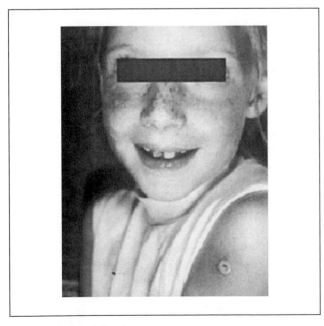

FIGURE 42-1

VACCINIA VACCINE ADVERSE EVENT. AUTOINOCULATION
Note the primary vaccine lesion on the left upper arm. The child scratched the arm then rubbed the face and eye. Notice the lesions around the right orbit.

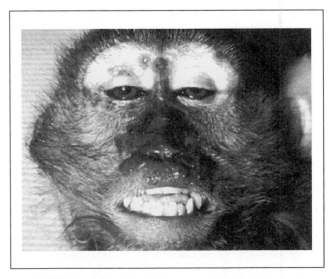

FIGURE 42-2

MONKEYPOX INFECTING PRIMATE IN THE CONGO

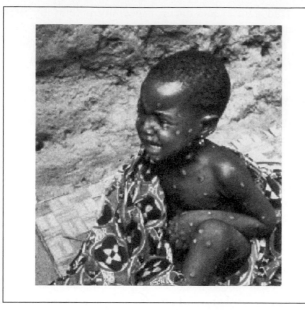

FIGURE 42-3

MONKEYPOX INFECTING CHILD IN THE CONGO

Unvaccinated children are most vulnerable and deaths have resulted from infection with monkeypox. Large outbreaks have occurred and controversy as well as concern persists surrounding the actual ability for person-to-person transmission. It appears to have a lower overall secondary attack rate than smallpox. The recent appearance of monkeypox in the United States underscores the problem of dissemination of pathogens outside their endemic area as well as the threat of animal importation in addition to the emergence of travel-related illness and global biological threats. Moreover the importance of early diagnosis cannot be overstated, not only to contain a potential outbreak but because of the impact upon immunosuppressed individuals. Monkeypox can be accidentally transmitted to humans and lead to small epidemics, even death. Given the relatively more common nature of monkeypox, its availability raises concern about the criminal introduction of this poxvirus which, given its transmissibility through prairie dogs, as well as person-to-person, makes it a potential bioweapon.

Clinical

Monkeypox can cause a febrile illness with vesiculopustular eruptions. Presumptive diagnosis can be made based upon clinical presentation, immunohistochemical evidence of poxvirus infection in skin lesion tissues (Table 42-1). Virus can be recovered in cell cultures. Monkeypox specific DNA sequences can be used to identify the virus. ELISA results correlate with virologic polymerase chain reaction (PCR) and viral culture results. If a poxvirus is suspected, respiratory precautions must be initiated immediately. In addition,

local public health must be notified to initiate a CDC response, including advice and access to advanced laboratory capabilities, as well as countermeasure support that may include antivirals, immunoglobulin, and vaccines. Like smallpox, there is a lengthy list of differential diagnosis (Table 42-2).

Presumptive diagnosis is made based upon clinical presentation, history of illness, and epidemiology (Table 42-1—CDC case definition).

Management

Limited data exist on the effectiveness of smallpox vaccination for preventing monkeypox. Data suggest preexposure smallpox vaccination is highly effective at >85% in protecting persons exposed to monkeypox from developing disease. The effectiveness of postexposure vaccination requires further study. Data suggest smallpox vaccination following exposure to smallpox is effective at preventing or ameliorating disease; given the similarity among orthopoxviruses, smallpox vaccination should confer similar benefit against monkeypox. Given the mortality rate from monkeypox ranges from 1 to 10%; the risk of death from smallpox vaccine is approximately 1–2 per million vaccinees. It is important to carefully screen potential vaccines for precautions and contraindications (Table 42-3). Persons without a successful vaccine "take" should be revaccinated within 2 weeks of the most recent exposure to monkeypox.

Rash illnesses suspected to be monkeypox should be confirmed by laboratory evaluation; such laboratories should have the capability to test varicella, vaccinia, and other similar viral infections.

No data are available concerning the benefit of VIG as treatment of monkeypox complications. It is unknown if a patient with severe monkeypox infection will thus benefit from treatment with VIG; its use however might still be considered. VIG can be considered for prophylactic use in person exposed to monkeypox who has severe T-cell function immunodeficiency where smallpox vaccine would be contraindicated. VIG could be obtained under an investigational new drug (IND) protocol. Physicians should contact their state health department; subsequently referred to the CDC clinical information line: 1.877.554.4625.

Cidofovir has demonstrated anti-monkeypox viral activity in animal and in vitro studies. The benefit to patients with severe infection is unknown. Nevertheless, one should consider using Cidofovir in such instances (See "Cidofovir" in smallpox section). Realizing the toxicity potential of Cidofovir, safety considerations suggest it should be utilized as a treatment for severe monkeypox but not as prophylaxis. It is licensed for use in the treatment of cytomegalovirus (CMV) retinitis in HIV patients. However if it was used in the treatment of monkeypox, vaccinia vaccine, or smallpox, it would be under the restrictions of an IND protocol. Clinical consultation is available concerning the use of VIG and Cidofovir from the CDC at 1.877.554.4625.

TABLE 42-1

UPDATED INTERIM CASE DEFINITION FOR HUMAN MONKEYPOX—CDC JANUARY 2004

Clinical Criteria

Rash

Macular, popular, vesicular, or pustular: generalized or localized, discrete or confluent

Fever

Subjective or measured temperature of >= 99.3°F (>= 37.4°C)

Other signs and symptoms

- Chills and/or sweats
- Headache
- Backache
- Lymphadenopathy
- Sore throat
- Cough
- Shortness of breath

Epidemiologic Criteria

- Exposure to an exotic or wild mammalian pet obtained on or after 4/15/03 with clinical signs of illness (e.g., conjunctivitis, respiratory symptoms, and/or rash)
- Exposure to an exotic or wild mammalian pet with or without clinical signs of illness that has been in contact with either a mammalian pet or a human with monkeypox
- Exposure to a suspect, probable, or confirmed human case of monkeypox

Laboratory Criteria

- Isolation of monkeypox virus in culture
- Demonstration of monkeypox virus DNA by polymerase chain reaction (PCR) testing of a clinical specimen
- Demonstration of virus morphologically consistent with an Orthopoxvirus by electron microscopy in the absence of exposure to another Orthopoxvirus
- Demonstration of presence of Orthopoxvirus in tissue using immunohistochemical testing methods in the absences of exposure to another Orthopoxvirus

Case Classification

  Suspect Case

- Meets one of the epidemiologic criteria
  and
- Fever or unexplained rash
  and
- Two or more other signs or symptoms with onset of first sign or symptom <21 days after last exposure meeting epidemiologic criteria

  Probable Case

- Meets one of the epidemiologic criteria
  and
- Fever
  and
- Vesicular-pustular rash with onset of first sign or symptom <21 days after last exposure meeting epidemiologic criteria
  or
- If rash is present but the type is not described, demonstrates elevated levels of IgM antibodies reactive with Orthopoxvirus between at least 7–56 days after rash onset

  Confirmed Case

- Meets one of the laboratory criteria

From: Guidelines and Resources. Updated Interim Case Definition for Human Monkeypox, January 2004. Centers for Disease Control (CDC), Dept. of Health and Human Services 4/4/06.

TABLE 42-2

DIFFERENTIAL DIAGNOSIS SMALLPOX
(SIGNIFICANT DIFFERENCES)

- Varicella (rash distribution, general appearance of patient)
- Monkeypox
- Disseminated herpes zoster (dermatomal rash distribution, history of illness, patient appearance generally not ill, usually afebrile)
- Impetigo (limited rash, appearance of patient, development of rash)
- Drug eruptions (history, appearance of rash and patient, distribution of rash—often pruritic, wheal and flare)
- Contact dermatitis (history, occupational risks, patient appearance—generally not ill)
- Erythema multiforme
- Enteroviral infections
- Disseminated herpes simplex
- Scabies
- Insect bites
- Molluscum contagiosum (immunocompromised patients)
- Secondary syphilis
- Rickettsial diseases

Smallpox (Variola)

The threat of Variola virus (smallpox)—the leading cause of infection—related death in history—has returned, and once again smallpox has become a household word. Smallpox infections have been recognized as far back as ancient Egypt, affecting Pharaohs and peasants. Unlike decades ago when smallpox was a naturally occurring infection, concerns are emerging that smallpox may become intentionally spread as a bioweapon. Intelligence sources suggest Iraq and other terrorist-friendly nations may have access to or already weaponized Variola. Rumors persist that scientists in the former Soviet Union were trying to develop an Ebola/Variola hybrid virus.

Smallpox is an Orthopoxvirus, which consists of the infectious agents that cause camelpox, smallpox, monkeypox, and cowpox. Immunity to one member of this family confers protection against others, hence the use of vaccinia (cowpox) virus to immunize against Variola. Vaccinia is a virus with minimal pathogenicity except in immune-compromised patients. Smallpox is a painful, disabling, febrile disease.

Variola occurs as primarily two strains—variola major (smallpox) and the less pathological version variola minor, which causes a milder febrile rash, and is sometimes referred to as alastrim. Smallpox presents a particularly serious risk because of a high case fatality rate estimated at 30–50% depending upon the strain, naive vaccine status of the exposed population, and inconsistent availability of appropriate health care to prevent secondary bacterial infection. It is a highly pathogenic virus; it is estimated <10–100 smallpox virions are necessary to cause human illness! Bioterrorism experts consider smallpox to be a significant threat because it is relatively easy to produce once starting material is obtained, the aerosol infectivity—contagiousness, widespread susceptibility of nonimmunized or underimmunized populations. Contagion results from transmitting virus in airborne droplets or by contact with lesions. Primary portal of entry is the respiratory tract so population density, overcrowding, as well as immune status affect the extent of spread. No significant subclinical carrier state is believed to exist, nor are there known animal reservoirs. Infected people are contagious from the onset of illness until the last crusts of the dermal lesions are gone. The smallpox virus is relatively

TABLE 42-3

SMALLPOX VACCINATION IS CONTRAINDICATIONS FOR THE FOLLOWING PATIENTS

1. Persons who have severe immunodeficiency in T-cell function, defined as
   a. HIV-infected adults with CD4 lymphocyte count less than 200 (or age appropriate equivalent counts for HIV-infected children)
   b. Solid organ, bone marrow transplant recipients or others currently receiving high-dose immunosuppressive therapy (i.e., 2 mg/kg body weight or a total of 20 mg/d of prednisone or equivalent for persons whose weight is >10 kg, when administered for >2 weeks)
   c. Persons with lymphosarcoma, hematological malignancies, or primary T-cell congenital immunodeficiencies
2. Persons with life-threatening allergies to latex or to smallpox vaccine or any of its components (polymyxin B, streptomycin, chlortetracycline, neomycin)

These persons have a risk of severe complications from smallpox vaccination that may approach or exceed the risk of disease from monkeypox exposure.

NB: In persons with close or intimate exposure within the past 2 weeks to a confirmed human case or probable or confirmed animal case of monkeypox, neither age, pregnancy, nor a history of eczema are contraindications to receipt of smallpox vaccination. These conditions are precautions, not contraindications. However active eczematous disease is more concerning, but in instances when the potential vaccine has had true close or intimate exposure, the risk of monkeypox likely is greater than the risk of smallpox vaccine-related complications. Appropriate vaccine site care should be used to prevent transmission of smallpox vaccine (vaccinia virus).
Source: Centers for Disease Control (CDC), Department of Health and Human Services 6/25/03.

resistant to environmental conditions; infections have occurred from Africa to North America. The last case of smallpox occurred during the 1940s in the United States, and the last naturally acquired case occurred in Somalia in 1977. Most clinicians have never seen this illness, so experienced diagnosticians are uncommon. Routine vaccination stopped almost 30 years ago.

Initial Presentation

Smallpox progresses through three phases: incubation, prodrome, and pox (Tables 42-4, 42-5, and 42-6, and Fig. 42-4). The incubation period on average is 7–17 days postexposure. The individual is asymptomatic and not considered contagious during this period. Typically smallpox victims will then experience a prodrome characterized by fever (100°F to 105°F), vomiting, headache, body ache, or backache; this period lasts for several days (usually 2–4) and the patient is extremely ill (Table 42-4). Some consider this stage potentially contagious. Appearance of a rash marks the third stage; this period lasts from 14 to 17 days. The rash appears as small red dots in the mouth and on the tongue then develop into sores (oropharyngeal enanthem) that rupture and release virus into the upper respiratory system. This is the most contagious stage. Patients will be prostrated and may continue to complain of severe headache, chills, backache, malaise, nausea, and vomiting. At about the same time as the oral lesions rupture, the typical skin rash—the

TABLE 42-4

CLINICAL DIAGNOSIS—SMALLPOX (FIGURE 42-5)

Entry—Airway
Incubation—12 days
Acute-onset febrile illness with prostration
Classic rash
• Appears 2–3 days after onset of fever
• Synchronous development of lesions
• Starts at head, hands, feet then progresses toward trunk
Death
• 30–50% case fatality rate depending upon strain
• Usually occurs between days 11 to 15
Laboratory Diagnosis
• Rule out chickenpox (PCR)
• Specimen of choice is lesion material from pustules
• Contact your state public health laboratory for guidance
Electron microscopy of vesicular scrapings = characteristic virions
• Light microscopy-Guarnieri bodies
• Gispen's modified silver stain = cytoplasmic inclusions appear black
• Characteristic growth on chorioallantoic membrane
• PCR

TABLE 42-5

BIODROME

Dermatologic manifestation *Hallmark Rash
*Centripetal distribution of lesions
Start at head, hands (palms), feet (soles)
Subsequent migration to trunk/legs/arms
*Nodular—dermal—hard to touch
*Lesions progress from papules to pustules in synchronous fashion
*All lesions on given body area of same developmental stage
*Febrile illness >101°F
Patients tend to look sick/prostrated
Mental status changes N
Neurological involvement (not common with other look alikes)
Significant constitutional symptoms (support severity of illness)
Headache
Backache
GI complaints
Fatigue

*Presumptive diagnosis of smallpox

exanthem usually appear, staring most often on the hands and face, spreading to the arms and legs then to the feet (Figs. 42-5, 42-6). The lesions evolve from macules to papules to vesicles to pustules and finally the lesions crust, which may take 1–2 weeks. All the lesions develop in a similar stage at any given time often referred to as "synchronous" development. The initial lesions usually appear on the palms of the hands, soles of the feet, feel firm, nodular to palpation. The distribution of smallpox lesions is centrifugal (Figs. 42-5, 42-6, 42-7)—extremity first, then trunk in contrast to the most similar disease in the differential diagnosis—chickenpox, whereupon the rash starts centrally on the trunk and works toward the periphery (Figs. 42-5, 42-8). Smallpox lesions often are on the extensor surfaces and are deep with firm multiloculated vesicles. After the crusting phase, scarring occurs and may cause severe disfigurement. Patients who have oral lesions are contagious, as are those who develop skin rashes. Dentists and others who may be called upon to examine complaints of a febrile illness and mouth sores should be sensitized to the potential of smallpox. Patients are contagious until *all* scabs have fallen off.

Types of Smallpox Illness

There are four types of smallpox illness identified by the pattern of rash.

Classic Smallpox Smallpox lesions in the classic presentation are deep and dermal. The lesions are synchronous

TABLE 42-6

KEY "LOOK ALIKE" AND KEY DIFFERENTIATORS

Varicella/Zoster (chickenpox)—Key differentiators

Rash

- Asynchronous development of lesions
    - Lesions in different stages papules and pustules on same region
- Centrifugal distribution (trunk then extremities)
- Not usually involving palms of hands or soles of feet
- Superficial skin involvement—soft to touch (not dermal/nodular)
- Rash usually pruritic

Patient Appearance

- Patients don't usually look very sick, just uncomfortable
- Febrile illness

Patients

- Usual patients are children. Adults, especially unvaccinated and without a history of chickenpox, may become infected.

Shingles (Zoster)

Rash

- Usually limited to dermatomal distribution
- May appear as popular cluster; similar in appearance to chickenpox
- Lesions are usually painful, itchy or patient complains of tingling/burning
- Generally present in older patients especially under stress with history of chickenpox

Patient Appearance

- Patients don't usually look sick, just uncomfortable
- Discomfort from localized lesions may keep patients awake
- Non-febrile or low grade fever

Molluscum contagiosum

Rash

- Multiple pearly white nodules (2–5 mm diameter with central umbilication)
- **Painless**
- Distribution usually anogenital region, but possible anywhere on the body

Patients

- Common in AIDS patients (lesions may be larger/atypical and severe in comparison with presentation involving non AIDS patients)
- Children, sexually active adults and sports involving close person-to-person contact or patients with impaired cellular immunity

in their development—whatever location of the body a cluster of lesions appears on, they appear similar. The lesions progress from macula, papule, vesicle, pustule (pox), and ultimately to scabs. The time from exposure to symptoms ranges from 7 to 17 days. Chickenpox (Varicella) lesions are asynchronous in development—some are umbilicated, others are newly emerging, while the remainder may be ready to fall off. Varicella lesions are often found on flexor surfaces. Unlike smallpox, chickenpox rarely affects the soles and palms. Other illnesses that may simulate chickenpox on cursory appearance include coxsackievirus, leprosy, and syphilis. Monkeypox also resembles smallpox (Figs. 42-2, 42-3).

The key distinguishing features between each illness is the history and differences in the rashes (Tables 42-4 to 42-6). Coxsackievirus usually affects adolescents and young adults, the patients do not appear ill, and the rash is superficial not dermal. Leprosy lesions are more confluent except in the tuberous version, with possible neurologic symptoms, a clear history of the ailment. Again, especially if the patient has been treated, he/she will not appear ill. Smallpox patients will appear very sick and prostrated. Syphilis patients will have lesions that tend to remain localized on the palms and soles, and may recollect a history of prior genital illness. Again such patients usually do not appear significantly ill. Rickettsialpox, a mite-borne disease that

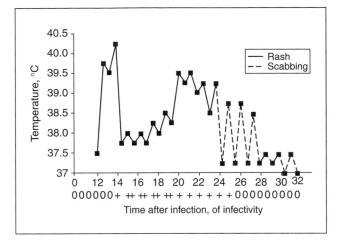

FIGURE 42-4

APPROXIMATE TIME OF APPEARANCE EVOLUTION OF THE RASH AND MAGNITUDE OF INFECTIVITY RELATIVE TO THE NUMBER OF DAYS AFTER ACQUISITION OF INFECTION

Source: From Henderson DA, Inglesby TV, O'Toole T (eds). Bioterrorism: Guidelines for Medical and Public Health Management. Chicago: AMA Press, 2002, p. 102 with permission from the author.

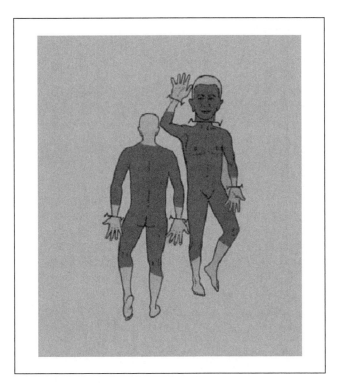

FIGURE 42-5

VARIOLA (SMALLPOX)

Smallpox exanthem would initially appear on the face, hands, and feet (white area) in contrast to where chickenpox rash would initially appear (dark area). Other hand-foot rashes: Syphilis, hand/foot/mouth, Coxsackie, mercury. Note the distribution of chickenpox in the shaded area. In contrast smallpox would originate in the white areas first, then progress toward the trunk regions.

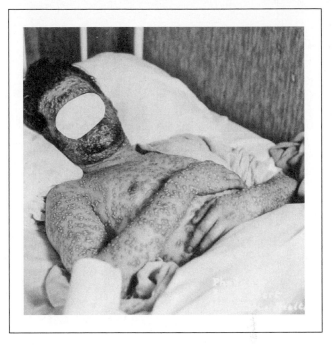

FIGURE 42-6

CLASSIC SMALLPOX (VARIOLA MAJOR)

Note the lesions are at the same developmental stage on the same region of the body. They also appear dense and embedded. Note the lesions: they are in the same stage of development per region. They appear nodular and deeper. The patient appears ill.
Source: Photo courtesy of the U.S. Army Medical Corps.

belongs to the spotted fever group of rickettsioses, is not a poxvirus. However it can cause fever and a papulovesicular eruption. Although the associated dermal manifestation may somewhat mimic smallpox, clinically it often causes an asymptomatic vesicle that rapidly ulcerates to become an eschar. Moreover rickettsialpox is an uncommon disease that occurs in urban populations in the eastern United States as well as globally. Patients often complain of fever and malaise, including headache and fatigue. Patients generally do not appear sick, unlike smallpox patients who often are prostrated and appear quite ill. Also, unlike smallpox, which generally results in multiple lesions, localized rickettsialpox has a primary lesion developing at the bite site within 48 hours that may result in lymphadenopathy and one or two eschars that resolve within 4 weeks. Generalized cutaneous eruptions have occurred however, and can appear on the face, trunk, and extremities with no specific sequence or involvement of palms and soles, bearing greater similarity to chickenpox than smallpox, which classically starts at the extremities and works towards the trunk and do include those latter areas. An enanthem is possible on the tongue, tonsils, uvula, or pharynx but is uncommon.

Approximately 15% of smallpox victims will have delirium. Encephalitis is possible.

Hemorrhagic Smallpox An atypical form of smallpox, the hemorrhagic variety, sometimes referred to as purpura

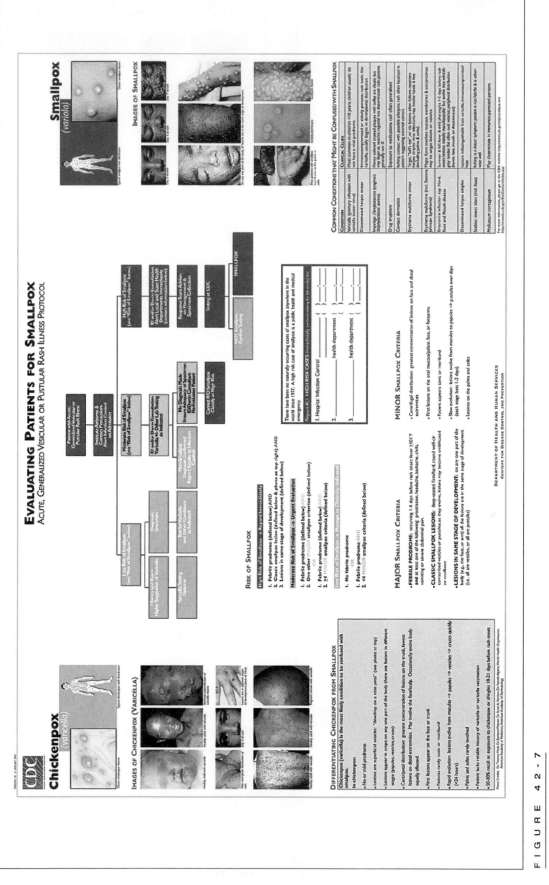

FIGURE 42-7

CDC SMALLPOX DIAGNOSIS CHART

A larger poster sized color version may be obtained directly from the CDC(available at www.cdc. gov); the reader is encouraged to request one.

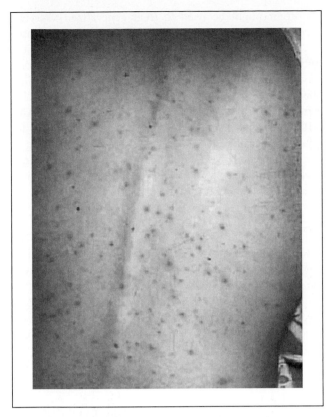

FIGURE 42-8

CHICKENPOX (VARICELLA)
Note the lesions are at different developmental stages on the same region of the body. They also appear superficial. Look at the lesions. Are they similar or in different stages of development? Are they nodular or superficial in appearance? What area of the body is this? Does it matter? How does the patient look? Other symptoms? Signs?
(*Photo courtesy of the U.S. Army Medical Corps.*)

variolosa, which is usually always fatal. It tends to occur more often in pregnant women or persons with significantly compromised immune response, and presents with epistaxis, hematemesis, hemoptysis, hematuria, subconjunctival hemorrhages, petechiae, ecchymosis, and bloody pustules on the skin and mucosa.

Flat/Confluent Smallpox Flat (malignant) smallpox where a dense confluent macular rash occurs. This version, like hemorrhagic smallpox, carries a high mortality rate. A deficiency in cellular immunity may be associated with this rare version, which occurs more often in children and is characterized by severe toxemia. The skin lesions develop slowly, become confluent, and remain flat, never developing into pustules. Some have described the lesions as "velvety" to the touch. Sections of the skin may slough off.

Modified or Subacute Smallpox Most often occurs in previously immunized patients. The lesions may be fewer in number and more superficial than classic smallpox. The

prodrome stage may include severe headache, backache, and fever, albeit it might be shorter. Once lesions appear, they usually evolve and crust over quicker.

Medical Management

Control of Exposure Rapid recognition and isolation of an individual suspected of smallpox infection is critical. Institute universal precautions, identify all individuals in contact with the patient, and contact the local health department.

Diagnosis Presumptive diagnosis is based upon the clinical picture; laboratory testing confirms the presence or absence of smallpox. The CDC provides a free, highly useful chart via the Internet (*www.cdc.gov*) or by mail, either of which should be prominently posted in the emergency department and clinical areas (Fig. 42-7). Although the differential diagnosis of smallpox appears a lengthy list (Tables 42-2, 42-6), true variola patients appear sick—and their disease usually follow the typical biodrome. If the diagnosis of smallpox (or monkeypox) is considered, immediate isolation must be initiated. All patient contacts should be identified. While laboratory confirmation with silver impregnation or fluorescent antibody staining of smears taken from skin lesions is possible, CDC involvement, biosafety level considerations, and other precautions must be taken. Contact public health, hospital laboratory about presumptive diagnosis; initiate lab precautions, obtain appropriate samples based upon laboratory capabilities, public health and infectious disease recommendations.

Laboratory Testing Early suspicion, collaboration with experts from the health department and CDC to identify or rule out smallpox with subsequent contact tracing, vaccination and containment strategies are essential to contain a mass incident from this highly contagious disease. Estimates of per person transmission rates vary from 8 to 30 depending on the computer models utilized and the environment. Studies suggest that health-care facilities are most likely to exhibit the highest transmission rates. Quarantine laws will probably be implemented under public health direction. Symptomatic and supportive care is essential. Prevention of secondary infections is critical. If such exigency occurs, antibiotics must be quickly initiated. Because smallpox is spread from airborne droplets, respiratory and fluid precautions using appropriate personal protective equipment (PPE) are necessary. Patient isolation in negative pressure rooms equipped with special filter systems is important.

Vaccines

Postexposure vaccination within 72 hours with vaccinia vaccine should confer significant protection for health-care workers and others who have been exposed.

VIG should be readily available to treat adverse events associated with the vaccine. Vaccinia vaccine was generally considered a safe vaccine when given in the 1960s and 1970s, with relatively low adverse events recorded. Unfortunately with the increased number of immunosuppressed persons who have HIV, transplants or chronic illnesses, and an aging society, there are subpopulations that may be at increased risk of adverse outcomes from the vaccine. Although rare, encephalitis and death can occur. The most common adverse event is autoinoculation (Fig. 42-1)—the patient scratches the vaccine site, then rubs his or her eye, subsequently developing a lesion. Patients with eczema are more likely to experience eczema vaccinatum. Eczema vaccinatum can occur when a person with atopic dermatitis receives the vaccination. Atopic dermatitis results from an immunological deficiency resulting in a skin abnormality. Untreated eczema vaccinatum can be fatal; treatment with VIG must be immediate. VIG is not considered effective in the treatment of postvaccination encephalitis or meningoencephalitis; rare, but life-threatening events with CFR of 25%. Generalized vaccinia results from the systemic spread of the virus from the vaccine site; usually a benign, self-limited complication of primary vaccination in healthy individuals. Realize that the risk of smallpox to these special populations is greater than the threat of vaccinia once exposure to variola occurs. As of April 2003, vaccinations have been halted in many regions due to concerns over unexpected cardiac-related deaths. Further studies reveal there was a small subset of European patients in the 1970s who also experienced cardiac reactions; usually they were minor. Some of those patients were treated with immune globulin; most of whom recovered. The patients with cardiac-related adverse events in 2003 were not treated with immune globulin; perhaps this should be considered as an intervention if mass vaccination resumes. Further studies should identify those individuals at risk or the precise mechanisms by which such deaths have occurred. Up-to-date information on smallpox vaccination, contraindications and news can be found at *www.cdc.org*: smallpox fact sheet.

Antivirals

Cidofovir (Vistide (r))[(S)-1-(3-hydroxy-2-phosphonylmethoxypropyl) cytosine] (HPMC) is an antiviral used for the treatment of CMV retinitis, especially in HIV patients (Fig. 42-9). Currently it is under clinical trials evaluating potential systemic treatment of AIDS. Cidofovir has demonstrated significant in vivo and in vitro activity in experimental animals. Whether or not the use of Cidofovir confers benefit superior to immediate postexposure vaccination in human smallpox victims remains uncertain. Other antivirals for use against variola are under investigation. Studies suggest Cidofovir antiviral has some effectiveness against smallpox.

Cidofovir might be used to treat generalized vaccinia, eczema vaccinatum, or progressive vaccinia. It is not licensed to treat the problems caused by smallpox vaccine, so it is only available through a special protocol called an IND protocol. Use of cidofovir to treat smallpox vaccine, reactions should be evaluated and monitored by experts at the U.S. Army Research Institute of Infectious Diseases (USAMRIID), National Institutes of Health, and the Centers for Disease Control and Prevention. Recommended dosing in the treatment of CMV retinitis is based upon the patient's underlying kidney function as represented by creatinine clearance (Cl_{cr}).

Dosing Schedule—Cidofovir (Vistide)

Caveat: Use of Cidofovir for the treatment of monkeypox or smallpox is under an IND. Cidofovir is FDA approved for the treatment of CMV retinitis in HIV patients.

Mechanism: Cidofovir diphosphate suppresses CMV replication by selective inhibition of viral DNA synthesis. Incorporation of Cidofovir into growing viral DNA chain results in reductions in the rate of viral DNA synthesis.

Dosing must take into consideration creatinine clearance (Cl_{Cr}).

Dosing in the patient with normal renal function
Induction: 5 mg/kg IV over 1 hour once weekly for 2 consecutive weeks

Maintenance: 5 mg/kg over 1 hour once every other week

It is recommended to administer probenecid 2 g orally 3 hours prior to each Cidofovir dose and 1 g at 2 hours and 8 hours after completion of the infusion (total 4 g).

It is also important to hydrate the patient with 1 L of 0.9% NS IV prior to Cidofovir infusion. A second liter may be administered over a 1–3-hour period immediately following infusion, if tolerated.

Dosing adjustment in renal impairment If the creatinine increases by 0.3–0.4 mg/dL, reduce the Cidofovir dose to 3 mg/kg; discontinue therapy for increases >= 0.5 mg/dL or development of >= 3+ Proteinuria.

Patients with preexisting renal impairment: Use is contraindicated with serum creatinine >1.5 mg/dL. Clcr <55 mL/min or urine protein >=100 mg/dL (>=2+ Proteinuria). However the clinician must balance the threat of the infection against the risk and benefit associated with antiviral therapy.

Contraindications include history of severe hypersensitivity to probenecid or other sulfa-containing medications, serum creatinine >1.5 mg/dL. Clcr <55 mL/min or urine protein >=100 mg/dL (>=2+ Proteinuria) or use within 7 days of nephrotoxic agents. Fanconi syndrome may occur.

Dose-dependent nephrotoxicity requires dose adjustment or discontinuation. Neutropenia and ocular hypotony have occurred. Safety and efficacy have not been established in children or the elderly. Other adverse effects include but are not limited to chills, fever, headache, pain, iritis, decrease in intraocular pressure, uveitis, cough, dyspnea, metabolic acidosis, cardiomyopathy/tachycardia, photosensitivity reaction/skin discoloration, abdominal pain, and tremor. Cidofovir is a pregnancy category C risk. It was shown to be teratogenic and embryotoxic in animal studies, some at doses, which also produced maternal toxicity.

Prepare admixtures in a class 2 laminar flow hood, wearing PPE and appropriate disposal precautions.

Potential New Therapies

HDP-Cidofovir U.S. researchers reported promising results on hexadecyloxypropyl-cidofovir (HDP-cidofovir), an oral drug active against smallpox, at the 15th International Conference on Antiviral Research (Prague, Czech Republic; March 17–21). "Cidofovir itself is active against smallpox but has to be given intravenously which limits its usefulness," says researcher Karl Hostetler (Veterans Affairs Medical Center and University of California, San Diego,

CA, USA). "Provided it passes all the necessary toxicity and safety tests, HDP-cidofovir could be self-administered." And, he adds, "Because it is also active against cytomegalovirus and herpes, varicella zoster, and Epstein Barr viruses, the agent might also be of use in more common diseases."

Other antivirals similar to Cidofovir are being investigated. These include Adefovir (Hepsera), which is used in the treatment of chronic hepatitis B with evidence of active viral replication including patients with lamivudine-resistant hepatitis B. A nucleotide analog—Adefovir dipivoxil—has demonstrated antipoxvirus activity but is still under investigation as a potential therapy for Orthopoxvirus infection (Fig. 42-9).

Unlike Cidofovir (Vistide), Adefovir (Hepsera) is an oral medication. Usual dose is 10 mg once daily. Patients with Clcr 20–39 mL/min: 10 mg every 48 hours. Clcr 10–19 mL/min: 10 mg every 72 hours.

Adefovir is a pregnancy category C risk. Lactic acidosis and severe hepatomegaly with steatosis (sometimes fatal) have occurred. Safety in pediatric patients has not been established. Adverse events include but are not limited to rash, pruritus, nausea, vomiting, diarrhea, abdominal pain, fever, and headache.

AUTOPSY

A case of smallpox would likely be considered a criminal event as well as a public health alert. As such, Federal agents and law enforcement are likely to become involved. Such non-health care professionals may not be accustomed to biosafety protocols nor be proficient in the use of PPE or infection control measures.

An autopsy may subject prosectors, laboratorians, security and pathologists as well as others to blood-borne and aerosolized pathogens. Realize Variola can be a viable pathogen on Fomites, in the air or contact. These risks can be significantly reduced through preparation, PPE and biosafety measures. Advanced planning that includes logistics, availability of cold storage and handling mass numbers of the dead, including collaboration with DMORT and local coroners is essential. Understanding evidence chain of custody, implementing strict infection control procedures, cross training with other responder professionals before an event to acquaint them with proper protocols and PPE should allow for safe evaluation of smallpox or other poxvirus victims.

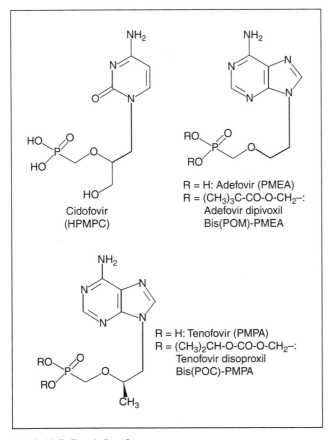

FIGURE 42-9

STRUCTURE OF CIDOFOVIR AND ANALOGUES
Source: From Erik De Clercq E. Clinical Potential of the Acyclic Nucleoside Phosphonates Cidofovir, Adefovir, and Tenofovir in Treatment of DNA Virus and Retrovirus Infections. Expert Rev Anti Infect Ther. 2003;1:23–24.

CONCLUSION

The poxviruses are a persistent health threat especially in Africa. In 2003 the first cases of monkeypox appeared in the United States and with it the realization that global pathogens can be imported through our borders. Smallpox and monkeypox pose an additional threat as potential biological weapons. There are numerous clinical "look alikes" to the poxviruses, especially varicella (chickenpox), which is a vaccine preventable disease. Preparedness efforts should emphasize varicella and other appropriate vaccinations, awareness of emerging pathogens, consistent training and updates, availability of antiviral medications and PPE, including practice with PPE, skills building exercises to test smallpox response plans, and close interaction with public health, infectious disease experts and preparedness officials.

Newer vaccines and antiviral countermeasures are being developed as is increased surveillance systems nationwide. Containing smallpox or other poxvirus infections depends upon early diagnosis, implementation of infection control measures, coordination of preparedness and response agencies, rapid administration of countermeasures, and effective communications with the public and across health-care and other emergency organizations. The CDC provides updates, preparedness guidance, and response assist; emergency departments should collaborate with local health departments in preparedness exercises and be familiar with procedures necessary to alert public health and the CDC.

Suggested Reading

Barclay L. Monkeypox Outbreak in the US: An expert interview with Cathy Roth, MD. Medscape Medical News 2003. Last accessed 5/18/06. *http://ww.medscape.com/viewarticle/457247*

Bioterrorism and Weapons of Mass Destruction 2004: Physicians as first responders. The DO. 2004; Mar Suppl:9–23.

Centers for Disease Control (CDC). Smallpox. *www.cdc.gov*

Diven DG. An overview of poxviruses. *J Am Acad Derm.* 2001;4(1):1–14.

Foster D. Smallpox as a biological weapon: implications for the critical care clinician. *Dimensions Crit Care Nursing.* 2003;22:2–7.

Goff A, Twenhafel N, Garrison A, Mucker E, et al. In vivo imaging of cidofovir treatment of cowpox virus infection. *virus res* 2007 May 22.

Halloran ME, Longini IM, Nizam A, et al. Containing bioterrorist smallpox. *Science.* 2002;298:1428–1432.

Henderson DA. *Emerging Infectious Diseases*—Special Issue—Smallpox: Clinical and Epidemiologic Features. *www.cdc.gov. ncidod/eid/vol5no4/henderson.htm*

Hirsch MS. ACP Medicine Online 2002; 10/02. Last accessed 5/18/06. *http://www.medscape.com/viewarticle/526732_print*

Ippolito G, Nicastri E, Capobianchi M, et al. Hospital preparedness and management of patients affected by viral haemorrhagic fever or smallpox at the Lazzaro Spallanzani Institute, Italy. *Eurosurveillance.* 2005; Mar 1–3;10:36–39.

Jones SW, Dobson ME, Francesconi SC, et al. *DNA Assays for Detection, Identification and Individualization of Select Agent Microorganisms; The Armed Forces Institute of Pathology, Division of Microbiology.* Washington, DC. Croatian Medical Journal 2005; 46(4):522–529.

Karupiah G, Panchanathan V, Sakala IG, Chaudhri G. Genetic resistance to smallpox: lessons from mousepox. Novartis Found Symp. 2007;281:129-36; discussion 136-40, 208-9.

Karem KL, Reynolds M, Braden Z, et al. Characterization of acute-phase humoral immunity to monkeypox: Use of immunoglobulin M enzyme-linked immunosorbent assay (ELISA) for detection of monkeypox infection during the 2003 North American Outbreak. *Clin Diag Lab Immunol.* 2005;(July)12(7):867–972.

Kern ER. In vitro activity of potential anti-poxvirus agents. *Antiviral Res.* 2003; Jan: 57(1–2):35–40.

Kim-Farley RJ, Celentano JT, Gunter C, et al. Standardized emergency management system and response to a smallpox emergency. *Prehospital Disaster Med.* 2003 Oct–Dec;18(4): 313–320.

Krugman S, Katz SL, Gershon AA, et al. Smallpox (variola_ and vaccinia, In: *Infectious Diseases of Children.* 9th ed. St. Louis, MO: Mosby, 1992, pp 457–462.

Lewis-Jones S. Zoonotic poxvirus infections in humans. *Curr Opin Infect Dis.* 2004 Apr;17(2):81–89.

McFee RB. Preparing for an era of weapons of mass destruction (WMD): Are we there yet? Why we should all be concerned. Part 1. *Vet Human Tox.* 2002;44(4):193–199.

Nalca A, Rimoin AW, Bavari S, et al. Reemergence of monkeypox: prevalence, diagnostics, and countermeasures. *Clin Infect Dis* 2005 Dec 15; 41(12):1765–71.

Nolte KB, Taylor DG, Richmond JY: Biosafety considerations for autopsy. *Am J Forensic Med Pathol,*. 2002;23(2):607–622.

Neff JM. Variola (smallpox) and monkeypox viruses. In: Mandell G, Douglas RG, Bennett J, eds. *Principles and Practice of Infectious Diseases.* 5th ed. New York, NY: Churchill Livingstone 2000, pp 1555–1556.

O'Byrne WT, Terndrup TE, Kiefe CI, et al. A primer on biological weapons for the clinician, Part I. *AdvStud Med.* 2003;3(2): 75–86.

Precopio ML, Betts MR, Parrino J, Immunization with vaccinia virus induces polyfunctional and phenotypically distinctive CD8+ T cell responses. *J Exp Med* 2007 May 29.

Reed KD, Melski JW, Graham MB, et al. The detection of monkeypox in humans in the Western Hemisphere. *N Engl J Med.* 2004 Jan 22;350(4):342–350.

Saini R, Pui JC, Burgin S. Rickettsialpox: Report of three cases and a review. *J Am Acad Derm.* 2004;51:S137–39.

Smee DF, Sidwell RW, Kefauver D, et al. Characterization of Wild Type and Cidofovir resistant Strains of Camelpox, Cowpox, Monkeypox and Vaccinia Virus. 2002 May; 46(5):1329–1335.

Sliva K, Schnierle B, From actually toxic to highly specific-novel drugs against poxviruses. *Virology* 2007, 4:8 http://www.virologyj.com/content/4/1/8. last accessed 6/4/07.

U.S. Army Medical Research Institute of Infectious Diseases. *USAMRIID's Medical Management of Biological Casualties Handbook.* 4th ed. 2001 Fort Detrick, Frederick, MD.

Yang G, Pevear DC, Davies MH, et al. An orally bioavailable antipoxvirus compound (ST-246) inhibits extracellular virus formation and protects mice from lethal orthopoxvirus challenge *J Urinol* 79(20):13139–49.

43

TULAREMIA

Kerstin Dostal and Daniel R. Rodgers

STAT FACTS

TULAREMIA

- Tularemia is a zoonosis caused by *Francisella tularensis*, a gram-negative coccobacillus.
- *F. tularensis* has the potential to cause severe disease by the airborne route with a low infectious dose.
- The most serious clinical manifestations are pneumonic and typhoidal tularemia while the most common is ulceroglandular disease.
- In a bioterrorism event, tularemia would most likely present as a clustering of acute, severe, respiratory illness in previously healthy adults.
- Definitive diagnosis is established with serologic testing as the organism is not present in large numbers in blood or sputum and is difficult to cultivate.
- In mass casualty situations, oral tetracyclines or fluoroquinolones should be used to treat adults, children, and pregnant women both for active disease and postexposure prophylaxis.

HISTORY

Discovery

Tularemia was first recognized in 1837 as a febrile illness characterized by generalized lymphadenopathy in people who had eaten infected rabbit meat. In 1912, GW McCoy isolated the causative organism from ground squirrels in Tulare County, CA. Public Health Officer Edward Francis isolated the bacteria from human blood in 1919; he named the blood-borne disease tularemia. Tularemia has also been known as rabbit fever, deerfly fever, and lemming fever.

Potential as a Biological Weapon

Between 1932 and 1945, Japanese germ-warfare units studied tularemia as a potential biologic weapon during the World War II occupation of Manchuria. In the United States, tularemia was maintained as a biologic weapon until an executive order terminated all biological warfare development in 1969. The Soviet Union also maintained stocks of weaponized tularemia with reports of strains engineered for resistance to antibiotics and vaccines. In his book *Biohazard*, former Soviet biologic weapons expert Dr Ken Alibek alleges the Soviet Union used tularemia against German troops during the battle for Stalingrad in 1942. Others believe that a naturally occurring outbreak, facilitated by the conditions of war, was a more likely explanation for the epidemic.

In 1969, the World Health Organization carried out a number of modeling studies to predict the effects of the airborne release of weaponized *Francisella tularensis*. They estimated that an aerosol dispersal of 50 kg of virulent *F. tularensis* over a metropolitan area with 5 million inhabitants would result in 250,000 incapacitating casualties, including 19,000 deaths with illnesses and relapses persisting for weeks to months.

PROPERTIES

Microbiology

F. tularensis is a small, aerobic, nonmotile, faintly staining, gram-negative coccobacillus. It has a thin lipopolysaccharide-containing envelope and is a hardy, nonspore-forming organism that survives for weeks at low temperatures in water, soil, animal carcasses, hides, and hay.

There are four major subspecies of *F. tularensis*: *tularensis, holarctica, novicida,* and *mediasiatica*. Strains of subspecies *tularensis* (Jellison Type A) are considered the most virulent in humans with an infectious dose of 10 bacteria when injected subcutaneously and 25 when inhaled as aerosol. It is the wild type found in North America. Strains of the subspecies *holarctica* (Jellison Type B) have a low mortality rate in humans and are found in Europe and Asia. Subspecies *novicida* and *mediasiatica* are not particularly virulent in immunocompetent humans.

Transmission

Zoonosis

Tularemia is a widespread zoonotic disease with isolation of the bacterium from at least 250 species of wildlife including rabbits, hares, beavers, and muskrats. The natural reservoir of *F. tularensis* is unclear with theories including aquatic mammals, ticks, amoebic cysts, and protozoa.

Human Infection

Blood feeding arthropods and flies are the most important vectors for tularemia in the US. Humans become infected through arthropod bites, contact with infectious animal tissues or fluids, direct contact with contaminated water or soil, or inhalation of infective aerosols. Person-to-person transmission has not been documented although illness may occur in families.

Ticks are responsible for approximately 75% of cases in the United States. In Eurasia, mosquito-borne infection regularly occurs in Scandinavian and Baltic regions.

EPIDEMIOLOGY

Geographic Distribution

Tularemia is endemic throughout much of the Northern Hemisphere between latitudes 30° North and 71° North. In Eurasia, tularemia is a rural disease and is most frequently seen in Sweden, Finland, and Russia.

Incidence

Worldwide incidence of tularemia is unknown, and the disease is probably underrecognized and underreported. During the 1990s, the United States reported an average of 125 cases per year. Persons in all age groups were affected, but most were children younger than 10 years and adults 50 years or older. Japan currently reports <10 cases a year. In Europe, most outbreaks occur in epidemics with no reported steady incidence.

Tularemia has a bimodal distribution with most cases occurring in spring and early summer secondary to arthropod bites. A second peak occurs during the winter months in association with hunting or other direct contact with infected animals.

CLINICAL MANIFESTATIONS

Tularemia's clinical appearance will vary depending on the site of inoculation, virulence of the organism, and number of infecting organisms. Skin and mucosal inoculations result in ulceroglandular or, more rarely, oculoglandular tularemia. Oral ingestion results in an oropharyngeal syndrome whereas inhalation causes tularemia pneumonia.

Tularemia is an illness characterized by several distinct forms; their clinical syndromes, as outlined in Table 43-1 have extensive overlap. The incubation period is usually 3–5 days with a range of 1–21 days. All are associated with the abrupt onset of vague constitutional symptoms including fever, chills, myalgias, fatigue, dry cough, and occasional pulse- temperature dissociation. All are associated with the abrupt onset of vague constitutional symptoms including fever, chills, myalgias, fatigue, dry cough and can also manifest pulse-temperature dissociation, also referred to as relative bradycardia. Without treatment, nonspecific symptoms can persist for several weeks causing progressive weakness, anorexia, and weight loss.

All forms of tularemia may lead to hematogenous spread and have been associated with meningitis, pericarditis, hepatitis, peritonitis, endocarditis, osteomyelitis, sepsis,

TABLE 43-1

CLINICAL PRESENTATIONS OF TULAREMIA

Presentation	Findings
Ulceroglandular	Cutaneous ulcer at site of inoculation
	Proximal lymphadenopathy, may suppurate
	Majority of naturally occurring cases
Glandular	Lymphadenopathy, may suppurate
	No evidence of cutaneous involvement (ulcer)
Oropharyngeal	Stomatitis, exudative or ulcerative pharyngitis tonsillitis
	Cervical lymphadenopathy
Pneumonic	Pulmonary involvement ± systemic findings
	Most likely presentation associated with aerosol exposure
Typhoidal	Febrile illness
	Systemic involvement without evidence of skin, mucosal, or lymphatic involvement
Oculoglandular	Ocular lesion, painful unilateral purulent conjunctivitis
	Cervical and preauricular lymphadenopathy

Source: Adapted from Cronquist SD. Tularemia: the disease and the weapon. Dermatologic Clinics. 2004;22:313–320. Reprinted with permission from Elsevier.

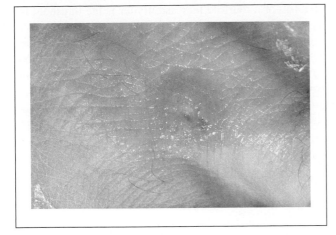

FIGURE 43-1

ULCER CAUSED BY FRANCISELLA TULARENSIS
Source: Courtesy of Dr Bachman, CDC.

septic shock with rhabdomyolysis, and acute renal failure. Children have similar presentations but have been reported to exhibit fever, pharyngitis, hepatosplenomegaly, and constitutional symptoms more often than affected adults.

Ulceroglandular

Ulceroglandular tularemia (Fig. 43-1) is the most common naturally occurring form of the disease and accounts for 75–85% of cases. It presents after inoculation from arthropod bites or after the handling of infected carcasses via previous cuts or abrasions. The most common sites of infection are the hands and distal extremities.

The infection begins as a tender, occasionally pruritic papule 2–5 days after exposure at the site of inoculation. The papule enlarges and ulcerates to a lesion (0.4–3 cm) with sharp demarcated borders, often covered by a thin layer of exudate. Gradually, the base of the ulcer becomes necrotic with a black eschar; this occurs when regional adenopathy is noted. Regional lymph nodes enlarge (0.5–10 cm), become tender with overlying erythema, and often suppurate. The original ulcer may persist for months before healing.

Glandular

Glandular tularemia (Fig. 43-2) is seen in 5–10% of naturally occurring cases. It is characterized by fever and tender lymphadenopathy without primary cutaneous findings.

Oropharyngeal

Oropharyngeal tularemia, a rare disease, is caused by the ingestion of infected soil, water, or inadequately cooked meat. It is characterized by exudative pharyngitis or tonsillitis with or without ulcerations. Cervical lymphadenopathy and stomatitis are frequently seen. Oropharyngeal tularemia may progress to more severe gastrointestinal disease. Symptoms range from mild but persistent diarrhea to an acute fatal disease with extensive ulceration of the bowel. In 2000, an outbreak of

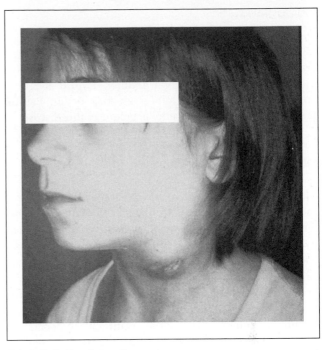

FIGURE 43-2

SUPPURATIVE LYMPHADENOPATHY IN A GIRL WITH TULAREMIA
Source: From Reintjes R, Dedushaj I, Gjini A, et al. Tularemia outbreak investigation in Kosovo: case control and environmental studies. Emerg Infect Diseases. 2002;8:69–73.

372 cases in Kosovo (former Yugoslavia) was traced to rodent infestation of food and water supplies.

Pneumonia

Tularemia pneumonia carries a high case fatality rate if untreated, is caused by direct inhalation of infected aerosols or by hematogenous spread of other primary forms of tularemia. Symptoms include fevers and nonproductive cough with possible dyspnea or pleuritic chest pain. Some patients may develop hemoptysis with mucopurulent sputum. Physical findings are similar to atypical pneumonias with diffuse or localized crackles. Pleural rubs are common.

Chest radiographic findings vary widely and may include apical or miliary infiltrates, single or multiple lobar infiltrates, bronchopulmonary infiltrates, pleural effusions, and cavitations. Hilar lymphadenopathy is commonly seen. The classically described triad of oval opacities, hilar adenopathy, and pleural effusions is rarely seen.

Typhoidal

Typhoidal tularemia is characterized by persistent high fevers and constitutional symptoms in the absence of an obvious site of inoculation or anatomic localization of infection. Patients typically appear toxic and may develop delirium, coma, and septic shock. Findings may include evidence of rhabdomyolysis, hepatitis, DIC, and advanced respiratory disease syndrome (ARDS).

Oculoglandular

Oculoglandular tularemia is a rare manifestation caused by direct inoculation of the eye. It is characterized by unilateral purulent conjunctivitis with chemosis and occasional discrete yellow conjunctival nodules. Eyelid swelling, corneal ulceration, and hypopyon may occur. Painful preauricular lymphadenopathy is unique to this disease.

DIFFERENTIAL DIAGNOSIS

The differential of glandular and ulceroglandular tularemia includes any disease with fever and acute regional lymphadenopathy: *Staphylococcus aureus* or *Streptococcus pyogenes* lymphadenitis, plague, cat-scratch disease, sporotrichosis, syphilis, anthrax, LGV, chancroid, deep fungal infection, atypical mycobacterial infections, or brown recluse spider bites. Oropharyngeal tularemia may resemble pharyngitis caused by β-hemolytic strep or diphtheria. Tularemia pneumonia is difficult to distinguish from many of the atypical pneumonias caused by *Mycoplasma* and *Chlamydia* species, legionellosis, Q fever, histoplasmosis, and viral pneumonias. Typhoidal tularemia must be differentiated from typhoid fever, other salmonelloses, brucellosis, and various rickettsial diseases.

LAB STUDIES NEEDED

Specimen Collection

The physician must notify the laboratory of any suspicion of tularemia as it is highly infectious. Routine diagnostic procedures can be performed in a biological safety level 2 laboratory under a biological safety cabinet. When tularemia is presumptively identified, specimens should be forwarded to a biological safety level 3 facility for further testing. The state public health department should be consulted immediately.

Blood, tissue, or fluid aspirates are collected for diagnosis. Biopsied tissue or ulcer scrapings are preferable to swabs of ulcerations.

Diagnostic Testing

Routine laboratory testing shows no abnormalities specific to tularemia. In a study of 88 patients with subspecies. *tularensis* infection, white blood cell counts ranged from 5000 to 22,000 with a median count of 10,400. The differential showed a slight lymphocytosis. Liver enzyme values were also somewhat increased.

The definitive diagnosis is established with serologic testing as the organism is not present in large numbers in blood or sputum. Tularemia tube agglutination testing is the most commonly used serological test. An acute phase titer of 1:160 or a fourfold increase in titer is the threshold for the diagnosis of tularemia. Unfortunately, diagnostic titers seldom develop until 11–21 days after the onset of illness.

Over the past decades, additional diagnostic methods have been used. They vary from enzyme-liked immunosorbent assay testing (ELISA/Western Blot) to a range of PCR products to directly identify the organism's DNA. Antigen fluorescence testing (DFA/TRF) may be performed directly on tissue specimens for diagnosis.

TREATMENT

Acute disease

Adults

In isolated cases of tularemia, streptomycin is the historically preferred treatment. The recommended dose is 1 g or 10 mg/kg IM twice daily for 10 days. Gentamicin is a more available and acceptable alternative. The recommended dose of gentamicin is 5 mg/kg IM or IV for 10–14 days. Chloramphenicol is another alternative.

In mass exposures of tularemia, tetracyclines and fluoroquinolones should be used. Treatment with tetracyclines, most commonly doxycycline 100 mg IV or PO twice daily, should last 14–21 days since high rates of relapse have been reported. Fluoroquinolones have recently demonstrated efficacy with ciprofloxacin at 400 mg IV or 500 mg PO twice daily for 10–14 days or streptomycin 7.5 – 10 mg/kg every 12 hours for 10–14 days as an acceptable treatment.

Special Populations

Children are treated with the same antibiotics as adults. Streptomycin at 15 mg/kg IM every 12 hours with a maximum dose of 2 g/day is the preferred treatment, but gentamicin may be used. In mass casualty situations, children should be treated with doxycycline or ciprofloxacin; the benefits of treating pediatric patients with these antibiotics outweigh the risks. Doxycycline is dosed at 100 mg twice a day for children over 45 kg and 2.2 mg/kg for children under 45 kg. Ciprofloxacin dosing recommendations are 15 mg/kg orally twice daily with a maximum dose limited to 1 g/day.

Pregnant patients should be treated with the same antibiotics as other adults. The preferred antibiotic is gentamicin since it has not been reported to produce fetal ototoxicity and nephrotoxicity. The benefits of using ciprofloxacin or doxycycline in a mass casualty situation outweigh the risks of treatment.

Disposition

Patients with typhoidal or pneumonic tularemia should be admitted to an intensive care unit setting. Other patients should be admitted to the hospital until a definitive diagnosis is made and until fever subsides. Only standard precautions are necessary as tularemia does not demonstrate person-to-person transmission.

Prognosis

With successful antibiotic treatment, most patients become afebrile in 2–3 days. Cutaneous lesions may take an additional 1–2 weeks to heal. If treatment is delayed for days to weeks, the response to treatment will take longer. Lymph node suppuration may occur regardless of successful response to treatment. Overall mortality is 1% with treatment.

If untreated, signs and symptoms typically last 1–4 weeks, but may even persist for months. Mortality may be as high as 30% in untreated cases of pneumonic or typhoidal tularemia.

Prophylaxis

Vaccination

In the 1960s, a live vaccine strain of *F. tularensis* was approved by the FDA for immunization of laboratory workers who were at risk of infection. The vaccine was then withdrawn for fear of possible reversion to full or partial virulence, especially in immunocompromised individuals. Though the search for a safe vaccine continues, there is currently no licensed vaccine for tularemia.

Postexposure Prophylaxis

Patients who have been exposed to an aerosol release of tularemia should be treated prophylactically with 14 days of oral ciprofloxacin or doxycycline and watched closely. If any fever or ulceration occurs, they would begin treatment for acute disease.

Postexposure prophylactic antibiotic treatment of close contacts of tularemia patients is not recommended since human-to-human transmission is not known to occur. Isolation of patients with tularemia is not necessary for the same reasons but standard precautions are recommended.

ENVIRONMENTAL DECONTAMINATION

F. tularensis may survive for extended periods in a cold, moist environment. Decontamination can be achieved by spraying a contaminated area with a 10% bleach solution. After 10 minutes, a 70% solution of alcohol can be used to further clean the area and reduce the corrosive action of bleach. Persons with direct exposure should wash body surfaces and clothing with soap and water. Standard levels of chlorine in municipal water sources should protect against waterborne infection.

SUSPICION OF BIOTERRORISM

The first indication of intentional tularemia release would follow recognition of a clustering of acute, severe, respiratory illness with unusual epidemiological features: the abrupt onset of large numbers of acute, nonspecific febrile illness in about 3–5 days with a variation from 1 to 14 days. A spectrum of respiratory disease from bronchitis to life-threatening pleuropneumonitis would develop in a significant number of previously healthy adults.

AUTOPSY

An autopsy subjects lab, pathology and other personnel to blood borne and aerosolized pathogens. Tularemia is a well recognized airborne risk to laboratory personnel. It is essential to notify laboratorians, pathologists and other HCF personnel who may become involved in the case about the risk of tularemia and the need for heightened biosafety as well as the need for appropriate PPE.

Suggested Reading

Cunha BA, Quintiliani R. The atypical pneumonia: A diagnostic and therapeutic approach. *Post Grad Med* 1979 Sep; 66(3): 95–102.

Cronquist SD. Tularemia: the disease and the weapon. *Dermatologic Clinics.* 2004;22:313–320.

Dennis DT. Tularemia, In: Strickland GT, ed. *Hunter's Tropical Medicine and Emerging Infectious Diseases, 8th ed.* Philadelphia, PA: W.B. Saunders Company, 2000; pp. 411–415.

Dennis DT, Inglesby TV, Henderson DA. Tularemia as a biological weapon. *JAMA.* 2001;285(21):2763–2773.

Ellis J, Oyston PCF, Green M, et al. Tularemia. *Clin Microbiol Rev.* 2002;15(4):631–646.

Martin GJ, Marty AM. Clinicopathologic aspects of bacterial agents. *Clin Lab Med.* 2001;21(3):513–548.

Nolte KB, Taylor DG, Richmond JY. Biosafety considerations for autopsy. *Am J Forens Med and Path* 2002;23 (2):107–122.

Oyston PCF, Sjostedt A, Richard WT. Tularemia: bioterrorism defense renews interest in Francisella tularensis. *Nat Rev Microbiol.* 2004;2:967–978.

Stocker JT. Clinical and pathologic differential diagnosis of selected potential bioterrorism agents of interest to pediatric health care providers. *Clin Lab Med* 2006 Jun; 26(2):329–44, viii.

Tarnvik A, Berglund L. Tularemia. *Eur Res J.* 2003;21:361–373.

Tularemia–a publication of the Office of Public Health, Louisiana Department of Health and Hospitals. 2004 – 21 Dec. www.infectiousdisease.loiusiana.gov. Last accessed 6/4/07.

44

HEMORRHAGIC FEVER

Jonathan Bankoff and Trevonne M. Thompson

STAT FACTS
HEMORRHAGIC FEVER

- Viral hemorrhagic fevers pose a significant threat as a terror weapon
  - Highly infectious
  - Extremely virulent
  - Low infectious dose
  - High morbidity and mortality
  - Few treatment options
- Primary features
  - Incubation period that ranges from 2 to 21days
  - Begins as a flu-like illness
  - Can progress to multiorgan failure
  - Bleeding manifestations common
  - Each etiologic agent has its own distinct clinical presentation
- Infection control is crucial
  - Prevent patient to patient transmission
  - Prevent patient to health-care personnel transmission

INTRODUCTION

A number of viruses are considered likely candidates for use as biological weapons: smallpox, viruses that cause encephalitis, and viruses that cause hemorrhagic fever. Some viruses, such as smallpox, have been a concern for years. Others, such as West Nile virus, are just emerging as threats to public health.

Viruses causing hemorrhagic fever (VHFs) poses a significant threat as terror weapons for several reasons. They are widely distributed in nature and are both stable and highly infectious by airborne means. They are extremely virulent, have a low infectious dose, and demonstrate a high rate of replication, potentially leading to high morbidity and mortality for both military and civilian populations.

The differential diagnosis for viral hemorrhagic fever (VHF) encompasses a wide variety of infectious organisms, making initial recognition of a VHF virus attack difficult to distinguish from other threats without sophisticated and time-consuming laboratory analysis. Most importantly, VHFs have limited therapeutic and prophylactic options and require intensive care support and monitoring, often impractical in the face of a mass casualty situation.

Epidemiologic Overview

VHFs are a group of febrile illnesses caused by RNA viruses from several viral families. The U.S. Army Medical Research Institute of Infectious Diseases lists four RNA viral families as the prime etiologic agents for VHFs in humans: (1) the Arenaviridae; (2) the Bunyaviridae; (3) the Filoviridae; and (4) the Flaviviridae. Despite the diverse taxonomy of this group, these viruses share some common characteristics (Table 44-1).

They are all relatively simple RNA viruses, and they all have lipid envelopes. This renders them relatively susceptible to detergents, as well as to low-pH environments and household bleach. Conversely, they are quite stable at neutral pH, especially when protein is present. Thus, these viruses are stable in blood for long periods and can be isolated from a patient's blood after weeks of storage at refrigerator or even at ambient temperatures. These viruses tend to be stable and highly infectious as fine-particle aerosols. These characteristics not only have great significance in the natural transmission cycle but also make nosocomial transmission a concern. Although human-to-human spread is possible, pandemics are unlikely.

Most hemorrhagic fever viruses that cause disease in humans occur in relatively localized areas of the world (notably sub-Saharan Africa and focal areas of South America). As a group, the viruses are linked to the ecology of their vectors or reservoirs, generally rodents or arthropods.

TABLE 44-1

MICROBIOLOGY OF HEMORRHAGIC FEVER VIRUSES

Family	Diameter, nm	Morphology	Presence of Envelope	Genome Size, kbp	Genome Nature*	Genome Configuration
Filoviridae	80	Bacilliform (filamentous)	Yes	19	Single-strand RNA (–)	Nonsegmented (1 – segment)
Arenaviridae	110–130	Spherical	Yes	11	Single-strand RNA (±)	2 ± Segments
Bunyaviridae	80–120	Spherical	Yes	11–19	Single-strand RNA (–)	3 – Segments
Flaviviridae	40–50	Spherical	Yes	10–12	Single-strand RNA (+)	Nonsegmented (1 + segment)

*Minus sign indicates negative-strand genome; plus sign, positive-strand genome; and plus/minus sign, ampisense genome.
Source: From Henderson DA, Inglesby TV, O'Toole T (eds). Bioterrorism: Guidelines for Medical and Public Health Management. Chicago: AMA Press, 2002, p. 199.

In that regard, most of these reservoirs tend to be rural, and a patient's history of being in a rural locale is an important factor to consider when reaching a diagnosis.

Cases of VHF in the United States are extremely rare and are usually found in patients who recently have visited endemic areas or among those with potential occupational exposure to hemorrhagic fever viruses. The major geographic location and general pattern of occurrence for each virus will be discussed in the context of their individual viral family.

The Arenaviridae

Arenaviruses are spherical or pleomorphic enveloped single-stranded bisegmented ambisense viruses (110–130 nm in diameter) that use virion ribonucleic acid (RNA)-dependent RNA polymerase for replication. All the arenaviruses are maintained in nature by a lifelong association with a rodent reservoir. Rodents spread the virus to humans, and outbreaks can usually be related to some perturbation in the ecosystem that brings man into contact with the rodents.

There are 18 arenavirus species, classified into the Old World and New World groups, with at least 7 causing hemorrhagic fever: (1) Lassa fever virus (Lassa fever), (2) Junin virus (Argentine hemorrhagic fever), (3) Machupo virus (Bolivian hemorrhagic fever), (4) Guanarito virus (Venezuelan hemorrhagic fever), (5) Sabia virus (Brazilian hemorrhagic fever with extensive hepatic necrosis), (6) Whitewater Arroyo virus (hemorrhagic fever with liver failure), and (7) Oliverous virus (hemorrhagic fever).

Lassa fever is a disease that has become endemic in West Africa over the past 30 years. Rodents are the primary reservoir for Lassa virus and, while nosocomial infections do occur, most Lassa virus infections can be traced to the carrier rodent, *Mastomys natilensis*, through contact with virus-containing aerosols of rodent excreta. The incidence of disease is highest during the dry season, although infections can occur year-round. An estimated 100,000–300,000 Lassa fever virus infections occur annually in West Africa, where it is associated with 10–15% of adult febrile admissions to the hospital and perhaps 40% of nonsurgical deaths. It is estimated to cause 5000 deaths annually, yielding an overall 1% mortality rate. In addition, Lassa fever is a common pediatric disease and the cause of high mortality in pregnant women.

New World hemorrhagic fever is caused by several different arenaviruses, most commonly Junin, Machupo, and Guanarito viruses. Most cases have occurred in regional areas of South America, although Whitewater Arroyo virus was recently identified as a cause of VHF in California. Similar to Lassa virus, these viruses appear to be transmitted via contact with rodents or virus-containing aerosols of rodent excreta. Despite recent sporadic outbreaks, New World hemorrhagic fever remains relatively uncommon and for some viruses (e.g., Sabia and Whitewater Arroyo virus), only a handful of cases have been recognized to date.

The Bunyaviridae

Bunyaviruses are a family of animal and plant viruses consisting of 51 species, divided into 5 genera. The bunyaviruses are spherical enveloped viruses (80–120 nm in diameter). The genome consists of a large, medium, and small single-stranded negative-sense RNA, and all members of the family contain viral sense RNA.

Among the bunyaviruses, the *Phlebovirus* genus is the most significant in regard to human pathogens and includes the Rift Valley fever (RVF) virus. RVF is a mosquito-borne disease primarily found in sub-Saharan and North Africa. Human illnesses generally are mild, although severe forms of disease (i.e., VHF, meningoencephalitis) occur in about 1% of cases. Outbreaks of RVF most often occur after heavy rainfalls, floods, and natural depressions. The flooding allows extensive hatching of the primary mosquito vector. RVF is also a disease of domestic livestock, and human infections have resulted from contact with infected animal blood, especially around slaughterhouses.

The *Nairovirus* genus consists of several tick-borne viruses, with Crimean-Congo hemorrhagic fever (CCHF) being the most prevalent and most severe. It has been associated with sporadic, yet particularly virulent, VHF in Europe, Africa, and Asia. CCHF has frequently occurred as small, hospital-centered outbreaks, owing to the copious hemorrhage and highly infective nature of this virus via the aerosol route. The Nairovirus can survive through various tick life-stages and from tick generation to generation.

The members of the *Hantavirus* genus, unlike the other bunyaviruses, are not transmitted via infected arthropods; rather, they infect man via contact with infected rodents and their excreta. The prototype virus from this group, Hantaan, is borne in nature by the striped field mouse, *Apodemus agrarious*. It is the cause of Korean hemorrhagic fever, as well as the severe form of hemorrhagic fever with renal syndrome (HFRS).

At least 3 subfamilies and 28 species of hantaviruses are associated with HFRS, including Puumala virus, which is associated with chronically infected bank voles (*Clethrionomys glareolus*). Recently in the southwestern United States, a new hantavirus (Sin nombre virus) has been associated with the hantavirus pulmonary syndrome (HPS), with a reservoir in the deer mouse, *Peromyscus maniculatus*. As many as 10 different hantaviruses with 10 different rodent reservoirs have been shown to cause HPS throughout North and South America.

The Filoviridae

The most notorious of the VHF viruses, Ebola and Marburg, make up the two genera of the Filoviridae. Both genera are enveloped, single-stranded negative-sense RNA viruses (80 nm in diameter). Ebola is bacilliform, bent pin-shaped; Marburg is filamentous-shaped. There are four species of Ebola virus (Zaire, Sudan, Reston, and Cote D'Ivoire) and one species of Marburg virus. The Zaire species of Ebola is the most virulent (60–90% case fatality rate) and the Reston species is the least virulent.

Ebola hemorrhagic fever is an important emerging infection in central Africa and has received much attention in recent years. Much is still unknown about Ebola virus transmission, natural reservoirs, disease pathogenesis, and treatment. Since the discovery of Ebola virus, a geographic pattern has emerged in which the Zaire strain affects predominantly central Africa, the Sudan strain affects East Africa, and the Ivory Coast strain affects West Africa. In some situations, human Ebola outbreaks have occurred in conjunction with outbreaks in animal species including gorillas, chimpanzees, and duikers (small antelopes).

Marburg hemorrhagic fever, like Ebola, is an emerging disease in sub-Saharan Africa, although Marburg appears to be less common. Similar to the situation with Ebola, the natural reservoirs and exact patterns of transmission have not been fully elucidated and pathogenesis and treatment have not been clarified. Case-fatality rates may be somewhat lower than those for Ebola virus infection. The case-fatality rate for the most recent, and largest, outbreak was 88%.

The Flaviviridae

The flaviviruses are spherical, enveloped, single-stranded, positive-sense RNA viruses (40–50 nm in diameter), consisting of three genera: (1) Flavivirus (dengue virus, Japanese encephalitis virus, Kyasanur Forest disease virus, Omsk hemorrhagic fever virus, St Louis encephalitis virus, tick-borne encephalitis virus, West Nile Fever virus, and yellow fever virus); (2) Hepacivirus (hepatitis C virus); and (3) Pestivirus.

The vectors for yellow fever virus include several mosquito species. Illness can range from mild to severe, with an overall case-fatality rate of 5–7%. Three cycles have been recognized:

1. A sylvatic, or jungle cycle, that primarily involves transmission between mosquitoes and nonhuman primates, with humans as incidental hosts.
2. An urban cycle that involves transmission between mosquitoes and humans in urban areas. The most important mosquito vector is *Aedes aegypti*. Urban outbreaks can involve hundreds to thousands of people and pose a substantial public health threat.
3. An intermediate cycle that is found in villages in humid and semihumid savannahs of Africa, where small epidemics occur. This form involves semidomestic mosquitoes that can infect both humans and nonhuman primates.

Kyasanur Forest disease and Omsk hemorrhagic fever are relatively rare forms of tick-borne VHF found in India and central Asia, respectively. Rodents, monkeys, muskrats, and other small mammals are the natural reservoirs. Outbreaks occur periodically and are usually signaled by epizootics in the local monkey population.

Pathogenesis

The pathogenesis of hemorrhagic fever viruses is not completely understood; however, key points include the following:

- Hemorrhagic fever viruses enter the bloodstream through various mechanisms (e.g., the bite of a mosquito or tick, inhalation, mucous membrane exposure, parenteral exposure), and all (except hantaviruses) cause disease during the period of viremia.
- The infectious dose for hemorrhagic fever viruses appears to be low (1–10 organisms).
- Endothelial infection occurs with most VHF viruses and may be limited or widespread, depending on the virus.
- Hemorrhagic manifestations occur as a result of thrombocytopenia or severe platelet dysfunction along with endothelial dysfunction.
- Increased vascular permeability is common and may result in periorbital edema and hemoconcentration. Vascular dysregulation also often occurs, manifested by flushing of the face and chest.
- Hemorrhagic fever viruses can cause necrosis and hemorrhage in most organs; however, hepatic involvement often is particularly prominent.
- Hantaviruses, New World arenaviruses, and Ebola, Marburg, and Lassa viruses cause cytokine activation. It is unclear whether the other hemorrhagic fever viruses cause cytokine activation. This cytokine activation, coupled with pronounced macrophage involvement, leads to increased vascular permeability and shock.
- Ebola, Marburg, yellow fever, and Rift Valley fever viruses have a marked cytopathic effect (highly destructive to the cells they infect), whereas arenaviruses appear to cause a loss of cellular function without any obvious signs of cellular damage (not cytopathic or cytotoxic).

Clinical Presentations

Although clinical features vary somewhat for the various hemorrhagic fever viruses, the clinical presentations overlap substantially. The exact nature of the disease depends on viral virulence and strain characteristics, routes of exposure, dose, and host factors. The target organ in the VHF syndrome is the vascular bed; correspondingly, the dominant clinical features are usually a consequence of microvascular damage and changes in vascular permeability.

All of the VHF agents cause a febrile prodrome. Other common presenting complaints, described as VHF syndrome, are fever, myalgia, and prostration. In mild or early exposure, clinical examination may reveal only conjunctival injection, mild hypotension, flushing, and petechial hemorrhages. Full-blown VHF, however, typically evolves to shock and generalized bleeding from the mucous membranes, and often is accompanied by evidence of neurological, hematopoietic, or pulmonary involvement. Hepatic involvement is common, but a clinical picture dominated by jaundice and other evidence of hepatic failure is seen in only a small percentage of patients exposed to specific agents. Renal failure is proportional to cardiovascular compromise,

except in HFRS caused by hantaviruses, where it is an integral part of the disease process. VHF mortality may be substantial, ranging from less than 5–10% with certain agents to approximately 90% or higher, as seen in more recent Ebola outbreaks.

Some of the major clinical characteristics that help define and distinguish the VHFs are included below:

- Ebola hemorrhagic fever has an incubation period of 2–21 days. It presents as abrupt onset of fever, severe headache, myalgias, conjunctival injection, mucocutaneous bleeding, and abdominal pain and diarrhea. It commonly has a maculopapular truncal rash, which evolves into petechiae over several days. As the disease progresses, bleeding manifestations worsen, with mucosal hemorrhage, hematemesis, bloody diarrhea, and venipuncture oozing. Eventually, patients develop DIC, severe metabolic acidosis, and shock. Mortality rates by Day 10 range from 60% to 90%.
- Marburg hemorrhagic fever has a similar appearance to Ebola, with the only differences being a shorter incubation period (2–14 days), a less virulent course, and a lower mortality rate (20–30%).
- Lassa fever has an incubation period from 7 to 14 days. The onset of the disease is gradual, with fever, malaise, and diffuse myalgias followed by exudative pharyngitis and conjunctival injection. As the disease progresses, bleeding manifestations may develop, along with facial and laryngeal edema, cyanosis, and shock. In as many as 30% of patients, pleural and pericardial effusions will develop. Specific to Lassa fever, up to 30% of patients will develop eighth cranial nerve damage leading to permanent sensorineural deafness. Patients with mild disease usually improve within 10 days, and most infections are thought to be mild or subclinical; only 5–10% of Lassa fever infections are considered severe. As a result, the overall mortality rate is between 1–2%, with the highest percentages seen in pregnant women and children.
- The clinical features of the New World hemorrhagic fevers (arenaviruses) are very similar to that of Lassa fever. The only significant differences are more severe neurologic findings and higher overall mortality rates. These patients are often more irritable, lethargic, and display muscular hypotonia, areflexia, difficulty ambulating, and fluctuations in level of consciousness. Untreated, as many as 15–30 % of these patients die.
- Rift Valley fever has a 2–6-day incubation period. The disease onset is nonspecific, with a self-limited febrile illness, headaches, and myalgias. Similar to the other VHFs, generalized rash, abdominal pain, and diarrhea are common, Unique to RVF, however, is significant ocular findings. Most patients have severe photophobia and retro-orbital pain, and as many as 10% of patients develop retinitis. Half of these patients have permanent visual impairment. Overall, the mortality rate is <1%.

- Congo-Crimean hemorrhagic fever has two distinct incubations: 1–3 days for tick bites and 5–6 days following contact with contaminated blood. Patients present with sudden onset of fever, chills, headache, neck pain, and myalgia. They have swollen, tender lymphadenopathy and hepatomegaly. As the disease progresses, patients develop severe gastrointestinal bleeding and DIC, followed by hepatic and respiratory failure. There is a 30% overall mortality rate.
- Hantavirus has two separate presentations: HFRS and HPS.
  - HFRS has an incubation period of 2–3 weeks. It has several distinct clinical phases: (1) febrile, (2) hypotensive, (3) oliguric, (4) diuretic, and (5) convalescent. The initial presentation is similar to a flu-like illness with myalgias and conjunctival injection. The bleeding manifestations are usually mild and transient, compared to the other VHFs. If untreated, 50% of the deaths occur during the oliguric phase.
  - HPS incubation is typically 1–2 weeks, with the prodromal stage usually occurring within 3–5 days. Patients have an abrupt onset of fever, myalgia, chills, and headache. As the disease progresses, there is significant prostration, abdominal pain, nausea, vomiting, and diarrhea. In severe cases, patients develop pulmonary edema and acute respiratory distress syndrome.
  - Overall mortality rates for both presentations are between 7% and 10%.
- Dengue fever is the most common VHF. It has an incubation period of 2–7 days. It presents with "break bone fever," a sudden onset of high fevers, severe muscle pains, headache, and prostration with facial flushing and conjunctival injection. More than half of patients have an early transient rash and mild hemorrhagic signs. There is often a long convalescent period for those with mild dengue. For those with more severe classical illness, the initial symptoms progress rapidly to shock, with diaphoresis, hypotension, restlessness, DIC, and respiratory failure. Mortality is 10% for dengue hemorrhagic fever, but may be reduced to 1% with aggressive fluid resuscitation.
- Yellow fever has an incubation period of 3–6 days. Most symptomatic infections are mild with gradual onset and patients recovering within 48 hours. Patients exhibit headache, myalgias, vomiting, abdominal pain, and relative bradycardia for the degree of fever (Faget's sign). For those with severe infection, the symptom presentation is more abrupt and leads to dehydration, jaundice, and mucocutaneous bleeding. Often, even these patients will experience a temporary recovery phase for 2–3 days, before rapidly deteriorating into shock and heart failure. Overall mortality is 5–7%, with more than 50% in those with severe infection.

Diagnosis

A wide range of conditions (bacterial, viral, and parasitic infections as well as noninfectious causes) should be considered in the differential diagnosis of VHF. However, most of these conditions do not cause bleeding manifestations as a primary feature and most are not likely to occur epidemiologically with simultaneous presentation of many cases. Primary agents to consider in the differential diagnosis are listed below:

- Septicemia caused by gram-negative bacteria
- Typhoid fever
- Meningococcemia
- Secondary syphilis
- Rocky Mountain spotted fever
- Gastroenteritis
- Ehrlichiosis
- Leptospirosis
- Influenza
- Malaria
- Hepatitis
- Hemolytic-uremic syndrome
- Thrombotic thrombocytopenic purpura
- Idiopathic thrombocytopenic purpura

The natural distribution and circulation of VHF agents are geographically linked with the ecology of the reservoir species and vectors. Therefore, elicitation of a detailed travel history is critical in making the diagnosis of VHF. Additionally, most clinicians in the United States have little or no clinical experience with the syndromes that characterize VHF; therefore, a high index of suspicion is needed to make an accurate diagnosis.

The diagnosis of VHF should be considered for any patient who presents with:

- Acute onset of fever (less than 3 weeks' duration)
- Severe prostrating or life-threatening illness
- Bleeding manifestations
  - At least two of the following: hemorrhagic or purpuric rash, petechiae (particularly in nondependent areas), epistaxis, hematemesis, hemoptysis, or blood in stool
- No predisposing factors for a bleeding diathesis

In naturally occurring cases, an appropriate travel or exposure history will usually be present. In the setting of a bioterrorism event, such a history will not be present and multiple patients will likely present simultaneously. Patients with arenaviral or hantaviral infections often recall having seen rodents during the presumed incubation period. Since the viruses are spread to humans by aerosolized excreta or environmental contamination, however, actual contact with the reservoir is not necessary. Large mosquito populations are common during the seasons when RVF virus and the flaviviruses are transmitted, but a history of mosquito bite is sufficiently common to be of little assistance in making a diagnosis. Tick bites or nosocomial exposure are of some significance when Crimean-Congo hemorrhagic fever is suspected. History of exposure to animals in slaughterhouses should raise suspicions of Rift Valley fever and Crimean-Congo hemorrhagic fever in a patient with VHF. When large numbers of military personnel present with VHF manifestations in the same geographical area over a short period of time, medical personnel should suspect either a natural outbreak (in an endemic setting) or possibly a biowarfare attack (particularly if the virus causing the VHF is not endemic to the area).

Laboratory findings can be helpful, although they vary from disease to disease and summarization is difficult. Leukopenia may be suggestive, but in some patients, white blood cell counts may be normal or even elevated. Thrombocytopenia is a component of most VHF diseases, but to a varying extent. In some, platelet counts may be near normal, and platelet function tests are required to explain the bleeding diathesis. A positive tourniquet test has been particularly useful in diagnosing dengue hemorrhagic fever, but this sign may be associated with other hemorrhagic fevers as well. Proteinuria or hematuria or both are common in VHF, and their absence virtually rules out Argentine hemorrhagic fever, Bolivian hemorrhagic fever, and hantaviral infections. Hematocrits are usually normal, and if there is sufficient loss of vascular integrity perhaps mixed with dehydration, hematocrits may be increased. Liver enzymes such as aspartate aminotransferase (AST) are frequently elevated. VHF viruses are not primarily hepatotropic, but there is hepatic involvement and an elevated AST may help to distinguish VHF from a simple febrile disease.

Definitive diagnosis in an individual case rests on specific virological diagnosis. Most patients have readily detectable viremia at presentation (the exception is hantaviral infection). Infectious virus and viral antigens can be detected and identified by a number of assays using fresh or frozen serum or plasma samples. Likewise, early immunoglobulin (Ig) M antibody responses to the VHF-causing agents can be detected by enzyme-linked immunosorbent assays (ELISA), often during the acute illness. Diagnosis by viral cultivation and identification requires 3–10 days for most (longer for the hantaviruses). With the exception of dengue, specialized microbiologic containment is required for safe handling of these viruses. Appropriate precautions should be observed in collecting, handling, shipping, and processing of diagnostic samples. Both the Centers for Disease Control and Prevention (CDC, Atlanta, GA) and the U.S. Army Medical Research Institute of Infectious Diseases (USAMRIID, Fort Detrick, Frederick, MD) have diagnostic laboratories operating at the maximum Biosafety Level (BL-4). Viral isolation should not be attempted without BL-4 containment.

Medical Management and Infection Control

Managing VHFs involves basic diagnostic, therapeutic, prophylactic, and infection control concepts, and a practical monitoring system for contacts. Patients with VHF syndrome require close supervision; some will require intensive care. Since the pathogenesis of VHF is not entirely understood and availability of specific antiviral drugs is limited, treatment is largely supportive. This care is essentially the same as the conventional care provided to patients with other causes of multisystem failure. The challenge is to provide this support while minimizing the risk of infection to other patients and medical personnel.

Patients with VHF syndrome generally benefit from rapid, nontraumatic hospitalization to prevent unnecessary damage to the fragile capillary bed. Restlessness, confusion, myalgia, and hyperesthesia occur frequently and should be managed by reassurance and other supportive measures, including the judicious use of sedative, pain-relieving, and amnestic medications. Aspirin and other antiplatelet or anticlotting-factor drugs should be avoided. Secondary infections are common and should be sought and aggressively treated. Intravenous lines, catheters, and other invasive techniques should be avoided unless they are clearly indicated for appropriate management of the patient. Attention should be given to pulmonary toilet, the usual measures to prevent superinfection, and the provision of supplemental oxygen. Immunosuppression with steroids or other agents has no empirical and little theoretical basis, and is contraindicated except possibly for HFRS. The diffuse nature of the vascular pathological process may lead to a requirement for support of several organ systems.

The management of bleeding is controversial. Uncontrolled clinical observations support vigorous administration of fresh frozen plasma, clotting factor concentrates, and platelets, as well as early use of heparin for prophylaxis of DIC. In the absence of definitive evidence, mild bleeding manifestations should not be treated at all. More severe hemorrhage indicates that appropriate replacement therapy is needed. When definite laboratory evidence of DIC becomes available, heparin therapy could be considered in the appropriate patient if appropriate laboratory support is available.

Management of hypotension and shock is difficult. Patients often are modestly dehydrated from heat, fever, anorexia, vomiting, and diarrhea. There are covert losses of intravascular volume through hemorrhage and increased vascular permeability. Nevertheless, these patients often respond poorly to fluid infusions and readily develop pulmonary edema, possibly due to myocardial impairment and increased pulmonary vascular permeability. Either colloid or crystalloid solutions should be cautiously given. Although it has never been evaluated critically for VHFs, dopamine would seem to be the agent of choice for patients with shock who are unresponsive to fluid replacement.

Two hemorrhagic fevers should be clearly separated from the other VHF diseases. Severe consequences of dengue infection are largely due to systemic capillary leakage syndrome and should be managed initially by brisk infusion of crystalloid, followed by albumin or other colloid if there is no response. Severe hantaviral infections have many of the management problems of the other hemorrhagic fevers but will culminate in acute renal failure with a subsequent polyuria during the patient's recovery. Careful fluid and electrolyte management is necessary for optimal treatment.

Patients with VHF syndrome generally have significant quantities of virus in their blood and, perhaps, in other secretions as well. Transmission within health-care settings has been noted for a number of hemorrhagic fever viruses, including Ebola, Marburg, Lassa, Machupo, and Crimean-Congo viruses. Well-documented secondary infections among contacts and medical personnel not parenterally exposed have occurred. Thus, caution should be exercised in evaluating and treating patients with suspected VHF syndrome. Appropriate isolation precautions for patients with suspected or confirmed VHF include a combination of airborne and contact precautions. Although airborne transmission of these agents appears to be rare, airborne transmission theoretically may occur; therefore, airborne precautions should be instituted for all patients with suspected VHF. According to the Working Group on Civilian Biodefense, the following precautions should be implemented for such patients/staff:

- Personal protective equipment for health-care providers, including N95 respirator or powered air-purifying respirator, double (leak-proof) gloves, impermeable gowns, face shields, goggles for eye protection, and leg and shoe coverings. (See Table 44-2 also.)
- Place the patient in a private room with negative air pressure, 6–12 air changes per hour, and restricted access of nonessential staff and visitors.
- Dedicated medical equipment for exposed patients and staff.
- Place all persons (including medical and laboratory personnel) who have had a close or high-risk contact with a patient suspected of having VHF during the 21 days following onset of symptoms under medical surveillance.
- If multiple patients with suspected VHF are admitted to one health-care facility, cohort them in the same part of the hospital to minimize exposure to other patients and health-care workers.

For more intensive care, increased precautions are advisable. Members of the patient care team should be limited to a small number of selected, trained individuals, and special care should be directed toward eliminating all parenteral exposures. The use of endoscopy, respirators, arterial catheters, routine blood sampling, and extensive laboratory analysis increase opportunities

TABLE 44-2

RECOMMENDATIONS FOR PROTECTIVE MEASURES AGAINST NOSOCOMIAL TRANSMISSION OF HEMORRHAGIC FEVER VIRUSES

- Strict adherence to hand hygiene: Health-care workers should clean their hands prior to donning personal protective equipment for patient contact. After patient contact, health-care workers should remove gown, leg and shoe coverings, and gloves, and immediately clean their hands. Hands should be clean prior to the removal of protective equipment (i.e., personal respirators, face shields, and goggles) to minimize exposure of mucous membranes with potentially contaminated hands, and once again after the removal of all personal protective equipment
- Double gloves
- Impermeable gowns
- N95 masks or powered air-purifying respirators, and a negative air-pressure isolation room with 6–12 air changes per hour, as required by the Healthcare Infection Control Practices Advisory Committee standards for airborne precautions*
- Leg and shoe coverings
- Face shields†
- Goggles for eye protection†
- Restricted access of nonessential staff and visitors to patient's room
- Dedicated medical equipment, such as stethoscopes, glucose monitors, and, if available, point-of-care analyzers
- Environmental disinfection with an Environmental Protection Agency–registered hospital disinfectant or a 1:100 dilution of household bleach
- If there are multiple patients with viral hemorrhagic fever in one health-care facility, they should be cared for in the same part of the hospital to minimize exposures to other patients and health-care workers

*These resources may not be possible in many health-care facilities or in a mass casualty situation. In this case, all other measures should be taken and would, in combination, be expected to substantially diminish the risk of nosocomial spread.

†Face shields and eye protection may be already incorporated in certain personal protective equipment, such as powered air-purifying respirators.

Source: From Borio L, Inglesby T, Peters CJ, et al. Hemorrhagic Fever Viruses as Biological Weapons. JAMA 2002; 287; 2391–2405.

for aerosol dissemination of infectious blood and body fluids, so judicious use is required.

The Working Group on Civilian Biodefense does not recommend prophylactic antiviral therapy for persons exposed to *any* hemorrhagic fever viruses (including Lassa virus) in the absence of clinical illness. Instead, the Working Group recommends that exposed persons be placed under medical surveillance. Specific recommendations from the working group include the following.

- Exposed persons include those with exposure to the initial bioterrorist release, and those who are close contacts of, or have high-risk exposure to, a patient with VHF.
- Exposed patients should monitor their temperatures daily and report any temperature of 101°F (38.3°C) or higher.
- Exposed persons should also report any other symptoms suggestive of VHF.
- If symptoms suggestive of VHF occur, or, if a temperature of at least 101°F (38.3°C) is documented by medical staff, ribavirin therapy should be initiated unless another diagnosis is confirmed or the etiologic agent is known to be a filovirus (Ebola, Marburg) or flavivirus (yellow fever, Kyasanur Forest disease, Omsk hemorrhagic fever).
- Surveillance should be continued for 21 days after the last exposure.

Specific pharmacologic antiviral therapy for VHF, in the form of ribavirin, has been recommended for Lassa fever and the other arenavirus hemorrhagic fevers, Rift Valley fever, CCHF, HFRS, and related viruses. Ribavirin is a nonimmuno-suppressive nucleoside analogue with broad antiviral properties. It reduces mortality from Lassa fever in high-risk patients, and presumably decreases morbidity in all patients with Lassa fever, for whom current recommendations are to treat initially with ribavirin 30 mg/kg, administered intravenously, followed by 15 mg/kg every 6 hours for 4 days, and then 7.5 mg/kg every 8 hours for an additional 6 days. Treatment is most effective if begun within 7 days of onset. Lower intravenous doses or oral administration of 2 g followed by 1 g/day for 10 days also may be useful. Ribavirin is contraindicated in pregnant women, but, in the case of definite Lassa fever, the predictability of fetal death and the need to evacuate the uterus may justify its use. Safety of ribavirin in infants and children has not been established. Small studies investigating the use of ribavirin in the treatment of Bolivian hemorrhagic fever and Crimean-Congo hemorrhagic fever have been promising, as have preclinical studies for Rift Valley fever. Conversely, ongoing studies conducted at USAMRMC predict that ribavirin will be ineffective against both the filoviruses and the flaviviruses. No other antiviral compounds are currently available for the VHF agents.

Passive immunization has been attempted for treatment of most VHF infections. This approach has often been taken in desperation, owing to the limited availability of effective antiviral drugs. For all VHF viruses, the benefit of passive immunization seems to be correlated with the concentration of neutralizing antibodies, which are readily induced by some—but not all—of these viruses. In the future, engineered human monoclonal antibodies may be available for specific, passive immunization against the VHF agents. The only established and licensed virus-specific vaccine available against any of the hemorrhagic fever viruses is yellow fever vaccine, which is mandatory for travelers to endemic areas of Africa and South America. For prophylaxis against Argentine hemorrhagic fever (AHF) virus, a live-attenuated Junin vaccine strain (Candid #1) was developed at USAMRMC and is available as an investigational new drug (IND). Candid #1 was proven to be effective in Phase III studies in Argentina, and plans are proceeding to obtain a new drug license. This vaccine also provides some cross-protection against Bolivian hemorrhagic fever in experimentally infected primates.

Two IND vaccines were developed at USAMRMC against Rift Valley fever: an inactivated vaccine that requires 3 boosters, which has been in use for 20 years; and a live-attenuated RVF virus strain (MP-12), which is presently in Phase II clinical trials.

For Hantaan virus, a formalin-inactivated rodent brain vaccine is available in Korea, but is not generally considered acceptable by American standards. Another USAMRMC product, a genetically engineered vaccinia construct, expressing hantaviral structural proteins, is in Phase II safety testing in U.S. volunteers. For dengue, a number of live-attenuated strains for all four serotypes are entering Phase II efficacy testing. However, none of these vaccines in Phase I or II IND status will be available as licensed products in the near term. For the remaining VHF agents, availability of effective vaccines is more distant.

The lack of an approved vaccine or proven prophylaxis and low survival rates of the most severely ill patients even with inpatient intensive care make VHF viruses potential bioterrorism agents with the intention of overwhelming society's resources. Mobilization of research is immediately needed for vaccine development, specific prophylactic and therapeutic interventions, strengthened public health response, and improved hospital infection control practices.

AUTOPSY

An autopsy may subject laboratory personnel, pathologists and prosectors as well as others to blood borne and aerosolized pathogens. Performing autopsies on persons who have died from a VHF poses significantly greater risks than typical illnesses. Prosectors have died from autopsy transmitted Marburg, Ebola and Lassa fevers. These infections were transmitted by direct cutaneous inoculation; aerosol risk must be considered as well. Absolute attention to safety, use of PPE and biosafety measures is critical. In a terrorist related VHF, persons unaccustomed to such precautions as PPE may become involved, such as law enforcement and federal agencies to investigate as well as preserve the evidence chain of custody.

SUMMARY

The VHF agents are a taxonomically diverse group of RNA viruses that cause serious diseases with high morbidity and mortality. Their existence as endemic disease threats or their use in biological warfare could have a formidable impact on public health.

The dominant clinical features of VHF are a consequence of microvascular damage and changes in vascular permeability. Patients commonly present with fever, myalgia, and prostration. Full-blown VHF syndrome typically evolves to shock and generalized mucous membrane hemorrhage, and often is accompanied by evidence of neurological, hematopoietic, or pulmonary involvement.

A viral hemorrhagic fever should be suspected in any patient who presents with a severe febrile illness and evidence of vascular involvement (subnormal blood pressure, postural hypotension, petechiae, easy bleeding, flushing of the face and chest, nondependent edema), and who has traveled to an area where the virus is known to occur, or where intelligence suggests a biological warfare threat.

Definitive diagnosis rests on specific virological diagnosis, including detection of viremia or IgM by ELISA at presentation. Diagnosis by viral cultivation and identification requires 3–10 days or longer and specialized microbiologic containment.

Appropriate precautions should be observed in collecting, handling, shipping, and processing of diagnostic samples. It is prudent to provide isolation measures that are as rigorous as feasible.

Patients with viral hemorrhagic fevers generally benefit from rapid, nontraumatic hospitalization. Aspirin and other antiplatelet or anticlotting-factor drugs should be avoided. Secondary and concomitant infections including malaria should be sought and aggressively treated. The management of bleeding includes administration of fresh frozen plasma, clotting-factor concentrates and platelets, and aggressive treatment to control DIC. Fluids should be given cautiously, and colloid or crystalloid solutions should be used. Multiple organ system support may be required.

Ribavirin is an antiviral drug with efficacy for treatment of the arenaviruses and bunyaviruses. Passively administered antibody is also effective in therapy of some viral hemorrhagic fevers. The only licensed vaccine available for VHF agents is for yellow fever. Experimental vaccines exist for Junin, RVF, Hantaan, and dengue viruses, but these will not be licensed in the near future.

Suggested Reading

Borio L, Inglesby T, Peters CJ, et al. Hemorrhagic fever viruses as biological weapons: medical and public health management. *JAMA.* 2002;287:2391–405.

CDC. Biological and chemical terrorism: strategic plan for preparation and response. *MMWR.* 2000;49:1–14.

CDC. Management of patients with suspected viral hemorrhagic fever. *MMWR.* 1988;37:1–16.

Centers for Disease Control and Prevention, National Institutes of Health. Biosafety in microbial and biomedical laboratories. 4th Ed. Washington, DC; US Dept. of Health and Human Services, US Gov't Printing Office, 1999.

Cleri DJ, Ricketti AJ, Porwancher RB, et al. Viral hemorrhagic fevers: current status of endemic disease and strategies for control. *Infect Dis Clin N Am.* 2006;20:359–393.

Dengue/Dengue haemorrhagic fever. Epidemic and Pandemic Alert and Responses (EPR). World Health Organization (WHO) 2007. Available at http://www.WHOint/CSR/DISEASE/DENGUE/EN. Last Accessed 5/30/07.

Franz DR, Jahrling PB, Friedlander AM, et al. Clinical recognition and management of patients exposed to biological warfare agents. *JAMA.* 1997;278(5):399–411.

Isaacson M. Viral hemorrhagic fever hazards for travelers in Africa. *Clin Infect Dis.* 2001;33(10):1707–1712.

Jahrling P. Viral hemorrhagic fevers. Chap 29. In: Zajtchuk R, Bellamy RF, eds. *Textbook of Military Medicine: Medical Aspects of Chemical and Biological Warfare.* Washington, DC: Office of the Surgeon General, Borden Institute, Walter Reed Army Medical Center, 1997.

Kortepeter M, Christopher G, Cieslak T, et al. Viral hemorrhagic fevers. In: *USAMRIID's Medical Management of Biological Casualties Handbook.* 4th ed. Fort Detrick, MD: Operational Medicine Department, US Army Medical Research Institute of Infectious Diseases; 2001. p 61–8.

Lopez Antonano FJ, Mota J. Development of immunizing agents against dengue. *Rev Pand Salud Publica* 2000; 7: 285-292.

McFee RB. Avian Influenza – The Next Pandemic? *Dis a Month.* 2007 (July) prepublication.

Nolte KB, Taylor DG, Richmond JY. Biosafety considerations for autopsy. *Am J Forens Med and Path* 2002; 23 (2): 107-122.

Peters CJ. Bioterrorism: viral hemorrhagic fever. In: Mandell GL, Bennett JE, Dolin R, eds. *Mandell Douglas, and Bennett;s Principles and Practice of Infectious Diseases, vol. 2.* 6th ed. Philadelphia, PA: Elsevier Churchill Livingston; 2005. pp. 3626–9.

Senanayake S. Dengue fever and dengue hemorrhagic fever. A diagnostic challenge. *Australian Family Phys* 2006; Vol 35 (8) 609–612.

Wilder-smith A, Schwartz E. Dengue in travelers. *N Engl J Med* 2005; 353: 924–932.

45

CDC CATEGORY B AGENTS

Andrea Carlson and Ejaaz A. Kalimullah

STAT FACTS

CDC CATEGORY B AGENTS

- Brucellosis is a granulomatous disease similar to tuberculosis that requires prolonged combined antibiotic therapy.
- Because no cases of glanders have been reported in the United States in the last 65 years, any case of glanders should suggest biological attack.
- Although most cases of Q fever resolve spontaneously, infection in pregnancy is associated with miscarriage, premature delivery, and stillbirth.
- An investigational vaccine for ricin is in development for use in the United States.
- Staphylococcus enterotoxin B causes a self-limited gastrointestinal illness when ingested, but if inhaled at high concentrations may cause septic shock and death.

INTRODUCTION

A number of common pathogens and biological toxins can be used as instruments of terror. The CDC defines such agents as Category B if they are moderately easy to disseminate, cause moderate morbidity but low mortality, and require specific enhancements of the CDC's diagnostic capacity and enhanced disease surveillance. A Category B agent may be selected for use when the primary goal is to incapacitate or cause panic, rather than to kill. Deaths from these agents would predominately occur in high-risk individuals, such as those with immunocompromise or at extremes of age. Many of these agents are easy to obtain and cultivate. Clinical manifestations of exposure and infection are often nonspecific and highly variable. At the present time, the CDC's list is limited to only a fraction of organisms and natural substances capable of causing disease. In the future, other agents may be manipulated by modern biology techniques to increase their ability to spread, cause disease, and resist antibiotic therapy.

SPECIFIC AGENTS

Brucellosis

Properties and Pathophysiology

Brucella species are gram-negative, aerobic, nonmotile, non-spore-forming, unencapsulated coccobacilli. Although zoonoses due to *Brucella* occur worldwide, infection is commonplace in the Mediterranean basin, the Arabian Gulf, the Indian subcontinent, and parts of Central and South America. Animal vaccines have eliminated much of infection in the United States. Roughly 100 cases are reported each year, with half of these occurring in California and Texas. Four species are capable of causing human disease. The most common human isolate is *Brucella melitensis*. Goats and sheep are this species' usual animal host. Other human pathogens include *Brucella suis* (swine), *Brucella abortus* (cattle), and *Brucella canis* (dogs and coyotes).

Brucella species are facultative intracellular pathogens. The bacteria are taken up by local tissue lymphocytes, transferred to regional lymph nodes in the circulation, and are then seeded throughout the body. They survive and multiply in polymorphonuclear leukocytes (PMNs) and monocytes, and thus concentrate in the lymphatic, hepatosplenic, and bone marrow systems. In animals the infection may be lifelong, and bacteria are harbored in reproductive tissues so milk, placental tissue, and urine are primary sources. Humans are most commonly exposed via contact with infected animal secretions. Direct contact may result in entry of the bacteria through abraded cutaneous or mucosal skin. Consumption of unpasteurized dairy products may result in foodborne illness. Inadvertent human inoculation by attenuated animal vaccines has occasionally produced infection. Inhalation is also a significant concern. *Brucella* is extremely infectious when inhaled; only 10–100 organisms are needed to cause disease. Microbiology lab workers have contracted *Brucella* via aerosolization of specimens.

The United States weaponized *Brucella suis* in 1954. This species was selected as a favorable agent of biological warfare due to its slow-growing nature and long incubation period (making diagnosis and recognition of exposure difficult), production of nonspecific symptoms, and resistance to treatment. At that time, experts estimated that release of an aerosolized form of these bacteria under optimal circumstances would cause 82,500 cases of brucellosis and 423 fatalities. In the present day, biological attack should be suspected if a case is without known contact risk.

Clinical Manifestations

Similar to tuberculosis, *Brucella* causes a chronic granulomatous disease. Acute or subacute infection manifests within 2 to 4 weeks of exposure. In its most common form, *Brucella* causes a nonspecific febrile illness. Undulant fever, malodorous sweats, malaise, anorexia, depression, headache, and backache are common. Gastrointestinal symptoms occur in up to 70% of patients. Cough and pleuritic chest pain is present in roughly 20% of cases. CNS manifestations other than depression and mental inattention are relatively rare (5–7%). The reproductive system is a common site of focal brucellosis. In 20% of infected men, this manifests as orchitis. Infection during pregnancy carries with it a substantial risk of spontaneous abortion.

Physical examination may reveal mild nonspecific lymphadenopathy and hepatosplenomegaly. Because *Brucella* has a predilection for the reticuloendothelial system, granulomatous hepatitis can occur. While the primary illness is rarely life-threatening, complications from *Brucella* contribute significantly to overall morbidity and mortality. Osteoarticular disease is the most common complication. Three distinct forms exist: a peripheral, nonerosive arthritis of the knees, hips, ankles, and wrists; sacroiliitis; and spondylitis. Endocarditis is rare (<2%) but causes the majority of fatalities due to *Brucella*. Acute pneumonia is also rare, but a variety of other pulmonary syndromes have been described. Reported abnormalities include pneumonitis, lung nodules, pleural effusions, and empyema (presumably due to rupture of pleural-based granulomas). Although CNS manifestations of acute infection are uncommon, complications such as meningitis and encephalitis have an ominous prognosis.

Lab Studies

In vitro growth of *Brucella* is slow, so cultures must be incubated at least 4 weeks before they can be declared negative. The rate of positive blood culture ranges between 15% and 70%. Bone marrow sampling results in higher culture yields. The bacteria are urease and oxidase positive. Catalase tests should not be performed as they may cause nebulization of particles, risking inhalation exposure in the laboratory.

Cases of suspected bioterrorism require an expedited diagnosis, which may be accomplished using serological testing. Serum agglutination test is widely available and thus the most popular method, but this modality is limited by some cross-reactivity with other bacterial species. A titer greater than 1:160 is diagnostic. Enzyme-linked immunosorbent assay (ELISA) testing carries a higher sensitivity and specificity but is more labor intensive. ELISA can also differentiate different antibody types to better characterize the stage of infection. IgM is the primary antibody present during the first week, while IgG titers begin to appear in the second week. Both antibodies peak during the fourth week, and may be present for almost a year. The presence of both IgG and IgA titers beyond 6 months suggests chronic infection. The use of antibiotic results in an overall decline in titers. PCR technology is being explored and may provide results as early as 10 days after inoculation. New rapid dipstick tests are also being developed.

In patients with pulmonary complications, chest radiography may reveal hilar and paratracheal lymphadenopathy, pneumonitis, lung nodules, or pleural effusions. Pathological specimens of the liver classically reveal noncaseating epithelioid granulomatous hepatitis.

Treatment and Disposition

Prolonged, combined drug therapy is required to treat *Brucella* infection. Current first-line therapy includes doxycycline 100 mg twice daily plus rifampin 600 mg once daily for at least 6 weeks. Streptomycin may be substituted for rifampin; studies suggest streptomycin may be slightly better at preventing relapse. The main disadvantage of streptomycin is that administration requires a 2–3-week inpatient stay. Other accepted regimens include TMP/SMX (trimethoprim/sulfamethoxazole) plus gentamycin, a fluoroquinolone plus rifampin, or a fluoroquinolone plus gentamycin. Rifampin is the drug of choice for pregnant women. To ensure adequate antimicrobial penetration into the CNS, ceftriaxone should be considered for cases of meningitis. Endocarditis and meningitis require longer therapy, with at least 6–9 months of treatment. Valve replacement may be required for endocarditis. Relapses are not uncommon even after long-term treatment. Mortality from *Brucella* is not affected by treatment; the death rate from infection is 5% with or without antibiotic therapy. Treatment is nevertheless indicated to prevent complications, which has a significant impact on overall morbidity.

Because human-to-human transmission of *Brucella* is unlikely, patients with very minor illness may be considered for discharge home on oral antibiotics with close follow-up pending laboratory confirmation of infection.

Decontamination, Personal Protective Equipment, and Prophylaxis

Surfaces contaminated with infected bodily fluids or specimens may be adequately decontaminated with 0.5% hypochlorite (bleach). Standard precautions are adequate to prevent exposure to *Brucella*. Respiratory precautions may be added during the handling of specimens in the laboratory, due to previous reports of lab workers contracting *Brucella* via inhalation in this setting. No human vaccine exists for *Brucella*. Postexposure prophylaxis is not generally recommended except in highly suspect cases (e.g., lab worker exposure, inadvertent injection with the animal vaccine, or apparent release as a bioterrorism agent). In such cases, treatment with a 3–6-week course of any one of the regimens is acceptable.

Clostridium Perfringens Epsilon Toxin

Pathophysiology

Clostridium perfringens is a gram-positive, anaerobic, spore-forming bacterium ubiquitous in soil, and also found in the GI tract of healthy humans and animals. There are five strains of *C. perfringens,* designated A through E. The bacteria elaborate twelve different protein toxins. Although the epsilon toxin is the only *Clostridium* toxin specifically classified as a Category B agent by the CDC, any one of the toxins could be produced, concentrated, and used as a weapon. For example, alpha toxin (produced by all five strains) is expected to be lethal if acquired by aerosol. This toxin can cause serious acute pulmonary disease, vascular leak, hemolysis, thrombocytopenia, and liver damage. Other toxins from the organism might be coweaponized to enhance effectiveness. The epsilon toxin deserves special mention because it is extremely potent, and because it is produced by only strains B and D, which do not usually infect humans. Thus, the finding of epsilon toxin in a human laboratory specimen strongly suggests foul play.

Clinical Manifestations

Illness from *C. perfringens* takes on one of three distinct forms: clostridial food poisoning; enteritis necroticans; or gas gangrene. There is little data available on the specific effects of epsilon toxin on humans; thus clinical consequences of aerosolizing epsilon toxin are not well-defined at this time. Most clinical information is extrapolated from animal studies. Epsilon toxin is known to be neurotoxic in animals, and has also been associated with development of pulmonary edema when injected. In mice, injection of epsilon toxin resulted in a significant decrease in dopamine levels in the brain. In vitro studies also show an increase in gastrointestinal and vascular permeability, potentially leading to vascular damage and edema in the brain, heart, lung, and kidneys.

Lab Studies

C. perfringens can be isolated from standard bacterial wound and stool cultures. Although a latex agglutination test has been developed, in most cases epsilon toxin will be detected using an ELISA assay. PCR can detect the epsilon toxin gene, if present.

Treatment

Treatment recommendations for epsilon toxin exposure are limited to supportive care measures. Animal studies suggest that medications that directly or indirectly inhibit release and receptors of dopamine may lessen the lethal effects of epsilon toxin. Chlorpromazine, trifluoperazine, butyrophenones, reserpine, diazepam, apomorphine, and γ-butyrolactone have all been offered as therapeutic options in this experimental setting. Unfortunately, thus far a protective effect has been demonstrated only in animals given these therapies *prior to* epsilon toxin exposure, so it remains unclear whether any of these agents would have any true clinical impact in a human exposure scenario.

Prophylaxis

Genetically engineered vaccinations against *Clostridium* induce the formation of antibodies against epsilon toxin in animals. From this technology, monoclonal antibodies have been produced and evaluated but none are available for clinical use at this time.

Glanders

Pathophysiology

Burkholderia mallei (formerly *Pseudomonas mallei*) is a small, gram-negative bacillus. This species is the cause of glanders, a disease of horses, mules, and donkeys. This agent was reportedly used as a biological weapon during the First and Second World Wars to incapacitate Russian mules and donkeys on the Eastern Front, thereby affecting movement of troops. Humans seldom acquire glanders, but sporadic cases have been reported worldwide. The disease has been mostly eradicated from the United States by destruction of infected animals. The last case of human glanders in the United States was in 1938. This involved a laboratory technician presumably exposed to a specimen containing *B. mallei*. Naturally occurring disease has not been seen in the United States in 65 years.

Exposure to *Burkholderia* may occur in many ways. The bacteria can enter via broken skin, or through mucous membranes of the nasopharynx, oropharynx, or conjunctiva. Ingestion of contaminated food or water may transmit the disease. Person-to-person spread is possible. Aerosolized release is also feasible. *B. mallei* is quite infectious via inhalation, resulting in severe disease with high mortality.

Due to the rarity of *B. mallei* in the United States, any domestic case of glanders should suggest biological attack.

Clinical Manifestations

Acute and chronic forms of glanders exist. Acute glanders presents in one of three ways: a local suppuration (also known as "farcy"); pneumonia; and septicemia. In farcy, a suppurative nodule forms after a 1–5-day incubation period. The nodule then calcifies or ulcerates and allows spread of the bacteria. Subacute farcy can affect the lungs, liver, spleen, or subcutaneous tissues. This may be associated with high spiking fevers. In the chronic form, cutaneous and intramuscular abscesses of limbs develop and are associated with regional lymphadenopathy. Hepatic and splenic abscess can also occur. Nasal discharge and ulceration may be seen in 50% of cases. The end result is extensive soft tissue destruction and scarring. Farcy can transform to acute septicemia at any time. Complications include osteomyelitis, brain abscesses, and meningitis.

As the most likely attack form of glanders would be inhalational, multiple cases of glanders pneumonia should raise suspicion. Ten to fourteen days after inhalation, pneumonia and pulmonary abscesses may develop and are associated with fever, rigors, sweats, myalgias, and pleuritic chest pain. The septicemic form presents with systemic symptoms similar to the pneumonia form, but also with diarrhea, photophobia, tearing, cervical lymphadenopathy, and splenomegaly. Erysipeloid lesions on face and limbs develop, followed by a generalized pustular eruption. Shock is common.

Lab Studies

Gram stain and tissue culture is diagnostic. Standard blood cultures are rarely positive until late in diagnosis. Serological and biochemical analysis of isolated cultures can also be performed. Agglutination tests may be positive in 7–10 days but are difficult to interpret. Paired tests performed in the second week of illness are considered positive when the titer is greater than 1:320. The complement fixation test, while specific when the titer is greater than 1:20, lacks sensitivity. PCR has been employed diagnostically. CXR may show miliary lesions, multiple lung abscesses, or bronchopneumonia.

Treatment and Disposition

Untreated acute glanders may be fatal within 7–20 days. Adequate antibiotic therapy has been demonstrated to reduce mortality of all forms of glanders. For mild localized disease outpatient therapy consists of: amoxicillin/clavulanate 60 mg/kg/dose divided TID; or TMP 4 mg/kg/dose with SMX 20 mg/kg/dose divided BID; or

tetracycline 40 mg/kg/d divided TID (for adults and children >8 years old). The duration of treatment should be 60–150 days.

For patients ill enough to require hospitalization, any of the above may be combined with imipenem. Another option is to use a combination of two of the above oral regimens for 30 days, followed by monotherapy with either amoxicillin/clavulanate or TMP/SMX for 60–150 days. If extra-pulmonary disease is present, therapy should continue for 6–12 months. Surgical drainage of abscesses may be required.

Severe cases will require 14 days of intravenous ceftazidime (40 mg/kg q 8 h) and TMP/SMX (2 mg/kg q 6 h) for the acute phase, to be continued 2 weeks or until a response is seen. After initial response, the patient may then be switched to doxycycline or TMP/SMX for 3–6 months for the eradication phase.

Decontamination, Personal Protective Equipment, and Prophylaxis

Application of a 0.5% hypochlorite solution will adequately decontaminate exposed surfaces. Standard and contact precautions will suffice for medical professionals attending to an infected patient. In the laboratory, Biosafety Level 3/droplet containment practices should be employed. Postexposure chemoprophylaxis may be tried with TMP/SMX, although efficacy, dose, and duration of therapy needed has yet to be determined. No vaccine is available for glanders.

Melioidosis

Pathophysiology

Burkholderia pseudomallei (formerly *Pseudomonas pseudomallei*) was first discovered in 1911. This motile, aerobic, non-spore-forming gram-negative bacillus is a close relative of *B. mallei*. It is a saprophyte that lives in soil and surface water throughout the world. Melioidosis is a common cause of fatal community-acquired bacteremic pneumonia in northern Australia. It is also highly endemic in Southeast Asia. In 2005, two human cases were reported in Florida. Both patients had traveled to Honduras before becoming ill. Disease occurs by inoculation of broken skin from contaminated soil or water, aspiration or ingestion of contaminated water, or inhalation of contaminated dust. An attack form of melioidosis would likely be aerosolized.

Clinical Manifestations

Melioidosis can be difficult to distinguish from glanders due to clinical and genetic similarities. Like glanders, acute and chronic forms exist. The disease exhibits a broad clinical spectrum, ranging from no symptoms to fulminant sepsis. In patients with subclinical disease, the infection may lie dormant for years, and become active if the patient develops immunocompromise. Minor illness presents with flu-like symptoms, or with localized suppurative disease affecting subcutaneous tissue and lymph nodes.

In its more progressive form, melioidosis leads to severe prostration and systemic symptoms. This will usually present along with severe pneumonia, which may be the primary diagnosis. Sputum is often purulent but rarely blood stained. Large or peripheral lung abscess may rupture into the pleural space to cause empyema.

Predisposing factors predicting more serious disease includes diabetes, chronic renal disease, emphysema, and alcoholism. In its most severe form, melioidosis presents as septicemia with multiple abscesses. Bacterial seeding can occur at any site. Most common abscess locations are the liver, spleen, skeletal muscle, and prostate. Renal abscesses can develop and are associated with calculi and urinary infection. CNS infections and endocarditis are rare. High fever, obtundation, shock, and pneumonia are typical. Untreated septicemia from melioidosis is fatal in 80% of cases.

Of the two U.S. cases reported in 2005, one patient (an elderly woman) died due to myocardial infarction and respiratory compromise early in the course of her illness. Her diagnosis was not known until 2 days after her death. The other patient, a younger male, survived but his clinical course was complicated with a spinal epidural abscess that required emergent decompression and caused residual paraplegia.

Lab Studies

B. pseudomallei grows readily on standard sheep's blood or chocolate agar and forms visible colonies within 24 hours. The bacteria resemble safety pins under the microscope. Broth blood cultures should be taken, as the rate of bacteremia may be as high as 50%. Throat cultures lack adequate sensitivity. Serological studies of urine or blood are useful, either via complement fixation, direct fluorescent antibody testing, or ELISA for IgG. PCR has also been employed.

Treatment and Disposition

The currently recommended therapeutic regimen for melioidosis is completed in two phases. For the initial phase, either ceftazidime 50 mg/kg q 6 hours, meropenem 25 mg/kg q 8 hours, or imipenem 25 mg/kg q 6 hours is infused with or without oral TMP 8 mg/kg with SMX 40 mg/kg given BID. The initial phase regimen is continued for 2 weeks, or until a clinical response is seen. This is followed by the eradication phase, using either oral TMP 8 mg/kg with SMX 40 mg/kg BID or doxycycline 2 mg/kg BID for 60–150 days. Other treatment options for melioidosis include chloramphenicol, third generation cephalosporins, carbapenems, tetracycline,

and amoxicillin-clavulanate. *B. pseudomallei* has demonstrated resistance to other penicillins, first- and second-generation cephalosporins, macrolides, colistin, and aminoglycosides.

Decontamination, Personal Protective Equipment, and Prophylaxis

Application of a 0.5% hypochlorite solution will adequately decontaminate exposed surfaces. Standard and contact precautions will suffice for medical professionals attending to an infected patient. In the laboratory, Biosafety Level 3/droplet containment practices should be employed. Postexposure chemoprophylaxis may be tried with TMP/SMX, although efficacy, dose, and duration of therapy needed has yet to be determined. No vaccine is available for melioidosis.

Psittacosis

Pathophysiology

Chlamydia psittaci causes psittacosis, a disease primarily of birds. Human infection occurs by inhalation of infected droppings or secretions, or by bird bites. A large community outbreak in Queensland in 1995 was not associated with bird contact, but time spent lawn mowing and in the garden. The CDC includes psittacosis as a Category B agent, with presumable aerosolized release, or possible water threat.

Clinical Manifestations

The incubation period of psittacosis is usually 4–14 days, but may be 3 weeks or longer. Symptoms consist of an influenza-like illness with high fever and headache. Hepatosplenomegaly and relative bradycardia are more specific findings. The disease untreated carries a 15–20% mortality rate; antibiotic therapy reduces this to less than 1%.

Lab Studies

The white blood cell count is usually normal or slightly elevated with demargination; CRP and ESR may be elevated. Liver function tests are often mildly abnormal; hyponatremia and/or mild renal insufficiency may also be seen. The most common radiographic lung findings in psittacosis are lobar consolidation or interstitial infiltrates. *C. psittaci* can be isolated from respiratory secretions. Acute and convalescent serology should be performed at least 14 days apart. A fourfold or greater increase in antibody against *C. psittaci* by complement fixation or microimmunofluorescence (MIF) to a reciprocal titer of greater than or equal to 32 or the presence of IgM antibody against *C. psittaci* by MIF to a reciprocal titer of greater than or equal to 16 is diagnostic. Alternatively, a single titer of 1:128 or higher can be considered positive. Antibody rise is delayed or diminished by antibiotic treatment. PCR has been employed diagnostically.

Treatment and Disposition

Doxycycline 100 mg BID orally for 10–14 days will adequately treat psittacosis. Prompt response to treatment is seen; fever resolves within 36 hours. Erythromycin is less effective and has reported treatment failures, but is nonetheless the only appropriate alternative for pregnant women and children, and those with allergies to tetracyclines.

Decontamination, Personal Protective Equipment, and Prophylaxis

Application of a 0.5% hypochlorite solution will adequately decontaminate exposed surfaces. Standard precautions will suffice for medical professionals attending to an infected patient. Postexposure prophylaxis is not indicated, as person-to-person spread has not been demonstrated. No vaccine is available for psittacosis.

Q Fever

Pathophysiology

First described in 1937, "Query fever" (meaning fever due to unknown infection) is a worldwide zoonosis caused by *Coxiella burnetii*. This spore-forming pleomorphic coccobacillus has gram-negative cell wall, and is a strictly intracellular organism. Once intracellular, it hides in acidic vacuoles, affording it resistance against antimicrobial therapy. Spores can remain viable in soil for up to 150 days. Q fever is a common disease of sheep, goats, cattle, dogs, cats, some wild animals, ticks, and birds. Infection in animals is not usually clinically apparent. Humans may contract Q fever by inhalation of dust from infected tissue, or by direct contact with infected animals. *C. burnetii* is extremely infectious; reportedly, inhalation of 1–10 organisms can cause illness. Q fever may also be foodborne, via ingestion of raw milk or fresh goat cheese. Less commonly, transmission may occur by percutaneous route, vertical transmission, and rarely, from blood transfusion. After Q fever became nationally reportable in 1999, 255 Americans Q fever cases (averaging 51 per year) have been reported between 2000 through 2004.

C. burnetii has been studied by military of many countries including the United States, weaponized, and stockpiled before 1971. It is considered an incapacitating agent. During the Second World War, British and American troops suffered an outbreak of Q fever while in Florence, Italy. Within 3 weeks, 300 soldiers became ill, as well as 20 lab personnel who handled the specimens in Naples. In total, 1000 cases were reported, with no confirmed deaths. During the same year, German troops developed the "Balkan grippe" while in Greece; specimens later analyzed showed *C. burnetii*. Possible attack routes include an aerosolized form, or contamination of food and possibly water.

After inhalation, bacteria multiply in lungs, and then disseminate into the bloodstream. Cell-mediated immunity can effectively control many cases of Q fever, but eradication of the organism is difficult. Chronic disease is possible.

Clinical Manifestations

Presentation of illness depends on route of entry, virulence of strain, and host immune factors. Asymptomatic seroconversion occurs in up to 50% of some populations. Following an incubation period of 2–14 days, the most common clinical syndrome of acute Q fever is a self-limited febrile illness, with high fever, chills, headaches, myalgias, and sweats. Atypical pneumonia may also develop, with pleuritic chest pain and rales on chest examination. Granulomatous hepatitis can occur with an increase in liver enzyme levels. Jaundice and abdominal pain are unusual. Neurological involvement has been described occasionally (2.2%) and seems to correlate with strong environmental exposure. Severe headache associated with meningeal syndrome is the most common presentation. Aseptic meningitis, encephalitis or encephalomyelitis, Guillain-Barre, peripheral neuropathy, extrapyramidal signs, multiple cranial nerve involvement, and neuro-ocular abnormalities have all been reported. Behavior and psychiatric disturbances are common. The prognosis of patients with meningoencephalitis is excellent; death is rare and the majority of patients recover in days to weeks. Overall, incapacitating illness may be present for 2–3 weeks, but Q fever is rarely fatal.

Endocarditis is a rare (1%) but worrisome complication, as it worsens prognosis. This most often presents as culture-negative endocarditis in patients with valvular heart disease, osteoarticular infections, chronic hepatitis, vascular or intrauterine infections. A case series of patient with Q fever–related endocarditis (1997–2001) documented a 16% mortality rate. Often patients will need cardiac valve surgery.

C. burnetii infection during pregnancy deserves special mention. The bacteria readily colonize the placenta, uterus, and mammary glands. Q fever during pregnancy is a serious disease. Infection can result in miscarriage, premature deliveries, and stillbirths. Illness in the first trimester significantly increases the risk of a poor outcome.

Less commonly, cases of prolonged fever, rash, myocarditis, pericarditis, and meningoencephalitis have also been reported. A chronic form of Q fever exists and can occur 1–20 years after the initial infection as a reactivation infection in those who develop immunocompromise. Serological profiles and treatment for chronic illness differ from acute infection.

Lab Studies

Aside from elevated liver function studies, routine labwork is often nonspecific. CSF findings may be normal, or may reveal an increase in mononuclear cells. Chest x-ray often demonstrates pleural based opacities or small pleural effusions. *C. burnetii* is difficult and hazardous to culture. Lab visualization requires Gimenez stain. Antibodies appear in the second week of illness and persist for up to 1 year. ELISA assays for these antibodies are available but labor intensive. Indirect fluorescent antibody (IFA) becomes positive 7–15 days after onset of symptoms; this modality can differentiate IgM, IgG, and IgA. *C. burnetii* phase II titers of 1:200 (IgG) or of 1:50 (IgM) are considered positive. High level titers against phase I suggest chronic infection. Complement fixation is specific but not sensitive and detects illness later in the course than ELISA or IFA. Microagglutination can be performed but requires more antigens than ELISA or IFA. All serological studies can cross-react with Legionella and Bartonella. Pathological analysis demonstrates "doughnut granulomas" (central clearing with a fibrin ring) that are nearly pathognomonic of Q fever.

Decontamination

Gross contaminated patients should have clothing removed and skin should be washed with soap and water. Low-level surface exposures may be decontaminated with 0.5% hypochlorite, 1% Lysol, 2% formaldehyde, or 5% H_2O_2. For high-level exposures at least 30-minute exposure to 70% ethanol, 5% formaldehyde, or 5% Enviro-Chem is required. Material, which can be autoclaved, can be disinfected at 350°F and 21 psi for 15 minutes or gas sterilized in 12% ethylene oxide in Freon-12 for 17 hours.

Treatment and Disposition

Most cases of Q fever resolve spontaneously, with untreated mortality only 1–2%. Treatment with doxycycline 100 mg BID or tetracycline 500 mg QID is recommended as this decreases mortality to less than 1%. Antibiotics have also been shown to reduce the risk of complications. Other choices include fluoroquinolones, erythromycin, chloramphenicol, cotrimoxazole, and ceftriaxone. Neurological involvement requires a fluoroquinolone to penetrate the CNS. For pregnant women, cotrimoxazole should be given throughout the duration of pregnancy. This antibiotic is only bacteriostatic, so it must be followed after delivery by 1 year of doxycycline and hydroxychloroquine. Breastfeeding should be discouraged, as Q fever has been isolated in breast milk. Patients with valvular heart disease have a 1 in 3 risk developing endocarditis; recommended treatment includes 12 months of doxycycline plus hydroxychloroquine 600 mg/d. For patients with endocarditis treatment should be extended to 3 years. The patient may ultimately need valvular replacement. Treatment of children under age 8 remains problematic as tetracycline and fluoroquinolones are contraindicated. Macrolides or TMP/SMX have been used but efficacy is unknown. Quarantine of patients is not needed; those with minor illness may be considered for outpatient management.

Personal Protective Equipment and Prophylaxis

Person-to-person transmission of Q fever is rare; universal precautions are adequate to prevent secondary exposure. In laboratories Biosafety Level 3 (BSL3) containment practices are needed. A formalin-inactivated whole cell vaccine ("Q-vax") is available in Australia. In the United States, there is an investigational vaccine in development. Skin testing is needed prior to vaccination due to severe local reactions in those with natural immunity. A 5-day course of doxycycline or tetracycline is given prophylactically 8–12 days after exposure; if given sooner it is less effective and may prolong the onset of disease. Doxycycline and alternative fluoroquinolones are part of the planned national pharmaceutical stockpile.

Ricin Toxin

Properties and Pathophysiology

Ricin is a glycoprotein derived from the beans of the castor plant (*Ricinus communis*). The plant is ubiquitous to subtropical and temperate climates throughout the world, and grows uncultivated in the southwestern United States. Ricin has gained recent notoriety as a bioterrorism agent after being found in a South Carolina mail facility in 2003 and on a mail-sorting machine in Senator Bill Frist's office building in 2004.

The oblong beans of the castor plant are light brown with dark brown or white speckles and are thought to contain approximately 1–5% ricin, 40% oil, and 0.3–0.8% ricinine. The yellowish castor oil is extracted for a variety of purposes including use in lubricating oils, varnishes, and paints. Castor oil itself does not contain ricin. The alkaloidal toxin ricinine can be coextracted in small amounts along with ricin from the beans, but has not had reported use as a human poison.

Purified ricin is a soluble white powder that is stable over a wide pH range. While ricin can be inactivated by heating, the degree and duration of heating required is variable depending on the quality and purity of the preparation. Ricin has a molecular weight of ~60–65 kDa and is composed of A and B polypeptide chains. Similar to other A-B type toxins, the B chain is a lectin that binds to cell surface glycoproteins and glycolipids to facilitate the entry of ricin via endosomal uptake. After reaching the cytosol, the A chain removes an adenine from position 4324 in the 28S rRNA component of eukaryotic 60S ribosomal subunits.

The modified ribosomal subunits are unable to bind protein elongation factors, causing protein synthesis to cease. Ricin's structure and mechanism of toxicity have led to its classification as a Type II ribosome-inactivating protein.

Toxicokinetics and Clinical Manifestations

Three routes of exposure have been described for ricin: ingestion, inhalation, and parenteral. Oral ingestion typically requires substantially higher doses to produce toxic effects due to limited systemic absorption of intact toxin from the gastrointestinal tract. The ingestion of unchewed castor beans is unlikely to produce toxicity. There are no published reports of human poisoning by ingestion of purified ricin. The lethal oral dose in humans following castor bean ingestion ranges from 1 to 20 mg ricin/kg. Clinical reports describe the number of beans ingested rather than well-quantified ricin doses. Symptoms have been reported following the ingestion of amounts ranging from 0.5 to 30 beans. Per animal data, ricin is systemically absorbed within 2 hours after ingestion and preferentially accumulates in the liver and spleen. About 20–45% is eliminated unchanged via the feces. Oropharyngeal pain, abdominal pain, nausea, vomiting, and diarrhea usually occur within 4–6 hours, although symptoms may be delayed for 10 hours or more. Patients may develop dehydration, significant electrolyte imbalances, and shock.

Toxicity following inhalational exposure is heavily influenced by particle size. Low micron-sized particles penetrate deeper into the bronchial tree and can also remain aerosolized in undisturbed air for several hours. In a primate model involving exposure to 1–2 μm particles, subjects developed respiratory distress within 20–24 hours following doses of 21–42 μg/kg. In addition to dyspnea, victims may report fever, cough, chest discomfort, and arthralgias as early as 4–8 hours after exposure. Patients may also exhibit IgE-mediated allergic responses following chronic exposure.

Parenteral exposure to ricin is not as well-described. The LD_{50} in mice following injection is 5–10 μg/kg with a minimum lethal dose of 0.7–2 μg/kg. Urinary excretion is the primary route of elimination following injection and usually occurs within 24 hours.

The clinical manifestations of parenteral exposure mimic those of sepsis with fever, nausea, anorexia, abdominal pain, malaise, and hypotension appearing within 10 to 12 hours. Localized tissue swelling as well as regional lymphadenopathy may be noted.

Laboratory

Laboratory findings may include leukocytosis, elevated liver transaminases and creatinine kinase, electrolyte imbalances, hyperbilirubinemia, anemia, myoglobinuria, renal insufficiency, and hyperamylasemia. While there are no commonly available commercial assays for detecting ricin in clinical specimens, radioimmunoassay and ELISA techniques have been used to detect ricin in blood or bodily fluids. Radioimmunoassay is able to detect concentrations as low as 50–100 pg/mL and concentrations of 0.1–1 ng/mL can be demonstrated by ELISA. In cases of suspected ricin exposure, clinicians should obtain serum and urine samples and contact their state public health agency or the CDC for information regarding confirmatory testing. In addition to the above methods, researchers have also used urine ricinine assays to detect ricin exposure, as well as PCR and time-resolved immunofluoresence methods to confirm the presence of ricin in environmental samples.

Treatment and Disposition

There are no specific antidotes for ricin poisoning. Treatment is supportive and consists of volume repletion and electrolyte replacement in the case of oral ingestion. Initial laboratory studies should include a complete blood count, serum electrolyte levels, urinalysis, renal and liver function tests. Patients with severe toxicity following oral or parenteral exposure may require the administration of vasopressors despite volume repletion. Such patients are at risk for developing multiorgan failure and may benefit from arterial blood gas analysis, lactate determination, and coagulation studies. After inhalational exposure, patients may require supplemental oxygen, bronchodilators, and even endotracheal intubation for positive-pressure ventilation. Patients may have infiltrates on chest x-ray, but will likely worsen in spite of empiric antibiotic therapy. Tetanus status should be updated following parenteral exposure.

All symptomatic patients should be admitted to the hospital for monitoring. Individuals with significant respiratory symptoms or hemodynamic instability warrant ICU admission. Patients who remain asymptomatic 12 hours after oral or inhalational exposure can be discharged home with appropriate instructions as they are unlikely to develop toxicity. There is a theoretical possibility of delayed toxicity in respiratory exposures up to 24 hours later. All cases of suspected ricin poisoning as well as illness outbreaks consistent with ricin exposure should be reported to local poison control centers as well as appropriate public health and law enforcement agencies.

Decontamination, Personal Protective Equipment, and Prophylaxis

First responders arriving at the scene of a suspected aerosolized ricin attack should wear level B personal protective equipment (PPE). Patients should be decontaminated away from the site of exposure in designated hazardous material (hazmat) decontamination areas. After addressing immediate life-threats, garments and jewelry should be removed, and double-bagged. The skin should be cleansed with soap and water for 5–6 minutes. All PPE should be washed with water prior to removal to prevent resuspension of ricin particles. Nondisposable PPE should be soaked in 0.1% sodium hypochlorite for 30 minutes and rinsed with soapy water to inactivate any residual ricin.

In the case of ingestion, gastrointestinal decontamination should be performed in nonvomiting patients via a single dose of activated charcoal. Activated charcoal is unlikely to benefit a vomiting patient and poses an aspiration risk. Local excision of retained foreign bodies may be warranted for parenteral exposures. Following decontamination, universal precautions alone are sufficient. Ricin poisoning is not contagious and health-care workers are not at risk for secondary contamination.

The investigational vaccine, RiVax, safely elicited ricin-neutralizing Abs human volunteers, and exhibited a dose-response effect. Recently completed Phase I trials show promising results. Development of this vaccine continues.

Typhus fever

Pathophysiology

Typhus fever, also known as epidemic typhus, is caused by *Rickettsia prowazekii*. Transmission of the disease is vector-borne via the human body louse (*Pediculis humanis*), or by inhalation of infected louse feces. Outbreaks of epidemic typhus occur during wartime, most likely due to compromised sanitation and living conditions. Outbreaks are also common in third world countries. Sporadic cases occur in the United States from contact with animal reservoirs, mainly flying squirrels, in the squirrel's natural distribution east of the Mississippi River. The mortality rate is 10–25% for untreated cases. As a vector-mediated act of bioterrorism would be difficult to orchestrate, terrorist attack would most likely involve aerosolization of the organism.

Clinical Manifestations

After an incubation period of 14 days, patients develop sudden onset of high fever with headache, limb pains, and vomiting. Epistaxis and dry cough may be seen. The classic rash appears on the third day of illness and consists of irregular pink macules, which darken and coalesce but are not hemorrhagic. The rash is located on the trunk and proximal limbs. Paralytic ileus manifests as constipation. Splenomegaly and lymphadenopathy may be detected on physical exam. Neural involvement is common, often presenting as some form of meningoencephalitic syndrome. This may include meningismus, tinnitus and hyperacusis, deafness, dysphoria, agitation, and/or coma. Survivors may develop hemiparesis, transverse myelitis, or peripheral neuropathy. Other complications include secondary bacterial infections (pneumonia, parotitis, or otitis media), myocarditis, peripheral gangrene, and venous thromboembolism.

Lab Studies

CSF analysis may reveal pleocytosis with predominant lymphocytes. The Weil-Felix test, demonstrating heterophile antibodies to strains of *P. mirabilis* has been used but is falsely negative in up to 50% cases. A group-specific agglutination test, species-specific immunofluorescent antibody test, or ELISA IgG-specific titers performed in both acute and convalescent phases can be diagnostic. PCR has also been employed.

Treatment and Disposition

Louse-infected individuals should be treated with pediculocides containing pyrethrins piperonyl butoxide, crotamiton, or lindane. Several applications may be needed. Specific treatment for typhus fever consists of oral doxycycline until afebrile for at least 3 days; usual duration is 5–10 days. Patients with mild illness who have been adequately decontaminated may be discharged. Those manifesting neural involvement or intractable vomiting will require admission for supportive care.

Decontamination, Personal Protective Equipment, and Prophylaxis

R. prowazekii can remain viable in a dead louse for weeks. A thorough decontamination of patient care areas is important. Standard precautions will suffice for medical professionals attending to an infected patient. Doxycycline is offered as postexposure prophylaxis by some clinicians. No vaccine is available.

Staphylococcus Aureus Enterotoxin B (SEB)

Properties of Exposure

Enterotoxin B is one of seven enterotoxins produced by strains of coagulase-positive *Staphylococcus aureus* bacteria. This heat-stable, pyrogenic toxin is the most common cause of classic food poisoning. In humans, illness is food-borne through ingestion of contaminated milk and milk products containing the preformed toxin. SEB possesses many properties making it desirable as a weapon for terrorism. It can be mass produced and is stable as aerosol. It is soluble in water, resistant to temperature fluctuations, and can withstand boiling for several minutes. In a freeze-dried state, it can be stored for more than a year. Inhalation of large quantities of SEB would cause shock and death. For aerosol exposures the effective dose, or ED_{50} (dose capable of incapacitating 50% of the exposed human population), is 0.0004 mcg/kg, and the lethal dose, or LD_{50}, is 0.02 mcg/kg. Intentional contamination of food and water would also be easy to accomplish, and could result in large-scale incapacitation.

Pathophysiology and Clinical Manifestations

SEB causes illness by acting as a "bacterial superantigen" and interacts with the host's immune system. The toxin binds to the major histocompatibility complex class II molecules that stimulate T cells. This causes massive release of cytokines including interferon gamma, interleukin 6, and tumor necrosis factor alpha. When ingested, the toxin triggers histamine and leukotriene release from mast cells.

Time to onset after ingestion of the toxin is short, with illness manifesting in 3–12 hours. Symptoms begin with abrupt onset of nausea, vomiting, cramping abdominal pain, and diarrhea. Most cases resolve in 8–24 hours. Inhalational exposure results in even more sudden onset; symptoms are seen within 1 to 6 hours. Headache, high fever lasting 2–5 days, myalgias, nonproductive cough, chills, and shortness of breath are possible. Lung auscultation may reveal fine rales. High-level inhalational exposure can result in septic shock and death. Hemodynamic compromise ranges between mild postural hypotension and profound vasodilatory shock. The clinical course usually progresses rapidly to a relatively stable level but patients can be incapacitated and coughing for weeks.

Lab Studies

Enterotoxin B may be isolated from stool and/or blood and may be detected serologically via ELISA. In cases of suspected inhalation, toxin may be identified in nasal swabs from persons exposed to respiratory aerosol for at least 12–24 hours. Chest radiography may be normal, or may show interstitial edema.

Treatment and Disposition

Patients with gastrointestinal illness may be treated symptomatically, with antiemetics and IV hydration as needed and discharged once clinically improving. In contrast, patients with symptoms suggesting significant inhalational exposure will most likely require brief admission, as ventilatory assistance and hemodynamic support may be required. In all cases, treatment of SEB is limited to supportive measures.

Personal Protective Equipment and Prophylaxis

Once the patient has been removed from the exposure site, standard precautions should suffice for protection of medical personnel. There is no chemoprophylaxis or vaccine available for SEB.

Viral Encephalitis

Properties of Exposure

The equine encephalomyelitis (EE) viruses are members of the genus *Alphavirus*. Venezuelan (VEE), Eastern (EEE), and Western (WEE) are the three most common species.

Humans are an accidental host via mosquito vectors. Horses and birds serve as amplifying hosts for EEE and WEE, while VEE has been linked to rodent hosts. EEE is the most virulent species, with a mortality rate of 30–40%. Between 1964 and 2004, 220 confirmed cases of EEE have been reported in the United States. Yearly, there is an average of five cases nationwide, mostly occurring in focal sites along the eastern seaboard, the Gulf Coast, and some inland Midwestern locations of the United States. The most recent cluster of EEE reported to the CDC occurred in 2005 in New Hampshire and Massachusetts. Eleven human cases were reported in total; of these, four patients died. Since 1964, 639 cases of WEE have been reported. Mortality from WEE is much lower, averaging 3%. Of the three species, VEE produces the fewest deaths; less than 1% of VEE infected humans will die. In fact, it is possible for some humans infected with VEE to show no symptoms whatsoever. In Southern Mexico, this virus is considered endemic with a seroprevalence of 18–75%. A VEE epidemic occurred in the fall of 1995 in Venezuela and Colombia with an estimated 90,000 human infections. Cases are clustered in Central and South America, but have occurred as far north as Texas. An aerosolized form of any of these viruses would be highly infectious. As they grow easily in cell cultures, all are reasonable candidates for weaponization.

Pathophysiology and Clinical Manifestations

Equine encephalitis viruses cause illness by seeding the brain and spinal cord. Following exposure, symptoms may develop within 3–10 days. Often there is a febrile prodrome of 1–5 days duration that occurs during viral replication. Infection of man with VEE virus is less severe than with EEE and WEE viruses. Adults usually develop only an influenza-like illness, and overt encephalitis generally occurs only in young children. Most WEE infections also present as mild, nonspecific illness. Patients usually have a sudden onset with fever, headache, nausea, vomiting, anorexia, and malaise, followed by altered mental status, weakness, and signs of meningeal irritation. Children, especially those under 1 year old, are affected more severely than adults and may be left with permanent sequelae, which is seen in 5–30% of young patients. The clinical course of EEE is most concerning. These symptoms begin with a sudden onset of fever, myalgias, and a headache of increasing severity. Varying degrees of neurological involvement follow. Meningismus, hyper or hyporeflexia, and altered mental status are common with EEE, and can progress to status epilepticus, spastic paralysis, loss of airway reflexes, and death. Those who recovered often suffer permanent neurological sequelae.

Lab Studies

Aside from mild lymphopenia, routine bloodwork is usually normal. When signs of meningitis are present, typical CSF findings include elevated protein, as well as pleocytosis. For patients with EEE, the finding of either high CSF white cell counts or severe hyponatremia portends a poor clinical outcome. Definitive testing includes viral culture of serum or CSF, or antibody (IgM) detection through ELISA. Neutralizing antibody testing of acute- and convalescent-phase serum may also be useful. CT or MRI imaging may demonstrate focal lesions in the basal ganglia and thalamus.

Treatment and Disposition

Similar to most viral illnesses, supportive care is the mainstay of treatment. Given the potential for significant neurological decompensation, admission for observation is warranted. This is especially true when EEE is suspected. In such cases, close attention should be given to control of core body temperature and airway management. Aggressive control of seizures may be needed.

Prophylaxis

Although equine vaccines are available and have proven effective, there are not yet vaccines approved for human use. The effectiveness of investigational live-attenuated human vaccines for VEE and WEE have been studied recently using animal models. Preliminary results show favorable antibody production, but less than complete effectiveness (50–85%), and a limited duration of immunity (perhaps less than a year).

Suggested Reading

Audi J, Belson M, Patel M, et al. Ricin poisoning: a comprehensive review. *JAMA.* 2005;294(18):2342–51.

Bossi P, Tegnell A, Baka A, et al. Bichat guidelines for the clinical management of glanders and melioidosis and bioterrorism-related glanders and melioidosis. *Euro Surveill.* 2004;9 (12):E17–8.

Clarke SC. Bacteria as potential tools in bioterrorism, with an emphasis on bacterial toxins. *Br J Biomed Sci.* 2005;62(1): 40–6.

Cowan G. Rickettsial disease: the typhus group of fevers—a review. *Postgrad Med J.* 2000;76(895):269–72.

Deresiewicz RL, Thaler SJ, Hsu L, et al. Clinical and neuroradiographic manifestations of Eastern Equine encephalitis. *NEJM.* 1997;26(336):1867–74.

Greenfield RA, Drevets DA, Machado LJ, et al. Bacterial pathogens as biological weapons and agents of bioterrorism. *Am J Med Sci.* 2002;3232(6):299–315.

Kagawa FT, Wehner JH, Mohindra V. Q fever as a biological weapon. *Semin Respir Infect.* 2003;18(3):183–95.

Karwa M, Bronzert P, Kvetan V. Bioterrorism and critical care. *Crit Care Clin.* 2003;19:271–8.

Pappas G, Akritidis N, Bosilkovski M, et al. Brucellosis. *N Engl J Med.* 2005;352:2325–36.

Spivak L, Hendrickson RG. Ricin. *Crit Care Clin.* 2005;21(4): 815–24.

Voskuhl GW, Cornea P, Bronze MS, et al. Other bacterial diseases as a potential consequence of bioterrorism: Q fever, brucellosis, glanders and melioidosis. *J Okla State Med Assoc.* 2003;96(5):214–7.

White NJ. Melioidosis. *Lancet.* 2003;361:1715–22.

46

CDC CATEGORY C AGENTS

Melissa L. Givens

STAT FACTS

CDC CATEGORY C AGENTS

Category C Agents

- Emerging pathogens with potential use as bioweapon: Availability, ease of production and dissemination, potential for high morbidity and mortality rates, and major health impact

Nipah Virus

- Family: Paramyxovirus
- Vector: Pigs
- Incubation period: 4–18 days
- Clinical findings: Influenza-like illness, encephalitis
- Treatment: Supportive care
- Mortality: 50%
- Personal Protection: Avoidance of infected tissue and secretions

Hantavirus

- Family: Bunyaviridae
- Vector: Rodent
- Incubation period: 2–6 days
- Clinical findings: Hantaviral fever with renal syndrome, Hataviral pulmonary syndrome
- Treatment: Supportive care, ribavirin (HFRS)
- Mortality: 50–60% (HPS), 1–10% (HFRS)
- Personal protection: Avoidance of infected rodents, respiratory filter (N-100)

INTRODUCTION

Category C diseases/agents are defined by the Centers for Disease Control and Prevention (CDC) as the "third highest priority agents to include emerging pathogens that could be engineered for mass dissemination in the future because of (1) availability, (2) ease of production and dissemination, and (3) potential for high morbidity and mortality rates and major health impact."

Based on the above criteria, certain viruses have been identified as potential threats because large quantities can be propagated in cell culture, they are transmissible as aerosols, and there are limited resources for prevention and treatment of infection. Currently the CDC lists Nipah virus and Hantavirus as Category C agents. There are many other agents/diseases that can also be considered as possible threats such as pandemic influenza, yellow fever, viral hemorrhagic fevers such as Crimean-Congo hemorrhagic fever, severe adult respiratory syndrome (SARS), and rabies. For the purposes of this discussion, only the agents specifically listed by the CDC will be explored in detail.

Hantavirus

Hantavirus, from the family Bunyaviridae, causes human infection, which can be classified as hantaviral fever with renal syndrome (HFRS) or hantaviral pulmonary syndrome (HPS). There are several well-described Hantaviral infections to include the Sin Nombre virus isolated from the deer mouse in the southwestern United States; the Seoul virus, which causes an Asian hemorrhagic fever; and Hantaan virus known to cause HFRS in China, Russia, and Korea.

Hantavirus makes an attractive option as a bioweapon because it exists worldwide and is fairly simple to replicate in a laboratory setting. Immunity in the general population is likely to be low, as several strains exist and cross-protection is unlikely. Viruses such as Sin Nombre can be dispersed in aerosol form and production of a vehicle for dispersion would be easy to design but widespread dissemination would be difficult. Although high fatality rates (up to 60%) from HPS suggest that this virus has potential to be a significant bioterrorist threat, the virus is less likely to be used as a bioweapon for several reasons. (1) The virus is difficult to produce. The virus is hard to isolate and poses a significant risk to personnel involved in the isolation. The life cycle of human viremia is short making it difficult to capture. (2) Transmission of Hantavirus is limited by the short period of infectivity in rodents. Once infected, rodents quickly develop neutralizing antibodies, thus limiting the usefulness of blood as a source for virus capture. Once antibodies develop, virus capture is limited to a few excretory organs and rodent excreta. (3) Hantavirus infections are preventable and treatable.

Nipah Virus

Nipah virus, named for the town of Sungai Nipah where the first outbreak was identified, is a novel virus from the family Paramyxoviridae that is closely related to the Hendra virus. From September 1998 into early 1999, 265 people in Malaysia developed febrile encephalitis and 111 of those affected died. This outbreak was linked to human contact with infected secretions of pigs. However, the potential of the Nipah virus to affect a variety of hosts and subsequently cause significant human disease with high mortality and few treatment options raises concern that this virus has potential as a bioweapon. This virus falls to a Category C because human-to-human transmission does not occur and droplet spread is limited.

PATHOPHYSIOLOGY/PROPERTIES OF EXPOSURE

Hantavirus

Hantavirus occurs in a worldwide distribution. Currently there are more than 20 sero/genotypes worldwide. Close contact with infected rodents is a precursor for disease transmission. Transmission to humans from rodents is through respiratory secretions, urine, and saliva. The Sin Nombre virus requires inhalation of urine or aerosolized feces but rodent bite transmission has been described for other hantaviruses in rare circumstances. Human-to-human transmission was first reported in an outbreak in Argentina in 1996 but other outbreaks have not demonstrated person-to-person spread.

The pathophysiology of hantaviral infection centers on vascular dysfunction. The vascular permeability that is the hallmark of infection appears to be immune mediated rather than a direct cytopathic affect of the virus. Elevated levels of tumor necrosis factor (TNF) and γ-interferon are noted in HPS and are probable mediators of pulmonary endothelial permeability. TNF likely mediates the fever, myalgias, and hypotension. Histopathologic findings in HFRS are mainly

hemorrhagic necrosis of the renal medulla with tubular degeneration. HPS hallmark histopathologic changes consist of interstitial pneumonitis transudative edema and mononuclear cell infiltration and areas of hyaline membrane formation with preserved respiratory epithelium.

Nipah Virus

Fruit bats, distributed across Australia, Indonesia, Malaysia, and the Philippines, are believed to be the natural hosts of the Nipah virus. The mode of transmission from bats to animals has yet to be identified and there is no evidence of bat to human transmission when looking at bat handlers. Human infection appears to require close contact with contaminated animal tissue or body fluids, with pigs being the source of outbreak in the Malaysian epidemic. Other infectious sources such as dogs and cats cannot be excluded, as the virus has been cultured in these animals.

The incubation period of Nipah virus is between 4 and 18 days. Once infection occurs, the virus spreads systemically, with primary central nervous system (CNS) involvement. Affected tissues demonstrate vasculitis-induced thrombosis and microinfarction. Histologic examination of infected tissues reveals intracytoplasmic viral inclusion and Nipah antigens in endothelial and parenchymal cells of the brain, lung, heart, and kidneys.

PERSONAL PROTECTIVE EQUIPMENT/DECONTAMINATION

Avoidance of close contact with infected rodents and their excrement is the primary method of protection against hantaviral disease. Use of a respiratory filter such as the N-100 will likely prevent inhalation of the virus when working in known contaminated areas. Nipah virus transmission can likely be prevented by avoidance of contact with infected tissue and body fluids. Although the virus has been identified in respiratory secretions, there is no documented person-to-person transmission. All patients directly exposed in a known bioterrorist attack should be decontaminated with soap and water. Standard universal precautions are indicated when caring for infected humans. Like other enveloped viruses, hantaviruses are inactivated by heat, detergents, organic solvents, and hypochlorite solutions. Decontamination is based on guidelines extrapolated from recommendation made by the CDC for viral hemorrhagic fever agents. Steam sterilization is likely the most effective method of decontaminating infected material. For those objects not amenable to steam sterilization, the CDC recommends a 1:100 dilution of household bleach or any of the standard hospital disinfectants registered with the U.S. Environmental Protection Agency.

CLINICAL MANIFESTATIONS/ DIFFERENTIAL DIAGNOSIS

Hantavirus

Hantaviral infection manifests with clinical diversity but can be simplified into the two described syndromes, HFRS and HPS. HPS generally progresses through three phases: prodromal, cardiopulmonary, and convalescent. The prodrome manifests as a short-lived influenza-like illness with fever, myalgias, and headache followed by the cardiopulmonary phase with hypoxia and shock associated with increased capillary permeability and noncardiac pulmonary edema. Rhabdomyolysis in the setting of HPS is common. Renal failure is not typical of the HPS caused by the Sin Nombre and New York hantaviruses but has occurred in association with the Bayou, Black Creek Canal, and Andes HPS. HFRS in the severe form as caused by the Hantaan and Dobra viruses progresses through five phases of illness: febrile, hypotensive, oliguric, diuretic, and convalescent. The febrile prodrome usually lasts 3–7 days and is associated with headache and myalgias. The hypotensive phase follows and may last from hours to days and it is at this stage of the disease that hemorrhagic complications tend to occur. Upon return of a normal blood pressure, the patient then enters the oliguric phase, which may persist for 3–7 days before urine output returns. This is followed by the diuretic phase in which the patient may have several liters of urine output per day, lasting up to several weeks. Lastly, the convalescence phase may last for several months until the patient feels back to baseline. The HFRS caused by the Seoul virus is similar to the Hantaan virus but is distinguished by the presence of hepatitis in a significant proportion of patients. Puumala virus causes a milder illness, without the hemorrhagic complications and hypotension associated with the more severe forms of HFRS. Clinical outcomes of HFRS are more favorable than outcomes associated with HPS. HPS has a case mortality rate of 50–60% while HFRS mortality ranges from 5% to 10% with Hantaan virus and as low as 1% with Puumala virus infection.

Early infection may be difficult to identify as clinical symptoms may mimic influenza with myalgias and gastrointestinal complaints or even atypical pneumonia when dealing with HPS. However, the laboratory findings described below help steer the clinician toward consideration of hantaviral infection.

Nipah Virus

Nipah virus appears clinically about 2 weeks after infection. Illness is characterized by fever, myalgias, headache, dizziness, and vomiting. Encephalitis manifesting as altered mental status with rapid progression to coma may occur in up to half of those infected with the virus. Physical findings include hypertension and tachycardia and abnormal neurologic findings to include decreased or absent reflexes, abnormal papillary response, myoclonus, and generalized tonic-clonic seizures. Magnetic resonance imaging (MRI) of the brain may show focal lesions in the subcortical and deep white matter.

The illness has been described to last from 3 to 31 days with a mean duration of 7 days. Patients with normal levels of consciousness can be expected to have a full recovery but those with altered mental status carry a poor prognosis.

LAB STUDIES

Hantavirus

Nonspecific laboratory findings occur in hantaviral infections to include thrombocytopenia, leukocytosis, and hemoconcentration. Laboratory markers associated with rhabdomyolysis such as myoglobinuria, elevated creatine kinase, hyperkalemia and hypocalcemia, and increased BUN and creatinine may be seen. For definitive diagnosis, viral serologic identification is required. Indirect immunofluorescence with native virus grown in E6 cells is the most commonly used test. Reverse transcriptase polymerase chain reaction with genus-or type-specific primers has been successfully used to identify HPS and has the advantage of being able to screen for multiple pathogens. Serologic identification using enzyme immunoassays remains the mainstay of diagnosis. Antigen detection in neutrophils and peripheral blood mononuclear cells with polyclonal and monoclonal antibodies has also reported to be useful in early HFRS and can also be used for postmortem tissue analysis. Isolation of Hantavirus is difficult, often taking several weeks and is therefore not useful clinically. Additionally virus isolation poses a potential threat to laboratory workers.

Nipah Virus

Laboratory findings in Nipah virus are also nonspecific and include leukopenia, thrombocytopenia, elevated aspartate aminotransferase, and alanine aminotransferase. Abnormalities in blood urea, creatinine, and electrolytes have not been noted in previous cases. Cerebrospinal fluid (CSF) analysis may reveal elevated white blood cell counts and elevated protein. However, there is no correlation between abnormal CSF findings and the severity of disease. Nipah virus can be cultured from body fluids (CSF, urine, and tracheal aspirates) and diagnosis can be made by identification of IgM antibodies in either blood or CSF. Serum or CSF samples may also be positive for antibodies against Hendra virus.

TREATMENT

Treatment is largely supportive for both Hantavirus and Nipah virus. Hantavirus requires intravascular volume maintenance and possibly even inotropic support. In the setting of HFRS, hemodialysis or peritoneal dialysis may be required. Nipah virus has less of an effect on circulatory issues but the CNS depression can result in respiratory compromise. In the case outbreak in Malaysia, half of the patients required ventilatory support. Ribavirin inhibits viral replication in laboratory animals but human results have been inconclusive. Ribavirin has shown clinical effectiveness in HFRS if given within the first 5 days of illness onset, reducing mortality, presence of oliguria during renal failure, and the risk of hemorrhage. However, the results have not been as promising in HPS. Ribavirin, aspirin, and pentoxifylline were also used in the Malaysian outbreak of Nipah virus with no significant effect on morbidity or mortality. Ribavirin is most effective if used within 7 days of the onset of symptoms. Current dosing recommendations by the CDC are to treat initially with ribavirin 30 mg/kg intravenously, followed by 15 mg/kg every 6 hours for 4 days, then 7.5 mg/kg every 8 hours for an additional 6 days. Ribavirin use may result in a dose-related, reversible hemolytic anemia.

PROPHYLAXIS

Currently the U.S. Army Medical Research Institute of Infectious Disease (USAMRIID) offers an investigational vaccinia-vectored Hantaan vaccine to laboratory personnel and there is an inactivated vaccine used in Asia against HFRS. No vaccine is available for Nipah virus.

FORENSIC ISSUES

Because Nipah virus is transmitted through contact with infected tissues, measures to prevent close contact with infected tissues and secretions should be taken.

Suggested Reading

Bronze MS, Huycke MM, Machado LJ, et al. Viral agents as biological weapons and agents of bioterrorism. *J Med Sci.* 2002;323(6):316–25.

Chapman LE, Mertz GJ, Peters CJ, et al. Intravenous ribavirin for hantavirus pulmonary syndrome: safety and tolerance during 1 year of open label experience. Ribavirin study group. *Antiviral Ther.* 1999;4(4):211–9.

Goh KJ, Tan CT, Chew NK, et al. Clinical features of Nipah virus encephalitis among pig farmers in Malaysia. *N Engl J Med.* 2000;342:1229–35.

Hooper JW, Li D. Vaccines against Hantaviruses. *Curr Top Microbiol Immunol.* 2001;256:171–91.

Lam SK. Nipah virus—a potential agent of bioterrorism. *Antiviral Research.* 57(102):113–9.

McCaughey C, Hart CA. Hantaviruses. *J Med Microbiol.* 2000;49:587–99.

Peters CJ, Khan AS. Hantavirus pulmonary syndrome: the new American hemorrhagic fever. *Clin Infect Dis.* 2002;34:1224–31.

47

EMERGING PATHOGENS

Robin B. McFee

S T A T   F A C T S

EMERGING PATHOGENS

Worldwide there are numerous viral, bacterial, parasitic, and fungal infections *not* common to the U. S. but increasingly likely to occur as immigration, global travel, occupations (laboratorian, researcher, Peace Corps) sets the stage for importing emerging diseases. Moreover, both globally and in the U. S. pathogens can adapt into selected highly virulent strains such as multidrug resistant TB.

Consider:

- Common presentations of uncommon infections (i.e. not well established in the U. S.)
- Uncommon presentations of common infections.

Highly worrisome pathogens that persist in causing global morbidity and mortality as well as increased incidence in certain parts of the world:

- Tuberculosis (multidrug [MDR TB] and extremely drug resistant [XDR TB] strains)
- Dengue
- Malaria
- Plague

Moreover, the astute provider will plan for numerous biopsychosocial morbidities, including unusual infectious diseases, from U. S. Military returning from overseas deployments, especially in the Middle East which harbors many desert illnesses including several vector borne illnesses.

The alert clinician should be aware of and inquire about the following risk factors:

- Occupation
- Travel
- Military
- Recent immigration to the U. S.
- Exposure to large groups (especially at risk groups—volunteers in prisons, working with homeless and undocumented populations)

Of concern are patients, especially young, previously healthy patients, including more than one case, present with the following:

- **Rapidly progressive symptoms**
  - High fever (>38°C/>101°F)
  - Patient states this is the worst he/she has ever felt
  - Especially short time from onset of illness to symptoms
  - Cascade of multisystem symptoms unexpected with common/community acquired illnesses
  - Severe symptoms per system
    - Shortness of breath
    - Chest pain
    - Significant gastrointestinal symptoms
  - Prolonged and/or rapidly progressive symptoms
  - CNS involvement
- **Categories of emerging pathogens**
  - Viral
  - Parasitic
  - Bacterial
  - Fungal
- **Routes of infection**
  - Deliberate
  - Food borne
  - Inhalation
  - Vector borne
  - Wound/percutaneous

The preliminary diagnosis of emerging pathogens is clinical with laboratory as confirmation. Alert laboratory when considering an unusual pathogen.

Involve infectious disease, public health and health care facility laboratory early for guidance.

The CDC Emergency Operations Center: 1.770.488.7100. The reader should complete the following and post in a readily available location:

Infectious Disease Consult:_____

Local health dept:_____

INTRODUCTION

"The single greatest threat to man's continued existence on earth is the virus."

—Joshua Ledeberg, Nobel Laureate.

The terrorist attacks of September 11, 2001, demonstrated that the United States is no longer isolated from a dangerous world or protected by its geography. Oceans and borders can be readily crossed, making the United States as vulnerable as other nations to acts of terrorism. Geoglobal and societal factors have combined to create conditions that facilitate the emergence and spread of previously unknown clinical entities such as severe acute respiratory syndrome (SARS), emerging pathogens not common to the United States but endemic to other regions such as West Nile virus, relatively harmless viruses evolving into highly lethal pathogens such as the HPAI H5N1 strain of avian influenza as well as the intentional release of biological weapons. Increased globalization, climate changes, encroachment of previously untouched natural habitats, worldwide food distribution, human population growth, overcrowding, and travel all favor the spread of infectious diseases—especially ones not commonly seen in the United States.

The former Soviet Union employed over 60,000 scientists at their bioweapon institute Biopreparat. Many of these scientists are now working for other countries. Estimates suggest that more than 20 countries have some form of bioweapons program. Tens of thousands of our servicemen and servicewomen will be returning from the Persian Gulf—many of whom may be infected with diseases endemic to the region or the result of undetected bioweapons. Certain "desert illnesses" as well as brucellosis, mosquitoborne diseases can present with central nervous system, behavioral and mental status changes. Will we diagnose them correctly or will their return be marked by another "Persian Gulf Syndrome?" This syndrome in the early postwar years became synonymous for post-traumatic stress disorder (PTSD). In reality, it represented a variety of etiologies ranging from chemical exposure, desert illnesses, as well as PTSD. Therefore the threat of biological weapons or uncommon illness is no longer the stuff of Robin Cook novels but the reality of our future practices. The ED physician should remain alert for such exigencies.

If the intentional use of anthrax in 2001 taught us anything it was that an astute physician could save lives. Equally, physicians who do not know the common signs of deadly, albeit uncommon illnesses will lose lives. Emerging infectious diseases can pose a significant threat to our communities, and may also be utilized in an intentional spread as a biological weapon.

Over the last few years, we have seen the appearance of monkeypox in the United States as the result of animal importation, plague patients diagnosed in New York (contracted it in the Southwest), SARS in nearby Canada, and avian flu affecting humans in Eurasia. Avian influenza remains a worrisome pathogen. Outbreaks of various viral hemorrhagic fever viruses from dengue to Ebola remain as persistent health threats. Each can be transported into the United States; recognition of their respective biodromes will make early recognition easier and thus increase the likelihood of rapid containment and improved survivability.

The optimism of the "antibiotic era" and our so-called victory over pathogens should be tempered by the realization that 5.7 million annual deaths are the direct result of TB, AIDS, and malaria, according to the World Health Organization (WHO). This represents approximately one-fourth of the deaths worldwide per year—the result of three infectious diseases. Multidrug-resistant tuberculosis (MDR TB) and extremely drug-resistant TB (XDR TB) are on the increase and pose a significant threat worldwide, including the United States where in certain regions and among certain risk groups remains a significant health problem.

The emergency department (ED) is situated at the crossroads between medicine, public health, and the forces responsible for rapid spread of infectious diseases. A safety net provider for many, the ED is a frontline center for disease surveillance and will be called upon for early identification of outbreaks. Recognition of the clinical syndromes associated with emerging pathogens—whether those previously unknown, pathogens spread to new areas by global forces, or biological weapons—as well as rapidly implementing containment and treatment measures will largely rest upon the clinical acumen of the ED physician. Maintaining an index of suspicion for relatively uncommon illnesses—this includes the common presentations of here to for nonendemic (to the United States) infections, staying abreast of trends in travel-related illness and emerging patterns of disease will be critical to make an early diagnosis. Realizing travelers can inadvertently import illness into countries where such entities are not endemic, thus making it essential to inquire about travel and occupation.

While the incidence of imported infectious disease presenting to HCF is not well-defined, it is well-known that significant numbers of patients present to medical facilities upon return from traveling with a variety of complaints, including respiratory infections. Studies suggest clinicians do a poor job of obtaining a travel history, including a general lack of awareness by physicians concerning the potential for nonendemic disease in the population that they attend. In one such study evaluating whether a travel history was recorded in patients, a travel history was recorded in only 2% of all patients presenting to this emergency department (ED) although among total number of patients presenting to the ED, 5.3% actually had the potential for a travel-related illness. Thus there remains the risk that imported diseases such as avian influenza may be undiagnosed in the acute setting, lead to possible spread before containment can be effected and delay treatment.

The two chapters of this book that discuss avian influenza and SARS should serve as an introduction to emerging pathogens, an approach to their diagnosis as well as demonstrating a need to remain vigilant for important infectious agents abroad that though historically uncommon to the United States have the potential and are likely to arrive in our ED given global forces.

Suggested Reading

Agarwal R, Shukla SK, Dharmani S, et al. Biological warfare—an emerging threat. *J Assoc Physicians India.* 2004 Sep;52: 733–8.

Henderson DA. *Emerging Infectious Diseases*—Special Issue—Smallpox: Clinical and Epidemiologic Features. Last accessed 4/19/03 *www.cdc.gov.ncidod/eid/vol5no4/henderson.htm*

McFee RB, Bush L, Boehm K. Avian influenza: critical considerations for the primary care physician. *Johns Hopkins Adv Studies In Med.* 2006; Nov/Dec:

McFee RB. Bioterrorism and weapons of mass destruction 2004: Physicians as first responders. *The DO.* 2004 March (Special BT Issue), 9–23.

McFee RB. Preparing for an era of weapons of mass destruction (WMD)—are we there yet? Why we should all be concerned. Part 1. *Vet Human Tox.* 2002.

O'Byrne WT, Terndrup TE, Kiefe CI, et al. A primer on biological weapons for the clinician, Part I. *Adv Stud Med.* 2003;3(2): 75–86.

Poison Perspectives For Health Care Professionals: Bioterrorism—Part 1. The Long Island Poison and Information Center. *http://www.winthrop.org* Last accessed 2/1/0

Saks MA, Karras D. Emergency medicine and the public's health: emerging infectious disease. *Emerg Med Clin N Am.* 2006; 24:1019–1033.

Stienlauf S, Segal G, Sidi Y, et al. Epidemiology of travel-related hospitalization. *J Travel Med.* 2005;12:136–141.

USAMRIID's *Medical Management of Biological Casualties Handbook.* 4th ed. 2001. Fort Detrick, Frederick, MD. *www.usamriid.army.mil* Last accessed 1/0.

Van Herck K, Van Damme P, Castelli F, et al. Knowledge, attitudes and practices in travel-related infectious diseases: the European airport survey. *J Travel Med.* 2004;11:3–8. *www.bt. cdc.gov* Last accessed 11/06

48

AVIAN INFLUENZA

Robin B. McFee

AVIAN FLU (H5N1)

Increasing numbers of young, previously healthy patients with rapidly progressive respiratory symptoms associated with other extrapulmonary symptoms.

The preliminary diagnosis of avian influenza is clinical. Treatment and preventive measures *should not* be delayed while waiting for laboratory confirmation.

H5N1 = STAT contact infectious disease, public health and health care facility laboratory

Avian influenza alerts and updates are available from the World Health Organization (WHO) www.who.int and the Centers for Disease Control www.cdc.gov

The CDC Emergency Operations Center: 1.770.488.7100. The reader should complete the following and post in a readily available location:

Infectious Disease Consult:_____
Local health dept:_____

Clinical

H5N1 follows an unusually aggressive clinical course: rapid deterioration, high fatality.

Incubation period: 2–8 days or as long as 14–17 days.

Illness: Early illness begins with fever—Fever spike usually >101°F [initial >38°C (>100.4°F)] and constitutional symptoms not normally associated with seasonal flu.

- Difficulty breathing—almost universal symptom of avian flu/always—occurs early in illness (worrisome and warrants work up even if not avian flu!)
- Respiratory distress, a hoarse voice, and a crackling sound when inhaling
- Sputum production is variable and sometimes bloody.
- Other features: CNS involvement—seizures/ encephalopathy

Testing

Presumptive diagnosis is clinical based upon a thorough travel (affected areas, interaction with sick birds)/occupational history, and symptom cascade (biodrome).

Chest X-Ray (CXR) Any of the following is associated with clinical deterioration:

- Extensive infiltration bilaterally
- Lobar collapse
- Focal consolidation
- Interstitial lung infiltrates (less common)

Laboratory

General

- Lower total peripheral white blood cell counts—more often lymphopenic
- Impaired renal function (~30% of H5N1 cases)
- Abnormal liver function tests (associated with pneumonia)

Specific H5N1

- Influenza A/H5 (Asian lineage) Virus Real-Time RT-PCR Primer and Probe Set can provide preliminary results on suspected H5 influenza samples within 4 hours (Laboratory Response Network test = contact CDC or local health department).
- RT PCR using nasopharyngeal aspirate or bronchial alveolar lavage followed by nasopharyngeal or throat swab placed in viral transport medium.
- Contact health care facility laboratorian for updated information and to warn of suspected H5N1 re: precautions and also guidance on sample handling.

Treatment

Patients can deteriorate rapidly; within 3–6 days. Early treatment with aggressive supportive care is essential to confer a chance of survival.

Oseltamivir

Adults and Adolescents >13 years: Twice daily dose of 75 mg by mouth is being recommended for avian influenza for 7–10 days or longer guided by patient's clinical course.

NB: Severely ill patients w/GI involvement may not effectively absorb Oseltamivir.

Children:

- >1 year = twice daily oral dosing based upon weight:
  - 30 mg/dose if weight is <= 15 kg.
  - 45 mg/dose if 15–23 kg

- 60 mg/dose if 23–40 kg
- 75 mg/dose >40 kg

Prophylactic use: Oseltamivir can be used as prophylactic chemotherapy for persons exposed to avian influenza. WHO recommends healthcare workers receive 75 mg orally once a day for at least 7 days with vaccination against seasonal influenza.

Infection Control

CDC recommends universal precautions: treat as airborne risk: respiratory precautions Screen patients upon intake, isolate and/or cohort patients once diagnosed

- Waiting room prompts/advisory to:
  - Notify receptionist if symptoms/travel risks consistent with H5N1
  - Wear mask (provide them) if coughing

BACKGROUND

The term "influenza" describes an acute viral disease of the respiratory tract caused by viruses that belong to the orthomyxovirus family, which includes the genera of influenza virus A, B, and C as defined by the antigenicity of the nucleocapsid and matrix proteins. Generally influenza A viruses are associated with more severe human illness, epidemics, and pandemics. Influenza A virus is a negative sense, single-stranded RNA virus, with an eight-segment genome that encodes for 10 proteins. Influenza A virus is further subtyped by two surface proteins—hemagglutinin (H), which attaches the viral particle to the host cell for cell entry, and neuraminidase (N), which facilitates the spread of progeny virus. It is the latter, which is a target for the class of antiviral therapy referred to as neuraminidase inhibitors, which will be discussed shortly.

There are 16 H and 9 N subtypes, which make up all the subtypes of influenza A by various combinations. The term "antigenic drift" refers to the various mutations and changes in surface antigenicity of these surface proteins as a response to host immunity. This is why every year, usually in February, World Health Organization (WHO) decides the strain of viruses to be incorporated into the annual influenza vaccine. More worrisome is the potential for "antigenic shift;" an event that can lead to the creation of a novel virus against which humans have little or no immunity. This can occur because influenza has a segmented genome—shuffling of gene segments can occur if two different subtypes of influenza A virus infect the same cell. If a human flu virus, such as H3N2 and an avian H5N1 virus coinfect a human or pig, a new virus "H5N2" could emerge—a hybrid that could bring the high virulence and case fatality rate of H5N1 with the efficiency of human to human transmission found in the "parent" human virus.

Studies suggest this is what happened in the 1957 and 1968 influenza pandemics. A pandemic is considered an epidemic that crosses continents. Of note, while Mother Nature has demonstrated its capacity to do this, such viral reassortment also could be accomplished in a laboratory for bioterrorism purposes. Therefore bioterrorism preparedness, increased surveillance, and efforts to enhance physician training in unusual or emerging diseases is of significant importance.

Unlike usual patterns of mortality associated with seasonal flu, namely the very young and old, both the 1918 pandemic and what is currently occurring with H5N1 involved all age groups. Once avian influenza A H5N1 becomes a more human-like virus with the ability to efficiently cause person-to-person spread, in the absence of an effective, prepositioned, widely available vaccine, a pandemic could rapidly develop. Illnesses can traverse the country given we must consider our nation is highly susceptible with little to no immunity. Most scenarios describe a significant number of people becoming quite sick over a relatively short period of time. The ability to contain such a public health crisis may well rest on the community physician who will be called upon to rapidly diagnose, treat, and, provide care to a potentially overwhelming number of patients (and protect his or her family, too)!

There are many genotypes of H5N1—the predominant one is "Z," which is associated with high virulence for a wide range of animals from poultry to felines. It appears to be stable in the environment for up to 6 days, but can be transmitted, albeit inefficiently, from person to person.

Influenza virus (the "seasonal" forms, which have caused significant respiratory illness for centuries), remains a major, global public health problem, which continues to result in millions of cases of severe illness, as well as approximately 500,000 deaths worldwide and 36,000 deaths in the United States annually. Yet it is a vaccine preventable disease.

An influenza pandemic occurs when (1) a new flu virus emerges for which people have little or no immunity, (2) the virus spreads readily from person to person, and (3) no vaccine is available. Avian influenza virus A H5N1 is a virus that has resulted in the death of over 140 million birds, is continuing to mutate, and, unlike other strains of flu, has demonstrated an ability to cause significant pulmonary damage. Avian flu, for the moment, passes easily from bird to bird. It infects birds via the intestinal tract, which allows the virus to be found in feces. Of note, the more ordinary strains of avian flu usually infect migratory birds and do not result in disease; the H5N1 is killing these very animals suggesting the virus has adapted and thus increased its virulence and capacity to kill. This persistence in the ground promotes contamination to people, other animals as well as a risk to water. Avian flu infects people via the respiratory tract, which can be accomplished by fomites, inhaling the virus, or getting it on hands and then contacting the pulmonary mucosa (Fig. 48-1). Currently H5N1 affects domesticated poultry (chickens, ducks, turkey) as well as migratory birds (wild ducks, geese, swans); it is the latter, which do not honor borders, are not readily contained thus enhancing the global spread. Fortunately people cannot get avian flu from eating properly cooked poultry. Eating raw eggs, poultry blood, or undercooked bird meat are modalities that one could become infected and are practices in countries where human avian flu cases have been recorded. The virus is demonstrating an ability to infect other species like cats and people.

The following must occur before avian flu can cause human pandemics the way it has caused bird pandemics: (1) avian flu must be able to infect humans, (2) it must be virulent, and (3) it must spread easily from person to person. Avian flu already has demonstrated the first two factors, but it has not quite achieved the last factor. While data suggest there have been a few cases resulting from human-to-human transmission, we have been fortunate that the infection stopped at the second person, usually a family member.

As of this writing, H5N1 is inefficient at person-to-person transmission unlike the highly contagious nature of the seasonal flu virus (actually viruses) in general.

POTENTIAL MAGNITUDE OF A PANDEMIC

However if avian influenza virus A H5N1 mutates into a more human-like influenza, (i.e., develops the ability to be as contagious as seasonal flu), is then likely to spread very rapidly in a sustained fashion across the globe and result in thousands, perhaps millions of deaths similar to the flu pandemic of 1918 (which resulted in deaths estimated at between 20 and 50 million people worldwide), some experts suggest upwards of 2.5% of the world's population could be affected in a matter of months while others pose more dire projections. Estimates suggest an influenza pandemic could sicken upwards of 90 million people in the United States, including over one-third of the health-care workforce. Federal officials are concerned at least 10 million influenza patients could require hospitalization at least for one night including almost 1.5 million requiring intensive care and possibly 750,000 needing ventilator assistance. Given the persistent problem of diminished surge capacity, hospital overcrowding from the emergency department to the ventilated beds in the critical care units is inevitable when a pandemic occurs. Overall poor infection control practices within health-care facilities in addition to health-care workers (HCW) demonstrating low vaccine rates, inconsistent hand-washing and deficiencies in other respiratory hygiene practices are the building blocks to promote rapid spread of an emerging contagion.

The exact impact of a global pandemic remains unknown in spite of numerous projection models. WHO leaders are concerned that it is not a matter of if, but when avian influenza breaks loose, not only arriving in the West, but becoming more efficient at person-to-person transmission. If that occurs, primary care physicians will likely be on the front lines, (perhaps even diagnosing the index case), clearly providing guidance to the worried well, treating the sick, and working with public health and other organizations in an attempt to contain the outbreak. It is a daunting task, especially in the absence of a widely available vaccine and few antivirals (of which each must be administered early in the course of illness). In a world without borders, unusual emerging pathogens from SARS to H5N1 can arrive on passenger airliners or many other entry points.

If seasonal influenza is a predictable killer, the avian flu has the potential to be a true killing machine. Despite the efforts of the international health community to contain the avian influenza epidemic that emerged in Southeast

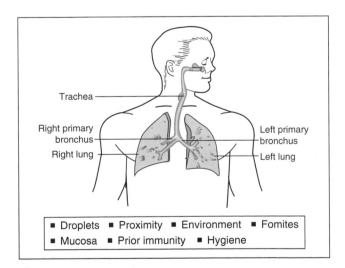

Trachea

Right primary bronchus

Right lung

Left primary bronchus

Left lung

- Droplets ■ Proximity ■ Environment ■ Fomites
- Mucosa ■ Prior immunity ■ Hygiene

FIGURE 48-1

SPREAD OF RESPIRATORY INFECTIONS

HUMAN CASES OF AVIAN INFLUENZA A H5N1 WORLD WIDE BY NATION

Location	Total # of Human Cases	Total Deaths
Azerbaijan	8	5
Cambodia	7	7
Djibouti	1	0
Thailand	25	17
Vietnam	93	42
Indonesia	98	78
China	25	16
Turkey	12	4
Egypt	34	14
Iraq	3	2
Total as of 6/04/07	**306**	**185**

Source: From World Health Organization (WHO), www.who.org WHO confirmed human cases—Updated 4 June 2007.

Asia in 2003/2004, sporadic cases of human influenza A H5N1 infection are still reported—and carry a high case fatality rate (Table 48-1). Never before has an avian influenza strain killed so many hundreds of millions of birds, traveled so far so fast, and posed the potential to simultaneously affect Asia, Europe, and other continents.

CLINICAL

Epidemiology

Unlike usual patterns of mortality associated with seasonal flu, namely the very young and old, both the 1918 pandemic and what is currently occurring with H5N1 involved all age groups, especially ages 20–40 who are confined together, such as the military and universities. The case fatality rate of H5N1 is >50% depending upon the country.

Pathogenesis of Avian Flu

H5N1 induces proinflammatory cytokines (such as interferon gamma inducible protein and tumor necrosis factor [TNF] alpha) in human macrophage cells, which may lead to a cytokine storm and death without extrapulmonary viral dissemination. The hemagglutinin of this influenza virus also may attach to respiratory epithelium to cause inhibition of epithelial sodium channels leading to pulmonary edema, alveolar flooding, and early acute respiratory failure—events that rarely accompany seasonal flu.

For the moment, the most important route of acquisition for avian influenza H5N1 infection is through contact with infected birds or their excreta. However, hospital-acquired infection was revealed in a retrospective study.

HCW exposed to patients with H5N1 infection were more likely to be seropositive and this was not attributable to animal exposure. It is reasonable to assume that the route of infection for avian influenza patients, like most flu patients, will be from inhalation of infective respiratory secretions and/or contact with virus-laden secretions and subsequent contact with mucous membranes (Fig. 48-1). Studies also suggest airborne transmission is possible, which would explain the occasional numerically explosive nature of influenza epidemics.

Clinical Presentation (Table 48-2)

Avian flu (H5N1) presents with a rapid onset of severe illness including a fever spike of over 101°F and often respiratory symptoms—nearly universal is dyspnea. Significant symptoms include muscle aches and generally feeling poorly, cough, headache, **shortness of breath, chest pain, and/or difficulty breathing**. The latter symptoms are not common to seasonal flu (especially in younger people), which seem to be increasingly affected by avian flu. *Avian flu illness is not subtle*; it will not present like the common cold or the average case of seasonal flu. Of those who present for medical attention, the illness is rapidly progressive with patients often complaining of chest pain and shortness of breath. True dyspnea is rarely associated with seasonal flu, especially in young, otherwise healthy, patients. Shortness of breath under most circumstances is worrisome and should be properly evaluated, but in the context of a rapid rise in temperature should raise an alarm for avian flu or other serious infection such as *Legionella* pneumonia. Furthermore, avian flu can have an extrapulmonary impact, including the central nervous system resulting in encephalopathy, seizures in addition to severe headache. Of note, while gastrointestinal (GI) symptoms may be more common among children with seasonal flu, **young adults and other age groups may experience abdominal pain, nausea, vomiting, or diarrhea before or during the development of respiratory symptoms from avian flu**, which is not common with seasonal flu in this age group. Unlike seasonal flu deaths, which often result from secondary infections such as pneumonia, avian influenza seems to cause direct pulmonary damage that can result in noncardiogenic pulmonary edema and pneumonia.

The differential diagnosis includes *Legionella* pneumonia and severe gram-negative pneumonias. *Legionella* pneumonia causes severe community-acquired pneumonia often requiring admission to an intensive care unit. Patients often have a nonproductive couth, pleuritic chest pain, diarrhea, and GI symptoms, not unlike the biodrome of avian influenza. A valuable clinical clue includes the finding of relative bradycardia as well as hyponatremia among Legionella patients. A recent study suggests *Legionella* is significantly underdiagnosed. Numerous clinical tests are available but each has limitations in time, sensitivity, or availability.

TABLE 48-2

KEY DIFFERENTIATING SYMPTOMS: AVIAN INFLUENZA COMPARED WITH SEASONAL FLU AND INFLUENZA-LIKE ILLNESSES/UPPER RESPIRATORY INFECTIONS

Is it? Number of "+" indicates strength of association`	Avian Flu (H5N1)	Seasonal Influenza (Flu)	Upper Respiratory Infection	Common Cold
Elevated temp	+++/++++	++	++	+/-
Fever/Chills	++++	++++	++++	
Cough	+++	+++	+++	+++
Shortness of breath	++++	+/-	+/-	
Chest discomfort	+++	++	++	
Sore Throat	+/-	+++	+++	++
Vomiting/nausea	++	+	+	
Diarrhea	++	+ (young children)	+/-	
CNS/Encephalopathy/Seizures	++	-	-	
Malaise/Fatigue	+	+++	+	
Runny nose/watery eyes	+/-	+	++	+++
Headache/Muscle Ache	++	+++	++	+/-
Young healthy at risk for serious illness	+++	+/-		

Source: With permission from McFee RB. Bush LM, Boehm KM. Avian influenza:Critical considerations for the primary care physician. Adv Stud Med 2006;6(60):432–440.

Polymerase chain reaction (PCR) for *L. pneumophilia* is available in some reference laboratories and can detect the organism in sputum, bronchoalveolar lavage (BAL) fluid and blood. *Legionella* species are not detected in routine cultures; physicians should specifically request culture for *Legionella* if it is suspected.

Tests

Presumptive diagnosis is clinical and based upon identifying the biodrome (symptom pattern recognition) (Table 48-2). Critical to diagnosing a potential case of avian flu include awareness in terms of most recent locations of avian influenza, asking your patient about recent travel (within 14 days) especially to countries suspected of having H5N1, an occupation history in addition to a thorough history of present illness and careful examination. However, certain initial tests can guide the clinician, especially with early infection control and treatment while initiating contact with specialized laboratories for confirmation.

Chest X-Ray

Major findings on chest x-ray (CXR) include extensive infiltration bilaterally, lobar collapse, focal consolidation, and less commonly interstitial lung infiltrates. Pleural effusion and widened mediastinum may be observed. Clinical deterioration associated with this is common.

Blood Work

Several patients had lower total peripheral white blood cell counts that are more often lymphopenic and associated with

fatality. Many patients presenting with pneumonia associated with H5N1 also had abnormal liver function tests. Over 30% of patients exhibited impaired renal function.

RT-PCR has superior sensitivity and specificity compared to antigen detection. Commercial immunochromatographic membrane enzyme immunoassay tests are not specific for H5 and only has a 70% specificity compared with viral culture. Nasopharyngeal aspirate or BAL followed by nasopharyngeal swab or throat swab placed in viral transport medium (VTM) should be collected with airborne precautions in patients suspected of having avian flu. A stool or rectal swab also placed in VTM should be considered. If H5N1 is suspected, the health department should be alerted for guidance as well as the laboratory to remind them to take proper precautions.

The Food and Drug Administration recently approved a laboratory test to diagnose patients suspected of being infected with avian influenza A/H5 viruses. The test is referred to as influenza A/H5 (Asian lineage) virus real-time RT-PCR primer and probe set. This test can provide preliminary results on suspected H5 Influenza samples within 4 hours once sample testing begins at the lab. This is a major advance given previous technology required 2–3 days for similar results. If the H5 strain is identified, further testing is required to determine the specific subtype (such as N1, etc). The test will be distributed nationwide to laboratory response network (LRN)-designated laboratories in order to enhance surveillance and diagnostic capabilities. There are approximately 140 LRN laboratories throughout the 50 United States. The CDC recommends *if a clinician suspects a patient may be infected with avian influenza, it is important to contact the local or state health department for assistance in accessing the LRN capabilities.* These laboratories can be accessed by calling 1.404.639.2790.

Management

CDC recommends respiratory/airborne precautions in addition to droplet and contact and standard precautions as infection control practices for HCW and health-care facilities. The period of communicability of H5N1 remains understudied but can last for up to 3 weeks in children.

Management strategies include identifying and isolating potential respiratory contagious patients, promoting the use of seasonal flu vaccines—especially among health care providers, maintaining adequate stocks of oseltamivir and zanamivir, universal and respiratory precautions, ample fitted N95 respirators, and personal protective equipment (PPE) that employees have been trained when and how to safely use. New antivirals and H5N1 vaccines are being evaluated but not currently available to the public.

Current Antivirals

There are two classes of antivirals available to treat influenza virus: the neuraminidase inhibitors oseltamivir (Tamiflu) and zanamivir (Relenza) (Refer to selected monographs.) The former is approved for influenza A and B viruses, and the M blockers amantadine (Symmetrel) and rimantadine (Flumadine). (Refer to selected monographs.) Each is designed to take advantage of influenza viral structure. While both classes can treat influenza viruses, avian flu H5N1 is already resistant to amantadine and rimantadine owing to several possible factors. The present circulating H5N1 has the genotype "Z," which confers a residue on the M2 protein—making avian flu intrinsically resistant to the M blockers. Some experts suggest the Chinese practice of administering amantadine to poultry may also have contributed to the antiviral resistance. At least for the moment, the neuraminidase inhibitors remain effective against both seasonal and avian flu but should be administered early—ideally within 48 hours of onset of illness. Oseltamivir when administered for seasonal flu is usually given at a dosage of 75 mg by mouth twice daily for 5 days. A higher dose (150 mg orally given twice daily) has been recommended in clinical trials and associated with a larger reduction in viral load and shorter duration of illness. Whether a higher dose given over a longer duration would confer benefit in avian influenza remains to be further evaluated but should be considered in patients with significant pulmonary and GI symptoms. Children older than 1 year of age can receive twice daily oral dosing based upon weight: 30 mg per dose if 15 kg or less, 45 mg if 15–23 kg, 60 mg for 23–40 kg and 75 mg for those over 40 kg. Unfortunately resistance to oseltamivir is emerging. Dosage may need to be adjusted in adults with renal impairment. There are insufficient human data to determine the risk to a pregnant woman or developing fetus (Pregnancy Category C). The most commonly reported adverse effects include nausea, abdominal pain, and vomiting. As with other antimicrobials, attention to early symptoms of anaphylactic/anaphylactoid risk is important.

The neuraminidase inhibitor oseltamivir can be used as a prophylactic chemotherapy for persons exposed to avian flu. WHO recommends HCW exposed to H5N1 receive 75 mg orally once a day for at least 7 days and may be required for 6 weeks; duration of protection lasts for the period of dosing. Vaccination against seasonal flu should be obtained if the HCW has not been immunized.

Zanamivir (Relenza) is an inhaled neuraminidase inhibitor, and has little systemic absorption; it may not be useful if extrapulmonary disease occurs. Data are lacking in terms of the effectiveness of Zanamivir against H5N1 either for acute treatment or as chemoprophylaxis, although experts consider it of value given the class effect of neuraminidase inhibitors.

Newer Treatments

Studies are underway evaluating a new neuraminidase inhibitor—Peramivir that in early studies, when compared to other neuraminidase inhibitors, showed promise against influenza. Other drugs being investigated to treat both seasonal and avian influenza include long-acting neuraminidase inhibitors, the antiviral Ribavirin and interferon alpha.

Other Modalities

It is important to avoid aspirin-containing products as a precaution against Reyes syndrome, in patients younger than 16 years of age. It should be noted, Reyes syndrome has been reported, albeit rarely, in adults as well. In addition to early administration of antiviral therapy, respiratory support and intensive care are critical during the acute stage of H5N1 pneumonic illness.

INFECTION CONTROL

Infection control for avian flu involves a two-tier approach: (1) Universal precautions, which apply to *all* patients at *all* times, including those who have HPAI H5N1, and (2) additional measures, which include droplet precautions, contact precautions, and the use of a high-efficiency (HE) mask (N95 or higher respirator) and negative pressure room if possible. Place patient in single room; cohort confirmed and suspected cases in designated areas. The distance between beds should be at least 1 m and separated by a barrier. Anyone entering the room must wear appropriate PPE: mask respirator, gown, face shield or goggles, gloves.

Transportation of Patients

If transportation is necessary from the isolation room, the patient should wear PPE, especially HE mask.

Waste Disposal

All waste generated in the isolation area should be treated as clinical/infectious waste. Handlers should also wear appropriate PPE. Liquid waste can be safely flushed into the toilet.

Cleaning and Disinfection

The survival time for the influenza virus is

- 24–48 hours on hard, nonporous surfaces
- 8–12 hours on cloth, paper, and tissue
- 5 minutes on hands

The virus is inactivated by 70% alcohol and by chlorine. Cleaning of environmental surfaces with neutral detergent followed by a disinfectant solution is recommended.

As an aside, it is very persistent in the environment, especially in farm soil in the presence of infected birds.

DISPOSITION OF THE DEAD

Continued use of universal precautions including HE mask is necessary. The body should be fully sealed in an impermeable body bag prior to transfer to the morgue/mortuary. The outside of the bag must be clean and free of liquid. A postmortem may be performed with caution given the lungs may still be filled with virus. Full PPE is recommended. Avoiding techniques that promote aerosolization of tissue is encouraged. Staff of the funeral home should be informed that the deceased had HPAI H5N1 and encouraged to follow universal precautions. Embalming may be conducted. Hygienic preparation of the deceased is permissible.

Vaccination Strategies

While an avian flu H5N1 vaccine is not available to the public, as of 2006, several are under clinical investigation worldwide. The U.S. government is conducting clinical tests on a vaccine that is based upon the Vietnamese H5N1 strain with early data suggesting the vaccine is both safe for human use and effective against the strain it was based upon.

Clinicians should encourage all patients to obtain seasonal flu vaccines immediately. While it is unknown if cross-protection for H5N1 is possible, and probably unlikely with the current batch of flu vaccines, seasonal flu remains a consistent killer and cause of significant morbidity annually.

POSTEXPOSURE PROPHYLAXIS

Individuals exposed to avian influenza should begin Oseltamivir. Prophylaxis should begin immediately or within 2 days—75 mg tablet each day for 7 days although therapy may continue upwards of 6 weeks according to WHO.

TRAVEL RECOMMENDATIONS

Persons planning to travel overseas for work, recreation, or humanitarian outreach should be able to do so relatively safely if precautions are taken. Vaccines against diseases endemic to the new host region may need weeks to evoke an immune response. Special precautions should be taken when contemplating visiting countries where avian flu infections are reported in birds, other animals, or people. This includes avoiding crowded places and farms, marketplaces that have poultry and/or kill chickens on demand, and changing clothes if visiting any of the above. No matter where the person visits, frequent hand-washing and respiratory hygiene should be stressed. Just as referral to a cardiologist for a patient with significant cardiac history is standard of care, so should referral to a travel medicine clinic or physician who specializes in travel medicine. These would be physicians with experience in emerging infectious diseases and the appropriate background such as infectious diseases, occupational medicine, medical toxicology, tropical medicine with additional specialized training in travel-related health issues that include not only pathogens but safety, nutrition, and other relevant topics. The U.S. Department of State provides important information about most countries with timely alerts on emerging threats, political instability or other risks for U.S. citizens. The CDC publishes the Yellow Book—a wonderful travel health resource. Recommendations about vaccines appropriate to foreign destinations can be obtained through CDC as well. The WHO publishes an updated screening and assessment algorithm for the management of returning travelers and visitors from countries affected by H5N1 presenting with febrile respiratory illness.

Autopsy

The risk of infectious disease transmission has long been recognized as a threat to prosectors, laboratorians and pathologists. Planning for large numbers of dead – ensuring adequate PPE, cold storage and logistics considerations for managing the dead – such as DMORT, is critical and an essential component for avian flu preparedness.

Suggested Reading

Avian flu/Pandemic flu. National Institutes of Health. *www.nih.gov* Last accessed 3/7/06.

Avian influenza—information for physicians. Centers for Disease Control and Prevention (CDC) *www.cdc.gov/flu* Last accessed 3/7/06.

Avian Influenza—Pandemic Preparedness. Mass Dept. of Health Projections March 2006.

Beigel JH, Farrar J, Han AM, et al. Avian influenza A (H5N1) infection in humans. *N Engl J Med.* 2005;353:1374–1385.

Bridges CB, Kuehnert MJ, Hall CB. Transmission of influenza: implications for control in health care settings. *Clin Infect Dis.* 2003;37:1094–1011.

Chen XJ, Set S, Yue G, et al. Influenza virus inhibits ENaC and lung fluid clearance. *Am J Physiol Lung Cell Mol Physiol.* 2004;287:L366–373.

Cheung CY, Poon LI, Lau AS, et al. Induction of proinflammatory cytokines in human macrophages by influenza A H5N1 viruses; a mechanism for the unusual severity of human disease? *Lancet.* 2002;360:1831–1837.

deJong MD, Bach VC, Phan TQ, et al. Fatal avian influenza A H5N1 in a child. *N Engl J Med.* 2005 Feb 17; 352(7):686–91.

Fouchier RA, Munster V, Wallensten A, et al. Characterization of a novel influenza A virus hemagglutinin subtype H16 obtained from black headed gulls. *J Vio.* 2005;79:2814–2822.

Gupta NE. Everything you should know about virulent avian flu. *Cortlandt Forum.* 2005 December 20:26–34.

HHS, FDA approves new laboratory test to detect human infections with avian influenza A/H5 viruses. 2006.02.03.

Highly Pathogenic Avian Influenza (HPAI) Inerim Infection Control Guidelines for Health Care Facilities—World Health Organization 18 February 2004.

Improving Influenza Vaccination Rates in Health Care Workers: Strategies to Increase Protection for Workers and Patients. National Foundation for Infectious Diseases, 2004 Washington, DC.

Infectious Diseases Society of America *www.idsociety.org*

Influenza A (H5N1): WHO interim infection control guidelines for health care facilities 2004. World Health Organization. *http: //www.who.int/csr/disease/avian_influenza/guidelines/ infectioncontrol1/en/*

Knight V, Gilbert BE. Ribavirin aerosol treatment of influenza. *Infect Dis Clin North Am.* 1987;441–57.

Krug RM. The potential use of influenza virus as an agent for bioterrorism. *Antiviral Res.* 2003;57:147–50.

Kunzelmann K, Beesley AH, King NH, et al. Influenza inhibits amiloride-sensitive NA+ channels in respiratory epithelia. *Proc Natl Acad Sci USA.* 2000;97:10282–7.

Langmuir AD. Changing concepts of airborne infection of acute contagious diseases; a reconsideration of classic epidemiologic theories. In: Kundsin RB, ed. *Airborne contagion.* New York, NY: Annals of the New York Academy of Sciences 1980;353:35–44.

Lederberg J, Shope RE, Oaks SC. Institute of Medicine Committee on Emerging Threats to Health. *Emerging Infections: microbial threats to health in the United States.* Washington, DC: National Academy Press. 1992.

Legionella pneumophila. In: *Infectious Diseases. Lexi-Comp Online.* Last accessed 5/20/06 *www.online.lexi.com/crlsql/ servlet/crlonline?a=doc&bc=idh&id=121387&mid=45264 &mn=*

Madren LK, Shipman C, Jr. Hayden FG. In vitro inhibitory effects of combinations of anti-influenza agents. *Antivir Chem Chemother.* 1995;6:109–113.

McFee RB Preparing for an era of weapons of mass destruction (WMD): are we there yet? Why we should all be concerned. Part I. *Vet Human Tox.* 2002;44(4):193–199.

McFee RB. Avian Influenza – The Next Pandemic? *Dis a Month.* 2007 (July) prepublication.

McFee RB, Bush LM, Boehm K. Avian influenza: Critical considerations and key strategies for the primary care physician. *Adv Stud Med.* 2006; 6(10):431–440)

Murdoch DR. Diagnosis of Legionella infection. *Clin Infec Dis.* 2003;36(1):64–69.

National Immunization Survey 2004. *MMWR.* 2006 *www. medscape.comviewarticle/522862_print* Last accessed 3/11/06.

Nolte KB, Taylor DG, Richmond JY. Biosafety considerations for autopsy. *Am J Forens Med and Path* 2002;23(2):107–122.

Osterholm MT, Emerging Infectious Diseases—A real public health crisis? Postgraduate Medicine online—1996 Nov; 100 (5). *http:// www.postgradmed.com/issues/1996/11_96/ed_nov.htm* Last accessed 2/16/06.

PandemicFlu.gov, AvianFlu.gov—Department of Health and Human Services (HHS). *http://ww.pandemicflu.gov/vaccine* Last accessed 3/7/06.

Preventing the flu. Influenza (Flu). CDC Key Facts About Flu Vaccine. *www.cdc.gov/flu/protect/keyfacts.htm* Last accessed 3/7/06.

Sidwell RW, Smee DF. Peramivir (BCX-1812, RWJ—270201): Potential new therapy for influenza. Expert Opinion. *Investig Drug.* 2002;11(6):859–869.

Silka A, Geiderman JM, Goldberg JB, et al. Demand on ED resources during periods of widespread influenza activity. *Am J Emerg Med.* 2003;21:534–539.

Singer AC, Nunn MA, Gould EA, Johnson AC. Potential risks associated with the proposed widespread use of Tamiflu. *Enviro Acad* 2007;115(1):102–106.

Smith SM. Where have you been? The potential to overlook imported disease in the acute setting. *Eur J Emerg Med.* 2005 Oct;12(5):230–3.

Stienlauf S, Segal G, Sidi Y, et al. Epidemiology of travel-related hospitalization. *J Travel Med.* 2005 May–Jun;12(3):136–41.

Taisuke H, Kawaoka Y. Influenza: lessons from past pandemics, warnings from current incidents. *Nat Rev Microbiol.* 2005;3:591–600.

Tran TH, Nguyen TL, Nguyen TD, et al. World Health Organization International Avian Influenza Investigative team. Avian influenza A H5N1 in 10 patients in Vietnam. *N Engl J Med.* 2004;350:1179–88.

Ungchusak K, Auerwarakul P, Dowell SF, et al. Probable person to person transmission of avian influenza A H5N1. *N Engl J Med.* 2005;352:333–340.

Ver Herck K, Van Damme P, Castelli F, et al. Knowledge, attitudes and practices in travel—related infectious diseases: The European airport survey. *J Travel Med.* 2004 Jan–Feb; 11(1):3–8.

World Health Organization. WHO interim guidelines on clinical management of humans infected by influenza A (H5N1). *http://www.who.int/csr/disease/avian_influenza/ guidelines/ Guidelines_clinical%20management_H5N1_rev.pdf*

World Health Organization: Algorithm for the management of returning travellers from countries affected by H5N1 presenting with febrile respiratory illness: recognition, investigation and initial management. *http://www.hpa.org.uk/infections/ topics_az/influenza/avian/algorithm.htm* Last accessed 5/20.06.

World Report. Nations set out a global plan for influenza action. *Lancet.* 2005; November 12;366. *www.thelancet.com* Last accessed 3/3/06.

Yuen KY, Wong SSY. Human infection by avian influenza A H5N1. *Hong Kong Med J.* 2005;11(3):189–199.

Zigmund J. No more room; overcrowding blamed for ambulance diversions. *Moderhealthcare.com* February 13, 2006. *www. modernhealthcare.com/printwindow.cms?articleId=38689 & pageType=article* Last accessed 3/11/06.

49

SARS: SEVERE ACUTE RESPIRATORY SYNDROME

Robin B. McFee

S T A T   F A C T S

SARS: SEVERE ACUTE RESPIRATORY SYNDROME

- Severe acute respiratory syndrome (SARS) is a highly contagious, severe febrile respiratory illness that can cause death.
- Case fatality rate (CFR) is 10%, but *can exceed 50% in the patients over 60* years old.
- Global travel = risk for nonendemic illnesses; be alert; consider in differential diagnosis.
- If SARS is suspected, involve infectious disease, public health, and the laboratory early for guidance on disease control, specimens, and newly released interventions if available.
- Be aware of SARS alerts from World Health Organization (WHO) and Centers for Disease Control (CDC)—Figs. 49-1 and 49-2.
- CDC Emergency Operations Center: 1.770.488.7100
- Local public health department _____, Extension Inf. Dis _____

Clinical

- Incubation period = 2–10 days (median 5)
- Early illness begins with fever, often 38°C (100.4°F) and associated with constitutional symptoms
  - Headache
  - Sore throat
  - Malaise
  - Myalgia
  - Chills
  - Rigors
- After 3–7 days as illness progresses, lower respiratory symptoms develop:
  - Dry/nonproductive cough

  - Dyspnea (always warrants further investigation and aggressive management)
  - The patient may deteriorate rapidly, experiencing respiratory distress, respiratory failure, and hypoxemia
- Extrapulmonary symptoms have developed in 20–60% (depending upon when the patient presented and the comprehensiveness of inquiry) most notably
  - Diarrhea

Testing

Chest X-Ray (CXR)

- By day 7, most SARS patients demonstrate abnormalities on CXR, including:
  - Focal interstitial infiltrates
  - Generalized patchy, interstitial infiltrates
  - Areas of consolidation

Laboratory per WHO/CDC (Suggest Laboratorian/Public Health Contact CDC Reference Lab)

- CDC-recommended specimens: blood (serum/plasma), upper respiratory (wash or O/P swabs), lower respiratory (sputum, BAL, tracheal aspirate, pleural fluid), stool or tissue (fixed during fatality)
- Nucleic acid tests: RT-PCR from at least two different clinical specimens or the same specimen collected on two or more different occasions
- ELISA seroconversion
- Virus isolation in cell culture from any clinical specimen and identification of SARS-CoV

Treatment

- Currently there is no specific, approved antiviral medication to treat SARS.
- Aggressive symptomatic and supportive care is necessary and may include ventilatory support.
- The clinical presentation of SARS is compatible with other etiologies of atypical and pneumonia and severe respiratory illnesses; empiric treatment regimens have included a variety of antibiotics to aggressively/presumptively treat known bacterial illnesses in the differential diagnosis.

Prevention

- Respiratory and hand hygiene measures should be routine in health-care facilities.
- Respiratory, droplet, and universal precautions should be implemented.
- Containment strategies should be coordinated early with public health and the health-care facility infection control team. These may include
  - Patient isolation
  - Use of masks (N95 that are fit-tested and used properly)
  - Negative pressure rooms
  - Segregation of well from patients presenting with respiratory symptoms

CDC Defined Probable SARS

- Early illness
  - Two or more: Fever, chills, rigors, myalgias, sore throat, headache (usually severe), rhinorrhea
- Severe respiratory illness of unknown etiology
- Clinical findings consistent with SARS
  - Temperature of 100.4°F or higher
- One or more respiratory findings
  - Cough
  - Shortness of breath/difficulty breathing
  - Hypoxia
- And at least one of the following:
  - Radiologic evidence of pneumonia
    Or
  - Respiratory distress syndrome
    Or
  - Autopsy findings
- Epidemiologic criteria for exposure
  - Travel to area with known SARS
  - Exposure to other SARS patient
- Lab can confirm
  - Antibody to SARS-CoV
  - Isolation of SARS-CoV in cell culture
  - Detection of SARS-CoV RNA molecular

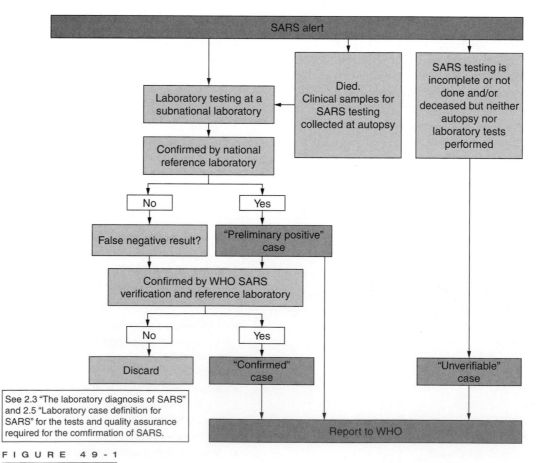

See 2.3 "The laboratory diagnosis of SARS" and 2.5 "Laboratory case definition for SARS" for the tests and quality assurance required for the comfirmation of SARS.

FIGURE 49-1

SARS ALERT ALGORITHM
(From WHO 2004)

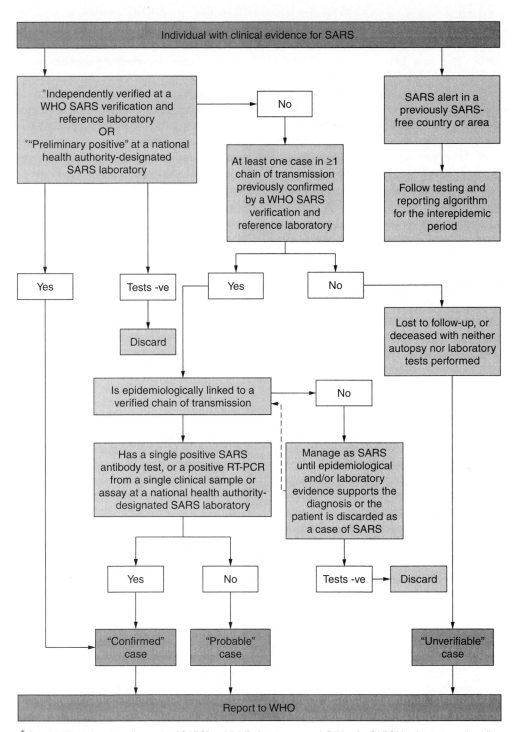

* See 2.3 "The laboratory diagnosis of SARS" and 2.5 "Laboratory case definition for SARS" for the tests and quality
assurance required for the confirmation of SARS.

FIGURE 49-2

ALGORITHM FOR INDIVIDUAL WITH CLINICAL EVIDENCE FOR SARS
(From WHO 2004)

Severe acute respiratory syndrome (SARS) became recognized as a global threat in 2003 when the World Health Organization reported a multicountry outbreak of severe atypical pneumonia. The first known cases of SARS occurred in Guangdong province, China, in November 2002. Subsequently SARS infections have been reported in Asia, and North America. As of March 21, 2003, the majority of patients identified as having SARS have been previously healthy adults between 25 and 70 years of age. Few suspected cases of SARS have been reported among children.

By July 2003, the international spread of SARS-CoV resulted in 8098 SARS cases in 26 countries (Fig. 49-3), with 774 deaths. Most cases were from China, Hong Kong, Taiwan, Singapore, and Canada. Areas affected by SARS suffered from significant social and economic disruption, with estimates in millions of dollars in lost revenue as a result of its impact on the travel industry as international travel plummeted, health services, commerce, conference cancellations, and the like. It is estimated that the direct and indirect cost of SARS was $100 billion. WHO reported that the last human chain of transmission of SARS in that epidemic had been broken on July 2003.

Since July 2003, there have been four occasions when SARS has reappeared. The most recent was reported in China in April 2004. Three of these incidents were attributed to breaches in laboratory biosafety and resulted in one or more cases of SARS (Singapore, Taipei, and Beijing); one of these incidents resulted in secondary transmission outside of the laboratory. One incident resulted in a cluster of nine cases, one of whom died, in three generations of transmission affecting family and hospital contacts of a laboratory worker. For this reason, WHO strongly urges countries to conduct an inventory of all laboratories working with cultures of live SARS-CoV, as well as other potentially contagious, deadly biologicals, in addition to caution in storing clinical specimens actually or potentially contaminated with SARS-CoV. Global case counts are available at *http://www.who.int* WHO and other preparedness experts also recommend that each country ensures that the correct biosafety procedures are followed by all laboratories working with the SARS Coronavirus and other dangerous pathogens, whether potential biological weapons or highly pathological H5N1, and that appropriate security, monitoring, and investigation of illness in laboratory workers is undertaken.

Thus the resurgence of SARS leading to an outbreak remains a worrisome possibility; preparing for such an exigency, whether SARS or pandemic influenza, is a prudent measure. In the interepidemic period, all countries should enhance surveillance and response capacity to detect and respond to the reemergence of SARS, avian flu, and other emerging pathogens.

While much has been learnt about this syndrome since March 2003, our knowledge about the epidemiology and ecology of SARS-CoV infection and of this disease remains incomplete. Ongoing research is underway to identify potential antiviral medications, effective vaccines, and rapid testing methods.

From a bioterrorism preparedness perspective is the concern that nations place sovereignty and national interests over global health. Were it not for the international media, WHO, and real-time electronic communications projects such as Global Outbreak Alert and Response Network (GOARN) and Global Public Health Intelligence Network (GPHIN) transmitted via the Internet or World Wide Web, information about infectious diseases would rest largely from voluntary reporting by countries influenced by concerns over commerce, tourism, or other issues of self-interest. Without GOARN and others, the lack of full access to data related to growing numbers of deaths due to an unknown respiratory illness in China, and delayed disclosure by the Chinese Ministry of Health, increased surveillance throughout Asia might have been also further delayed. This lack of disclosure can jeopardize disease containment and set the stage for wider spread of emerging pathogens. Preparedness within the United States will continue to depend, at least in part upon forces outside our control, and thus warrant clinicians to remain alert to emerging threats abroad.

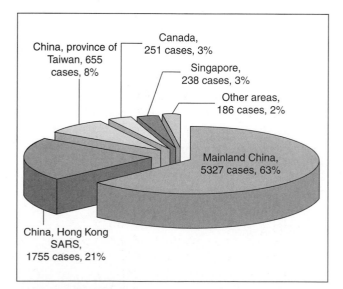

FIGURE 49-3

PIE CHART SHOWING THE INTERNATIONAL SPREAD OF SARS-COV RESULTING IN 8098 SARS CASES IN 26 COUNTRIES BY JULY 2003
(*Abstracted from WHO Data*)

MICROBIOLOGY

The etiological agent is SARS Coronavirus (SARS-CoV) (Fig. 49-4), believed to have been an animal virus that crossed the species barrier to infect humans. A number of wildlife species—the Himalayan masked palm civet (*Paguma larvata*), the Chinese ferret badger (*Melogale moschata*), and the raccoon dog (*Nyctereutes procyonoides*)—consumed as delicacies in southern China have shown laboratory evidence of infection with a related

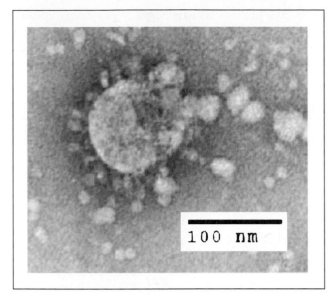

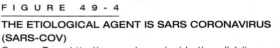

FIGURE 49-4

THE ETIOLOGICAL AGENT IS SARS CORONAVIRUS (SARS-COV)
Source: From http://www.cdc.gov/ncidod/sars/lab/images.htm

Coronavirus. Domestic cats in Hong Kong were also found to be infected with SARS-CoV. More recently, ferrets (*Mustela furo*) and domestic cats (*Felis domesticus*) were infected with SARS-CoV experimentally and found to efficiently transmit the virus to previously uninfected animals housed with them. These findings indicate that the reservoir for this pathogen may involve a range of animal species. It was thought, given the ever increasing encroachment of previously uninhabited territories, that recent ecological changes increased opportunities for human exposure to the virus perhaps along with virus adaptation, enabling human-to-human transmission.

First isolated from chickens in 1937, coronaviruses cause a large proportion of cold-like illnesses in humans. Coronavirus particles contain RNA, are irregularly-shaped, are approximately 60–220 nm in diameter, and have an outer envelope bearing distinctive, "club-shaped" peplomers approximately 20 nm long and 10 nm wide. The name Coronavirus (Corona = crown in Latin) refers to the projection of these peplomers around the virus. When viewed with electron microscopy, the projections give the appearance of a "corona" around the virus.

The Coronavirus envelope contains two glycoproteins: a spike glycoprotein (S), which participates in receptor binding and cell fusion, and a membrane glycoprotein (M), which participates in budding and envelope formation. Genetic material of coronaviruses consists of a single-stranded (+) sense RNA, approximately 27–31 kb in length. The entire 29,736 nucleotide sequence has been identified. The genome is associated with a basic phosphoprotein (N). The polymerase gene is the most highly conserved portion of the Coronavirus genome. The prototype strains HCoV 229E and HCoV OC43 are primarily associated with

common cold syndrome. Reinfections with coronaviruses appear to occur throughout life, implying multiple serotypes (at least four are known) and/or antigenic variation, which may limit the possibility of successful vaccine development. Analysis of the genome by PCR and sequencing has demonstrated that SARS is caused by a novel Coronavirus, which has not been previously identified in humans.

Clinically, most Coronavirus infections result in a mild, self-limited disease, typically resembling classic "cold" symptoms, in which growth appears to be localized to the epithelium of the upper respiratory tract, in contrast to SARS-CoV infection, which encompasses the lower respiratory tract, and results in a much higher severity of symptoms. Unlike the mild infections associated with most coronaviruses, SARS is associated with significant mortality.

EPIDEMIOLOGY

Coronaviruses are transmitted by aerosols of respiratory secretions, by the fecal-oral route, and by mechanical transmission. Viral replication occurs primarily in epithelial cells; however, infection of other cell types including macrophage, liver, kidneys, and heart have been described. Coronavirus infection is very common and occurs worldwide. A strong seasonal relationship (greatest incidence in children during the winter months) is present for most Coronavirus infections.

CLINICAL DIAGNOSIS

Generally the initial clinical signs and symptoms of SARS-CoV illness are nonspecific. As the disease process advances, the severity of the respiratory illness becomes manifest. The differential diagnosis therefore may include a wide range of common respiratory pathogens including influenza virus, parainfluenza viruses, respiratory syncytial virus (RSV), *Haemophilus influenzae, Mycoplasma pneumoniae, Chlamydia* species, *Legionella* species, and *Coxiella burnetii*. Each of these illnesses has important clinical distinctions, which the clinician should be aware of, and thus it is important to include appropriate inquiry during history-taking. Additionally, there are no widely available rapid office tests or laboratory tests that reliably diagnose SARS in the early onset of illness.

Clinicians and public health professionals should be familiar with the epidemiology of other diseases that have presentations similar to the symptoms and signs of SARS, including the common causes of community-acquired and hospital-acquired respiratory illnesses.

Caution should be exercised in diagnosing nonspecific viral pneumonia without detailed inquiry to ascertain risk factors for SARS in the 10 days before the onset of illness. These include determining whether other family members and/or other close social or occupational contacts have had a similar illness (particularly in a laboratory or hospital setting), or a relevant history of travel to an area at risk of SARS-CoV transmission from animal reservoirs or a recent outbreak of SARS.

Establishing an alternative diagnosis should not delay the triggering of a SARS alert and the timely implementation of patient isolation and stringent infection control measures if a SARS diagnosis cannot be confidently excluded. Indications for testing during a SARS Alert are given in later sections of this chapter.

CLINICAL SYNDROMES

In humans, coronaviruses may cause a variety of clinical syndromes, including respiratory infections (primarily cold-type illnesses), enteric infections (primarily in infants), and rare neurological syndromes. These are generally self-limiting. New attention has focused on this family following the description of severe lower respiratory tract infections (SARS).

SEVERE ACUTE RESPIRATORY SYNDROME

The incubation period for SARS is typically 2–7 days and may be as long as 10 days.

A prodrome has been described, consisting of high fever (>100.4°F [>38.0°C]), possibly associated with chills, rigors, and other flu-like symptoms (headache, myalgia, malaise). Mild respiratory symptoms may be present at the onset of illness. Rash, neurologic symptoms, or gastrointestinal disturbances are typically absent, although diarrhea during the febrile prodrome has been reported.

After 3–7 days, a second phase—the respiratory phase—involving the lower respiratory tract begins. Symptoms include a dry, nonproductive cough and/or dyspnea, which may progress to hypoxemia. Shortness of breath is uncommon in influenza-like illnesses, is always worrisome regardless of etiology and warrants aggressive clinical attention. Of note, most biological weapons that target the respiratory tract, as well as significant infectious illness can cause shortness of breath.

In a substantial proportion of patients, the respiratory phase is characterized by early focal interstitial infiltrates. These frequently progress to generalized, patchy, interstitial infiltrates. Consolidation may be observed in some patients during the late stages of SARS. In some cases, chest radiographs remain normal during the prodrome and throughout the course of the illness.

Laboratory findings may include thrombocytopenia and leukopenia. Early in the respiratory phase, elevated creatine phosphokinase levels (CPK) (as high as 3000 IU/L) and elevated hepatic transaminases have been noted.

The severity of illness appears to be highly variable, ranging from mild illness to death. Respiratory compromise requiring intubation and mechanical ventilation may occur in 10–20% of cases. The case-fatality rate among persons with illness meeting the current WHO case definition of SARS is approximately 3%. Some close contacts, including healthcare workers, have developed similar illnesses.

DIAGNOSIS

The Centers for Disease Control (CDC) has provided the following SARS case definition criteria:

Revised CST SARS Surveillance Case Definition (Summary of Criteria) (available at *http://www.cdc.gov/mmwr/preview/mmwrhtml/mm5249a2.htm*)

Clinical Criteria

Early Illness

- Two or more of the following: Fever, chills, rigors, myalgia, headache, sore throat, rhinorrhea
- Mild-to-moderate respiratory illness
  - Temperature >100.4°F, *and*
- One or more clinical findings of LRT illness (e.g., cough, SOB, difficulty breathing)

Severe Respiratory Illness

- Meets clinical criteria of mild-to-moderate respiratory illness, *and*
  - radiographic evidence of pneumonia
  - acute respiratory distress syndrome
  - autopsy findings consistent with pneumonia or acute respiratory distress syndrome

Epidemiological Evidence

Possible exposure to SARS-associated Coronavirus (SARS-CoV): One or more of the following in the 10 days before symptoms:

- Travel to a location with recent transmissions of SARS, *or*
- Close contact with a person with LRT illness and the aforementioned travel history

Likely exposure to SARS-CoV: One or more of the following in the 10 days before symptoms:

- Close contact with a confirmed case of SARS-CoV disease, *or*
- Close contact with a person with LRT illness for whom a chain of transmission can be linked to a case of SARS-CoV in the 10 days prior to symptoms

Special Populations

Atypical presentations such as afebrile illness or concurrent bacterial sepsis or pneumonia have been observed as particularly problematic in the elderly. This holds true for other biological weapon-related illness where the normal physiologic and anatomic changes of aging can confound commonly expected symptoms. Underlying chronic illness and medications, as well as frequent reliance upon the health-care facility may contribute to unrecognized nosocomially transmitted events or early diagnosis of SARS and other aggressive respiratory pathogens.

SARS during 2003 was observed less frequently and presented as a milder illness among pediatric patients. Of the cases affecting pregnant women, data suggest in increase in fetal loss during early pregnancy and possibly increased risk for maternal mortality during later pregnancy.

THE LABORATORY DIAGNOSIS OF SARS

Laboratory Findings

Currently there are no specific biochemical or hematologic tests specific for SARS-CoV. During the 2003 outbreak, patients exhibited the following:

Hematologic findings:
- Lymphopenia is common and progressive
- Thrombocytopenia may occur along with prolonged APTT

Biochemical findings:
- LDH is frequently high. In some patients this was associated with a poor prognosis
- AST and CPK elevation may occur but less frequently than LDH changes
- Abnormal serum electrolytes have been reported upon presentation and during illness, including
  - Hyponatremia
  - Hypokalemia
  - Hypomagnesemia
  - Hypocalcemia

MICROBIOLOGY

The Coronavirus responsible for SARS has several unusual properties, including growth in cell culture (most coronaviruses cannot be cultivated).

The following tests are recommended for the laboratory diagnosis of SARS. A single test result is insufficient for the definitive diagnosis of SARS-CoV infection because both false negative and false positive results are known to occur.

NUCLEIC ACID TESTS

Reverse transcription polymerase chain reaction (RT-PCR), positive for SARS-CoV using a validated method from:

1. At least two different clinical specimens (e.g., nasopharyngeal and stool).
   or

2. The same clinical specimen collected on two or more occasions during the course of the illness (e.g., sequential nasopharyngeal aspirates).
   or

3. Two different assays or repeat RT-PCR using a new RNA extract from the original clinical sample on each occasion of testing.

Seroconversion by ELISA or IFA

Negative antibody test on acute sate serum followed by positive antibody test on convalescent phase serum tested in parallel.
or
Fourfold or greater rise in antibody titer between acute and convalescent phase sera tested in parallel.

Note: Virus neutralization should be conducted to exclude serological cross-reactions with other human and/or animal coronaviruses. Virus neutralization should only be conducted in a specialized laboratory under the appropriate biosafety level (BSL3). It is recommended in the interepidemic period and for at least one case in each new (independent) chain of human transmission when an outbreak is being verified to exclude serological cross-reactions. Once SARS-CoV transmission is well-established, virus neutralization will not usually be required but may be used when the results of RT-PCR and serology are difficult to interpret.

Virus Isolation

Isolation in cell culture from any clinical specimen and identification of SARS-CoV using a validated method such as RT-PCR.

The Interpretation of Laboratory Results for SARS-CoV

The reliability of the results of diagnostic tests for SARS-CoV infection depends crucially on the type of clinical specimens collected, the time of collection, and the method of collection. WHO has established a network of international reference and verification laboratories for SARS to assist with independent verification of testing in national laboratories and for primary diagnosis if requested. Guidance on the clinical specimens for the laboratory diagnosis of SARS-CoV and the timing of their collection can be found in *WHO SARS International Reference and Verification Laboratory Network: Policy and Procedures in the Inter-Epidemic Period.*

Serological testing is improving, although quality assurance has indicated a significant level of missed positive specimens and of false positive results. Where acute and convalescent phase sera show a fourfold or greater rise in titer when tests are carried out in parallel, but no PCR product is available or virus isolated, viral neutralization assays should be performed. This test should be performed by the national reference laboratory and, depending on whether the case occurs in the interepidemic period or during an outbreak, by a WHO SARS International Reference and Verification Laboratory for final confirmation and to ensure that the rising titer is not due to a second human Coronavirus.

In the interepidemic period, WHO strongly recommends that all countries seek verification of laboratory-confirmed cases of SARS ("preliminary positive" cases), preferably by an external laboratory which is part of the WHO SARS International Reference and Verification Laboratory Network.

Virus isolation and sequencing should be undertaken wherever possible to monitor the evolution of SARS-CoV in human populations and the frequency of interspecies transmission. Virus isolation requires BSL3 conditions and practices. The United States Laboratory Response Network is undergoing ongoing advancements, and are closely aligned with the CDC and state public health authorities. WHO will facilitate testing at one of the Network laboratories for national health authorities without their own SARS-CoV testing facilities. All laboratories should adhere to the biosafety levels recommended for diagnostic work on clinical specimens actually or potentially infected with SARS-CoV and research on SARS-CoV. Biosafety guidance for handling SARS-CoV safely is found in *Laboratory Biosafety Manual,* third edition, and the *WHO Biosafety Guidelines for Handling of SARS Specimens.*

Clinical Evidence for SARS

The following clinical criteria for SARS, presented in Table 49-1, are used for public health (surveillance) purposes only. Clinicians are advised to refer to the clinical case description for further details of the symptoms and signs of SARS (Table 49-1).

Laboratory Criteria (Not Completely Established)

- Detection of antibody to SARS-CoV, *or*
- Isolation of SARS-CoV in cell culture, *or*
- Detection of SARS-CoV RNA molecular methods and subsequent confirmation

Diagnostic Test/Procedures

Consult the clinical microbiology laboratory for advice and information regarding specimen selection, collection, and transport *before* selecting, collecting, and transporting specimens for the laboratory diagnosis of SARS (Table 49-1).

HEALTH-CARE MANAGEMENT

Treatment

Treatment generally involves aggressive supportive treatment only, including hemodynamic and ventilatory support. A variety of experimental and current antiviral agents are currently being evaluated. Oseltamivir (Tamiflu) and Ribavirin have been given empirically to SARS patients without clear efficacy. In addition, steroids have been administered orally or intravenously in combination with Ribavirin. The efficacy of these agents has not been confirmed.

Although no specific agent against SARS-CoV is available; drug development is ongoing based upon different molecular targets on the SARS-CoV. These include compounds that block the S-protein-ACE 2-mediated viral

TABLE 49-1

CDC-RECOMMENDED SPECIMENS FOR EVALUATION OF POTENTIAL CASES OF SARS

Specimen	Outpatient	Inpatient	Fatal
Blood	• Serum (acute and convalescent >28 days post onset) • Plasma	• Serum (acute and convalescent >28 days post onset)	• Serum • Plasma
Upper respiratory	• N/P wash/aspirate • N/P or O/P swabs	• N/P wash/aspirate • N/P or O/P swabs	• N/P wash/aspirate • N/P or O/P swabs
Lower respiratory	• Sputum	• Bronchoalveolar lavage (BAL), tracheal aspirate, pleural fluid • Sputum	• Bronchoalveolar lavage (BAL), tracheal aspirate, pleural fluid
Stool Tissue	Yes	Yes	Yes • Fixed from all major organs • Frozen from lung and upper airway

Source: www.cdc/gov/ncidod/sars/guidance/f/app4.htm

entry, SARS-CoV M (pro), papain like protease 2 (PLP2), SARS-CoV helicase, as well as compounds that are active but have unspecified targets. Research is also being conducted on other aspects of viral replication and host entry.

Studies in animal models demonstrated efficacy of SARS-CoV-specific monoclonal antibodies, pegylated interferon –a, and other RNA focused compounds. Some researchers suggest the use of interferons be considered should SARS-CoV or other Coronavirus emerge. As of this writing, none are specifically approved for the treatment of SARS but may, nevertheless, be worth considering in consultation with CDC or WHO for updated information on countermeasures released after the printing of this text.

In the United States, clinicians who suspect cases of SARS are requested to report such cases to their state health departments. CDC requests that reports of suspected cases from state health departments, international airlines, cruise ships, or cargo carriers be directed to the SARS Investigative Team at the CDC Emergency Operations Center (telephone 770-488-7100). Outside the United States, clinicians who suspect cases of SARS are requested to report such cases to their local public health authorities. Additional information about SARS (e.g., infection control guidance and procedures for reporting suspected cases) is available at *http://www.cdc.gov/ncidod/sars*

PREVENTIVE STRATEGIES

Personal protective equipment and respiratory precautions and infection control should be implemented immediately upon first suspicion of SARS to reduce the risk of contagion. During the 2003 epidemic, health-care workers were not only particularly susceptible to SARS infection but early on, prior to implementing effective respiratory protections, became a source of illness transmission. Attention to proper use of PPE (prior instruction/practice, fit testing, proper disposal), isolation of suspected patients, and adherence to strict infection control are essential. Close interaction with public health officials for contact tracing is important to contain SARS in the early stages of reemergence.

Early suspicion of any potentially contagious respiratory pathogen must be communicated immediately to implement appropriate facility containment strategies as well as an appropriate public health response. Contact information for the CDC, local/state public health, infection control and laboratory should be prominently displayed.

During influenza season and when an alert about a potential outbreak may be imminent, health-care facilities should increase surveillance and preventive measures. These include highly visible prompts to alert patients and visitors to employ respiratory hygiene, provision of hand sanitizers and masks to reduce contact and airborne spread respectively, and whenever possible, separation of well and potentially contagious patients in visiting and common areas.

During the SARS epidemic of 2003, technologies were being sought out that could identify a potential SARS victim using distance thermal imaging (Fig. 49-5) and other approaches. While the notion of "arms length" detection to identify ill patients before they arrive within the airport or health-care facility is attractive, unfortunately there are limitations to the performance capabilities of these technologies, undermining the practicality of their use. The expected plus or minus error rate at normal body temperatures equates to a 1.4°C variance. Most thermal detector manufacturers term the error rate as ±2% or 1°C, "whichever is the greater." Many manufacturers actually state a minimum 2°C variance. This variance could effectively negate patients meeting the CDC threshold of 38°C or over-read a normothermic patient as febrile. These detectors are also effected by environmental factors; health-care and airport facilities generally cannot establish adequate environmental controls to meet the performance window of most of the detectors.

A large number of people with fevers could slip through on the minus side and an equally large number of people could be indicated as having a fever. Noncontact thermal imaging simply does not have the finite qualitative and quantitative resolution to act as a SARS screening device.

Thus it is imperative to train intake personnel on key questions, signs, and symptoms that can be communicated to appropriate health-care personnel before the patient is introduced to a large waiting area where contagion can be facilitated.

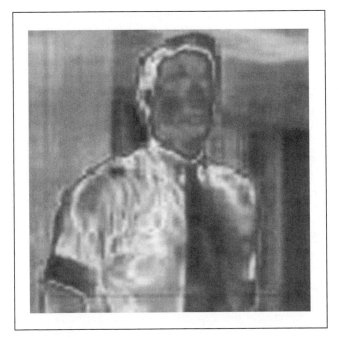

FIGURE 49-5

THERMAL IMAGING

CONCLUSION

SARS has been referred to as the first pandemic of the twenty-first century, having originated in southern China as an unusual respiratory disease during 2002, subsequently appearing in Hong Kong, and other Pacific Rim nations. During 2003, WHO reported an outbreak of acute respiratory syndrome in China, suggesting it was highly contagious through close person-to-person contact and rapidly spread through air travel as a respiratory pathogen. SARS subsequently emerged in Canada during 2003. The potential for reemergence was manifest in 2004 when a case of SARS from Guangdong was reported, resulting in widespread slaughter of animals considered able to harbor the virus, including 10,000 civet cats and other mammals. Laboratory-related cases have also occurred.

SARS is a progressive febrile, respiratory illness that can cause respiratory distress or failure and death, especially among the elderly which experience a higher CFR (50%) than younger adults (~10%). Severe cases rapidly develop respiratory distress and oxygen desaturation, with approximately 20% requiring intensive care. Currently no antiviral medication is available to specifically treat SARS. While combinations of antiviral medications have been tried, none have demonstrated significant or consistent clinical value, nor are they approved for SARS. However, several are under development. Some suggest the use of interferons. Management consists of aggressive symptomatic and supportive care.

Owing to the rapidly progressive, highly contagious nature of the illness, early presumptive diagnosis, access to public health, implementation of infection control measures and aggressive management, which may include ventilatory support and intensive care are essential. Moreover, without prior planning for adequate resources, training and PPE, an inadequate response may occur. Familiarity and ongoing collaboration with public health, infectious disease as well as developing and revising response plans are essential to address SARS or other emerging pathogen. The use of infection control and diagnostic prompts—important tools—should be prominently displayed (Figs. 49-1 and 49-2).

Given the relatively nonspecific nature of the early disease, it is critical to obtain a good travel, occupational, and exposure history in addition to careful scrutiny of signs and symptoms in order to arrive at a presumptive diagnosis. Early suspicion of SARS is essential to initiate appropriate response and containment strategies to stop the transmission of infection before it becomes an outbreak. Lessons learned from the outbreak of 2003 included misuse of PPE and inadequate containment measures that posed an early problem in Canada until remedied.

The diagnosis of SARS depends upon history, clinical, and ultimately the appearance of virus antibody, which usually occurs unfortunately during the later stage of infection. Of interest, SARS-related antibodies were found in serum samples collected in mid-2001 indicating exposure prior to the 2003 outbreak.

Of interest from a global preparedness perspective, of the 1315 reports of an infectious disease outbreak presented to WHO from 2001 to October 2004, 61% came from unofficial, mostly electronic sources including the media. Only 39% originated from ministries of health. While some nations persist thinking emerging pathogens are the exclusive purview of their sovereignty to control the attendant information, the global risk of diseases that do not honor borders requires broader information sharing and reminds us in the West, where respiratory illnesses such as influenza and SARS will ultimately arrive, to be alert to global infection trends and realize global travel brings to our shores (and the Heartland) nonendemic illnesses that we should consider in our differential diagnosis.

Suggested Reading

Antia R, Rogoes RR, Koella JC, et al. The role of evolution in the emergence of infectious diseases. *Nature.* 2003;426:658–661.

Biosafety and SARS Incident in Singapore, September 2003. Report of the review panel on new SARS case and biosafety. *http://www.moh.gov.sg/corp/sars/pdf/Report_SARS_Biosafety.pdf*

CDC SARS 2004. *http://www.cdc.gov/mmwr/preview/mmwrhtml/mm5249a2.htm*

CDC Severe Respiratory Syndrome, 2006. *http://www2.ncid.cdc.gov/travel/yb/utils/ybGet.asp?section=dis&obj=sars.htm* Last accessed 12/25/06.

Centers for Disease Control and Prevention. Update: severe acute respiratory syndrome—worldwide and United States. *MMWR.* 2003;52:664–665.

Cyranoski D, Abbott A. Virus detectives seek source of SARS in China's wild animals. *Nature.* 2003;423:467.

Data submitted by Bio Economic Associates of Cambridge, Massachusetts.

Drosten C, Gunther S, Presser W, et al. Identification of a novel coronavirus in patients with severe acute respiratory syndrome. *New Engl J Med* 2003;348:1967–1976.

Guan Y, Zheng BJ, He YQ, et al. Isolation and characterization of viruses related to the SARS coronavirus from animals in southern China. *Science.* 2003;302: 276–278.

Haagmans BL, Osterhaus ADME. Coronaviruses and their therapy. 2006.

HE JF, Peng GW, Zheng HZ, et al. An epidemiological study on the index cases of severe acute respiratory syndrome which occurred in different cities in Guangdong province (English Abstract). In: *Collection of papers on SARS published in CMA Journals.* Beijing: Chinese Medical Association, 27 May 2003, p 44.

Heymann DL. SARS and emerging infectious disease: a challenge to place global solidarity above national sovereignty. *Ann Acad Med Singapore.* 2006;35:350–353.

Johnson A, Howe JL, McBride MR, et al. Bioterrorism and emergency preparedness in aging (BTEPA): HRSA-Funded GEC collaboration for curricula and training. *Gerontology Geriatrics Ed.* 2006;26(4):63–86.

Ksiazek TG, Erdman D, Goldsmith CS, et al. A novel coronavirus associated with severe acute respiratory syndrome. *New Engl J Med.* 2003;348:1953–1966.

Lashley FR. Emerging infectious diseases at the beginning of the 21st century. *Online J Issues Nursing.* 2006;11(1): Last accessed 1/2/07 *www.nursingworld.org/ojin/topic29/tpc29_1.htm*

Marina BE, Haagmans BL, Kuiken T, et al. Virology: SARS viral infection of cats and ferrets. *Nature.* 2003;425:915.

McFee RB, Leikin JB, Kiernan K. Preparing for an era of weapons of mass destruction (WMD)—are we there yet? Why we should be concerned. Part II. *Vet Human Toxicol.* 2004;46: 347–351.

NG SKC. Possible role of an animal vector in the SARS outbreak at Amoy Gardens. *Lancet.* 2003;362:570–572.

Nolte KB, Taylor DG, Richmond JY. Biosafety considerations for autopsy. *Am J Forens Med and Path* 2002;23(2):107–122.

Normile D. Viral DNA match spurs China's civet roundup. *Science.* 2004;303:292.

Peiris JSM, Lai ST, Poon LLM, et al and the SARS Study Group. Coronavirus as a possible cause of severe acute respiratory syndrome. *Lancet.* 2003;36:1319–1325.

Skowronski DM, Astell C, Brunham RC, et al. Severe acute respiratory syndrome (SARS): a year in review. *Ann Rev Med.* 2005;56:357–381.

Sorensen MD, Sorensen B, Gonzalez-Dosal R, et al. Severe acute respiratory syndrome (SARS): development of diagnostics and antivirals. *Ann NY Acad Sci.* 2006 May;1067:500–505.

Svoboda T, Henry B, Shulman L, et al. Public health measures to control the spread of severe acute respiratory syndrome during the outbreak in Toronto. *New Engl J Med.* 2004;350: 2352–2361.

Tsang KW, Ho PL, Ooi GC, et al. A cluster of cases of severe acute respiratory syndrome in Hong Kong. *New Engl J Med.* 2003;348:1977–1985.

Vu TH, Cabau JF, Nguyen NT, et al. SARS in Northern Vietnam. *New Engl J Med.* 2003;348:2035.

World Health Organization (WHO). Summary of probable SARS cases with onset of illness from 1 November 2002 to 31 July 2003 based on data as of the 31 December 2003. *http://www.who.int/csr/sars/country/table2004_4_21/en/*

World Health Organization. China's latest SARS outbreak has been contained but biosafety concerns remain. Update 7, 18 May 2004. *http://www.who.int/csr/don/2004_05_18a/en/*

World Health Organization. Consensus document on the epidemiology of severe acute respiratory syndrome (SARS). WHO/CDS/CSR/GAR/2003.11. *http://www.who.int/csr/sars/en/WHOconsensus.pdf*

World Health Organization. SARS: one suspected case reported in China, 22 April 2004. *http://www.who.int/csr/don/2004_04_22/en/*

World Health Organization. Severe acute respiratory syndrome (SARS) in Singapore, 10 Sept 2003. *http://www.who.int/csr/don/2003_09_10/en/*

World Health Organization. Severe acute respiratory syndrome (SARS) in Taiwan, China, 17 December 2003. *http:///www.who.int/csr/don/2003_12_17/en/*

World Health Organization. Summary of the discussion and recommendations of the SARS laboratory workshop. 22 Oct 2003. *http://www.who.int/csr/sars/guidelines/en/SARSLabmeeting.pdf*

Wu W, Wang J, Liu P, et al. A hospital outbreak of severe acute respiratory syndrome in Guangzhou, China. *Chinese Med Journal (English).* 2003;116:811–818.

Wu YS, Lin WH, Jsu JT, et al. Antiviral drug discovery against SARS-CoV. *Curr Med Chem.* 2006;13(17):2003–2020.

50

AGROTERRORISM

Edward M. Bottei

AGROTERRORISM

- There are seven different phases of food production and the contamination of food may occur during any phase.
- Accidental contamination of the food supply is a very common occurrence.
- Deliberate food contamination happens much less frequently.
- Either accidental or deliberate contamination may cause illness or death.
- The presenting signs and symptoms of an outbreak will depend upon which biological, chemical, or radiological agent is used in the attack.
- Recognition of a foodborne disease outbreak may be difficult because (1) some agents have a delayed onset of symptoms, (2) different patients may develop symptoms at different times, and (3) patients may become geographically dispersed.
- Clinicians need to have a high degree of suspicion in order to achieve early detection of a foodborne outbreak.

INTRODUCTION

The human food supply has always been vulnerable to natural diseases, animal predators, and either accidental or deliberate contamination by humans. Humans can take advantage of the modern food processing and delivery systems to cause deliberate contamination of foodstuffs to harm people. The potential goals of an agroterrorist attack are several: (1) destruction of the food supply, (2) creation of distrust in the safety of the food supply, or (3) the use of food as a vehicle to cause death, illness, or panic in humans. All three of these effects will likely also cause economic upheaval for the agriculture market. The direct destruction of the food supply, via diseases such as

bovine spongiform encephalopathy (BSE, "mad cow disease") or late blight of potato, is beyond the scope of this chapter.

This chapter will review the system of how food is grown, processed, and distributed. Specific examples of accidental and deliberate contamination of food with biologicals, chemical, or radionuclides will be presented. The discussion will then focus on recognition of such an outbreak and how to assist in the management of such an outbreak.

THE FOOD SUPPLY SYSTEM

An understanding of the food supply system is necessary so that health-care professionals investigating a food-related outbreak can figure out how extensive an outbreak might be. Food's pathway from farm to table can be broken into seven distinct phases:

1. Prefarm: seeds and feeds
2. Agricultural production and harvesting (farms)
3. Storage and transport of raw materials
4. Processing at a processing plant
5. Storage and transport of processed materials
6. Wholesale and retail distribution
7. Human consumption (individual or food service preparation)

There are distinct vulnerabilities in each phase and certain poisons are better suited for contamination at certain steps. How many people and how much food will be affected is also dependant upon which step in the food chain is attacked.

In the prefarm phase, there is the possibility of contaminated animal feed being a starting point for chemicals or diseases entering into the food chain. In 1997, it was discovered that certain chicken feeds, which contained ball clay as a flowing agent, were contaminated with 2,3,7,8-tetrachlorodibenzo-p-dioxin (TCDD). Analysis of processed chicken products associated with this contaminated feed had levels of TCDD in the nanogram per kilogram range. While there were no immediate human illnesses associated with this event, it did create a scare that people who had consumed chicken products may develop medical problems in the future.

In Iraq in 1971 nearly 100 tons of methylmercury-treated wheat and barley seeds were distributed around the country to be used for planting. Instead, much of this was ground into flour and consumed. Over the next several months, thousands of people developed signs and symptoms of methylmercury toxicity. Some reports tallied 6530 people hospitalized and 459 deaths, with the actual death toll likely to be much higher than this figure.

On farms, a high level of security may not be achievable because of the large land area involved. However, since crops are typically spread out during the growing season, contaminating a large amount of crops in the field can be very difficult. If the goal is to cause human suffering, then crops would have to be contaminated close to harvest time in order to get the product into the food chain. In contrast to field crops, animals are typically concentrated in a smaller geographical area. If access can be gained to the animals' confinement area, a biological or chemical could be easily introduced into the food chain.

With regard to storage and transportation, if there is inadequate security of the containers, a contaminant can easily be added to the product. How contamination in this step affects people depends upon the quantity and potency of contaminant added, and the possible dilution-factor of the processing phase.

Processing facilities have the benefit and the drawback of being central collecting and processing points. If contaminated food from one location comes in to be processed, it is possible that mixing the contaminated food with food from other sources could dilute down the contaminant to the point where the contaminant may not be harmful to an individual. However, if the foodstuff is heavily contaminated or contaminated with a very potent poison, the contaminated foodstuff may contaminate everything it is mixed with or comes into contact with. Thus, everything that leaves the plant may be contaminated with the poison, magnifying the scope of the problem. Processing facilities also have the vulnerability that food can be directly contaminated in the facility (as in fecal contamination in a slaughter house), or can be poorly processed (undercooking, etc), leading to contamination.

Once the product makes it to retail markets, the foodstuff has typically been broken down into more manageable quantities (cans, bags, etc), so large-scale contamination may be more difficult. Also, the use of tamper-resistant and tamper-evident packaging makes contamination of foodstuffs more difficult and more detectable.

In the consumption stage, there are two different focuses. With individual preparation, large-scale contamination is extremely unlikely; typically families or small gatherings are affected. In contrast, a busy food service establishment may affect many people if they distribute a locally contaminated product. This scenario could occur in a busy restaurant, at a sporting event or at a convention.

FOOD CONTAMINATION AS VIEWED THROUGH FSIS RECALLS

Vulnerabilities to contamination in the food industry are highlighted by the U.S. Department of Agriculture's (USDA) Food Safety Inspection Service (FSIS) recalls. From 2002 through 2005, a total of 293 food product recalls were issued. Fifty-five percent of the food recalls were for bacterial contamination with *Listeria monocytogenes* (34%), *Escherichia coli* (18%), or *Salmonella* (3%). Other reasons for recall included undeclared allergens in the food (e.g., eggs, peanut oil, etc); contamination with glass, metal, or plastic; mislabeling; undercooking; unsanitary conditions; and contamination with chemicals or heavy metals. In total, over 71 million pounds of food were recalled; four large recalls accounted for 54 million pounds of these recalls. While this is a very large quantity of food, there are other food recalls handled by other agencies, which are not in the FSIS total. For example, in 2002, the FDA recalled 4080 cans of refried beans because of possible *Clostridium botulinum* contamination.

BIOLOGICAL FOOD CONTAMINATION

Accidental Contamination

An outbreak of listeriosis in the northeastern United States in 2002 led to the largest food recall in USDA history. Approximately 52 people came down with culture-confirmed listeriosis and 7 people died. Some estimates are as high as 120 people made ill and 20 deaths. Two different companies recalled a total of approximately 31.5 million pounds of ready-to-eat chicken and turkey products. Also in 2002, there were two separate incidents of fresh and frozen beef products becoming contaminated with *E. coli* leading to at least 25 people being hospitalized and 5 developing hemolytic-uremic syndrome. Over 22.5 million pounds of beef were recalled from across the country.

Intentional Contamination

The best known and most widely repeated story of deliberate bacterial food contamination occurred in Oregon in late 1984. The Bhagwan Shree Rajneeshee cult owned a ranch in Wasco County, OR. The cult used biological attacks in an attempt to control the local governing body so as to pass laws favorable to the cult. In August 1984, the cult infected a judge and two county commissioners by giving them *Salmonella*-tainted water when the three visited the compound. In an attempt to sway the November 1984 elections, the cult members infected salad bars in ten restaurants in The Dalles, OR, the county seat of Wasco County. At least 750 people contracted salmonellosis and 45 were hospitalized, but none died.

In October 1996, a laboratory worker in a Dallas, TX, hospital deliberately contaminated muffins and donuts with *Shigella dysenteriae* type 2. She then left the food for her coworkers in the communal break room. Approximately 45 persons became ill and 5 were hospitalized. There were no deaths.

While best known for their March 20, 1995, release of the nerve agent sarin in the Tokyo subway system, the Aum Shinrikyo cult attempted to assassinate an attorney by placing botulinium toxin in his drink. The attempt failed because the cult failed to obtain the correct strain of *Clostridium*.

CHEMICAL FOOD CONTAMINATION

Accidental Contamination

At a wedding reception in Ankeny, IA, in March 2003, approximately 140 guests became ill with dizziness, headaches, weakness, and dyspnea after drinking a punch, which had a peculiar taste. The diagnosis of methemoglobinemia (MetHb) was made and MetHb levels ranged from 1.7% to 60.3%. Thirty-seven guests were treated for MetHb with methylene blue; twenty guests were hospitalized. A sample of the dry punch mix was found to have sodium nitrite concentration of 5000 ppm while the liquid punch's nitrite concentration was 500 ppm. It was later determined that sodium nitrite was accidentally substituted for sodium citrate in the manufacture process of the dry powder punch base. The Environmental Protection Agency's (EPA) maximum contaminant level (MCL) for nitrites in drinking water is 1 mg/L (1 ppm).

In two separate incidents in Japan and Taiwan in the late 1970s, rice oil used for cooking was accidentally contaminated with a mixture of polychlorinated biphenyls (PCBs) and polychlorinated dibenzofurans (PCDFs). Over 4000 people were affected and manifested symptoms of chloracne, skin, and mucous membrane hyperpigmentation, abnormal finger nails, and endocrine disorders. An association was made with these exposures and impaired cognitive development in children with in utero exposure.

In 2005, 389,000 lb of poultry products were recalled because of potential contamination with the organophosphate insecticide ronnel. There were no reported human effects. There have also been FSIS recalls for food contaminated with cleaning detergents, lead, hydraulic fluid, oil, and chlorfenvinphos, an organophosphate insecticide.

Deliberate Contamination

The best reported incidents of deliberate chemical contamination of food typically involve food contaminated in the retail distribution or consumption phases.

In early 2003, approximately 111 people in the town of Byron Center, MI, became ill with nausea, vomiting, diarrhea, and diaphoresis after eating contaminated ground beef. A disgruntled employee of a local supermarket mixed Black Leaf 40 into approximately 250 lb of ground beef. Black Leaf 40 is an insecticide, which contains 40% nicotine as its active ingredient. Analysis of the beef found a nicotine concentration of 300 mg/kg. With a lethal dose of nicotine for an adult being ~50 mg, ingestion of ~6 oz of meat could have been lethal.

In 1988, a 41-year-old waitress and her family from Alturas, FL, were poisoned by their next-door neighbor. The neighbor, irritated because of noise problems, contaminated an 8-pack of pop with thallium nitrate and placed it in the victims' house. The waitress died while two of her sons were hospitalized but survived.

RADIOLOGICAL FOOD CONTAMINATION

Accidental Contamination

While the explosion of the nuclear power plant in Chernobyl, Ukraine, on April 26, 1986, was an environmental disaster, the incident resulted in the most widespread accidental radioactive contamination of foodstuffs in history. Within days of the explosion, there were concerns over external contamination of foodstuffs and radioactive contamination of the milk supply. Liquid milk harvested in early May 1986 revealed a radioactivity content of 900 Bq/L (**) while powdered milk made from the same milk source had a content of 3000 Bq/kg. The safe level for radiation content in food in Europe has been set at 600 Bq/kg. Some samples of powdered milk from Europe were contaminated as high as 8000 Bq/kg. Tens of thousands of tons of contaminated powdered milk had to be disposed of.

Even today, there are concerns about radioactive contamination of foodstuffs grown or processed within areas of Europe, which suffered heavy radioactive contamination from the Chernobyl disaster. A wild boar killed in France in February 1997 had a radioactivity level of 1709 Bq/kg. Bulgarian mushrooms stopped at the French border in September 1999 had a radioactivity level of 2470 Bq/kg.

Deliberate Contamination

In 1995, there were two well-publicized incidents in which radioactive phosphorus-32 (P-32) was used maliciously to contaminate food. The first instance involved a 31-year-old female scientist at the National Cancer Institute who was

17 weeks pregnant at the time. She ingested approximately 300 microcuries (µCi) (**) of P-32 on June 28, 1995. The P-32 was placed in her lunch, which was kept in a refrigerator outside of the laboratory in which she worked. Her contamination was discovered the next day when she set off a Geiger counter during a routine radiation sweep of her lab. Twenty-five other coworkers ingested smaller amounts of P-32 that had been placed into a communal water cooler. The Nuclear Regulatory Commission has set the Annual Limit of Intake (ALI) for P-32 at 600 µCi.

(**) 1 becquerel (Bq) = 1 disintegration per second; 1 microcurie (µCi) = 37,000 Bq.

The second incident occurred on August 14, 1995, at the Massachusetts Institute of Technology. A postdoctoral researcher ingested approximately 580 µCi of P-32 that was deliberately placed into his food or drink that was kept in a break room adjacent to the lab. His contamination was not discovered until August 19 when he preformed a routine radiation survey on himself after handling other radionucleotides.

While neither of these scientists, nor the first scientist's child, was believed to have suffered permanent harm, these two cases clearly show how easily food can be contaminated with large quantities of radioactive material.

CONFIRMING THE THREAT

A foodborne disease outbreak may or may not be difficult for the clinician to detect. In the case of the nitrite-contaminated punch, recognition of an outbreak was prompt. However, with many biological, radiological, and chemical agents, the onset of symptoms may be significantly delayed from the time of ingestion. It is this time-delayed effect that makes use of these agents desirable to a terrorist. In addition to a delayed onset of symptoms, having a small number of patients present to different hospitals at different times can make detection of an outbreak difficult. The dispersal of patients over large distances can be quite prominent if the food contamination occurred at a convention or at an airport restaurant and those who consumed the food become dispersed across the country.

SYMPTOMS/LABORATORY/MEDIACAL MANAGEMENT

The patients' presenting symptoms, the laboratory requirements, and the medical management of a foodborne disease outbreak will depend upon what the suspected contaminant is.

WHO TO REFER TO AND WHEN

Whenever a clinician suspects a foodborne disease outbreak, that clinician needs to contact their local public health department. In many jurisdictions, public health is charged with the task of conducting the epidemiological investigation and may be able to provide management advice. Since many local public health agencies in small or rural counties have a small staff, a moderate-sized outbreak could easily overwhelm the local public health resources. In these instances, assistance from the state health department or the Centers for Disease Control and Prevention (CDC) may be requested. For the clinician managing the patient, consultations with various specialists may be helpful: an infectious disease specialist for infectious agents, or a medical toxicologist for chemical agents. The Department of Energy's (DOE) Radiation Emergency Assistance Center/Training Site (REAC/TS) has numerous physicians experienced in the management of radiation-related injuries. REAC/TS can be reached by calling (865) 576 1005 and asking for REAC/TS.

FORENSIC ISSUES

If an outbreak is believed to be deliberate, law enforcement agencies become involved. The clinician will need to save the appropriate clinical samples and ensure that the appropriate chain-of-custody procedures are followed. Good documentation of the patient's history, signs and symptoms, physical exam, and treatment may provide important information needed to reconstruct the events of the attack.

Suggested Reading

Centers for Disease Control and Prevention, Diagnosis and management of foodborne illnesses: a primer for physicians and other health care professionals. *MMWR Recomm Rep.* 2004;53(RR-4):1–33.

Crutchley TM, Rodgers JB, Whiteside HP et al. Agroterrorism: where are we in the ongoing war on terrorism? *J Food Prot* 2007 Mar; 70 (3): 791–804.

Cupp OS, Walker DE, Hillison J. Agroterrorism in the US: Key security challenge for the 21st century. *Biosecur Bioterr* 2004; 2 (2): 97–105.

Iowa State University, Center for Food Security and Public Health; *http://www.cfsph.iastate.edu/*

Khan AS, Swerdlow DL, Juranek DD. Precautions against biological and chemical terrorism directed at food and water supplies. *Public Health Rep.* Jan–Feb 2001;116(1):3–14.

Levin J, Gilmore K, Nalbone T, Sheperd S. Agroterrorism workshop; engaging community preparedness. *J Agromedicine* 2005; 10 (2): 7–15.

Schier JG, Schrug RH, Patel MM et al. Strategies for recognizing chemical associated food borne illness. Mil Med 2006; 171:1174–1180.

Sobel J, Khan AS, Swerdlow DL. Threat of a biological terrorist attack on the US food supply: the CDC perspective. *Lancet.* March 9, 2002;359(3909):874–880.

United States government Center for Food Safety; *http://www. foodsafety.gov/*

VI

IONIZING RADIATION

INTRODUCTION

The medical response to radiation—whether radiological warfare, terrorism, occupational accident, or radiated patient in the hospital remains one of the least taught among all segments of medical education in spite of a generation raised on the Cuban Missile Crisis! Few health-care professionals possess the knowledge or skills to identify, let alone treat a radiation victim. While many remember bomb shelters, few can effectively describe the risks attendant to radiation, let alone the rationale behind such shelters! The current Iran and North Korean threats notwithstanding, the widespread availability of radioactive materials from medical and commercial sources, in addition to the proliferation of nuclear materials and technology make the likelihood of acquiring and using ionizing radiation as a weapon much more likely. Add to this the potential threat associated with the enormous tonnage of radioactive waste being transported across the country to facilities that may include the Texas—New Mexico Border and Yucca Mountain in Nevada. Most are not aware of the daily use of radioactive materials within their communities or the variety of threats such activities pose.

Beyond the persistent lack of awareness concerning the threat of radioactive materials, and as a result of inadequate training, there remains a perception that our response capabilities, especially in terms of treatment options are limited. Such is not the case! The treatment of radiation casualties is possible and newer countermeasures and medical interventions are highly effective. Therefore it is essential that we become more engaged in our radiation response capabilities.

In the chapters that follow, we will introduce the critical information you need to diagnose and manage victims of a radiation event, prepare your facility to identify vulnerabilities in preparedness such as training gaps, as well as radioactive materials that might be easily stolen. We'll discuss the various threat scenarios likely to involve radiation, introduce important definitions associated with radioactivity, help you identify the types of expertise as well as resources and agencies that must be contacted before or during a radiation emergency, equipment and other supplies including antidotes and other countermeasures necessary to prepare your facility and respond to radiation victims including detection technologies you should obtain and practice with. As with other sections of *Emergency Bioterrorism* you will note STAT Facts start out each chapter in this Radiation Section to guide you as a review or checklist to prepare.

51

A PRACTICAL BASIS FOR EARLY MANAGEMENT OF RADIOLOGICALLY INJURED OR ILL PATIENTS: IONIZING RADIATION PHYSICS AND INSTRUMENTATION, RADIATION PROTECTION, CONTAMINATION CONTROL, DOSIMETRY, AND RADIOLOGICAL/NUCLEAR (R/N) TERRORISM

Doran M. Christensen, Steve Sugarman, A. Seaton Garrett, Otis W. Jones, and Albert L. Wiley, Jr.

STAT FACTS

A PRACTICAL BASIS FOR EARLY MANAGEMENT OF RADIOLOGICALLY INJURED OR ILL PATIENTS: IONIZING RADIATION PHYSICS AND INSTRUMENTATION, RADIATION PROTECTION, CONTAMINATION CONTROL, DOSIMETRY, AND RADIOLOGICAL/NUCLEAR (R/N) TERRORISM

- Most radioactive materials and radioactivity are relatively easy to locate with detection instruments, an advantage not available for chemical and biological hazards.
- Once located, radioactive materials and radioactivity can be managed methodically and safely using some fairly simple and intuitive rules. Many of them are already used by health-care providers for other kinds of hazards: universal precautions and appropriate personal protective equipment.
- The basics of physics, instrumentation, radiation protection, contamination control, principles of "ALARA"

(keeping radiation doses As Low As Reasonably Achievable), and dosimetry only appear formidable. The principles can be understood and used by almost anyone with minimal time and effort spent in training.

- Health physicists (HP) need to be integrated into preparations for R/N incident response and consequence management *prior* to an incident not *during*.
- Historically, the provision of health care to radiologically injured or ill patents is relatively low risk. There is no known history of significant exposure to ionizing radiation (IR) to health-care workers who have provided medical care to R/N victims.
- Disaster planning must take into account how to communicate with and divert potential patients from the emergency department (ED) who have only a perception of radiation-induced injury/illness and those who may be contaminated but uninjured. The misinformation/misperceptions about radiation with the resulting fear and anxiety

may well result in the ED being overwhelmed with numbers of "patients" who don't need medical care.

- Irradiated and contaminated patients can be managed in the ED or elsewhere in hospital. Access needs, not be denied.
- *Local* decontamination is recommended for smaller areas of contamination. Total body decontamination like showering is usually not required for localized areas of contamination. In fact, total body decontamination for localized radioactive materials can make a situation more difficult to manage because of spread to other parts of the body that will then have to be decontaminated. Widespread contamination may require total body decontamination. Biological and chemical contamination may require total body decontamination. In fact, the presence of biological and chemical contamination and the risks they represent may actually provide the basis for decontamination decisions.

INTRODUCTION TO BASIC IONIZING RADIATION PHYSICS, RADIATION PROTECTION, AND CONTAMINATION CONTROL

The following primer is provided as a basis for understanding the medical management of radiation-induced injuries and illnesses presented in Chap. 52.

Basic Atomic Structure

The atom has a central nucleus containing protons (p) and neutrons (n), sometimes collectively called "nucleons." Protons have a positive charge. Neutrons have no charge. Both have approximately the same mass. Surrounding the nucleus is a cloud of electrons. Electrons carry a negative charge. In a stable and electrically neutral atom, the number of protons in the nucleus equals the number of negative electrons surrounding the nucleus.

Radiological Nomenclature

The "Z" number of an element is the *atomic number*, which is equivalent to the number of protons in the nucleus. The Z number defines the element. The "N" number of an element is equivalent to the number of neutrons in the nucleus. The "A" number of an element is equivalent to the *atomic mass number* or the total number of protons and neutrons in the nucleus.

The atomic mass number is

$$A = Z + N$$

The standard notation with "E" as the abbreviation for an imaginary "element" is

$$^A_Z E_N \quad \text{or} \quad ^A E$$

Note that the atomic mass number A is not the same as the chemical atomic weight noted on most periodic tables of the elements. The chemical atomic weight is a weighted average of all natural isotopes of an element based upon their relative abundance.

Examples: Hydrogen or ^1H (= Hydrogen-1 or just Hydrogen) is hydrogen with only one proton and no neutrons. This element is stable and nonradioactive. Deuterium or ^2H (= Hydrogen-2) is hydrogen with one proton and one neutron in the nucleus. Deuterium is also stable and nonradioactive. Tritium or ^3H (= Hydrogen-3) is hydrogen with one proton plus two neutrons in the nucleus. Tritium is radioactive.

The atomic number or "Z" number for uranium is always 92, that is, Z determines the identity of the element. If it were not 92, it would be another element. Uranium therefore always has 92 protons in its nucleus but the number of neutrons can vary. In nature, uranium has various atomic mass numbers or A numbers, such as U-233, U-234, U-235, U-238, and others, depending upon how many neutrons are in the nucleus. These are called "isotopes" of uranium. Isotopes have the same Z number but different A and N numbers. All isotopes of uranium are radioactive and are called "radioisotopes." Generically, radioactive materials are sometimes called "radionuclides."

Standard notation is, for example, U-238

$$^{238}_{92}U_{146}$$

Nuclear Disintegration

Nuclear stability depends largely upon the ratio of protons to neutrons in the atomic nucleus. Unstable atoms attempt to become stable by disintegrating. Disintegration results in the release of various kinds of radiation. The A number or Z number of the radionuclide may change as the nuclei disintegrate depending upon the mode of decay. For example, U-238 disintegrates with the release of an α-particle. As below, an α-particle is equivalent to 2 protons and 2 neutrons. With the release of this α-particle, U-238 then becomes thorium-234. The A number changes because of 2n and 2p being emitted. The name of, that is, the identity of the element changes with the number of protons (p).

What is Radiation

Radiation is the emission and propagation of energy through space or through a medium in the form of waves or particles that in some ways behave like electromagnetic waves. There are a number of different kinds of radiation in the electromagnetic spectrum most of which do not have sufficient energy to cause ionization. Most radiations in the spectrum are nonionizing such as microwaves, visible light, ultraviolet light, infrared light, to name a few. Deposition of their energy can cause damage by creation of heat but not by ionization.

What is Ionizing Radiation

Ionizing radiation is energy that has the potential to remove electrons from other atoms. By stripping a negative electron from an atom, an "ion pair" is created—an electron and a positively charged atomic remnant.

- Ionization creates instability in molecules, the most important of which is cellular genetic material made up of deoxyribonucleic acid (DNA).
- Another mechanism of cell damage from ionizing radiation is by hydrolysis of water to form "free radicals."
- Free radicals are very reactive and can create potentially destructive chemical reactions in other atoms.
- The differences among types of ionizing radiation relate to energy and charge.
- These properties determine
  - how deeply ionizing radiation can penetrate cells, tissues, or organs, and,
  - how they deposit energy along their tracks.
- The range of penetration by ionizing radiation also depends upon the nature of the absorber. This is the basis for shielding.
- Ionization is the primary basis for locating radioactivity and radioactive materials.
- "Spectrometry" is used to identify the energy of the radiation allowing it to be compared to a known spectrum. This tool is required for identification of specific radionuclides. Each radionuclide has a unique energy spectrum much like every human has unique fingerprints.

Types of Ionizing Radiation

Alpha, beta, and neutrons are the primary types of *particulate* ionizing radiations. Gamma and x-rays are the primary types of *electromagnetic* ionizing radiations, or "photons." There are relatively large numbers of other subatomic particles that currently are not as biologically important as these five. Very briefly

Alpha particles (α)

- Are equivalent to Helium-4 (= ^{4}He) nuclei, which consist of 2 protons (p) and 2 neutrons (n)
- Have significant kinetic energy
- Have a +2 charge
- Generally cause direct ionization of other atoms or molecules—largely because of their size and charge
- Have little penetrating power—cannot penetrate a sheet of paper or the epidermis of skin. Shielding is therefore relatively easy
- **CAVEAT: Water, blood, tissue, or many other materials will shield alphas making detection impossible. Samples of body fluids that may contain alpha-emitting radioactive materials should be dried on a cotton-swab or 4 × 4 before concluding that an alpha-emitting material is not present**
- Alpha emitters are only a hazard when they are inhaled, ingested, or otherwise taken into the body

Beta particles (β^-)

- Are identical to electrons
- Have a negative charge
- Have very little mass—about 1/2000th the mass of a proton or neutron
- Are generally less energetic than α-particles
- Shielding can be accomplished with a piece of tinfoil or perhaps 20 sheets of paper or other such light materials
- Can penetrate the epidermis and cause skin injury
- Beta emitters pose internal and external hazards

Gamma (γ) and x-ray electromagnetic waves

- Commonly called "photons," which can be thought of as "packets" of electromagnetic energy
- Depth of penetration in tissues depends upon their energy
- Shielding is usually accomplished with *high* atomic weight elements, such as the heavy metals: lead or depleted uranium
- Gamma emitters pose internal and external hazards

Neutrons (n)

- Originate from atomic nuclei
- Are generally fairly energetic over a range
- Require special shielding
- Are differentially absorbed by *low* atomic weight nuclei like hydrogen, carbon, and oxygen

- Water is therefore a good absorber of neutrons and is commonly used to shield neutrons
- Would normally be present following an incident only if a "criticality" has occurred, which is very rare (see Chap. 52), or a neutron-emitting radionuclide, for example, californium-252, is present
- Are the only kind of radiation that can make other materials "radioactive" by changing the proton to neutron ratio in target nuclei

Health Physicists

Health physicists (HP) are specialists in radiation protection and contamination control. Their skills will be critical to the guidance of medical management of radiation injuries and illnesses discussed in the next chapter. HPs can help:

- "Reconstruct" an incident, which may provide an estimate of the radiation dose and the identity of radioactive materials or radiation(s) involved.
- Incident reconstruction is equivalent to the physician's identification of the "mechanism of injury" following physical trauma. Radiological *and* medical histories are essential to medical diagnosis, treatment, and management.
- Determine the nature and extent of exposures—assist with "dose estimates" or assessments of "radiation-absorbed dose."
- With environmental contaminations and control of radioactive materials and is equivalent to "irradiation."

Medical physicists (MP) are also physicists but apply their discipline in different ways. They generally assist radiation oncologists with calculations of radiation doses used in radiotherapy (RT) for treatment of cancers.

What is Exposure

For present purposes, "exposure" means being in the presence of ionizing radiation as one might be "exposed" to heat, cold, or the measles and is equivalent to "irradiation."

What is Radiation Dose

Dose refers to the absorption of radiation energy per unit mass of absorber. The conventional U.S. dose unit is the rad. 1 rad = 100 erg/g. The SI unit is the gray (Gy). 1 Gy = 1 Joule/kg. 1 Gy = 100 rad. An easy way to remember the conventional unit for dose is **R**adiation **A**bsorbed **D**ose = "rad."

What is Dose Equivalent

Dose equivalent refers to the biological damage and long-term risk that may result from various kinds of radiation when compared to photons. The conventional U.S. unit of dose equivalent is the rem. The SI unit is the sievert (Sv). 1 Sv = 100 rem. An easy way to remember the conventional unit for dose equivalent is **R**adiation **E**quivalent **M**an = "rem."

A dose equivalent is calculated by multiplying a dose by a "quality factor" (QF).

$$\text{Dose Equivalent} = \text{Dose} \times \text{Quality Factor}$$

The QF relates the amount of biological damage, and resulting risk, caused by any type of radiation to that caused by the same absorbed dose of photons. The QF for photons and β-particles is 1. Alphas have a QF of 20 (internal only). Neutrons have varying QFs from 3 to 20 depending upon their energy.

Caveat: For the intent and purpose of acute care, roentgens are equivalent to rads which are equivalent to rems. These two chapters (Chaps. 51 and 52) deal with radiation-induced injuries or illnesses that result from relatively acute or short-term exposures occurring over seconds to hours. Therefore, doses expected to cause short-term effect should be discussed in grays or rads. Acute doses that may be expected to cause late effects such as cancers should be discussed in sieverts or rems. (See Table 51-1.)

What is "Activity"

Disintegrations of radioactive materials are detected and counted as a basis for determining the "activity" of radioactive sources. Activity is the number of disintegrations in a unit of time, for example, disintegrations per minute or disintegrations per second (dpm or dps). The U.S. conventional unit for activity is the curie, which is equivalent to 37 billion (3.7×10^{10}) disintegrations per second or 2.22 trillion (2.22×10^{12}) disintegrations per

TABLE 51-1

RADIOLOGICAL UNITS OF MEASUREMENT

Quantity	Measures	Conventional Units (United States)	SI Units
Exposure	Ionization	roentgen (R)	coulomb/kg
Absorbed dose	Energy deposition	rad	gray (Gy) (= 100 rad)
Dose equivalent	Biological damage/risk	rem	sievert (Sv) (= 100 rem)

minute. A disintegration per second is called a "becquerel" (Bq) in the SI (International System or Systéme Internationale) method of nomenclature.

"Irradiation" *versus* "Contamination"

Understanding the difference between these terms is absolutely critical to medical management:

- "Irradiated" patients have been "exposed" to ionizing radiation like patients who have had diagnostic x-rays.
  - They are not radioactive and pose absolutely no risk to others.
- "Contaminated" patients have radioactive materials in them or on them, called "internal contamination" or "external contamination."
  - Patients may be externally contaminated with radioactive materials on clothing or skin.
  - Patients may also be internally contaminated with radioactive materials by inhalation, ingestion, percutaneous absorption, or penetration.
  - Contaminated patients *may* pose a risk to others.
  - That risk depends upon the type and quantity of radioactive material present.
  - Hospital personnel safely handle patients on a daily basis who have had nuclear medicine scans who are internally contaminated with injections of radioactive materials.

Detection of Radiation and Radioactive Materials

The ability to detect, locate, and quantify radioactive materials is a major advantage not afforded by other hazards like biological or chemical agents. Geiger-Muller counters or so-called "Geiger counters" are used to detect ionizations. There are a number of other kinds of detectors available for use but these are the most common and easiest to use.

"Survey meters" are used to detect radiation in which case they are used to count ionizations in counts per minutes (cpm). Another like piece of equipment is used to *quantify* radiation levels, in which case, they are usually referred to as "dose-rate meters." They read in roentgens per hour, milliroentgens per hour, microroentgens per hour, etc.

It may not be known immediately after an incident or even by the time patients arrive at the ED that an incident has involved radioactive materials. First-responders in the emergency medical services (EMS) system and public safety (fire, police) and first-receivers may be unknowingly irradiated and/or contaminated; therefore, it is wise to have such detectors in constant use in the field.

They are relatively easy to operate and anyone can learn to use them. Almost every hospital nuclear medicine department will have personnel familiar with this equipment. These personnel may be used as a resource for teaching others how to use the equipment. Immediately after an event, HPs and other very knowledgeable technicians may not be available; therefore, health-care workers should learn how to use the equipment *before* an incident occurs. *Interpretation* of the level of radioactivity present will require assistance from HP. Such experts need to be identified and integrated into ED response plans *before* an incident occurs.

A common instrument used to detect/measure radioactive contamination is a pancake probe attached to a survey meter. See Fig. 51-1.

Just as with any medical equipment, certain precautions must be taken to prevent a failure to detect or prevent inaccurate results. Radiation detectors

- Should be calibrated on at least a yearly basis
- Need batteries checked or replaced at regular intervals to ensure that power is available from corroded contacts, deterioration with age, and so on
- Batteries should always be checked prior to each use
- Should be checked with a "check source" of radiation prior to use to ensure that it is operating properly

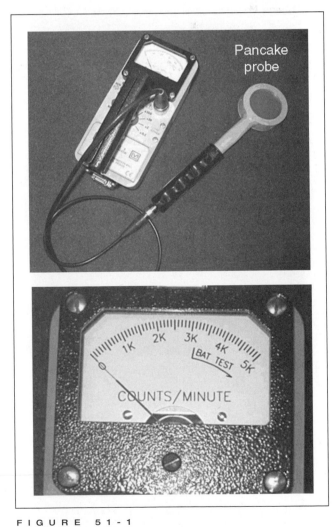

FIGURE 51-1

GEIGER-MULLER COUNTER WITH PANCAKE PROBE
Note the scale reading in counts per minute.

Prior to use, background radiation levels must be checked in the area where patients from a radiological incident will be evaluated and treated. Background levels vary with geographical area. For example, in Oak Ridge, TN, background levels are generally on the order of 20–40 counts per minute (cpm). Higher levels may generally be found in areas at higher elevation but may vary by locale because of other factors. (See Figs. 51-1 through 51-4.)

These devices are read just like a tachometer in a car. The reading on the face of the meter is multiplied by a

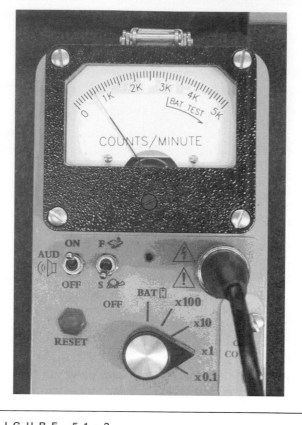

FIGURE 51-3

SURVEY METER READING

Scale Reading (cpm)	Range Multiplier (×100, ×10, etc.)	True Reading (cpm)
700	1	700

700 cpm x 1 = 700 cpm

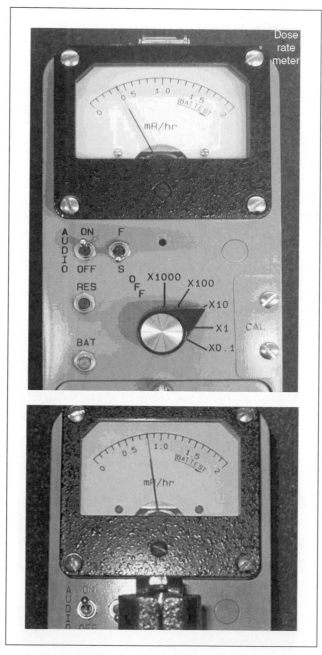

FIGURE 51-2

DOSE-RATE METER

Note scale reading in mR/h or milliroentgens per hour. For all practical purposes, it can be read as millirads per hour.

multiplier chosen with a switch under the dial, just as the number on a tachometer is multiplied by 1000. The multipliers on various meters can vary.

Identification of Radioactive Materials

Geiger counters can be used to detect and locate radioactive materials. They cannot be used to *identify* radiation and radioactive sources, although with a basic understanding of ionizing radiation, pancake probes can be used to distinguish between α, β, and γ radiations. This ability can be very useful when trying to decide how to proceed with medical management.

For example:

- Hold the probe about half inch (1 centimeter) from the source;
- Move the probe away 2 inches (5 centimeters)—if counts disappear, it's probably an alpha-emitter;

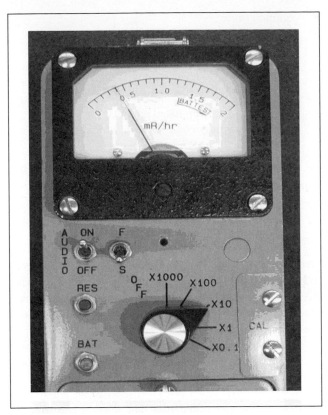

FIGURE 51-4

DOSE-RATE METER READING

Scale Reading (mR/h)	Range Multiplier (×1000, ×100, etc.)	True Reading (mR/h)
0.4	10	4

0.4 mR/h × 10 = 4 mR/h

- Turn the probe back to detect position and return the probe to a half inch from the source;
- Turn the probe back over with metallic side facing the source—if counts are still detected, it's probably a gamma source;
- If counts disappear, it's probably a beta-emitter.

Two inches of air is usually sufficient to shield α-particles. Beta particles are shielded by the metal casing on the back of the detector. Gammas will penetrate both.

HPs will help convert counts per minute or "cpm" mathematically to disintegrations per minute (dpm), which is a measurement of radioactivity. The history of an incident may give clues to the identity of radioactive materials and types of radiation(s) involved.

Spectroscopy

One piece of equipment for *identification* of radioactive material is a gamma spectrometer. This is a relatively sophisticated piece of equipment that may be located only at fairly specialized facilities. The facilities that can provide identification services need to be identified, located,

and included in the ED response plan *before* an incident. Some portable spectrometers are available on the market but even they may require HP assistance for interpretation.

Dosimetry

Unless an incident occurs in a radiation-controlled environment, such as in radiological or nuclear industries, most victims will not have worn "dosimeters." A "physical" dosimeter is a device that can be used to determine how much radiation is absorbed at the location on the body where the device is worn. These devices are designed to detect some, but not necessarily all, radiations, and they must be properly selected in advance according to likely scenarios. HPs need to be consulted for decisions about devices to be used in EDs in advance of an incident. They may also be needed for consultation about devices that might have been worn by victims during an R/N incident and their interpretation.

Some dosimeters must be "developed" after the fact by a special process and will be of no immediate help with dose assessment. Thermoluminescence dosimeters (TLD) worn by radiology department personnel or optically stimulated luminescence dosimeters (OSLD) must be developed after the fact by a special process. "Ring" dosimeters may be worn by personnel handling radiation sources with their hands, such as during extraction of a piece of shrapnel or other surgical procedures. See Fig. 51-5.

Dosimeters may be "direct-reading" that can give some assistance in determination of dose to a person or a part of a

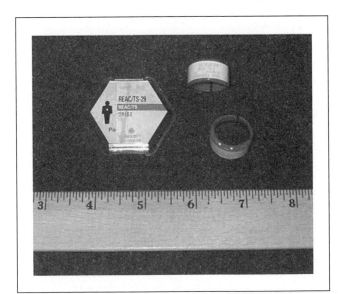

FIGURE 51-5

On the left is an optically stimulated luminescence dosimeter (OSLD) usually attached to clothing between the shoulders and waist. On the right are two views of ring dosimeters. Both types must be "developed" by a special process to determine dose absorbed in the area where the dosimeter is worn.

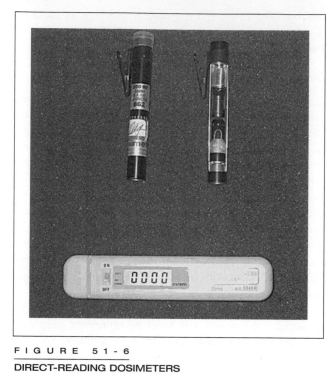

FIGURE 51-6

DIRECT-READING DOSIMETERS
At the top are "pen" or "pencil" or "pocket" dosimeters from which photon doses can be read directly by looking through the device to see a reading of dose to the dosimeter. At the bottom is a digital direct-reading dosimeter.

person where a dosimeter is located. Direct-reading "pen," "pencil," or "pocket" dosimeters may be worn by health-care personnel during management of patients. See top of Fig. 51-6. They respond to photons, not alphas or betas, and can be read directly after or during patient management. These dosimeters must be "zeroed" or its reading noted prior to use. There are some electronic devices that will directly report dose rates or radiation doses absorbed by the devices in measurable quantities in real-time. See Fig. 51-6.

Radiation Protection and Contamination Control

Protection from radioactive materials and radioactivity is not much different than protection from biological or chemical agents. It is relatively easier to provide protection from radiological materials because of the ability to detect them. Contamination control is the most important way to prevent exposures. A very basic level of understanding of physics, how radioactive materials behave, and how to control radioactive contamination is all that is needed by health-care providers.

Personnel can help protect themselves by using

- universal precautions
- sterile techniques

- common sense
- appropriate personal protective equipment (PPE)—surgical scrub suit and gown or Tyvek or other impermeable body suit, double gloves, surgical face mask, rarely N95 masks, splash shields, booties. For a presentation of donning and doffing appropriate dress for managing contaminated patients, see *http://orise.orau.gov/reacts/guide/procedures.htm*
- principles of "ALARA"—see below

The level of personal protective wear should be appropriate for the hazard. Particular attention should be to worker safety and the potential for heat stress in the ED.

Decontamination

Decontamination is not complicated but the process needs to be methodical and systematic. It also needs to be practiced in advance of an incident. Contamination is nothing more than dirt with radioactive atoms mixed in, so remove the dirt and the radioactive materials that go with it. Decontamination efforts should not be too aggressive because abrading the skin may increase the risk of absorption. Priorities for decontamination should be given to open wounds first, then body orifices in particular nose and mouth, or any other area that may be a portal for radioactive materials to enter the body. For detailed instructions, see *http://orise.orau.gov/reacts/guide/procedures.htm* See also the decision-support algorithm in Fig. 52-1 in the next chapter.

Isolated areas of contamination with radioactive materials should be decontaminated locally. Total body showering is generally not necessary unless there is widespread skin contamination or there is a mass casualty incident with insufficient resources to survey patients for radiological materials. Because of the relative inability to localize biological and/or chemical contamination, total body decontamination like showering may be necessary even with the presence of radioactive materials. In many cases, biological or chemical hazards may be more hazardous than radiological materials therefore management of those contaminants will dictate the best method of decontamination.

Body hair, including beards and eyebrows, should not be shaved because microabrasions may allow absorption and internalization. Shaved eyebrows may not regrow. Removal of contamination can be accomplished simply with soap and water, shampoos, shaving cream, industrial nonsolvent grease removers, and any number of other types of cleansers. Degreasers or other solvents should not be used because defatting of the skin may damage the skin enough to allow percutaneous absorption of radioactive and other materials.

The supplies needed for external decontamination of radioactive materials can be purchased at reasonable prices at any grocery store and many other such retailers. No other special supplies above and beyond the usual hospital soft-goods will be needed. A very helpful item though is water-proof sheets to place under patients. A few should be placed on a gurney before patient placement for treatments and decontamination.

Decontamination of wounds with IV fluids and spring-loaded syringe is a very helpful technique for wound management. For a demonstration, see *http://orise.orau.gov/reacts/ guide/procedures.htm* Wound care, debridement, and repair can generally proceed as usual. Generally, if a medical intervention should be done in the absence of radioactive materials, the intervention can usually be done with the presence of radioactive materials.

KEY POINTS RELATED TO CONTAMINATION CONTROL AND DECONTAMINATION

- Contamination control of radioactive materials is not that much different than control of biological or chemical agents.
- Simple removal of all clothing will generally remove 60–90% of contamination but, of course, depends upon what the patient was wearing at the time of the incident.
- Pay particular attention to areas that were not covered during an incident, particularly head, neck, face, and hands.
- Care should be taken to survey the face and wounds early because these areas may provide a direct route of intake for radioactive materials.
- Early identification of facial or wound contamination may allow early intervention with specific therapies for radionuclides. See Chap. 52 for treatment of internal contamination.
- *Local* decontamination is preferable to *total* body attempts to decontaminate like showering.
- If an incident involves *only* radioactive materials, showering will *rarely* be required.
- The presence of other toxic biological or chemical agents may dictate decontamination efforts.

Counting needs to be repeated after each effort at decontamination but the distance between a radiation source and the pancake probe must be the same for each survey. Failure to ensure consistency of distance from the source with each survey can result in confusion and improper decisions about decontamination. For example, if the probe is held 2 inches from a contaminated area on the survey and after decontamination the probe is held half inch from the area, the number of counts will be higher, giving an impression that contamination is becoming worse. Learning the technique to maintain consistency requires some practice.

"ALARA" Principles

ALARA principles = keeping exposures to radiation or radiological/nuclear materials "as low as reasonably achievable."

- Minimize *time* spent around or near sources of ionizing radiation
- Maximize *distance* from sources. The inverse square law defines the effect of distance upon dose. If the distance is doubled, the dose will be quartered. If the distance is halved, the dose will be four times higher
- Maximize *shielding* from sources
- Minimize *amounts* of radioactive materials handled

RADIOBIOLOGY

Ionizing radiation causes damage to living cells by ionization of atoms and molecules, the most important of which is DNA. Cells have enzymatic processes in place to repair damage to DNA. Generally, the effects of radiation injury *at survivable doses* are delayed by hours, days, and sometimes weeks. Even death from large radiation doses is delayed, unlike deaths from physical trauma or thermal burns, which can be immediate. In fact, *immediate* deaths from serious radiological or nuclear incidents, including nuclear detonations, are always from various types of physical trauma, thermal insults and *not* radiation. See incident scenarios in Chap. 52.

What Radiation Causes—"Deterministic Effects"

The amount of damage to an organism is related to

- Dose—the total amount of energy deposited
  - Deterministic effects have a threshold dose at which an effect appears, that is, the dose determines the effect.
  - Above that threshold as radiation dose increases, the effects become worse.
- Dose rate—the time over which ionizing radiation energy is deposited. The shorter the time period of delivery, the greater the effects.
- Volume of cells or tissues absorbing the dose—the larger the volume of tissue irradiated, the greater the effects.
- Function of the cells receiving the dose.
- Schedule of dose delivery—if a dose is delivered in smaller divided doses or is *fractionated versus* the entire dose given at one time, greater effects will be seen with the single acute dose.
  - Fractionation allows some repair of damage between doses.
- Type and quality of radiation.
- Age—the young and old are more susceptible to radiation injury and illness.
- Presence of other injury or illness, for example, combined injuries defined as radiation injury with trauma and/or thermal burns increase morbidity and mortality.

- Individual variations in susceptibility. No two persons are alike in their ability to withstand any kind of insult whether it be radiation, chemical toxicants, biological toxins, trauma, or thermal.

What Radiation Causes—"Stochastic Effects"

"Stochastic effects" have "no lower threshold" (NLT) at which the effects are seen. They are random or probabilistic "events" rather than "effects." For example, number of cancers generated, or cancer incidence, increases with increasing radiation dose to a population but the various types of cancer that develop do not become "worse." For purposes of emergency care, a thorough understanding of stochastic effects is not necessary but will be necessary for patient counseling after an incident.

Radiosensitivity

The "law" of Bergonie and Tribondeau (1906) states that:

- Cells that are less differentiated are generally more radiosensitive than more differentiated cells. Stem cells or precursor cells are generally more sensitive to radiation than more differentiated cells, for example, red blood cells, sperm, striated muscle cells, neurons, to name a few.
- Cells that are actively dividing are generally more radiosensitive than those that are not actively dividing, for example, hematopoietic cells in marrow are very actively dividing and are more sensitive *versus* nervous system tissues that are not rapidly dividing.

Sensitivity is also differential depending upon the point in the organism's life. The embryo and fetus are more sensitive than later development in utero. Children are more radiosensitive than adults. Some organs are more radioresistant than others, for example, the thyroid gland is more radiosensitive than the liver.

Linear Energy Transfer

Some radiations, called "high linear energy transfer" or "high LET" radiations, can cause direct ionization of DNA. Alpha and neutron radiations, are generally high LET that deliver a large amount of energy, sufficient to cause ionization along their track through cells. Other radiations called "low LET" radiations can cause indirect damage to DNA by creation of free radicals from hydrolysis of water, which then can combine with electrons from atoms in DNA. Free radical formation is a by-product of normal cellular respiration and fatty acid metabolism but it is significantly increased with ionizing radiation exposure. Some living cells have evolved mechanisms for scavenging

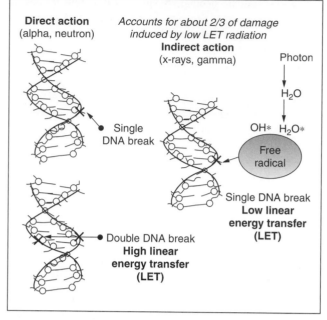

FIGURE 51-7

HIGH VERSUS LOW LINEAR ENERGY TRANSFER (LET) RADIATIONS AND PRIMARY MECHANISMS OF DNA DAMAGE BY IONIZING RADIATION

free radicals. Glutathione, and vitamins A, C, and E, among others, are free radical scavengers. (See Fig. 51-7.)

Mitotic Cell Death

Radiation can cause cellular death by two primary mechanisms: (1) mitotic death or (2) apoptosis (programmed cell death or PCD), which will be discussed below. Ionization of DNA can cause single-, double-, or multiple-strand breaks in DNA, either of which can undergo a certain amount of repair. The latter are much more resistant to repair than single-strand breaks. Accurate repair of breaks may result in no net effect on cellular division. Symmetrical exchange of DNA after a break, if repaired properly, may still result in normal or near-normal cellular function. Inaccurate repair at the break(s) may result in impaired function or cell death. (See Fig. 51-8.)

Symmetrical exchanges of equivalent strands of DNA can result in normal or perhaps subnormal functioning of the DNA. Such exchanges are simply called translocations. (See Fig. 51-9.)

Asymmetrical or Nonequivalent DNA Exchange

Double-strand breaks can result in an "asymmetrical" exchange of DNA between sister chromatids shortly after DNA duplication. This asymmetrical exchange may result

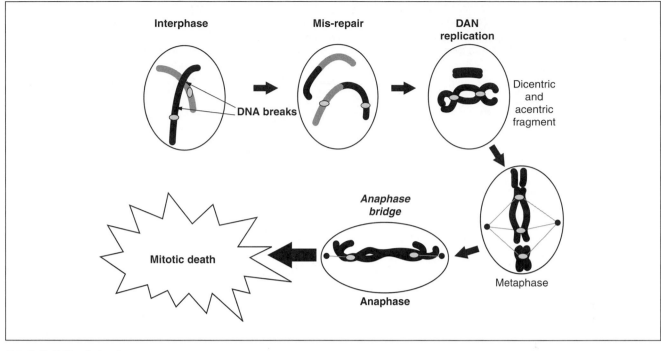

FIGURE 51-8

DICENTRIC AND ACENTRIC CHROMOSOMAL ABERRATIONS RESULTING IN MITOTIC DEATH
The chromosomes cannot divide because of the (2) centromeres.

in what is called a "dicentric" chromosome aberration. This occurs because of a DNA exchange that results in both centromeres of the two chromatids ending up on only one chromosome. The other chromosome has no centromere, that is, it is "acentric" or is an "acentric" fragment. Such asymmetric chromosomal "aberrations" will result in failure of cells to divide at anaphase. This method of cell death is called a "mitotic" death. (See Fig. 51-10.)

For purposes of this discussion, these asymmetrical chromosomal aberrations are pathognomonic of radiation injury. If certain blood cells, such as circulating peripheral lymphocytes

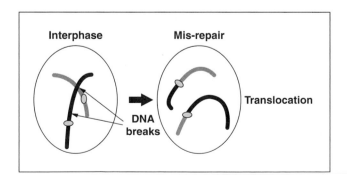

FIGURE 51-9

A TYPE OF SYMMETRICAL BUT EQUIVALENT EXCHANGE OF DNA BETWEEN CHROMOSOMES
Translocations may allow for complete or partial repair that may result in normal or near-normal cellular functioning.

are stimulated to mitosis Fig. 51-10 in cell cultures then stopped at metaphase, the numbers of dicentric and acentric forms of chromosomal aberrations can be counted. Dose-response curves can then be developed for various radiations. The "dicentric assay" can then be used as a "biodosimeter." The dicentric assay is the "gold standard" of ionizing radiation biodosimetry against which all other types of dosimetry may be compared. See the discussion of "clinical," "laboratory," and "cytogenetic" biodosimetry in Chap. 52.

Apoptosis

The second major method of cell killing by ionizing radiation is called apoptosis, sometimes called "programmed cell death (PCD)." Apoptosis is really a normal biological function required for development and maturation. Apoptosis accomplishes removal of obsolete or unneeded cells from the organism. A good example is the loss of the tail from the tadpole of a frog. The cells in the tissue of the tail have the molecular biological apparatus that "knows" that it is time to die in the maturation process. Another example is the formation of fingers and toes from an amorphous cellular mass in mammalian embryos. Ionizing radiation can cause the activation of very complex but systematic molecular biological processes. The efficiency and efficacy of this kind of cell killing is regulated by cascades of enzymatic processes that can be upregulated, downregulated, or otherwise modulated.

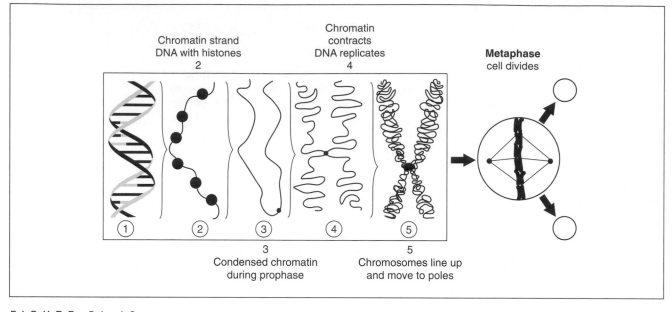

FIGURE 51-10

NORMAL MITOSIS

SUMMARY

Health-care providers need a basic, but not necessarily extensive, understanding of ionizing radiation physics, radiation protection, contamination, instrumentation, dosimetry, and radiobiology to effectively manage radiation-induced injuries and illnesses. This understanding will provide the basis for methodical, systematic, and safe medical management of the consequences of a radiological or nuclear incident. Key, however, is planning, education, and training in *advance* of an ionizing radiation incident.

Acknowledgments

From the Radiation Emergency Assistance Center/ Training Site (REAC/TS), Oak Ridge TN, Oak Ridge Institute for Science and Education (ORISE), of the US Department of Energy (DOE). This document describes activities performed under contract number DE-AC05-06OR23100 between the US Department of Energy and Oak Ridge Associated Universities (ORAU).

Suggested Reading

Gollnick DA. *Basic Radiation Protection Technology*. 4th ed. Altadena, CA: Pacific Radiation Corporation; 2000.

Hall EJ, Giaccia AJ. *Radiobiology for the Radiologist*. 6th ed. Philadelphia, PA: Lippincott; 2005.

Mettler FA, Upton AC. *Medical Effects of Ionizing Radiation*. 2nd ed. New York: Elsevier Science; 1995.

Sources and Effects of Ionizing Radiation, United Nations Scientific Committee on the Effects of Atomic Radiation (UNSCEAR) Report to the General Assembly, United Nations, New York; 2000.

52

DIAGNOSIS AND MEDICAL MANAGEMENT OF RADIATION INJURIES AND ILLNESSES

Doran M. Christensen, Steve Sugarman, A. Seaton Garrett, Otis W. Jones, and Albert L. Wiley, Jr.

STAT FACTS

DIAGNOSIS AND MEDICAL MANAGEMENT OF RADIATION INJURIES AND ILLNESSES

- Emergent medical and surgical conditions take relative priority over radiological concerns. Once those emergent conditions have been stabilized, radiological issues may be addressed.

- At survivable doses of ionizing radiation, symptoms and signs of radiological illness are usually delayed unlike many other biological, chemical, or traumatic insults.

- Incident history is as critical to management of radiation injuries and illnesses as is the medical history. Incident history is one basis for accurate ionizing radiation dose assessment that will help guide diagnosis and management.

- In the absence of a history of a radiological or nuclear (R/N) incident, the challenge for the clinician is to determine if radiation could be causal or a contributor to the clinical findings. Radiation injuries and illnesses may look like other conditions.

- The human body can be used as a "biological dosimeter" or "biodosimeter" to help guide medical management. Knowledge about the relative radiosensitivity of various cell types is the basis for understanding the onset and duration of symptoms and signs of the acute radiation syndrome (ARS).

- Health physics support and psychosocial resources need to be identified and integrated into the emergency department (ED) response to R/N incidents in advance.

- In the absence of significant medical/surgical conditions or thermal burns, the $LD_{50/60}$ for acute whole body irradiation (WBI) can be pushed from about 3.5 Gy (350 rad or cGy) to almost 7 Gy (600–700 rads or cGy) with aggressive supportive care; prophylactic antibiotics for viral, bacterial, fungal, and parasitic infections; treatment of specific infections; treatment of bleeding disorders and anemia; cytokine use; specific antidotes and toxicological management; decorporation and other management of internal contaminations; and stem cell transplants.

- Surgeries should be performed within the first 24–48 hours if at all possible. Emergency surgery will have to be performed at the time it is deemed necessary based upon standards of surgical care. Otherwise, surgery should be delayed until other systemic injury such as ARS is successfully managed.

- Decisions to amputate for traumatic injuries should be performed as needed based upon standards of surgical care. Decisions to amputate for radiation injury are very problematic; must be made with considerable deliberation; require expert health physics input and incident/dose reconstructions; require radiation medicine expert consultation; and unfortunately the decisions cannot usually be made within 24–48 hours.

- Combined injuries, defined as the presence of mechanical trauma and/or thermal burns *with radiation injury*, significantly increase morbidity and mortality.

OVERVIEW OF EARLY MANAGEMENT OF RADIOLOGICAL/NUCLEAR CASUALTIES IN THE EMERGENCY DEPARTMENT

The following is a very brief summary:

- The management of patients who are *irradiated only* and who are *not contaminated* requires no special area within the treatment facility.
- Prepare a special area for receipt, evaluation, and treatment of contaminated patients.
- Use the Radiation Patient Treatment algorithm in Fig. 52-1 to guide medical management and prioritize decontamination efforts.
- **Caveat: Manage urgent or emergent medical and surgical conditions *first*, and then deal with radiological issues.**
- "Combined injuries" are defined as radiation injuries/illnesses *plus* trauma and/or thermal burns.
  - Combined injuries significantly increase morbidity and mortality.
  - Morbidity and mortality from radiation injuries and illnesses will usually be delayed unlike some traumatic and thermal injuries.
- As soon as possible after medical and surgical conditions have been stabilized, survey face, mouth, nose, and open wounds and collect swabs from nose and mouth to survey for contamination. See Fig. 52-1 for decontamination priorities.
- **Caveat: Priorities for decontamination are open wounds, then body orifices, and then intact skin. Decontamination must be accomplished to prevent or minimize internal contamination and begin specific antidotes for some radioactive materials.**
- Essentials:
  - ED personnel should be able to perform initial surveys for radiation and radioactive contamination.
  - History of the incident—document.
  - **Caveat: The history of a radiological or nuclear incident is as essential as the medical history is to the medical diagnosis and management of patients.**
  - History of the incident—document.
  - History of mechanism of injuries—document.
  - History and times of onset and duration of symptoms—document.
  - Call for health physics support for assistance with:
    - Patient radiation surveys.
    - Incident history and reconstruction may give clues to identification of radioactive materials and dose.
    - Radiation dose estimates—accurate radiation dose estimates—will help guide medical management.
    - The process of incident history and dose estimation will usually need to be repeated, sometimes many times, to help guide medical management.
- Complete physical examination including vital signs, temperature, weight, and so on— document.
- Both radiological and health-care personnel should be identified, trained, and integrated into ED processes *prior* to an incident.
- Call for psychosocial, pastoral, and other support.
  - Psychosocial support personnel need to be identified, trained, and integrated into ED processes *prior* to an incident
  - **Caveat: The general lack of knowledge about R/N matters, and the general anxiety, even fear, about all things radiological, may well result in a magnified or exaggerated response from patients, families, coworkers, and others, including health-care providers.**
  - **Therefore, expect far larger numbers of patients with the *perception* of radiation injury or illness than those who actually may have *real* significant radiation exposures or contamination.**
- Laboratories that can identify and quantify radioactive materials on clothing, dressings, or in- body fluids (bioassays) need to be identified *prior* to an incident.
- Save and double-bag contaminated clothing and dressings as samples for further radiological analyses— keep clothing separate for return.
- Suspicious incidents will almost certainly be complicated by the necessity for police involvement and need for collection of forensic samples. Therefore, be aware in advance of the need for scrupulous attention to proper collection, containment, and identification with patient name, patient identifier, date, and time of collection and name of collector.
- Laboratories that can perform cytogenetic biodosimetry need to be identified *prior* to an incident. Special handling and packaging are required. Usually, only one lithium-heparin tube is needed.
  - Most cytogenetic laboratories that perform chromosomal analyses do so for genetic disease diagnosis and counseling rather than dose assessments.
  - Most cytogenetic laboratories are not set up to perform chromosomal analyses for radiation biodosimetry.
  - Two federally funded cytogenetic biodosimetry laboratories currently exist in the United States: the Armed Forces Radiobiology Research

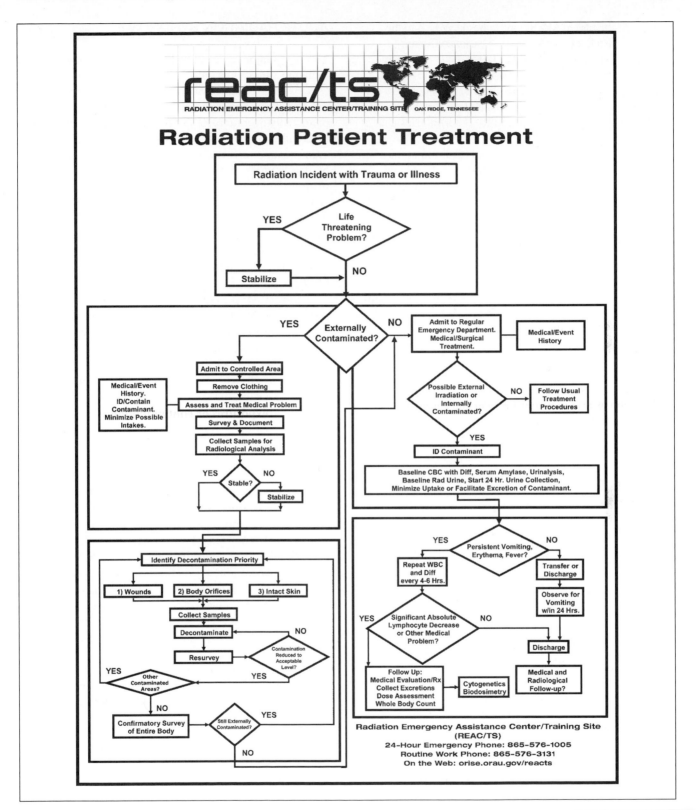

FIGURE 52-1

PRINCIPLES OF MANAGEMENT OF RADIATION INJURY, ILLNESS, AND CONTAMINATION—AN OVERVIEW OF MEDICAL MANAGEMENT

Source: From the Radiation Emergency Assistance Center/Training Site (REAC/TS), Oak Ridge Institute for Science and Education (ORISE), Oak Ridge, TN. Used by permission.

Institute (AFFRI) in Bethesda, MD, and the Radiation Emergency Assistance Center/ Training Site (REAC/TS) at the U.S. Department of Energy's Oak Ridge Institute for Science and Education (ORISE) in Oak Ridge, TN.

- Draw all laboratory specimens and perform diagnostic testing as required for other injuries and illnesses.
- Laboratory specimens and special studies that may be required for evaluation of radiological injuries and illnesses depending upon the history of the incident are the following:
  - Complete blood count (CBC) with absolute lymphocyte counts (ALC) and absolute neutrophil counts (ANC) every 6 hours for the first 24 hours than every 12 hours for 2 days, then daily thereafter.
  - Check initial urine specimen for radioactivity with a Geiger counter. This is identified as "rad urine" on the Radiation Patient Treatment decision support algorithm in Fig. 52-1.
    - Some high-energy photons like those from cesium-137 might be detected in urine depending upon how soon after an event the initial spot urine is checked.
    - Alpha and beta radiations cannot be detected in urine.
    - Negative initial spot urine radiation surveys are meaningless—only positives that indicate internal contamination are significant.
  - Begin 24-hour urine and fecal collections for "radiobioassays." Such laboratories need to be identified *prior* to an incident.
  - Serum amylase initially, then at 24 hours
    - Significant irradiation of the salivary glands can result in high amylase levels.
    - Interpret high amylase levels with caution with face, head, neck, chest, or abdominal trauma.
  - Type blood
    - Cross match only if needed for other medical or surgical conditions.
  - Draw blood for HLA tissue typing.
  - Draw one lithium-heparin tube for cytogenetic biodosimetry.
  - Cultures of wounds, blood, or other body fluids as indicated.
    - **Caveat: Severely neutropenic patients, particularly those who are also anemic, may not mount normal inflammatory responses, for example, urinary tract infection without pyuria, pneumonia without chest x-ray infiltrate, or skin infection without typical cellulitis.**
  - Baseline chest x-ray and other special studies as needed.

ACUTE RADIATION SYNDROME

The first major topic related to medical management of radiation illnesses is called the acute radiation syndrome (ARS). ARS is a spectrum of radiation-induced illnesses, the symptoms and signs of which will appear somewhat predictably over time. At survivable doses, however, symptoms and signs may not appear for days or weeks, sometimes even months. ARS and its subsyndromes are characterized by development of groups of symptoms and signs that are manifestations of acute irradiation of the whole body or significant portions of it. The reactions of various tissues depend upon a number of factors including, but not necessarily limited to, dose, dose rate, volume of tissue irradiated, schedule of dose delivery, type and quality of radiation, age, other medical conditions, individual variations, among others.

Caveat: At survivable doses of acute whole body irradiation (WBI), the appearance of symptoms and signs are always delayed for hours to days, weeks, or even months. The time to onset of symptoms and signs becomes shorter as the radiation dose increases. The duration of clinical signs and laboratory findings also becomes shorter, that is, the injury or illness progresses more quickly as the dose increases.

Radiosenstivity and "Biodosimetry"

Methods of cell killing were discussed in Chap. 51. To continue, living cells are differentially sensitive to radiation, that is, are more or less "radiosensitive" or "radioresistant" based upon their embryonic origin along with other factors. Knowledge of such sensitivity is the basis for understanding the constellation of symptoms and signs that will appear as the dose of acute WBI increases.

The onset and duration of symptoms of the ARS and the hematopoietic, cutaneous, gastrointestinal, and cardiovascular/central nervous system (neurovascular) subsyndromes relate directly to the relative radiosensitivity or the obverse, the radioresistance, of various cells in the particular body system. The relative sensitivity of cells is related to a number of factors, including cell cycle, cell life span, differentiation, presence of a nucleus, mitotic activity, level of metabolism, and other factors.

There is a hierarchy of cellular sensitivity with circulating peripheral lymphocytes being among the most radiosensitive. This is an exception to the rule of Bergonie and Tribondeau discussed in Chap. 51. Lymphocytes are quite differentiated and they do not undergo mitosis but they can be killed by radiation in interphase. Many other cells are more sensitive at mitosis. Because of the sensitivity of lymphocytes to radiation injury, loss of these cells can occur relatively quickly, that is, within hours to days. This feature allows clinicians to use lymphocyte depletion kinetics as a biodosimeter.

Stem cells or precursor cells to sperm and blood cells (spermatogonia and myeloblasts) are fairly radiosensitive. Damage to these cells will not become manifest for some days to weeks after radiation injury. Tissues that make up body barriers such as skin, mucosal linings of the gastrointestinal system and respiratory tract, and small blood vessels are less radiosensitive. Significant damage to these cells appears much later, on the order of weeks to months, and at higher doses.

Osteocytes, spermatocytes, mature sperm, mature white blood cells, mature red blood cells (RBCs), fibrocytes, chondrocytes, muscle cells, and nerve cells are progressively more radioresistant. The appearance of damage to these cells occurs over weeks, months, or years, and at even higher doses.

The time of onset and duration of certain symptoms and signs can help determine the dose. Their time of onset and duration is roughly predictable at certain doses. The human body can thus be used as a "biological dosimeter" or "biodosimeter."

If certain details about an incident are known, some measure of prognostication can be done, although these prognostications are tenuous and may have to be revised many times over the clinical course. The incident history or manner in which the patient was irradiated, the source and source "term" (the radionuclide and its "activity"), and the position of the patient with respect to the source will help guide medical management. If the dose of ionizing radiation is not known, the human body will give clues to the dose. Three levels of biodosimetry can be used: clinical, laboratory, and cytogenetic biodosimetry (CB), discussed below. (See Table 52-1.)

Caveat: If it is known that an ionizing radiation incident has occurred, practitioners can be expectant of certain systemic illnesses related to radiation exposure. Patients presenting to hospital without a known history of a radiation incident could potentially be very confusing to unwary practitioners. Depending upon the nature

and timing of exposure(s), patients may present with mixed symptoms and signs of several of the subsyndromes. Radiation illness might therefore be kept in any number of differential diagnoses.

Phases of the Acute Radiation Syndrome

The ARS and its various subsyndromes may roughly be divided into four phases: the prodrome, latent phase, the period of manifest illness, and lastly, the period of recovery or death. The time to onset of each phase and the duration of symptoms and signs is determined by a large number of factors discussed above and in Chap. 51.

- **Prodromal phase.** In the prodrome, any signs and symptoms are generally "primitive" in nature such anorexia, nausea, vomiting, fatigue, and perhaps low-grade fever.
- **Latent phase.** No clinical signs are apparent at all. Significant doses will result in a more or less slow progression of cellular damage that will not be evident until the manifest illness phase.
- **Manifest illness phase.** Symptoms and signs of damage to specific cells and tissues will begin to appear based upon their radiosensitivity.
- **Period of recovery or death.** If the dose absorbed is not too high, recovery can be complete or can be incomplete with persistent or long-term sequelae.

Caveat: The greatest challenge to the clinician is to make a diagnosis of acute or chronic radiation-induced injury or illness in the absence of such a history. This difficulty arises because the various constellations of symptoms and signs of radiation injury and illness look much like more common injuries and illnesses.

What Radiation Does Not Cause

Understanding what ionizing radiation *does not* cause is as important as understanding what it does cause.

Caveat: At *survivable* doses, ionizing radiation does not cause *sudden* death, incapacitation, or burns. Fairly sudden loss of consciousness, seizures, hypotension, and other signs can occur with acute ionizing radiation exposure, but would indicate a lethal dose if the exposure is acute. Ordinarily, these severe symptoms and signs will have some other etiology. Even with lethal doses of ionizing radiation, death will not occur for many hours to days, sometimes even months.

Some very early "primitive" symptoms such as anorexia, nausea, vomiting, and low-grade fever may appear with significant *survivable* doses of ionizing radiation. But, at survivable doses, these are usually *transient*. They are merely a prelude or a prodrome to what is to follow.

TABLE 52-1

ACUTE RADIATION SUBSYNDROMES AND APPROXIMATE THRESHOLDS

Subclinical	<.75–1 gray (75–100 rad or cGy*)
Hematopoietic	>1–2 gray (>100–200 rad or cGy)
Cutaneous	>3 gray (>300 rad or cGy)
Gastrointestinal	> 6 gray (600 rad or cGy
Respiratory	> 6 gray (600 rad or cGy)
Cerebrovascular/Central Nervous System (CV/CNS) = Neurovascular	>30 gray (3000 rad or cGy)

*1 gray = 100 rad = 100 centigray (cGy)

Radiation Lethal Dose-50/60 (LD$_{50/60}$)

In humans, the LD$_{50/60}$ is approximately 3.5 gray (350 rads or cGy) for acute WBI without treatment. Fifty percent of a population uniformly exposed to such a dose of ionizing radiation will die within 60 days if not aggressively treated. The goal is to push the LD$_{50/60}$ to a higher dose.

Caveat: Aggressive supportive care; antibiotics; treatment of bleeding disorders and anemia; cytokines; specific antidotes; standard toxicological treatments; and stem cell transplants must begin early or at least: decorporation and other treatments for internal contamination; considered early in the clinical course in order to minimize morbidity and mortality. In the absence of significant medical/surgical conditions or thermal burns, the LD$_{50/60}$ for acute WBI can be pushed from ~3.5 gray (350 rad or cGy) to somewhere between 6 and 7 gray (600–700 rads or cGy). Some partial body exposures are somewhat more difficult to assess, diagnose, and predict prognosis.

Combined Injury

Combined injury is defined as radiation injury or illness plus trauma or thermal burns. Combined injuries significantly increase morbidity and mortality, that is, they significantly lower radiation LD$_{50/60}$.

Biodosimetry

A discussion of biodosimetry related to acute WBI will set the stage for a more detailed discussion of diagnosis and management of patients exposed to significant doses. (See Table 52-2.)

TABLE 52-2

SOME LOW DOSE DETERMINISTIC EFFECTS

Dose	Effect
0.1 Gy (10 rads or cGy)	No detectable difference in exposed *vs* nonexposed patients
>0.12 Gy (12 rads or cGy)	Sperm count decreases to minimum but is delayed to about day 45. Of no value for dosimetry.
0.2 Gy (20 rads or cGy)	Detectable increase in dicentric/acentric forms of chromosomal aberrations. See Chap. 51 and below. No clinical signs or symptoms.
~0.75–1.0 Gy (75–100 rads or cGy)	Detectable bone marrow depression. Persistent and unremitting nausea and vomiting in a small percentage of an exposed population. See Table 52-5.

Laboratory Biodosimetry

Lymphocyte Depletion Kinetics The decrease in the ALC will be one of the first signs of significant ionizing radiation exposure. Lymphocyte depletion kinetics can be used as a laboratory biodosimeter to further refine an initial dose estimate from an incident history (see Table 52-3).

Kinetics of other blood cell lines such as polymorphonuclear neutrophils (PMN), erythrocytes (RBC), and platelets can also be used as biodosimeters. They are not as helpful as lymphocyte depletion kinetics because their changes appear too late. In fact, changes in their numbers might be predicted with some variable accuracy as the dose is refined with lymphocyte depletion kinetics. It can be a helpful prognostic tool to guide medical management (See Table 52-4).

Caveat: Trauma and burns can cause confusing changes of lymphocyte and leukocyte numbers. Interpret blood cell kinetics cautiously with combined injuries.

Cytogenetic Biodosimetry

Analyses of chromosomal aberrations, especially the "dicentric assay," can also be used as a laboratory biodosimeter. Dicentric forms of chromosomal aberrations with their acentric fragments result from asymmetrical exchanges of DNA at mitosis and improper cellular repair of the damage. Counts of dicentric and acentric forms of lymphocyte chromosomal aberrations can be used for dose estimation.

Cytogenetic biodosimetry (CB) is the "gold standard" of radiation biodosimetry and is the standard to which all other forms of dosimetry can be compared. The process is time-consuming and requires at least 72 hours before results are available. It is also relatively expensive. CB can be indispensable for guiding medical management. It is also very helpful when counseling patients about effects of radiation injury.

Most cytogenetic laboratories in the United States exist for diagnosis of genetic diseases and genetic counseling rather than biodosimetry. Two U.S. government facilities can perform cytogenetic analyses for biodosimetric purposes: Armed Forces Radiobiology Research Institute (AFRRI) in Bethesda, MD, and the Radiation Emergency Assistance Center/Training Site (REAC/TS) in Oak Ridge, TN (routine phone: 865-576-3131 and emergency phone:865-576-1005). There are a number of laboratories available outside of the United States.

All living creatures are constantly bathed in a sea of radiations from outer space, soil, water, and food, therefore most humans will have 1–2 dicentric chromosomes per thousand lymphocytes. Dose-response curves can be developed for the various radiations allowing the dicentric assay to be used as a biodosimeter.

Clinical Biodosimetry

Some clinical symptoms and signs can also be used for dosimetry. Early symptoms and signs from significant

TABLE 52-3

LYMPHOCYTE DEPLETION KINETICS FOR ACUTE WHOLE BODY IRRADIATIONS (PHOTON EQUIVALENTS)

Dose (Gy)	Absolute Lymphocyte Count (ALC) ($\times 10^9$/liter) by Day					
	.5	1	2	4	6	8
0	2.45	2.45	2.45	2.45	2.45	2.45
1	2.30	2.16	1.90	1.48	1.15	0,89
2	2.16	1.90	1.48	0.89	0.54	0.33
3	2.03	1.68	1.15	0.54	0.25	0.12
4	1.90	1.48	0.89	0.33	0.12	.044
5	1.79	1.31	0.69	0.20	0.06	.020
6	1.69	1.15	0.54	0.12	0.03	.006
7	1.58	1.01	0.42	.072	.012	.002
8	1.48	0.89	0.33	.044	.006	<.001
9	1.39	0.79	0.25	.030	.003	<.001
10	1.31	0.70	0.20	.020	.001	<.001

Source: From the Radiation Emergency Assistance Center/Training Site (REAC/TS), Oak Ridge Institute for Science and Education (ORISE), Oak Ridge, TN. Used by permission.

ionizing radiation exposure include anorexia, nausea, vomiting, and low-grade fever. These "primitive" signs and symptoms are related to a primary inflammatory response.

Time-to-Emesis Data from the Radiation Emergency Assistance Center/Training Site (REAC/TS) Accident Registry in Oak Ridge, TN, has been used to determine how the time to vomiting or time-to-emesis can be statistically analyzed to help estimate dose. Vomiting can be a reliable sign of significant radiation exposure but must be interpreted cautiously and in the context of other biodosimetry because of the many etiologies of vomiting. Following acute WBI, as the time to appearance of nausea and vomiting increases, the possible acute WBI dose decreases—the shorter the period of time before their appearance, the higher the dose. The vomiting from acute radiation exposure is usually persistent and unremitting. Be aware that some people will vomit in response to other noxious stimuli, including the sights, sounds, and smells of other people vomiting, so-called "psychogenic" vomiting.

Persistent and unremitting vomiting within 1 hour of acute WBI may be the clue to a dose on the order of >6 Gy (600 rad or cGy) a poor prognosis, *if other causes are ruled out*. Vomiting that begins 4 hours or more after an acute WBI may mean that the dose is survivable and treatable (see Table 52-5).

Other Clinical Biodosimetry

There are a large number of signs of cellular, tissue, and organ damage that will help determine dose.

Caveat: Reliance should not be placed upon any one dosimetric parameter alone. All sources used for dose estimation should be evaluated in the context of the others. No one biodosimeter will be accurate 100% of the time.

Manifestations of the Acute Radiation Syndrome

Subclinical

Below 50–100 rads, CBC may help to determine effects upon the hematopoietic system. The dicentric assay from chromosomal aberration analyses may be required to determine doses below 100 rads (1 gray or Gy). There are generally no signs or symptoms until a dose of about 1 gray (100 rad or cGy) is reached. A small percentage or about

TABLE 52-4

CHROMOSOMAL ABERRATION ANALYSIS OF DICENTRIC/ ACENTRIC FORMS PATHOGNOMIC FOR ACUTE WBI (PHOTON EQUIVALENTS)

Dose (Gy)	Per 50 Cells	Per 1000 Cells
0	0.05–0.1	1–2
1	4	88
2	12	234
3	22	439
4	35	703
5	51	1024

Source: From the Radiation Emergency Assistance Center/Training Site (REAC/TS), Oak Ridge Institute for Science and Education (ORISE), Oak Ridge, TN. Used by permission.

TABLE 52-5

POPULATION TIME-TO-EMESIS BASED UPON ACUTE WHOLE BODY IRRADIATIONS (PHOTON EQUIVALENTS)

Dose (Gy)	%	Time (h)
0	—	—
1	19	
2	35	4.63
3	54	2.62
4	72	1.74
5	86	1.27
6	94	0.99
7	98	0.79
8	99	0.66
9	100	0.56
10	100	0.48

Source: From the Radiation Emergency Assistance Center/Training Site (REAC/TS), Oak Ridge Institute for Science and Education (ORISE), Oak Ridge, TN. Used by permission.

10% of the population will begin to vomit at around 1 Gy acute WBI. See Table 52-5 to use time-to-emesis as a biodosimeter.

Hematopoietic Syndrome

Acute WBI with doses from 1 to 2 gray (100–200 rad or cGy) cause progressive decrements in cells in marrow and peripheral blood as the dose increases. As a result, stem cells may be depleted. Leukopenia and sometimes pancytopenia may be seen. Infectious complications can be expected with hemorrhage, anemia, and impaired wound healing.

CBC should be drawn STAT and then every 4–8 hours in the first 24 hours following an incident then every 12–24 hours thereafter. Decreased ALC may occur within hours to days after a significant exposure. As the dose increases, the ALC will decrease sooner and drop to its nadir more quickly. See Table 52-3 for use of the ALC as a biodosimeter.

At roughly 1 Gy, absolute neutrophil counts will increase at about the same time as the ALC drops. At about 2–3 Gy, the neutrophils will drop just as the lymphocytes but will lag the nadir of the lymphocytes. There may be an "abortive rise" in the neutrophils some days later, then another drop occurs. As the dose increases above 2–3 Gy, the neutrophil nadir, just like the lymphocyte nadir, will occur earlier and will drop lower. As the dose increases, marrow becomes progressively more cytopenic.

Caveat: Beware of using the lymphocyte count and neutrophil count as biodosimetric tools in the face of mechanical trauma or thermal burns. Trauma or burns can cause changes in blood cell counts that will confound interpretation of blood cell kinetics.

Decrements in RBC and platelet counts occur much later than the decrements of lymphocytes and other leukocytes. Bleeding and anemia may be significant at higher survivable doses but do not occur for several weeks after irradiation.

Caveat: The following detailed descriptions of the various subsyndromes are not absolutely essential for emergency physicians to know. However, the information is presented to heighten awareness of short-term, intermediate-, and long-term manifestations and management of radiation illnesses. Everyone will know if a nuclear detonation occurs. Radiological incidents, however, may not be apparent and patients may present days or weeks following exposure with symptoms related to these various subsyndromes.

Treatment of the hematopoietic syndrome Management of the hematopoietic syndrome will require the assistance of hematologists, medical oncologists, radiation oncologists, and/or infectious disease specialists who have experience managing cytopenic patients.

Blood Products

Trauma or thermal burns may require the early use of blood products. If the emergency situation permits, these blood products should be leuko-reduced and irradiated to 25 Gray to prevent transfusion associated graft versus host disease. Do not withhold life-saving blood products. Packed RBCs and platelets for hematopoietic damage will not be required for several weeks at survivable acute WBI doses.

Immunosuppression and Infection Control

Loss of peripheral circulating lymphocytes and leukocytes as well as decrements in marrow stem cells result in an immunologically compromised patient who will be susceptible to an array of infectious events. This phase of the hematopoietic syndrome is almost identical to the clinical course of human immunodeficiency virus (HIV) infection. Infection control is a fairly complicated matter. Hematology/ oncology and infectious disease expertise will be needed.

Those patients with doses of >2 Gy (200 rad or cGy) acute WBI should be placed in reverse isolation in a general hospital. Patients with doses of 5–6 Gy (500–600 rad or cGy) and those with combined injuries will probably require treatment at a specialty hospital or medical center. Antibiotic prophylaxis and specific antidotes will be required. Antibiotic use should be directed toward specific foci of infection in non-neutropenic patients.

Control of infections in the neutropenic phase of the hematopoietic syndrome is critical, is the most difficult to manage, and is the major limiting factor for successful outcome in otherwise salvageable patients. Neutropenic patients with an ANC of $<0.500 \times 10^9$ cells/L should be given a broad-spectrum fluoroquinolone or a fluoroquinolone with coverage for *Streptococci.*

A febrile event in the neutropenic patient who has been given prophylaxis but without other focal evidence of infection should be interpreted as the beginning of gram-negative sepsis that can be rapidly fatal. Fluoroquinolones should be stopped and treatment of sepsis should begin. This treatment needs to include coverage for *Pseudomonas auruginosa*, in particular, as well as for organisms known to be opportunists in the particular hospital.

Gut decontamination has previously been recommended but is no longer thought to be beneficial except for patients with abdominal wounds or infection such as *Clostridium difficile* enterocolitis. Neutropenia and immunocompromise will allow mucosal overgrowth of *Candida* species, which may be partially controlled with fluconazole, 400 mg daily. Some *Candida* species, molds, and *Aspergillus* are resistant to fluconazole. The presence of these organisms requires special considerations beyond the scope of this work.

Disruption of cutaneous and mucosal barriers also help create a favorable environment for opportunistic infections. There are many special considerations for managing infectious complications of the ARS that will specialty consultation. Radiation-induced cellular damage creates an ideal medium for reactivation and growth of quiescent infectious agents such as *Herpes simplex* (HSV) and *Cytomegalo* viruses (CMV). Shortly after the nadir of lymphopenia, *Herpes simplex* virus (HSV) reactivation may occur in those patients who have previously been infected. Prophylaxis with acyclovir or one of its congeners will be required. Serologies for HSV are recommended, however, in the presence of mucositis, empirical treatment may be started. Stomatitis from these infections can look like radiation-related stomatitis. Similarly, the presence of *Pneumocystis carinii* pneumonia requires special considerations.

Cytokines

Growth factors or colony stimulating factors (CSF) are critical to management of the hematopoietic syndrome. Granulocyte CSF or granulocyte-macrophage CSF (G-CSF and GM-CSF respectively) and the pegylated form of G-CSF are three cytokines used to treat cytopenias in oncology patients. The rationale for their use in the medical management of patients from radiation incidents is based upon that experience.

Cytokines cause proliferation and differentiation of stem cells that lead to increased numbers of circulating blood cells. For optimal efficacy, they need to be administered early, preferably as soon as it is determined that there may have been an acute WBI of >1.5–2 Gy (150–200 rad or cGy).

Stem Cell Transplants

Pancytopenia and depletion of stem cells from higher radiation doses may eventually require stem cell transplants.

There are a number of methods for stem cell transplantation, however, this is not a matter for concern in the ED early in the clinical course. Blood for tissue typing should be drawn in the ED if possible, however. Later consultation with a specialist in hematology/oncology may be required to evaluate the necessity of using the valuable resource.

Gastrointestinal Syndrome

GI injury will become manifest at doses approaching 6–8 Gray acute WBI (600–800 rad or cGy). As with other cellular damage from ionizing radiation, symptoms and signs of acute injury heralding the onset of the GI manifestations can be delayed up to 2 weeks at survivable doses of WBI. Severe anorexia, nausea, and vomiting may begin within an hour of acute whole body irradiation at this level. Diarrhea that begins in less than a week can indicate a dose greater than 6 gray and a potentially lethal dose.

Damage to cells of the intestinal villi or intestinal crypt cells results in progressive thinning then sloughing of the intestinal mucosa. Diarrhea can be severe and becomes bloody as sloughing progresses. Complications may develop because of thrombocytopenia, fluid shifts, fluid loss, electrolyte imbalance, and malabsorption. Loss of the mucosal barrier allows passage of pathogens, therefore opportunistic infections are to be expected. These complications must be treated aggressively. Sepsis is common. Infectious disease consultation will be required. Other complications may include ileus, distention, renal failure, eventual cardiovascular failure, and/or death.

All of the management tools used for the hematopoietic syndrome will be required for the GI syndrome because the hematopoietic syndrome will also be present. Standard medications for diarrhea may be used. Standard antiemetics may be tried to help control vomiting, but occasionally serotonin (5HT3) antagonists such as granisetron or ondansetron might be required. Intravenous fluids and electrolyte management will be required.

Caveat: Instrumentation of the GI tract such as endoscopy is relatively contraindicated because of the potential for perforation.

Multiple organ failure, respiratory complications and vascular complications At about 6 Gy (600 rad or cGy) and higher acute WBI, multiple organ damage may become manifest. Of particular importance are damage to the lungs and the microvasculature. At these doses, acute respiratory distress syndrome (ARDS) may occur. ARDS from radiation exposure looks like ARDS from any cause, is treated in the same way, and unfortunately, has the same or greater mortality rate. Damage to the endothelium of smaller blood vessels is a basis for multiple organ damage and multiple organ failure (MOF). Multiple organ damage begins to appear at >6 gray and above from occlusion of these small vessels. Without adequate blood supply, to the tissues these vessels support will die.

Neurovascular Syndrome

Cerebrovascular (CV) and central nervous system (CNS) manifestations of the ARS, sometimes called the neurovascular syndrome (NVS), occur at much higher doses of acute WBI. This is the only subsyndrome of ARS that may have very early symptoms and signs of CNS disturbances, sometimes within minutes. At very high doses, confusion and disorientation may appear early. There may be cerebral edema, convulsions, and eventually coma. High fever may be present unlike the low-grade fever with much lower doses of ionizing radiation. At extremely high doses, death may occur within 1–2 days.

The basis for the NVS is probably related to a CNS inflammatory response, CNS cellular damage, vascular injury, and derangements of the neurotransmitter functions. Such neurotransmitter abnormalities relate to alterations in dopamine, serotonin, acetylcholine, and others.

There may be relatively early signs of prostration within minutes to hours of exposure in the prodromal period of the NVS. These symptoms and signs include anorexia, nausea, vomiting, and diarrhea. These manifestations are gastrointestinal and may occur because of damage to the GI system but may also occur because of CNS injury. At lower doses, these symptoms may be transient only to recur later in the course of the illness. As the dose increases, further evidence of CNS irritation, edema, and inflammation appear within hours to days with high fever, hypotension, and headache. Fever is usually much higher than at lower doses.

At 10 Gray and above, extreme nausea and vomiting actually begin to decrease with generalized CNS depression and incapacitation. Within hours to weeks, neurological signs of ataxia, dizziness, and fainting may occur. Effects on cognition may also appear relatively early at very high doses.

Treatment of internal contamination   This is a topic of major concern and is quite complex. Treatment of internal contamination essentially presents toxicological challenges. Cells process radioactive materials exactly as they do their nonradioactive relatives. For example, radioactive cesium is internalized, transported, metabolized, and excreted exactly like nonradioactive cesium. The pathology from internalization of Cesium-137 is related to its radiological toxicity. Nonradioactive cesium is relatively innocuous.

Routes of entry to the body may be by inhalation, ingestion, percutaneous absorption, or injection. By whatever route, a number of factors determine the fate of internalized radioactive materials. More soluble materials tend to be excreted via the renal system. More insoluble materials tend to be excreted via the GI system. These factors also help determine the urgency of treatment with specific antidotes, of which there are only a few. Standard toxicological principles and therapies apply. Poison control centers (PCC) may be very helpful because generally they employ

a number of nonphysician specialists in poison information (SPIs) and emergency physicians, many of whom are also medical toxicologists.

The intake, uptake, and incorporation of radioactive materials is relatively fast for some radionuclides such as radioiodines and radiocesium. Therefore, treatment should begin very quickly, that is, within hours.

Therapies are generally categorized into:

* Saturation and blocking, for example, the use of stable potassium iodide to prevent thyroid uptake and incorporation;
* Ion binding, for example, the use of Prussian blue (ferric ferrocyanate) for radiocesium and radio- and nonradioactive thallium;
* Displacement, for example, the use of calcium to compete with radiostrontium;
* Chelation, for example, the use of diethylenetriaminepentaacetate (DTPA or pentetate) for transuranics (primarily americium, curium, and plutonium);
* Isotopic dilution, for example, the use of high intakes of water for tritium that has H^3 or radioactive hydrogen as part of the water molecule.

The authoritative manual for treatment of internal contamination is the National Council on Radiation Protection and Measurements (NCRP) Report #65 (1979), *Treatment of Persons Accidentally Internally Contaminated with Radioactive Materials.* Incidentally, this reference is being updated and should be published sometime in 2007 and will be available from the NCRP, Bethesda, MD.

Cutaneous and local injury   Injury to the skin may be isolated without damage to deeper structures and there may be widespread injury to only the skin, usually called the "cutaneous syndrome." More circumscribed areas of injury with damage to deeper structures other than skin are sometimes called "acute local injuries." There is no standard for use of the term "acute local injury" so clarification will be needed when it is used.

THE SKIN

The skin or integument, as a major body organ, serves a number of functions critical to the integrity of the body as a whole. As a very large organ covering approximately 2 m², it serves:

* Against intrusions from the environment as one of three major bodily barriers. The other two are the linings to the gastrointestinal and respiratory systems;
* As a major component of the body's temperature regulation process along with the hypothalamus and vascular system;

- To provide sensory input to the nervous system related to temperature, touch, pain;
- An immune function.

The two major layers of the skin are the dermis and epidermis. The epidermis is relatively thin, on the order of 20–300 μm (or 0.02–0.3 mm), and is on average about 100 μm thick, depending upon the part of the body it covers. The epidermal cell type is stratified squamous epithelium. New epidermal cells are generated from the basal or germinal cell layer that rests upon a basement membrane. Basal stem cells gradually migrate to the surface. As they migrate outward, they become keratinized, to eventually die and slough off. The life span of the epithelium is about 14 days.

The dermis is separated from the overlying epidermis by a basement membrane. The dermis is much thicker than the epidermis, on average 1.25 mm thick. The dermal vascular plexus at the base of the dermis provides nourishment to the skin and to a great measure helps regulate body temperature. Hair follicles from the epidermis invaginate the dermis, and because of this are partly responsible for the skin's ability to regenerate following radiation injury. The dermis also contains various other structures related to other skin functions including sebaceous glands, sweat glands, melanocytes, fibrocytes, and other types of cells.

Penetration and Attenuation of Ionizing Radiation in Soft Tissue

The depth of penetration of ionizing radiations is determined by their energy. Alpha particles cannot penetrate the outer layers of epidermis. Alpha-emitters are an internal hazard only. They must be inhaled, ingested, or absorbed percutaneously to cause harm. Betas and some very low energy photons, can barely penetrate the thin epidermis into the dermis. They may be attenuated or absorbed at more shallow depths, unlike photon radiations, which may penetrate much deeper. Some photon radiations (x and gamma rays) may sometimes cause little cutaneous damage.

This feature of ionizing radiation contributes to the importance of incident reconstruction and dose estimates that are used to guide medical management. Despite their notorious inaccuracy, incident reconstructions can help clinicians plan for future medical management. In many cases, these dose estimations will have to be repeated many times as the clinical course progresses. Continual adjustments of dose estimates are the rule rather than the exception.

Radiosensitivity of the Skin

Signs of skin damage progress rather predictably depending upon dose and the physics of the radiation source. At lower acute doses, starting at about 3 Gy (300 rad or cGy), loss of hair or epilation may occur. Permanent loss of hair may occur at 7 Gy (700 rad or cGy). Erythema or redness of the skin may appear at about 6 Gy (600 rad or cGy). An early erythema can occur within hours to a day or two,

TABLE 52-6

APPROXIMATE RADIATION DOSE THRESHOLDS FOR SKIN INJURY

Sign	Threshold Dose
Epilation	3 Gy (300 rad or cGy)
Erythema	6 Gy (600 rad or cGy)
Dry desquamation	10–15 Gy (1000–1500 rad or cGy)
Wet desquamation	>20 Gy (>2000 rad or cGy)
Bullae formation	>25 Gy (2500 rad or cGy)
Ulceration/necrosis	>50 Gy (3000–5000 rad or cGy)

These thresholds as with others described in this chapter are only approximate and are dependent upon the physics of the radiation source and the delivery scenario.

depending upon the radiation dose. This early erythema is transient and is related to release of vasoactive amines in a primary inflammatory response. It will disappear only to reappear later in 2–3 weeks. An early erythema that persists is a sign of a larger acute dose to the skin. (See Table 52-6.)

Cutaneous Syndrome

Injury to the skin has a clinical course with prodrome, latent period, period of manifest illness then recovery just as the other subsyndromes of the ARS. There may be a prodrome with early erythema that may include dysesthesias, vague uncomfortable sensations of pinching or heat. A latent period may follow during which there appears to be nothing happening. A manifest period of injury may ensue with progression of skin damage.

Acute Local Injuries

Acute local injuries or injuries to much smaller circumscribed areas of skin may result in skin symptoms and signs only. Or, damage may be deeper including damage to dermal structures, vascular infrastructure, and subcutaneous structures. Even if an event reconstruction and dose estimate is done, the human body will eventually tell the clinician the extent of injury and the dose.

These are special cases that require special attention and may be quite complicated. Consultation with hand surgeons, plastic surgeons, burn surgeons, and others should be sought as early as possible. Surgeons familiar with radiation injuries are preferable and more likely to be found at cancer treatment centers.

Caveat: The ARS may accompany the cutaneous syndrome and acute local injury.

Although these conditions are discussed separately from the ARS, the ARS may be present depending upon factors already discussed. Dose estimates for skin injuries can be quite complex and will almost certainly require HP support. Dose reconstruction may have to be repeated multiple times as the clinical course progresses to help determine appropriate therapies. Expert health physics support must be identified prior to an R/N incident and should be engaged early following an incident.

Later Signs of Skin Injury

Other later signs of true radiation damage to the skin are sloughing, at first dry, then later wet desquamation, with progressive deeper loss of skin cells. Formation of blisters or bullae occurs at even higher doses. Damage to the supporting dermis and the microvasculature in the dermal vascular plexus is largely responsible for the more severe signs of skin damage including ulceration and necrosis. Desquamation, bullae formation, ulceration, and necrosis are usually delayed on the order of weeks. The earlier appearance of desquamation, bullae, and ulceration are grave signs that the skin dose is very high.

The delay in appearance of ionizing radiation injury accounts for the relatively greater difficulty in making a diagnosis and managing skin injuries as opposed to the diagnostic advantage afforded the ARS using lymphocyte depletion kinetics and time to emesis dosimetry. An incident reconstruction and dose estimate takes on even greater importance for cutaneous injury but is also more difficult than with the ARS.

Management of the Cutaneous Syndrome and Acute Local Radiation Injury

Initial incident reconstructions and dose estimates can be inaccurate following radiation exposure to the skin or contact with radioactive materials. The effective dose to skin and deeper structures can usually only be appreciated as wounds progress. The human body will tell clinicians what the effective dose to skin and deeper structures really is, that is, the human body becomes a "biological dosimeter" or "biodosimeter."

Historically, many cases of significant skin injury have been unsuspected even by patients who knew they were working with radiological equipment or radioactive sources. In some of the more recent cases, patients who are unwittingly exposed to radioactive sources may believe they have an infection, allergy, insect bite, or thermal burn. Likewise, clinicians may be fooled by the history, as well as the symptoms and signs of acute radiation injury that can look like much more common and familiar conditions. In some cases, radiation injury should be included in the differential diagnosis even in the absence of a history of a possible radiation exposure.

Caveat: If there are *immediate* signs of skin damage from a radiological or nuclear event, that is, within minutes to hours, they will probably be as the result of mechanical/physical trauma or thermal burns rather than radiation injury, unless the dose is extremely large.

The pathology of mechanical trauma or thermal burns is usually apparent early in the course of the insult, that is, instantaneously or within hours. This is not necessarily the case with radiation injuries except when the dose is extremely large. With smaller doses, some symptoms and signs such as numbness, tingling, and erythema may appear early, that is within hours, but they are transient, only to appear later. Early signs of skin injury that persist, as with early symptoms and signs of acute whole body radiation, are signs of serious injury. If the nature of the incident and type of radiation are known, it may be possible to determine a dose range but such estimations are notoriously inaccurate. The early appearance, within hours to days, and persistence of erythema, hair loss, desquamation, and blister formation, indicate a serious injury and significant radiation dose with poor prognosis. As with the ARS, early onset and shortened duration of the prodromal and latent periods portend serious injury.

Depth of radiation injury to skin and underlying structures will usually become apparent over weeks. Radiation damage to epidermis, dermis, microvasculature, and underlying structures can contribute to bleeding, infections, and failure of wounds to heal. Associated physical trauma and thermal burns must be treated in a manner consistent with standards of care for medical and surgical management. Combined injuries, that is, radiation injury associated with physical trauma and/or thermal burns, increase morbidity and mortality. Initially, the medical management for the cutaneous syndrome with widespread skin injury, or acute local injury to a more circumscribed area of the body, should be conservative. Pentoxifylline plus vitamin E analogue, in the form of α-tocopherol succinate, have demonstrated efficacy in treatment of radiation therapy patients with cutaneous injury. Topical or systemic corticosteroids have also been used for the cutaneous syndrome and acute local injuries.

Determination of Extent of Injury—Special Studies

Acute local injuries, that is, smaller and more circumscribed areas of skin injury, must be observed closely and documented thoroughly. Medical management will depend upon the nature and temporal factors related to radiation exposure. Management will also depend upon repetitive determinations of the depth and extent of skin and subcutaneous damage. Radiation injury to deeper structures or the potential for such injury to supporting subcutaneous tissues, vascular and neural tissues, muscles, tendons and bones, needs to be determined early to help guide medical and surgical management.

Serial color photographs are recommended in all cases. A medium blue background and inclusion of a sheet of white paper for later comparison and calibration of photographs is recommended. Digital photos are recommended because of their ease of electronic transmittal for tele-medical endeavors related to advice, consultation, and collaboration with experts at long distances. A measurement device should be included in the photos for comparison.

A number of special studies can be used to determine depth and extent of damage to skin, vascular, and other subcutaneous structures. These studies include: ultrasound (US, standard 7.5–20 MHz B scan), thermography, capillary microscopy, profilometry, magnetic resonance imaging (MRI), and histological studies. Three-phase bone scanning has been described as the method of choice for evaluating acute soft-tissue injuries using technetium-99m methylenediphosphonate (MDP). Magnetic resonance arteriography (MRA) has also been recommended to evaluate blood flow to injured areas.

Psychosocial Effects and Support

Psychosocial upheaval may interfere with medical management of patients involved in an R/N incident. The general lack of knowledge about radiation and radioactive materials, coupled with the general high level of anxiety, even fear, about all things radiological may result in exaggerated responses.

- Psychosocial support professionals need to be identified *prior to* an R/N incident and engaged early following an incident.
- Support personnel should include psychologists, pastoral care, social workers, public information officers, and others.
- Many patients will present to health-care facilities that only have the *perception* of significant exposure or contamination but are really without the need for medical care—their needs will be primarily for reassurance and psychological support.
- The real issue for first responders and first receivers is to determine who really have significant irradiation and thus the potential for significant radiation-induced injuries and illnesses.
- Planning and preparation for radiological/nuclear (R/N) terrorist incidents must take these factors into account in order to communicate with and control patients effectively after an incident.

Radiological and Nuclear Terrorism

Scenarios for terrorism with any hazardous material are limited only by the imagination. In some cases, they represent weapons of mass *disruption* rather than weapons of mass *destruction* (WMD); however, they run the gamut from relatively nonconsequential to disastrous. A few are of particular concern for emergency planners, public safety, and the health-care system. The history of an R/N event is necessary to help predict the nature and extent of human injury and illness. Such history may also help predict what radionuclides may have been involved. The identification

and quantification of the radionuclides will help guide medical management.

General Surgical Considerations

Surgical procedures should be performed very early in the course of a radiological insult, preferably within 24–36 hours. Surgical procedures performed after 36–48 hours from the time of the radiation injury may be complicated by failure to heal and a variety of infections. Tissue edema, leakage of fluids, and vascular damage make an ideal medium for growth of microorganisms. Immunocompromise from hematopoietic damage can also complicate management. Skin grafts, if performed too early in the course of a radiation injury, may be doomed to failure, especially if there is significant injury to the microvasculature supporting the skin.

Clearly, emergency surgery must be performed as medical standards of surgical care dictate but caution should prevail. Unfortunately, some of the cases of acute cutaneous syndrome and/or acute local injury were not known to be radiation-related early in their course. The presence of the ARS with hematopoietic syndrome, infection, immunocompromise, or other organ damage makes the prognosis for serious cutaneous injury much worse.

Treatment of radiation injury to the skin can proceed much as with thermal burns over weeks or months. Debridement that is normally performed prior to skin grafting can exacerbate underlying radiation damage and lead to acceleration of the injury. Pending skin grafting, appropriate gentle skin care, and/or artificial skin protection of the damaged areas are in order. Devitalized or necrotic tissue, however, must be carefully debrided and excised to remove this medium for infection.

Consultation with burn surgeons, plastic or cosmetic surgeons, radiation and medical oncologists, and infectious disease experts will probably be required. Some cases can be managed in local hospitals. Combined injuries may require care at burn centers or centers that have experience with management of complications from radiation oncology therapy. Pain control, infection prophylaxis, infection control, nutritional support up to and including total parenteral nutrition (TPN), fluid and electrolyte balance, along with psychosocial support, will be required just as for trauma and thermal burns.

Caveat: Most physicians and surgeons have little experience with management of radiation injuries. Most will be unaware of the need to perform surgery early in the face of significant radiation injuries and illnesses. If surgery cannot be performed within the first 24–36 hours, it should be delayed if at all possible until other systemic injury, in particular the ARS, has stabilized and the depth of radiation injury and its progression have been determined. Failure to heed these recommendations can result in poor wound healing, bleeding and infections, failure of surgery, and a more complicated clinical course.

Penetrating Wounds—Imbedded Radioactive Material

The health risk from imbedded radioactive materials can range from a very serious matter to nonconsequential. The impetus for removal of imbedded radioactive material may be physical or radiological. The location of imbedded materials near neurovascular structures or organs may be the impetus for removal. On the other hand, removal may be driven by the extent and nature of the radiological hazard.

Wound probes (radiological) can be used to locate radioactive materials if not palpable or visible. X-rays for foreign bodies may show radio-opaque materials. Larger shards or shrapnel can be removed in the same way that other nonradioactive shrapnel might be. "Punch" biopsy techniques can be used for material that is too small to isolate and remove by dissection and excision.

Health-care personnel can protect themselves by limiting the time spent removing the material or by using long-handled surgical instruments to maximize distance from the material. They should also wear finger or "ring" dosimeters, if available (nuclear medicine department, perhaps). Once removed, the material and any tissue should be placed in a lead "pig" for shielding until appropriate disposal can be arranged. These "pigs" are commonly used in nuclear medicine departments.

Depleted Uranium Shrapnel

Depleted uranium (DU) has been and is still used for armor-piercing ordnance. Depleted uranium has a lesser concentration of U-235 than found in nature. During wartime, a number of casualties have resulted from penetration with such material and their retention in the body. The radiation risk must be weighed against the physical risk from bodily retention of such material or its removal. In some cases, removal of shrapnel has presented a greater risk of physical harm from surgical procedures than the radiological risk. The radiological hazard from such materials may be of acceptably low risk; however, the toxicological hazard may be the impetus for removal. Making a decision to remove or excise the imbedded shrapnel requires consideration for surgical complications as well as the radiological risk of prolonged dose to the patient.

TYPES OF DEVICES

Some of the devices about which there is considerable concern are briefly described here.

Radiation exposure devices (RED) have been and could be used by terrorists to cause harm to individuals rather than populations. Radioactive materials that could be used for these devices are ubiquitous. The radioactive sources used for radiation oncology, industrial radiography, and any number of other applications in medicine,

industry, academia, research institutions, military, and other settings could be used as weapons. Likely sources would be Cobalt-60, Iridium-192, Cesium-137, Strontium-90, and others.

Some features of these devices are:

- Generally will result in irradiation only, therefore patients will pose no risk to others, however.
- Breech of containment shielding for a sealed source could pose risk of external and/or internal contaminations.
- Mass casualties from the terrorist use of such sources will be unlikely—small numbers of people will usually involve only those who handled or were exposed to a radioactive source.
- Surreptitious placement of a radioactive source in a high-traffic area could result in multiple radiological patients who will not have a history of exposure.
- A sealed source, if intact, could cause high levels of exposure to skin where it has been in close contact with the body.
- Depending upon the radionuclide involved and if exposure time is long enough, irradiation of internal organs could result in the acute radiation syndrome, cutaneous syndrome, or acute local injuries.

Radiological dispersal devices (RDD) are designed to spread radioactive materials. Materials used in an RDD could be in gas, aerosol, solid, particulate, liquid, or other form. A type of RDD of considerable concern is one that uses conventional explosives, for example, TNT, dynamite, plastic explosives, or others, to pulverize or vaporize, then spread radioactive materials. This is commonly called a "dirty bomb." Radioactive materials that could be used in such devices are the same as those that could be used in REDs above. These devices would be designed to cause physical injuries from explosive blasts or flying debris and shrapnel and thermal injuries.

Distribution of lower level radioactive hazards frequently found in fairly uncontrolled settings such as academia, medicine, and industry could also be used to create havoc. Their distribution without explosives by whatever method would still be an RDD, which could meet the purposes of terrorists.

Criticality and Nuclear Fission

The nuclear binding forces that hold protons and neutrons together are a source of tremendous potential energy. Absorption of neutrons by elemental nuclei such as U-235 or Pu-239, results in production of more neutrons with "fission" or fragmentation of the atom. Those "new" neutrons can then continue to bombard other nuclei, each of which will result in the production of more neutrons and additional fission fragments.

The fission of a nuclear fuel results in production of new elements with A numbers predominantly around 90 and 135, such as strontium, iodine, cesium, xenon, krypton, among others. Many of these new elements are themselves unstable and radioactive, such as strontium-90, iodine-131, and cesium-137.

If the generation of neutrons can be controlled at a steady level by carefully controlling neutron production, a self-sustaining nuclear fission, or "criticality," can be used for heat then electricity production. This is the basis for nuclear reactors. The heat produced by fission is used to heat water and produce steam to move turbines that turn generators to produce electricity.

Detonation of a nuclear weapon results from a "super-criticality." As with common explosives, a nuclear weapon detonation of explosive blast forces can cause direct physical damage to tissues from shock waves of sudden pressure changes. If detonated successfully in an urban area, it can result in hundreds to tens of thousands of deaths, and a similar number of sick and wounded, depending upon the size of the weapon just from the explosion itself rather than from ionizing radiation.

Improvised nuclear devices (IND) are devices that are considered relatively unsophisticated attempts to cause a supercriticality and a nuclear detonation. If designed properly to create a supercriticality, a nuclear detonation can result with the consequences as described above.

Even a small IND, if successful, could cause extensive damage, injuries, and contamination. On the other hand, because of the relatively unsophisticated nature of these devices, if an IND fails to result in a nuclear detonation, the detonation of conventional explosives needed to cause a criticality would essentially create the same scenario as with an RDD above.

Nuclear detonations may result from sophisticated **nuclear weapons (NW)** or **IND**. The term "nuclear weapons" usually refers to sophisticated weapons with complex design and structural features. IND technically are also nuclear weapons; however, if an IND fails to result in a nuclear detonation, the device would essentially be an RDD—see above.

Detonation of such devices in populated areas could result in multiple deaths. Physical trauma and thermal burns are the immediate hazards to life and limb. Immediate deaths will not be the result of exposure to ionizing radiation. Patients far enough away from the epicenter who might survive may require treatment for physical injuries, thermal injuries, as well as radiation-induced injuries and illnesses. The blast forces can cause ruptured tympanic membranes, pneumothorax, pneumomediastinum, "shock lung," and other air-membrane interfaces, some of which can result in significant medical/surgical attention, if not death. Medical management of such a scenario would require extensive radiological and medical triage of patients to ensure appropriate and efficient utilization of public health and emergency medical resources.

Although there are some prompt radiation effects, the *immediate* hazards to living creatures from a nuclear detonation are physical and thermal just as for common chemical explosives. The amount of explosives and the kind and amount of radionuclide(s) used in such devices will determine the extent of physical injuries from the detonation. These physical injuries will be blast injuries, blunt trauma, shrapnel injuries, thermal burns, etc. The immediate hazard is not ionizing radiation or radioactive materials. Most of the immediate deaths from a nuclear detonation will be from the blast and heat at or near the epicenter of a nuclear detonation.

Internalization of radioactive materials by inhalation, ingestion, or other mechanisms of internalization will also determine the extent of radiation injuries and illnesses. A large population could potentially be affected that could place significant burdens upon receiving centers; radiological personnel required for event history, radiological triage, and estimation of intakes; public safety and health infrastructure; medical/psychosocial support system; and supplies of medical materiel especially required for radiation-induced injuries and illnesses.

Other Human and Environmental Effects

The most likely route of exposure to humans and animals caught in an airborne plume of radioactive materials would be inhalation and/or ingestion. These materials could be particulates, vapors, mists, or gases. Eventually, particulate matter and cooled other materials will fall to the ground as "fall-out" and cause ground contamination.

On the ground, these materials can be metabolized by plants, ingested by animals, metabolized in animals, causing, for example, contamination of cows' milk, which in turn could be ingested by humans. Also, if the ground contamination is disturbed, it can again become airborne and present inhalation and ingestion hazards.

Isotopes such as iodine-131, strontium-90, and cesium-137 are of concern due to the yields (creation) of these radioisotopes in the fission process.

There would be widespread human, airborne, and environmental contamination requiring prophylactic thyroid blocking therapy with potassium iodide (KI). Early blocking of the thyroid gland, that is, within 6 hours of exposure with KI is an urgent need for those near the site or downwind of a plume of debris. See NCRP Report Number 65 for dosages and methods of delivery. Identification and quantification of internal contamination with various radionuclides is needed to guide chelation and/or other decorporation therapies.

Significant public infrastructure devastation will require mobilization of federal resources such as the Federal Radiological Monitoring and Assessment Center (FRMAC), a multiagency response contingency managed by the National Nuclear Security Administration (NNSA) of the U.S. Department of Energy. Emergency medications and supplies used for treatment of radiological injuries and illnesses are maintained by the Centers for Disease Control and Prevention (CDC) in the Strategic National Stockpile (SNS). Mobilization of the SNS may also be required for any significant R/N incident.

Blast Injuries

These forces can cause physical damage to areas where air meets tissue such as eardrums and lungs. Ruptured tympanic membranes can occur depending upon proximity to the epicenter. In the lung, such forces can cause pneumothorax, hemothorax, pneumomediastinum, air embolism, lung edema and hemorrhage, respiratory distress, and death. Such lung injuries are a primary cause of mortality with nuclear detonations. Their management is no different than for those same injuries received from conventional trauma. Their management differs only with management required for internal/external contamination and irradiation.

Such forces can also cause blunt trauma to other systems including musculoskeletal system, nervous system, cardiovascular system, and internal organs. These are also a primary cause of death from nuclear detonations. Treatment of these conditions is no different than those from conventional trauma. As above, their management differs only with that required for internal/external contamination with radioactive materials and radiation exposure.

Flying debris can result in penetrations, blunt trauma, or crush-type injuries. These are also a primary cause of death from nuclear detonations. Treatment of penetrating wounds and embedded shrapnel are discussed above. Shrapnel may be radioactive and may need to be removed as any other piece of embedded material.

Thermal Injuries

These injuries include direct heat injury, flame burns from clothing that is incinerated by intense heat, and flash burns from infrared (nonradioactive) radiation exposure. Emergency treatment of these conditions is generally the same as for any thermal burn. Wound and burn contamination must be managed.

Ionizing Radiation Injuries

Acute whole body irradiations may require the treatment of ARS depending upon the distance the patient was relative to the epicenter and therefore the extent of whole-body exposure. The presence of radioactive materials on the skin and external contamination from direct deposition or fallout of radioactive materials can cause radiation skin damage sometimes (but not technically correct) called "radiation burns." The skin may need to be decontaminated depending upon the contaminant and the extent of contamination. Such treatments may be complicated by the nature of other skin injuries like burns that may or may not require debridement.

Nuclear reactors and reactor incidents will be very unlikely to be *detonations*. Most reactors now have structurally hardened containment structures to prevent release of radiological materials from a reactor site should there be overheating of the reactor fuel core and a criticality or "meltdown." The creation of heat used to advantage steam to turn a turbine then a generator to produce electricity is a disadvantage if the necessary criticality is not controlled.

The most common type of incident of concern is disruption of the cooling for the reactor core of nuclear fuel. Loss of coolant accidents (LOCA) can result in failure to cool a reactor core allowing it to reach temperatures at which the nuclear fuel and associated assembly melts (hence the term "meltdown"). The cause may be a pipe break, valve failure, or pump failure that interrupts cooling. Reactors generally are now designed to avoid a LOCA by automatic insertion of control rods to shut down the criticality. LOCAs may result in the release of radioisotopes such as Sr-90, Cs-137, and I-131 to name a few. Medical management of workers or other individuals near the site of a reactor incident with release of radioactive materials may require immediate care for medical conditions, surgical conditions, and thermal burns.

If a plume were allowed to escape the reactor facility and containment structure, it would drift with the current wind conditions and direction. Airborne, ground, environmental, animal, and human contamination could occur in the plume's path as with a nuclear weapon detonation requiring considerations much as for a nuclear detonation above.

NCRP Report Number 138, Management of Terrorist Events Involving Radioactive Material, is an excellent resource for matters related to types of incidents, protection, response and other issues.

SUMMARY—MEDICAL MANAGEMENT OF RADIOLOGICAL INJURIES AND ILLNESSES

Symptoms and signs of significant irradiation are usually delayed for hours, days, even weeks, and sometimes months to years. Ionizing radiation does not cause *sudden* death, incapacitation, burns, or other immediate and obvious tissue damage except at extremely high doses of acute whole body irradiation. Early symptoms and signs in the prodrome of radiation-induced injury or illness are "primitive" and represent an acute and nonspecific inflammatory response, for example, anorexia, nausea, vomiting, and low-grade fever. If there is no history of an R/N incident, the systemic or cutaneous manifestations of radiation injury or illness may be indistinguishable from many other conditions. Furthermore, early symptoms and signs may disappear in a latent phase of the ARS, only to return later when they fully manifest themselves based upon the extent of cell, tissue, and organ damage.

An incident history, that is, an R/N event history and dose estimation are as critical to successful management of radiologically injured or ill patients as is the medical history and physical examination. Event histories, mock-ups, and recreations may have to be repeated many times to further refine the initial dose estimate. Patients involved with industrial, academic, medical, or military incidents may know what radionuclides have been involved in an incident or may be wearing some kind of dosimeter to help guide radiation dose estimation. In a mass casualty or terrorist R/N incident involving civilians, identification and quantification of radiological materials may be difficult and may require expert health physics (HP) support.

Radiation protection and contamination control techniques discussed in Chap. 51 will minimize the risk of irradiation or contamination of health-care providers. Treat patients and their medical/surgical conditions *first* then deal with radiological matters.

Early radiological triage and sampling from clothing, nasal smears, mouth swabs, wound swabs, urine, and blood are essential to a determination of whether internal contamination, uptake, and incorporation of radiological materials has occurred. Early identification and quantification of radionuclides involved in a radiation-induced injury or illness is essential for rapid and appropriate medical management including the use of chelators, ion-exchange pharmaceuticals, cytokines, stem cell transplants, and other treatment modalities.

Key to the diagnosis of radiation-induced injuries and illnesses is the understanding that no one parameter, including in particular dose estimates from incident histories, should be used alone. They must all be taken in context and in relationship to other methods of dose estimation.

To review, medical management of acute radiation injuries and illnesses may require:

- Aggressive supportive care—early and aggressive management of medical and surgical conditions, fluid resuscitation, treatment of shock, management of thermal burns, and management of other medical and surgical conditions are essential.
- Prophylactic antibiotics against viral, fungal, and bacterial infection related to immunosuppression and breech of normal barriers, that is, skin, intestinal mucosae, respiratory epithelium, and vascular endothelium:

Human intake and incorporation of other fission products will require decorporation therapy for transuranic radionuclides and alkalinization of urine to diminish renal toxicity from the excretion of uranium radioisotopes.

Significant public infrastructure devastation will require mobilization of federal resources such as the Federal Radiological Monitoring and Assessment Center (FRMAC), a multiagency response contingency managed by the National Nuclear Security Administration (NNSA) of the U.S. Department of Energy. Emergency medications and supplies used for treatment of radiological injuries and illnesses are maintained by the Centers for Disease Control and Prevention (CDC) in the Strategic National Stockpile (SNS). Mobilization of the SNS may also be required for any significant R/N incident. The following should be considered for any radiological/nuclear casualities.

- Acyclovir for viral prophylaxis and prevention of reactivation of *Herpes* viruses.
- A fluoroquinolone like ciprofloxacin for general bacterial prophylaxis if absolute neutrophil count (ANC) is <500 cells/mm^3.
- Fluconazole for prophylaxis against invasive fungal infections.
- Appropriate treatment of opportunistic infections and sepsis—an episode of febrile neutropenia with ANC <500 cells/mm^3 requires cessation of prophylactic fluoroquinolones and coverage for sepsis and treatment for *Pseudomonas auruginosa*, in particular.
- Treatment of bleeding from thrombocytopenia and treatment of anemia from damage to their precursor cells.
  - Blood products must be leuko-reduced and irradiated to 25 gray.
- Cytokines to stimulate proliferation and differentiation of hematopoietic stem cells—recombinant forms of
  - Granulocyte-colony stimulating factor (G-CSF, Neupogen, Amgen Inc.)
  - Granulocyte-macrophage-CSF (GM-CSF, Leukine, Berlex)
  - Pegylated form of G-CSF (Neulasta, Amgen Inc.)
- Early use of specific antidotes for internal contamination with certain radionuclides—pentetate or diethylamine-triamine-penta-acetate (DTPA), calcium salt 1 g IV initially, followed by zinc salt, 1 g IV daily. Prussian blue (PB) or ferric hexacyanoferrate for radiocesium or radiothallium— 1 g po tid.
  - DTPA and PB are managed under New Drug Application (NDA) status for the Food and Drug Administration (FDA) by the Radiation Emergency Assistance Center/Training Site (REAC/TS).
  - Smaller amounts of these pharmaceuticals may be obtained in emergencies from REAC/TS with U.S. Department of Energy (DOE) consent 24 hours per day, 7 days per week (emergency phone: 865-576-1005). Supplies are maintained by REAC/TS coinvestigators around the country.
  - The CDC maintains these and a number of other pharmaceuticals and supplies for incidents involving larger numbers of patients in their Strategic National Stockpile (SNS).

- Hospitals and other institutions may purchase and maintain these pharmaceuticals for emergency use.
- Generic antidotes and standard toxicological management of internalization of various materials whether or not they are radioactive, such as activated charcoal and cathartics.
- Use PCCs and the CDC's National Center for Environmental Health (NCEH) Emergency Response Center for toxicological support.
- Use the Radiation Emergency Assistance Center/ Training Site (REAC/TS) for advice and consultation on management of radiation-induced injuries and illnesses (Emergency phone: 865-576-1005).
- Use National Council on Radiation, Protection, and Measurements (NCRP) Report #65, *Treatment of Persons Internally Contaminated with Radionuclides*, to guide therapies for specific radioactive materials.
- Consider bone marrow or stem cell transplants. Use hematology/oncology specialists for guidance.

CONCLUSION

This chapter has provided a basic overview of medical management of the consequences of a radiological or nuclear incident. By and large, the management of R/N incident victims differs very little from other more common hazardous incidents. Emergent medical and surgical conditions take relative priority over radiological concerns. Management of the radiological issues only appear formidable. Early consultations with specialists in hematology/oncology, infectious diseases, and surgery are advised. Compare various kinds of dosimetry to help early diagnosis, prognosis, and medical management. When all else fails, the human body will be the biodosimeter that helps the clinician determine appropriate therapies.

Acknowledgments

From the Radiation Emergency Assistance Center/ Training Site (REAC/TS), Oak Ridge TN, Oak Ridge Institute for Science and Education (ORISE), of the US Department of Energy (DOE). This document describes activities performed under contract number DE-AC05-06OR23100 between the US Department of Energy and Oak Ridge Associated Universities (ORAU).

Suggested Reading

Berger ME, Christensen D, Lowry PC, et al. Medical management of radiation injuries: current approaches. *Occupational Medicine (London)*. 2006 May;56(3):162–72.

Daniak N, Waselenko JK, Armitage JO. The hematologist and radiation casualties. *Hematology Am Soc Hematol Educ Program*. 2003;473–96.

Fliedner TM, Friesecke I, Beyrer K. *Medical Management of Radiation Accidents: Manual on the Acute Radiation Syndrome*. London, British Institute of Radiology, 2001.

Flynn DF, Goans RE. Nuclear terrorism: triage and medical management of radiation and combined-injury casualties. In: Rush RM, Martin RF, Kiley KC, eds. *Surgical Clinics of North America: Surgical Response to Disaster*. Philadelphia, PA: Saunders; 2006:86(3):601–36.

Goans RE, Waselenko JK. Medical management of radiological casualties. *Health Phys*. 2005 Nov;89(5):505–12.

Gusev IA, Guskova AK, Mettler FA, eds. *Medical Management of Radiation Accidents*, CRC Press, Boca Raton, FL; 2002.

Harrison J, Leggett R, Lloyd D, et al Polonium 210 as a poison. *J Radiol Protection*. 2007(27):17–40.

Hughes WT, Armstrong D, Bodey GP, et al. 2002 guidelines for the use of antimicrobial agents in neutropenic patients with cancer. *Clin Infect Dis*. 2002 Mar 15;34(6):730–51.

Koenig KL, Goans RE, Hatchett RJ, et al. Medical treatment of radiological casualties: current concepts. *Ann Emerg Med*. 2005 Jun;45(6):643–52.

Leikin JB, McFee RB, Walter FG, Radiation Emergencies, A primer to nuclear incident. *JEMS* 2007(March):122–137.

NCRP Report No. 65, *Management of Persons Accidentally Contaminated with Radionuclides*, National Council on Radiation Protection and Measurements (NCRP), Bethesda, MD (1979).

NCRP Report No. 138, *Management of Terrorist Events Involving Radioactive Materials*, National Council on Radiation Protection and Measurements (NCRP), Bethesda, MD (2001).

McFee, Leikin JB, Radiation terrorism: the unthinkable possibility, the ignored reality. *JEMS* 2005(Apr):78–92.

Mettler FA, Upton AC. *Medical Effects of Ionizing Radiation*. 2nd ed. Elsevier Science, New York. 1995.

Ricks RC, Fry SA, eds., *The Medical Basis for Radiation Accident Preparedness II: Clinical experience and follow-up since 1979*—Proceedings of the second annual REAC/TS conference. Elsevier Science, New York. 1990.

Ricks RC, Berger ME, Fry SA, eds. *The Medical Basis for Radiation Accident Preparedness III: The Psychological Perspective*—Proceedings of the third annual REAC/TS conference. Elsevier Science, New York. 1990.

Ricks RC, Berger ME, O'Hara FM, eds. *The Medical Basis for Radiation Accident Preparedness: The Clinical Care of Victims*—Proceedings of the fourth annual REAC/TS conference. Parthenon, Boca Raton, FL. 2002.

Waselenko JK, MacVittie TJ, Blakely WF, et al. Medical management of the acute radiation syndrome: recommendations of the Strategic National Stockpile Radiation Working Group. *Ann Intern Med*. 2004 Jun 15;140(12):1037–51.

S E C T I O N

VII

EXPLOSIVES/INCENDIARIES

INTRODUCTION

The use of explosives remains the leading weapon of choice for terrorism accounting for over 85% of all terrorist events world wide, and usually involving improvised explosive devices (IED) often made from readily available components. While most such events occur in foreign lands, it is worth remembering that the Oklahoma City bombing was the work of US citizens, not international terrorists. The devastating destruction was the result of fuel oil and ammonium nitrate (fertilizer!). These bomb making ingredients remain easily obtained in quantities sufficient to inflict significant destruction.

The double edged sword—in the United States we are both fortunate and limited by having few events and little experience in the preparedness and response to terrorism and explosives. With information about creating IED still available on the Internet as well as through militia and other agenda group (domestic and foreign) pamphlets and training, it is critical to understand the impact explosives and incendiary devices can have. Moreover from an emergency responder perspective, it is important to realize secondary events can occur—these involve the use of IED to target health-care responders as they arrive at the primary event. In fact, responders are often targeted by terrorist to destabilize the capabilities of a community and demoralize the remaining staff members.

This section, written by one of the world's leading experts in both the medical management of explosives' victims as well as health-care facility (HCF) preparedness, is designed to present to the reader insights into the often complicated pattern of injury such victims present with. You will learn practical approaches such as resource adaptation—important and necessary in optimizing the staff and facilities to accommodate an onslaught of victims after a mass casualty event. Given a HCF can easily be overwhelmed given the general lack of surge capacity nationwide, this section offers a strategy for preparedness that has stood the test of time in a region that has had far too much experience with the threat *and* reality of terrorist use of explosives.

53

MEDICAL MANAGEMENT OF EXPLOSIVES

Pinchas Halpern

S T A T   F A C T S

MEDICAL MANAGEMENT OF EXPLOSIVES

- Brainstorm with all stake holders, develop threat assessment, and response strategy.
- Obtain management support for strategy, funding for equipment, system development, training, drilling.
- Prepare and disseminate 1–2-page response algorithm for bomb-related multiple casualty incidents in the ED.
- Ensure immediate, 24/7 availability of 1-page checklist for such events (see Table 53-1).
- Drill the ED staff in the basics of checklist use, ED evacuation, gate control, staff call-up and so on.
- Develop appropriate charts, forms, IT capability.

INTRODUCTION

Definitions

A mass casualty incident (MCI) is a sudden influx of multiple casualties into the medical facility. The absolute numbers of victims is not as relevant as how demands reconcile with the capacity of the receiving facility. MCI is a large number of casualties, generated over a short period of time, which can be appropriately managed with existing or extended resources. A mass casualty event (MCE) in contrast is a major medical disaster that overwhelms medical capacity in the response area, either because of the number, severity, or type of injuries (e.g., mix of many severe biological or chemical agent involvement, massive numbers of specific injuries such as burns, crush, etc.). The goal is thus not to plan for an overwhelming MCE, which is impossible by definition. However, a large MCI may locally overwhelm even the

most experienced trauma center, and the task of any ED is to realistically assess the potential threat, the maximum capability inherent in the emergency department (ED), and the methods to optimize that capability.

The Threat

Bombings employing conventional explosives, both standard military issue and improvised, comprise, at the present time, the vast majority of terrorism-related MCIs. The Memorial Institute for the Prevention of Terrorism (MITP, a U.S. Government funded, academic nonprofit research institute established after the Oklahoma bombing in 1995) estimated terrorist activity type breakdown in 2005 as bombings 2650, armed attack 1532, kidnapping 310, assassination 159, arson 114. An analysis of 44 mass-casualty, terrorist bombings found an overall 3% (1–14%) mortality, hospital admission rates of 34% (14–53%) and arrival times of first victims from 5 minutes to hours. While bombing of civilian targets by terrorist groups is not new, the events of 9/11 have resulted in a heightened awareness and interest in the medical management of MCEs. In the United States alone between 1980 and 1990, there were 12,216 intentional bombings. Explosions from intentional bombings are among the few instantaneous traumatic events that can produce massive numbers of casualties requiring immediate medical attention. Another review of 14 published studies of terrorist attacks that occurred between 1969 and 1983 involving a combined population of 3357 casualties demonstrated that the overall mortality at the scene was 12.6%, with 30% of the immediate survivors requiring hospital admission. Thus, the great majority of injuries suffered by immediate survivors of bombings are not life-threatening, resulting in the "walking wounded." However, with large MCEs, even a small percentage of critically injured victims can overwhelm the local and regional medical systems. Additionally the large number of "walking wounded" that often show up at local hospitals places further burden on the already overtaxed medical facilities and resources. The MITP indicates an annual death rate from terrorism related activity of 10,860 in 2004, 6200 in 2003, 7349 in 2002, 6403 in 2001.

Bombs need not be complex devices to be devastating. Both the 1993 World Trade Center bombing and the Oklahoma City bombings were done with different mixtures of ammonium nitrate obtained from common household fertilizer. Conventional terrorist bombs are usually solid. The compound combusts rapidly, producing an expanding sphere of hot dense gas pushed outwards at tremendous speed so as to produce a shock wave, propagating at the speed of sound in all directions. The destructive power of this shock wave as well as the thermal products of the explosion in conjunction with their effects on structures and personnel makes explosions ideal terror weapons. The effect of the shock wave varies tremendously with the location of the blast (open, semiclosed, or closed location), physical structures such as walls in the vicinity of the blast, the distance from the explosion, the number and type of embedded shrapnel in the bomb.

Proper medical management of terror attacks resulting in multiple casualties begins even before the event. Pre-event preparedness is crucial to optimize care. Extensive early planning for MCEs helps minimize chaos and improve outcomes. Frequent reassessments of the disaster plans and performance of multiple drills are vital to successful implementation of mass casualty plans. A good rule of thumb may be that a hospital should make itself capable of coping with a number of casualties equal to 20% of its inpatient bed capacity within 30 minutes of an event, and 60% within 12 hours. This is the Israeli model (PH, personal communication).

Blast injury

The detonation of a conventional explosive generates a blast wave that spreads out from a point source. The blast wave consists of two parts: a shock wave of high pressure, followed closely by a blast wind, or air in motion. The effects of blast on victims are multiple. Generally speaking, such effects are divided into four main types: (1) *Primary*: direct effect of blast overpressure on tissue. Primary blast injury affects air-filled structures such as the lungs, ears, and gastrointestinal tract (GIT), via the following mechanisms: spalling, for example, from lung parenchyma to alveolar space, causing tissue surfaces to explode geyser-like; shearing due to differential inertia (e.g., pulmonary vessels and air spaces, resulting in ruptured vascular and bronchial pedicles) implosion of flexible air spaces, which, after shock wave passes, rebound to greater than original size, resembling mini-explosions. (2) *Secondary*: due to flying objects, shrapnel. (3) *Tertiary*: the victim is propelled through the air and strikes stationary

objects. (4) *Quaternary or Miscellaneous*: all other injuries such as burns, smoke inhalation, chemical agent release etc.

The effects of a bomb blast are difficult to predict in the individual victim, as well as in the group. However, a number of important principles are known:

1. Distance of victim from explosion: the intensity of an explosion pressure wave declines with the cubed root of the distance from the explosion. A person 3 m (10 ft) from an explosion experiences nine times more overpressure than a person 6 m (20 ft) away. Proximity of the person to the explosion is an important factor in a primary blast injury.

2. Enclosed versus open space: the effects of an explosion in closed space (e.g., a room, bus, train) are much greater than in open spaces. Injuries are more severe, mortality is greater;

3. Surrounding environment (e.g., the presence of intervening protective barriers): blast waves are reflected by solid surfaces; thus, a person standing next to a wall may suffer increased primary blast injury.

4. Quantity of explosive: obviously, the greater the quantity of explosive the greater the potential for damage at any distance.

5. Type of explosive: high-order explosives (HE) undergo detonation, an almost instantaneous transformation of the original explosive material into gases occupying the same volume of space under extremely high pressure. These high-pressure gases expand rapidly, compress the surrounding medium, and produce a supersonic, overpressure blast wave. Examples of HE include dynamite, TNT, ammonium nitrate fuel oil, dynamite, and C-4 "plastic" explosives. In general, only HE explosions produce severe primary blast injury.

6. Embedded shrapnel: many terrorists purposefully embed multiple pieces of metal and plastic in the explosive, maximizing the number and severity of secondary injuries. From the point of view of medical care, shrapnel injuries are the most numerous, important, and potentially misleading.

PRINCIPLES OF COPING WITH BOMB-RELATED MCI/MCE IN THE EMERGENCY DEPARTMENT

MCIs Resulting From Terror Bombing Pose Special Problems

1. They present casualties with a multidimensional injury pattern (Kluger Y, Einav S), that results from the simultaneous primary, secondary, tertiary, and quaternary explosion injury mechanisms.

2. They often occur in urban settings, in close proximity to the ED, and EMS often practice "scoop and run" in these situations, leaving very little time for the ED to prepare before the first casualties start flooding the facility.

3. They often occur in semiclosed spaces (transportation stations, buses, restaurants, markets), allowing the benefit of rapid extrication and transportation of victims to medical care, but also producing very rapid casualty loading of the receiving hospitals (Einav S). Thirty-four percent of bombing related patients arrived within 10 minutes and 65% of the patients arrived within 30 minutes of time zero. The average arrival time of admitted patients was 24 ± 30 minutes.

4. They may occur at all hours, but typically in daytime, when on the one hand staff is available, but also the hospital is at its busiest (e.g., operating rooms are full).

5. Medical and nursing staff in most hospitals have very little training in handling explosion-related trauma in the individual patient and managing MCIs as such.

6. Hospitals are reluctant to invest time and resources into planning for what is often perceived as being a very remote possibility (A 2002 National Assessment of State Trauma System Development, Emergency Medical Services Resources, and Disaster Readiness for MCEs, *http://www.hrsa.gov/trauma/survey/table10.htm*, 42% had no plans for when capacity was exceeded and 64% had no plans for increasing capacity in disasters).

7. Physicians are usually poorly trained in managing bomb blast-related casualties.

Issues to be Decided Before Planning

There exists a list of issues that need to be addressed by the planner:

What is the *local* definition of an MCI (i.e., when to activate emergency plans)? It depends on the hospital's and the ED's capacity during working hours (e.g., number of ED beds, staff, surgical, intensive care and anesthesia staff and beds, CT and other diagnostic abilities), and also on the ability to respond to after hours events (staff numbers, staff response times based on geography and weather etc.).

Does one produce a single plan (and therefore, definition) or a range of definitions (e.g., "small MCI" up to n severe and m light casualties, "moderate MCI" up to x and y and a "full response" MCI thereafter)? We have concluded that in our medical center, we activate three separate plans: (1) A "minor" event is declared when fewer than 5 "red" and 5 "yellow" patients are anticipated; such an event is handled by on-call staff, with some augmentation. (2) Moderate events are defined up to 20–30 casualties, involving the activation of a beeper and cell phone short text messaging (SMS) systems, calling in dozens of extra staff. (3) A full response MCI results in the calling in of hundreds of staff. (4) MCE. If the expected caseload is more than 20% of the number of our hospital beds >240 casualties, full activation of the hospital staff and resources will be initiated including opening of special designated and equipped areas for casualty evaluation and management other than the ED.

What is the activation plan? Mass casualty protocols are initiated bearing in mind that this could be a false alarm, that is, that all patients are injured lightly, or that only few will arrive. Overdoing is preferred to underpreparedness.

NOT ALL BOMBINGS ARE THE SAME: FACTORS DETERMINING OUTCOME

Timing of the Event (AM/PM)

While a daytime event means everybody is in house, it also means that operating rooms are full, the postanesthesia care unit is busy, ED, radiology etc. are busy. It may take minutes to clear some of these critical sites, but not so for complex surgery, the movement of patients from the intensive care unit (ICU), etc.

Rapidity and Quality of Response of EMS

Modern EMS have highly trained staff, responding quickly to major incidents. The usual practice (except in parts of Europe) is to provide only life-saving and stabilization care on site and to transport the casualties as quickly as possible to EDs. Short reaction times, rapid patient ingress, result. The ED must therefore assume 10–30 minutes of preparation time in urban events, 1–2 hours in rural events.

Location: Urban or Rural

The event's location has major implications on the hospital's preparation plan and protocol activation. A remote site or difficult transport conditions imply prolonged evacuation. This allows the admitting hospitals more time to prepare and enables the hospital's command center to collect relevant data before the arrival of the first patient. Since the triage officer controls a remote MCE evacuation, it is expected that the severely injured arrive in the first wave and that those eventually evacuated first be severely injured.

Capacity of Adjacent Hospitals

There will be a huge difference in the way a hospital prepares if it is located within short transport distances from other significantly capable hospitals, or whether it is a relatively isolated facility (geographically or transportation-wise).

COMPONENTS OF THE PREPAREDNESS SYSTEM

Commitment by Management

While CBRN threats have received high visibility and funding, the more "mundane" threat of bombings has often been neglected, to a large extent based on the assumption that any ED capable of handling the daily type of accidents and emergencies may easily expand its response to care for the victims of a bomb. Unfortunately, this is far from obvious, and unless top management makes it a priority, the first (and possibly, only) event the ED will encounter may not be handled very well.

Involvement Of and Buy-In By All Relevant Players in Development of Concepts and Procedures

Management involvement is not sufficient if all potential players do not participate and bring in their respective areas of expertise.

Clearly Defined Concepts

Every ED and hospital is different. Planning starts with a concept that best suits the hospitals location, size, capacity, adjacent institutions, and so on.

Sequence of ED Activities in an MCI

1. *Initial announcement and confirmation*: Initial announcement may be received from bystanders, family members, the media, police, EMS, and so on.
2. *Decision to implement MCI protocol*: Confirmation is important, but should never delay timely preparations: Authority to declare an MCI condition should be predetermined and clear to all. When in doubt, in the interest of speed, responsibility may need to be taken by ED staff. False alarms are an opportunity for drilling.

PROTOCOL IMPLEMENTATION

Checklists

Checklists are critical for successful implementation of rarely used protocols. They should be concise, never more than 1–2 pages, and available in a location known to everybody 24/7. Complex flow charts are of little use, as is long-winded explanatory text (Table 53-1).

Assignment of Responsibility

Assignment of responsibility is generic (i.e., "charge nurse" rather than to specific persons, who will likely be away at the crucial moment).

Strict Perimeter and ED Entrance Control

Strict perimeter and ED entrance control should be achieved: no unauthorized persons allowed into the ED. Family members and the public are directed to the information center (see below). This is critical to minimize crowding and confusion.

ED Evacuation

A predetermined plan must exist. At the Tel Aviv Medical Center we achieve 5–7-minute evacuation times for 50–70

TABLE 53-1

CHECKLIST FOR BOMB-RELATED MULTIPLE CASUALTY INCIDENT

- Call back to check information
- Initiate log, activate emergency information systems
- Call MCI code (per ED senior physician and nurse; only if apparent time permits—consult with _____)
- Notify:
  a) Shift ED charge nurse
  b) Hospital matron
  c) ED chief
  d) ED head nurse
- Notify:
  a) All ED staff via overhead
  b) Hospital switchboard to activate call up system
  c) Hospital management
  d) Trauma chief
  e) Security
  f) ED admissions office
  g) OR
  h) Radiology
  i) Blood bank
  j) Lab
  k) Respiratory therapy
- Initiate ED evacuation plan
- Brief staff and distribute ID vests
- Assign staff to positions as they arrive
- Prepare and preposition equipment per protocol
- Prepare ambulance bay (gurneys, porters, security, traffic control)
- Man triage point (MD, RN, registration clerk, security)

patients via a simple method: a hospital charge nurse comes immediately to the ED with a current list of available beds in the nonsurgical departments, and requests every available porter to the ED; an ED physician and nurse determine those patients requiring intensive monitoring during and after transfer, and they are assigned appropriate staff and equipment (usually 2–5 such patients are in the ED at any moment in time); everybody else is given the choice to either self-discharge (e.g., minor trauma, all walk-in clinic patients) or to be taken to inpatient departments, where ward staff completes ED workup and discharges or admits as appropriate. Wards know they cannot, as a rule, send patients back to the ED even after the event, so they have an incentive to complete care quickly and make disposition decisions. Registration of patient movements in the hospital is kept to a minimum, and is often carried out in the receiving ward.

ED Entrance Preparation

ED gurneys, porters, and an authoritative official to manage patient and ambulance flow must exist. In our hospital, there is no medical presence in the ambulance bay.

Triage Point

Triage may be done in the ambulance bay or at the inside ED door. We prefer the second choice, because holding up the ambulances in the bay will likely result in rapid clogging of transportation routes. Patients are taken out of the ambulance by paramedics with hospital porter assistance, brought into the ED and triaged at the first physical choke point in the ED.

Triage

We have learned that initial overtriage occurs commonly, that such decisions in the initial ED encounter are not very critical because they may be rectified later in the ED, and that patients' condition changes rapidly anyway. Consequently, triage is performed by a senior resident or young attending (surgery or emergency medicine). It consists of a rapid inspection seeking determination of level of consciousness, obvious respiratory difficulty, obvious major trauma or burns or external bleeding, or the so called "Ask-Look-Feel" system. Such triage takes literally seconds, and is geared towards systematic (though thoughtful) overtriage. More complex, numbers-based triage protocols take 1–3 minutes, and with casualty inflows of several patients per minute, are in my opinion impractical (Table 53-2).

Registration

Prenumbered charts may be used. We use dedicated MCI charts (Fig. 53-1), which are sequentially numbered, in lieu of attempting to identify victims during the hectic event. These numbers are used for all identification purposes, including blood typing. Only after the initial receiving phase of the event is over, is a systematic transition to the conventional hospital identification and tracking system performed. Links to the MCI numbering system are maintained, to prevent errors. Computerized registration systems are being implemented. One such system, locally developed by us, is in use at 11 major institutions, using mobile computer terminals at the triage point, sequential numbers, and a minimal data set of (1) gender, (2) age group (e.g., infant, child etc.), (3) injury site(s), (4) triage severity, (5) indicated ED location. It takes 5–10 seconds to key in the data on a touch screen with no drop-down menus, and drills have shown it does not impede patient inflow.

Command and Control (C&C) and Staffing

MCIs are characterized by gradual accumulation of staff. The ED attending or senior present surgeon or physician is initially in charge, until senior ED and surgery staff arrive. Multiple transfers of command are avoided by determining, that only upon arrival of the most senior staff is official command handed over. Trauma/surgery chief and ED chief then share command: trauma/surgery chief is medical control, ED chief is logistics and comedical control (Table 53-3). A single person has difficulty controlling a large MCI in a large ED. Therefore, the ED is divided into control areas and area commanders are assigned, who report to the overall C&C team. Every bed is ideally assigned one physician and one nurse, according to staff availability. Importantly, staff is taught not to join other care teams unless specifically requested to, in order to maintain readiness to receive incoming patients at their own assigned posts.

Care Plans

Most emergency medicine and surgical residents have little experience of bomb blast injuries, and the confusion of an MCI degrades their abilities further. Senior personnel should serve as advisors, moving from one patient to another, advising, making key decisions, and moving on, rather than concentrating on the first or most severe casualties. Care plans should be succinctly charted, so that all involved may continue their implementation when, inevitably, the patient is transferred elsewhere.

Patient Care

Only immediately relevant procedures are carried out initially. Thus, no time is lost on plaster casts, but temporary splinting, traction, and dressings are used. Irrigation and disinfection of wounds is urgent and takes little effort, while their definitive debridement and closure may wait a few hours. Patients deemed fit for discharge need to have definitive care of their (obviously) minor injuries prior to discharge. Given the austerity of initial care and the propensity to miss important injuries, secondary and tertiary assessments of all casualties must be carried out. As patients are assigned to inpatient departments often not based on their primary injury but according to bed availability, a senior trauma and nursing team must see them all within a short period of time, ensure no missed injuries exist, and that appropriate care plans are laid out, recorded, and carried out. In-hospital transfers may occur subsequently, as the bed situation stabilizes and patients' main problems come into focus.

Secondary Transfers

Every institution has a limit to the number and severity of victims it can effectively care for. Based on the overall situation in other hospitals, transportation assets available, and the magnitude of the event, such a point may be reached in the judgment of the command staff. Regional and national authorities must have in place appropriate plans for the transfer of appropriate patients to more distant facilities. In extreme circumstances, when the hospital is totally overwhelmed with casualties, it may go into "Triage Hospital" mode. This concept entails the entire hospital becoming essentially an ED, receiving, triaging, stabilizing, and preparing casualties for further transfer. No definitive care is offered beyond immediately life-saving procedures.

TABLE 53-2

TRIAGE AND INITIAL REGISTRATION FORM

Date: _____

Sticker	Name	Adult/Child	M/F	Triage Severity	Apparent Main Injured System/s	Destination
		A	M	Green	Head Neck	Bay 1
		C	F	Yellow	Torso Vascular	Bay 2
				Red	Abdomen Back	
				Black	Limbs Other	
		A	M	Green	Head Neck	Bay 1
		C	F	Yellow	Torso Vascular	Bay 2
				Red	Abdomen Back	
				Black	Limbs Other	
		A	M	Green	Head Neck	Bay 1
		C	F	Yellow	Torso Vascular	Bay 2
				Red	Abdomen Back	
				Black	Limbs Other	
		A	M	Green	Head Neck	Bay 1
		C	F	Yellow	Torso Vascular	Bay 2
				Red	Abdomen Back	
				Black	Limbs Other	
		A	M	Green	Head Neck	Bay 1
		C	F	Yellow	Torso Vascular	Bay 2
				Red	Abdomen Back	
				Black	Limbs Other	
		A	M	Green	Head Neck	Bay 1
		C	F	Yellow	Torso Vascular	Bay 2
				Red	Abdomen Back	
				Black	Limbs Other	
		A	M	Green	Head Neck	Bay 1
		C	F	Yellow	Torso Vascular	Bay 2
				Red	Abdomen Back	
				Black	Limbs Other	
		A	M	Green	Head Neck	Bay 1
		C	F	Yellow	Torso Vascular	Bay 2
				Red	Abdomen Back	
				Black	Limbs Other	
		A	M	Green	Head Neck	Bay 1
		C	F	Yellow	Torso Vascular	Bay 2
				Red	Abdomen Back	
				Black	Limbs Other	

Analgesia

Oligo-analgesia (insufficient analgesia) in EDs has been documented often. While not specifically documented, oligo-analgesia is more pervasive in MCI situations. Chaotic states, insufficient information regarding patient status and potential contraindications to opiates, staff inexperience and focus on immediate life-saving care, all conspire to make analgesia administration seem like a secondary concern. As is true in everyday care, this is not so. There are few if any contraindications to judiciously used analgesics during an MCI. A simple protocol, such as: mild pain—2 acetaminophen tablets, with or without codeine; moderate pain—oral (e.g., oxycodone, tramadol solution 50 mg) or sublingual opiate (e.g. 0.2–0.4 mg buprenorphine) or injectable nonsteroidal anti-inflammatory drug (NSAID) (e.g., ketorolac); severe pain—IM/IV morphine, is easy to implement. It is

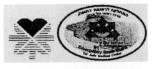

Tel Aviv Medical Center
<u>**Multiple Casualty Incident ED Casualty Treatment Chart**</u>

Mechanism fo injury: Explosion (enclosed space); explosion (open space); GSW, stab, chemical

Mode of arrival: ALS ambulance; BLS ambulance; private car; walk-in; helicopter

<u>**Externally visible injuries:**</u>

1. _____

2. _____

3. _____

4. _____

5. _____

6. _____

Time _____: **Primary survey**

A-airway:	normal	hoarse	aphonic	stridor	intubated
B-breathing:	normal	rapid	very rapid	slow	ventilated
C-circulation:	normal	mild hypovolemia	significant hypovolemia	shock	pulseless
D-disability:	alert	verbal	pain	unresponsive	intubated

Injury severity:

Time: _____ Mild	Moderate	Severe	Intubated	Dying	Dead
Time: _____ Mild	Moderate	Severe	Intubated	Dying	Dead

Doctor's name: _____   Nurse's name: _____

Time	BP	Pulse	SpO$_2$	Respirations	Pain 0–10

FIGURE 53-1

SAMPLE MCI PATIENT CHART

Physical examination:

Head Normal _____

Face Normal _____

Neck Normal _____

Chest Normal _____

Eyes Normal _____

Abdomen Normal _____

Back Normal _____

Upper limbs Normal _____

Lower limbs Normal _____

Genitalia Normal _____

Vascular Normal _____

Other _____

Care plan:

F I G U R E   5 3 - 1
(CONTINUED)

Time	Order	Doctor's name	Nurse's name	Time performed
	Intubation			
	Closed chest tube drainage right/left			
	FAST			
	Otoscopy			
	Fiberoptic laryngoscopy			
	Angiography of _____			
	X-rays of: _____ _____			
	X-rays of: _____ _____			
	CT of _____			
	Ophthalmology exam			
	IV/IM Atropine _____ mg IV/IM Atropine _____ mg IV/IM Atropine _____ mg			
	IV/IM Toxogonin _____ mg IV/IM Toxogonin _____ mg IV/IM Toxogonin _____ mg			
	IV/IM Midazolam _____ mg IV/IM Midazolam _____ mg IV/IM Midazolam _____ mg			
	Tetanus toxoid			

Valuables: Sent with pt in safe given to _____

Telephone numbers for contacts: _____

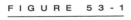

F I G U R E   5 3 - 1

(*CONTINUED*)

Tel Aviv Medical Center
Multiple Casualty Incident ED Casualty Discharge Chart

The patient was treated at the Tel Aviv Medical Center for injuries caused in a multiple casualty incident. The following is a brief summary of our findings and recommendations:

_____

_____

_____

_____

_____

_____

_____

Main diagnoses:

1. _____

2. _____

3. _____

4. _____

- ☐ Pt was seen by psychologist/psychiatrist/social worker
- ☐ Continued psychological support suggested
- ☐ Pt received Hepatitis B active immunization
- ☐ Pt must complete Hepatitis B immunization schedule
- ☐ Pt has NOT received Hepatitis B immunization because: _____
- ☐ Pt received Tetanus toxoid
- ☐ Pt must complete Tetanus immunization schedule
- ☐ Pt requires continued surgical follow up for wounds

Disposition:

Transfer to: CT   Angio   OR   ICU   Ward   Extension site

Admit to: _____   **Discharge** home

Doctor's name and signature: _____

Time: _____

FIGURE 53-1

(CONTINUED)

the incident commanders' job to ensure analgesia is a priority with care givers. Again, while strict science is scarce, large clinical experience clearly indicates that in patients without obvious cardiorespiratory or neurological compromise (of which there are usually only few in every incident), analgesia is safe and there is no excuse to withhold it.

Imaging

Utilize radiology sparingly, ideally only chest x-rays in shock room and skull x-rays for shrapnel localization (Fig. 53-2). Remember that visualization of a metal object in single-plane film is often inadequate for thorough evaluation, but it can direct the team to the need for urgent surgery or for additional imaging. Bedside FAST (focused abdominal sonography for trauma) does not unduly disrupt patient care and is used liberally. Skeletal x-rays are performed only after casualty admission has all but stopped. CT is _the_ major imaging resource, control by incident commander is essential (Einav et al found that more than one-third of the admitted patients were sent to CT scan directly from the ED.) Surprisingly, implementation of digital radiography has complicated radiology utilization by requiring that the physician be physically present at the viewing station rather than the film being brought to the bedside. Mobile, wireless viewing terminals may solve this problem in the near future.

TABLE 53-3
ROLES OF THE INCIDENT COMMANDERS

Medical Commander	Logistics Commander
Major clinical decisions (e.g., operative interventions, CT scanning, angiography)	Major logistic decisions (e.g., opening additional sites, calling in more staff, requesting external material and staff support)
Prioritizing and approving every patient movement out of the ED	Patient transfers
Instructing and consulting patient care teams	Staff assignment and management
Maintenance of the overall clinical picture	Maintenance of the overall casualty flow picture
Casualty disposition	Communication with hospital administration
Casualty reassessment	Communicating information to the media
	Information system management
	Resource management
	Blood bank issues
	Medical charting

Laboratory

We use no laboratory tests other than blood typing and cross-matching during the initial phase of the event. There is little use to serum chemistry or hemoglobin values in the early care of bomb blast victims. Elderly and obviously chronically ill patients may be an exception, and a CBC and serum glucose-sodium-potassium-creatinine panel may be warranted. Pulse oximetry may be useful to assess blast lung injury severity, and ventilated patients may be monitored with capnography and occasional venous or arterial blood gas determinations.

Special Populations

Children are cared for in the main treatment areas, attempting to keep them in proximity to their parents or accompanying adults. Dedicated bays in the ED may be reserved for children if possible, if the incident happens to include a large proportion of children. Pregnant women are cared for in the main treatment areas, but gynecologists and obstetricians are involved early and may assume full responsibility for the patients once significant maternal injuries have been ruled out or addressed.

Psychological Support

Psychological support is offered to patients in obvious distress, but no effort is made to debrief or counsel everybody. All patients discharged home are given telephone numbers to call for postevent psychological care.

Informatics

The importance of real-time information for event management cannot be overemphasized. Accurate records are critical for data analysis, study, and subsequent research. Every institution has its own systems. A practical system should focus on information that is relevant, practical to record by harassed and understaffed medical and surgical staff. Standardization of data reporting formats is beneficial for analysis of events where almost universally casualties are treated at a number of medical facilities. A special issue is the identification of unidentified victims and of information distribution across large

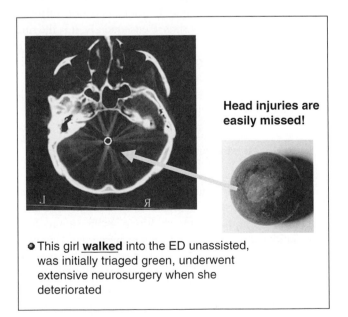

Head injuries are easily missed!

● This girl **walked** into the ED unassisted, was initially triaged green, underwent extensive neurosurgery when she deteriorated

FIGURE 53-2

PENETRATING WOUNDS: NOTE THE LOCATION OF THE SHRAPNEL
Source: Emergency Department, TelAviv Medical Center, Israel.

distances for the benefit of relatives living at a distance from the actual event. Web-based, digital photography and forensic data systems have been developed. The Israeli "Adam" system is operative and has been proven in many incidents (P. Halpern-personal communication).

Forensic Issues

Police and crime scene investigators, as well as counterterrorism and other security services have legitimate interests in securing forensic and other information. Efforts should be made to accommodate them, but never at the expense of medical care. Prior coordination with all relevant authorities should establish protocols, such as who and how many persons from these offices are allowed in, when, into which parts of the ED, how they are identified, who controls them and is empowered to limit their entry and work in specific locations and circumstances, and so on. These issues are probably best left to hospital security to work out. As a rule, however, while a terrorist event is a crime, experience shows that forensics in the hospital are of minor relevance compared to the actual crime scene, and other than interrogating lightly injured victims regarding the event and obtaining shrapnel taken out of victims' bodies, not much is urgent.

Dead Casualties

It is important to develop a coherent plan for the handling of dead casualties, both dead-on-arrival and died-in-the-ED victims. A secure location must be identified, appropriate documentation ensured (including copies for relevant authorities), facilities for relatives provided, family support ensured. Consideration must be given to the difficulty in identifying mutilated bodies, and errors prevented. In the Israeli system, only the Forensic Medical Institute is allowed to provide identification, and *all* dead victims are taken there, families directed there as well, and identification occurs there exclusively. DNA identification methods are routinely employed.

Information Center

As part of any MCI, an information center is activated. Such centers are ideally located in relative proximity to the hospital entrance, so that relatives may be easily directed there rather than having them wander around the campus. Social workers, psychologists, nurses, and at least one physician are permanently assigned there. Computer links, rest areas, telephones, refreshments must be provided.

Staff Safety

Issues of staff safety include (1) possible infiltration of the ED by perpetrators intent on causing second explosions or attacks in the hospital; (2) unexploded explosives inadvertently brought into the ED; (3) transmissible disease in the setting of inadvertent body fluid exposure or needle sticks during stressful, rapid work; (4) violence from relatives, patients unhappy with care, and so on. All satchels and bags brought into the ED from the site are examined by bomb-disposal experts. Maintain staff awareness, use security wisely, adhere to work safety principles.

Casualty Discharge

The apparently simple matter of discharging lightly injured and anxiety reaction casualties form the ED is very important to manage correctly. Missed injuries occur, unrecorded data is common, important postevent care information needs to be given out, and further opportunity to seek psychological support must be provided. A structured system, a designated location, team and forms, all are necessary.

Debriefing

Immediate debriefing of staff must be carried out after the incident, even though many participants may still be busy in the operating rooms, ICU, and so on. Impressions not immediately recorded may become colored by discussions with colleagues and by short-term memory. Structured, pre-prepared forms are very useful and should be available as part of the emergency response documents.

Infectious Disease

A report from Israel documents the presence of hepatitis B in bone fragments from suicide bombers, retrieved from the bodies of the bomb victims. Consequently, it is the rule now in Israel to provide active hepatitis B immunization in the ED to all bomb victims, unless they specifically indicate they are immunized. The issue of HIV transfer and consequent need for prophylaxis may need to be considered in locations with high HIV seropositivity prevalence.

Clinical Examination and Treatment of the Blast Victim

Advanced trauma life support (ATLS) and advanced cardiac life support (ACLS) protocol generally apply in MCI situations. However, the need to prioritize resources may lead to deviations from the protocol. For example, imaging may be delayed beyond normal routine because of the need to assign the resources to other, more severely injured casualties. Diagnostic peritoneal lavage has sometimes resurged as a useful method when scarce CT resources are outstripped. Operating rooms may be initially unavailable, laboratory tests are irrelevant, warming devices scarce, angiography suites busy, and so on. High-grade clinical expertise is therefore even more in demand than usual during MCIs, in order to allow optimal use of resources and minimize potential suboptimal decision-making under stressful conditions.

Respiratory System

Oxygen-resistant hypoxemia, hemorrhage, contusion (appearing as a bi-hilar "butterfly" pattern on chest radiographs), pneumothorax, hemothorax, pneumomediastinum, and subcutaneous emphysema are typical of pulmonary blast injury (Fig. 53-3). Lung tissue quickly becomes friable and susceptible to pressure-induced barotrauma. Physical examination if often is initially unremarkable. Pulse oximetry must be performed with the patient breathing room air, to detect shunt otherwise masked by oxygen supplementation. Assume that a patient's wheezing associated with a blast injury is from pulmonary contusion. Other causes of wheezing in this setting may include inhalation of irritant gases or dusts, pulmonary edema from myocardial contusion, and adult respiratory distress syndrome (ARDS). Blast lung injury is a very severe disease. Low-volume, low-inspiratory pressure, lung-sparing strategies of mechanical ventilation must be employed from the onset in ventilated patients. Pressure limited ventilation, inverse inspiratory/expiratory (I:E) ratio, ventilation, and permissive hypercapnia should be considered early on. Multiple pneumothoraces may be quickly caused by careless use of the ventilator. Extreme methods of oxygenation, such as extra corporeal membrane oxygenation (ECMO), intravascular oxygenation (IVOX), and so on may become necessary within hours of the injury.

Ears

Obtain a chest radiograph in the presence of tympanic membrane (TM) injury, since this may indicate exposure to significant overpressure. However, a patient with isolated

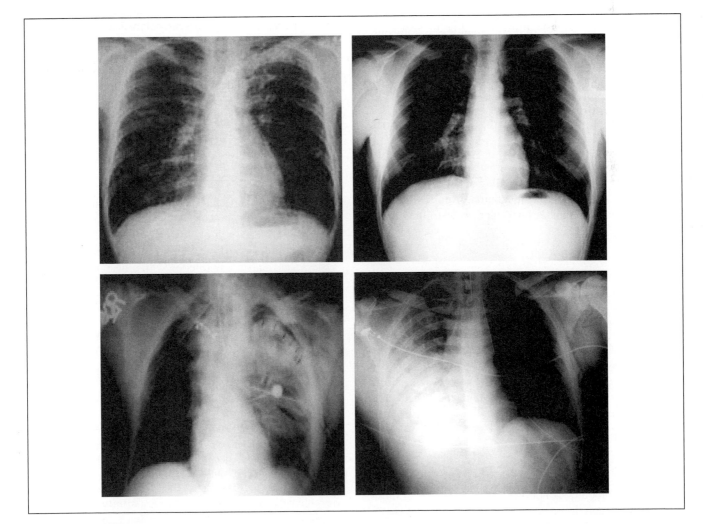

FIGURE 53-3

BLAST LUNG: RADIOLOGICAL PICTURE MAY CHANGE SIGNIFICANTLY
Source: Emergency Department, TelAviv Medical Center, Israel.

TM perforation but no other immediately identified injuries does not automatically require an extended period of observation. In a study by Leibovici, none of the 137 patients initially identified as having isolated TM rupture and well enough to be discharged developed later manifestation of pulmonary or intestinal blast injury. Conversely, intact TMs do not imply the absence of serious injury.

Abdomen

Abdominal injuries from explosions may be occult, and serial examinations are required. Reported rates are low. Air is a poor conductor of blast-wave energy, thus those who were subjected to enough energy to damage abdominal organs probably were situated near the explosive devices.

Neurological

The risk of air emboli to the brain exists and has been documented, but the likelihood of timely diagnosis in an MCI is small. Diagnosis is clinical (evidence of focal neurological lesions in the absence of direct brain trauma), funduscopy may theoretically reveal intra-arterial bubbles. Treatment consists of administration of 100% oxygen, hemodynamic support and, whenever feasible, emergent hyperbaric therapy.

Vascular

Shrapnel injuries may be very misleading. Small entry wounds may mask severe vascular and other damage. Careful assessment and documentation of pulses and perfusion in affected limbs is important, as is follow-up for delayed presentations.

Critical Resources

In this age of cost cutting and containment, just-in-time supplies are the norm and many hospitals have few supplies available beyond those required for the next few days of routine operations. Massive immediate needs and delayed supply capability may occur in an MCI, because many institutions demand the same type of equipment at the same time. However, a practical assessment of the immediate needs after an MCI indicates few special needs and fewer needs beyond any well functioning hospital's daily capability.

Blood

Surprisingly, blood does not often seem to be one of these limitations, though the situation may be changed by a single massive-transfusion casualty. Stocking blood for MCI is not feasible, but good communications with regional blood banks and the ability of such blood banks to rationalize distribution of their stocks to area hospitals is crucial. In-house ability to receive blood donations is useful, but may create issues of crowd control during the first few hours after the event.

Mechanical Ventilators

Critical injuries (usually indicating the need for mechanical ventilation) occur in 1–15% of casualties. Thus, in a 200-victim incident, up to 30 patients may need immediate mechanical ventilation and many more may need postoperative ventilatory support. Sufficient quantities of mechanical ventilators need to be planned for, either in the hospital or available rapidly from a nearby stock (e.g., county, state). Remember, that blast-injured patients require sophisticated mechanical ventilatory support and thus—ventilators. In our medical center we have trained 150 nonmedical staff (physiotherapists, radiology technicians, pharmacists, laboratory technicians, etc.) to bag-valve-endotracheal tube ventilate patients until mechanical ventilators become available. Training consists of 3 hours of didactics and manikin hands-on experience and a yearly refresher course, as well as participation in the hospital-wide drills.

Hepatitis B Active Vaccines

A stock of a few dozen ampoules is kept in the pharmacy or even ED. Cost is minimal.

CONCLUSION

The risk of encountering bomb-related trauma is increasing everywhere. A modern, well-prepared hospital should be able to provide high-quality care to many bomb-related victims simultaneously. Every hospital must have a plan, system, and staff ready to cope with a designated number and severity of casualties. Beyond that, a gradual degradation in the quality of care is to be expected. Only regional, state, and national systems working together may be able to cope with massive numbers of simultaneously generated casualties.

Suggested Reading

Arnold JL, Tsai MC, Halpern P, et al. Mass-casualty, terrorist bombings: epidemiological outcomes, resource utilization, and time course of emergency needs (Part I). *Prehospital Disaster Med.* 2003 Jul–Sep;18(3):220–34.

Drory M; Posen J, Vilner D, et al. An Israeli model of a hospital emergency information center. *Prehospital and Disaster Medicine.* 1999 Jan–Mar;14(1):13–16.

Einav S, Aharonson-Daniel L, Weissman C, et al. The Israel trauma group in-hospital resource utilization during multiple casualty incidents. *Ann Surg.* 2006;243:533–540.

Einav S, Feigenberg Zvi, Weissman C et al. Evacuation priorities in mass casualty terror-related events. Implications for contingency planning. *Annals of Surg.* 2004; (March); 239(3): 304–310.

Eshkol Z, Katz K. Injuries from biologic material of suicide bombers. *Injury.* 2005 Feb;36(2):271–4.

Halpern P, Tsai MC, Arnold JL, et al. Mass-casualty, terrorist bombings: implications for emergency department and hospital emergency response. *Prehospital Disaster Med.* 2003; 18:235–41.

Hirshberg A, Holcomb JB, Mattox KL. Hospital trauma care in multiple-casualty incidents: a critical view. *Ann Emerg Med.* 2001;37:647–52.

Leibovici D, Gofrit ON, Shapira SC. Eardrum perforation in explosion survivors: is it a marker of pulmonary blast injury? *Ann Emerg Med.* 1999 Aug;34(2):168–72.

Memorial Institute for the Prevention of Terrorism *(MIPT)* Terrorism Knowledge Base. *http://www.tkb.org/ ChartModule. jsp* Accessed Oct 14,2006.

RG DePalma, DG Burris, HR Champion, et al. Current concepts: blast injuries. *N Engl J Med.* 2005;352:1335–42.

Severance HW. Mass-casualty victim "surge" management. Preparing for bombings and blast-related injuries with possibility of hazardous materials exposure. *NCMJ.* 2002;63:242–246.

Singer AJ, Singer AH, Halperin P, et al. Medical lessons from terror attacks in Israel. *J Emerg Med* 2007 Jan; 32(1);87–92.

INTRODUCTION

The primary purpose of this section is to present to the reader the capabilities and associated agencies that exist beyond that of the hospital boundary for identification and limiting exposure/spread of such agents within a population. This is critical given a multidisciplinary approach is required for an effective response to an outbreak – planned or natural, or a terrorist release of a biological. Public health will become a key response partner from several perspectives: coordinating numerous agencies, communications, prophylaxis, surveillance and other services. Communications is usually an early victim in mass casualty events –introductions to, working with and understanding the critical response agencies beyond your health care facility, including who to call and when are essential. Understanding the lines of communication – from individual physicians, health care facilities or patients to public health organizations should be established as part of your facility preparedness planning to make the ultimate response more effective. Numerous other preparedness agencies will likely be called upon as well to collaborate. A familiarity with the roles, responsibilities and capabilities of these various agencies before an event is critical to successfully managing the event. Surveillance of disease through symptom recognition is a primary component of identification and may involve Emergency Departments, Poison Centers and Public Health Departments. Vaccine development has accelerated over the past decade, in large measure as a result of efforts by CDC and the Department of Health and Human Services (HHS), and is now looked upon as a key intervention in preventing the spread of biological agents – natural or planned, within a population. Public Health may play a pivotal role in mass vaccine implementation, providing primary prophylaxis as well as establish treatment and follow up centers if a biological event occurs. What follows is an introduction to the critical role public health may play and the potential assistance they may offer your facility as part of preparedness efforts.

54

POISON INFORMATION CENTERS

Michael S. Wahl and Jerrold B. Leikin

S T A T   F A C T S

POISON INFORMATION CENTERS

- Poison control centers are staffed primarily by health-care personnel who have received training in toxicology.
- In 2005, 2,424,180 human exposures were reported to the American Association of Poison Control Center Toxic Exposure Surveillance System by 61 poison control centers nationwide.
- Poison control centers can provide health-care professionals with treatment recommendations necessary to treat severely poisoned patients by chemical, biological, or radiation exposures.

In the early 1900s, toxicology was viewed as an esoteric field of medicine, was essentially ignored in medical schools, and not regarded as separate discipline. However, since 1953, when the first U.S. poison information hotline opened in Chicago, poison centers have emerged as an integral part of the nation's health-care system, and toxicology has developed into a recognized medical subspecialty.

As poison control centers began to flourish, The American Association of Poison Centers (AAPCC) was created in 1958 for the purpose of developing educational programs for health-care providers and, more importantly, standardizing the operation of poison control centers. The European Association of Poison Centers and Clinical Toxicology was formed in 1964. Currently, criteria for AAPCC designation as a regional poison control center include:

- A geographically defined region with a population base of 1–10 million people.

- Twenty-four hour a day availability to the general public and health-care providers.
- Written protocols to guide staff on triage criteria.
- The availability of specialists, including a medical director in toxicology, who have passed an AAPCC certifying examination.
- Regional data collection to be reported to Toxic Exposure Surveillance System (TESS) for identifying trends, epidemiology, and new and emerging poisoning hazards.
- Educational program for the general public and health-care professionals.

In the 1980s and 1990s, there was a marked decline in the number of poison control centers, from 107 in 1991 to 64 in 2003 in the United States (52 of which were certified by the AAPCC). An updated list of U.S. poison control centers can be obtained from the AAPCC website *www.aapcc.org,* while international poison centers can be accessed via *www.intox.org.* There are about 80 poison centers in Europe. Local poison centers can be accessed in the United States by a common phone number (800-222-1222). The United Kingdom's common number is 0870-600-6266.

TESS was developed in 1983 to function as a comprehensive toxicological database for the United States. Regulatory agencies along with industry rely on TESS data to monitor changes in regulations, packaging, and reformulation of drugs. Table 54-1 lists the standard data tables in each TESS tabular report. In 2005, the 61 regional poison centers responded to an average 8.2 human exposures per 1000 population served. Also in 2005, American poison centers reporting to the AAPCC's TESS system responded to 2,424,180 human exposures (with 1261fatalities) and there are over 40 million exposures totally in the TESS database. In addition to human exposure calls, poison centers also manage cases involving animal exposures, and supply information on poisons, poison prevention, drugs and drug identification, teratogenicity, as well as occupational, medical, and environmental concerns.

Beginning in March 2003, real-time active toxicosurveilliance of cases was initiated by all the U.S. poison centers (except for Puerto Rico). These cases are submitted within 20 minutes of occurrence and monitored by clinical toxicologists at AAPCC. Outliers are identified and additional information is thus obtained from the individual poison centers (Table 54-2). Surveillance currently centers on clinical effects that are suggestive for nerve agents, cyanide, arsenic, botulism, ricin, anthrax, irritant gasses, smallpox, arena virus, radiation and puffer fish ingestion. Recent enhancements to the system include GIS mapping

TABLE 54-1

STANDARD DATA TABLE IN EACH TESS REPORT

Acute vs. Acute-on-Chronic vs. Chronic
Reason
Exposure site
Exposure to multiple substances
Route of exposure
Distribution of clinical effects
Management site
Use of decontamination and therapeutic intervention
Decontamination (frequency distribution)
Other Therapies (frequency distribution)
Medical outcome
Duration of clinical effects by medical outcome
Age by gender
Reason by age categories (adults lumped)
Reason by age categories (adults in decades)
Clinical effects by age
Clinical effects by reason
Medical outcome by intentional vs. unintentional
Medical outcome by specific reasons
Medical outcome by management site
Reason by exposure chronicity
Management site by age
Treatment by management site
Decontamination by management site
Outcome by age categories (adults lumped)
Outcome by age categories (adults in decades)
Generic codes by category by age
Generic codes by category by reason
Generic codes by category by medical outcome
Generic codes by category by management site
Log of individual cases by medical outcome
Medical outcome by route of exposure

http://www.aapcc.org

TABLE 54-2

OUTLIERS IDENTIFIED FOR POTENTIAL PUBLIC HEALTH CONSEQUENCES

1. Significant increases in hourly call volume
2. Specific clinical effects
3. Carbon monoxide poisoning cases (daily)
4. Cases involving contaminated water
5. Food poisoning cases

and web-based software that will enable users to assess regional and national aggregate data.

Poison centers can also serve as a virtual information source following a biological event even if that event does not occur in the poison centers local area. For example, between October 4, 2001 and November 20, 2001, 22 cases of anthrax were identified on the eastern U.S. Coast. The Texas Poison Center received up to 31 anthrax calls daily during this period and over 500 such calls in the succeeding time period. Following a chlorine gas release in Bexar County in 2004, the first call into the Texas Poison Center Network was received about 35 minutes after the release with a total of 42 calls received over the next 10 days.

It is apparent that Poison Centers are in a unique position to monitor, validate and analyze information in a real-time capacity in order to recognize patterns, assess risk, and disseminate information. Certainly, the regional poison center is able to be the central resource for triage/treatment protocols along with accessing antidotes (and assessing antidotal supply) within its region.

Suggested Reading

Burda AM, Burda NM. The nations first poison control center: taking a stand against accidental childhood poisoning in Chicago: *Vet Hum Toxicol.* 1997;39:115–119.

Doyle CR, Akhtar J, Mrvos R, et al. Mass sociogenics illness— real and imaginary. *Vet Hum Toxicol.* 2004 Apr;46(2):93–5.

Forrester MB. Investigation of Texas poison center calls regarding a chlorine gas release: implications for terrorist attack toxicosurveillance, *Tex Med.* 2006:102:(5):52–57.

Forrester MB, Stanley SK. Call about anthrax to the Texas poison center network in relation to the anthrax bioterrorism attack in 2001. *Vet Hum Toxicol.* 2003 Oct;45(5):247–8.

Greenfield RA, Bronze MS. Symposium introduction: clinical aspects of terrorism. *J Okla State Med Assoc.* 2002 Sep; 95(9):583–6.

Harcock R. L., Koren G., Einarson. A., Unger W.J., The effectiveness of teratology information services (TTS). *Report Toxicol.* 2007:23:125–32

Hertzberg J. Disease registries for biologic and chemical terrorism. *Manag Care Interface.* 2001 Nov;14(11):58–9.

Klein KR, Herzog P., Smolinske, S., While Demand for Poisons control center Services "surged" during the 2003 blackout. *Clin Toxicol.* 2007: 45;248–5.

Krenzelok EP. The critical role of the poison center in the recognition, mitigation, and management of biological and chemical terrorism. *Prezegl Lek.* 2001;58(4):177–81.

LoVecchio R, Katz K, Watts D, et al. Media influence on poison center call volume after 11 September 2001. *Prehospital Disaster Med.* 2004 Apr–Jun;19(2):185.

Mathieu-Nolf M. The role of poison control centers in the protection of public health: changes and prespective. *Przegl Lek.* 2005;62(6):543–546

McFee RB, Leikin JB Kiernan K. Preparing for an era of weapons of mass destruction (WMD)—are we there yet? Why we should all be concerned. Part II. *Vet Hum Toxicol.* 2004;46(6):347–351.

Salem H. Issues in chemical and biological terrorism. *Int J Toxicol.* 2003 Nov–Dec;22(6):465–71.

Stewart CE. Chemical and biological warfare: improvisational agents. *Emerg Med Serv.* 2002 May;31(5):88–90.

Lai MW, Klein-Schwartz W, Rodgers GC, et al. 2005 Annual Report of the American Association of Poison Control Centers' national poisoning and exposure database, *Clin. Toxicol.* 2006:44:803–932.

Volans G.N. Karalliedde. L., Wiseman the Poisons Centers and the reporting of adverse drug events; the case for further development. *Drug Saf.* 2007:30(3);191–194.

Waring W.S., Palmer SR, Bateman D.N: Alerting and Surveillance Using Poisons Information Systems (ASPIS): Out comes from an International Working group. *Clin Toxicol.* 2007: 45(5):543–548

Young D. CDC Rolls Out Nerve-Agent Antidote Program. *Am J Health Syst Pharm.* 2004 Sep 15;61(18):1866–8, 1875.

55

BIOSURVEILLANCE

Michael Gillam, Craig Feied, Ed Barthell,
Mark Smith, and Jonathan Handler

STAT FACTS

BIOSURVEILLANCE

- National efforts are currently underway to coordinate surveillance efforts for chemical and biological agents exposure.
- Biosurveillance is most effective when data are shared across a region and if they can enhance early detection and intervention.
- Heterogenous data are needed for biosurveillance to be most effective.
- Combining environmental data with clinical data can be an efficacious approach.

INTRODUCTION

Communities throughout history have faced a continuing barrage of public health threats with the potential to cause catastrophic morbidity and mortality. In 1334, Hopei, a northeast province of China, was struck with an epidemic that would kill 90% of their population—almost 5 million people. This "Black Death" spread to Tartar forces at war with the Genoese. Before retreating, the Tartar forces, decimated by disease, catapulted plague-infested bodies into the sieged city of Kaffa. The Genoese quickly threw the bodies into the sea, but not quickly enough. Four Genoese trading ships brought the plague back to Italy and within 2 years, the plague would kill one-third of the European population. Today, we have antibiotics for the plague, but the risk for disease pandemics remains. Recent events, such as severe acute respiratory syndrome (SARS) and the anthrax attacks on the United States, have brought to the forefront of public consciousness the need for a coordinated system for surveillance and response.

National efforts are underway to coordinate national surveillance efforts for newly emerging diseases and agents of bioterrorism. These efforts fall into the realm of effort called biosurveillance whereas biothreat is the term given to the diseases and agents that are potential threats to public health.

A RECENT HISTORY OF BIOTHREATS

Recent events have focused the nation's attention on assessing the strength of the public health system to detect and respond to biothreats. Several specific recent incidents provide examples of how the current lack of an electronic network that allows data sharing between clinical caregivers and public health authorities is a problem, and how a future real time national surveillance system may be beneficial:

1. Milwaukee, WI, 1993—cryptosporidium contaminates regional water supplies causing significant morbidity and mortality over a period of months. Retrospective analysis of emergency records shows markedly increased numbers of diarrhea cases began weeks before the deaths but the problem was unrecognized.
2. Chicago, IL, 1995—a major summer heat wave leads to hundreds of deaths. A retrospective review suggests an emergency encounter surveillance system could have tipped off authorities of the impending disaster days in advance of the deaths.
3. Tokyo, Japan, 1995—Sarin gas chemical weapons attacks are perpetrated against the public. Most victims used private transportation to go to hospitals scattered across the region, where caregivers often had little or no understanding of the etiology of the symptoms they were trying to treat.

4. Hong Kong, China, 2003—World health leaders reported the emergence of a highly contagious respiratory disease naming it SARS. Case fatality rate would reach as high as 10%. Certain individuals infect vast numbers of people earning the name "super-spreaders." A single patient visiting a residential building, the Amoy Gardens, leads to 321 infected residents within 3–4 weeks. The epidemic spread quickly to health-care workers accounting for up to 65% of the SARS cases in Canada.

In 2001, while the nation faced biologic attacks with anthrax, emergency departments were inundated with patients. Cases ranged from credible exposures, to patients with worrisome symptoms but no clear exposure, to the worried well. Particularly challenging were patients with possible exposure risks and vague symptoms that could be attributed to common benign illness but could just as equally be the early signs of actual ominous disease. For some frontline physicians, the event was the beginning of the realization that emerging diseases, whether from bioterror agents or arising spontaneously in nature, could present like common disease, be initially misdiagnosed, and only be recognized after significant epidemiologic spread.

There is a close overlap between biosurveillance needs for emerging disease and bioterrorism. If SARS had become endemic in a war torn zone such as Iraq where infected insurgents could become vectors for biologic terrorism, the story of SARS containment could be quite different. The close overlap of biothreats and bioterrorism underscore the need to understand the diverse sources from which biothreats can emerge.

THE DIVERSE ORIGINS OF BIOTHREATS

The potential sources for biothreats are varied and range from newly emerging diseases range from the result of unintentional human activity to actual malevolence.

Newly emerging diseases, unchecked, can lead to pandemics of staggering mortality. In 1918, returning World War I veterans brought home to their countries, not only stories from the war, but the seeds for disease. The "Spanish flu" spread rapidly from soldiers to civilian populations propagated widely by the soldiers return to their home countries. The disease killed rapidly. Initially healthy victims could within hours die suffocating from their own respiratory secretions. With a mortality rate 25 times higher (2.5%) than previous influenza epidemics (0.1% mortality), the disease showed an unusual predilection for healthy young adults. Medical schools, public schools, and churches had to be closed. Third- and fourth-year medical students were put to work as physicians and nurses. Massive numbers of dead forced funerals to 15 minutes in length. The Spanish Flu killed 60 million people worldwide, including 675,000 Americans. The total number of deaths was 10 times higher than deaths attributable to combat casualties in World War I.

SARS had a mortality rate four times higher than the Spanish flu. That fact is a startling reminder that the risk of pandemics today is every bit as real today as it was in 1918.

Some public health threats emerge from human ignorance. In August of 2000, workers replacing old gas regulators in the greater Chicago area spilled mercury into homes resulting ultimately in forced inspections across 361,000 homes. Around 1361 homes had residential mercury contamination, some requiring evacuation of the inhabitants. The mass exposure was only uncovered after a resident of Mount Prospect, IL, happened to observe mercury spilled beneath a regulator. Other events have also been noted. In 1997, an unlicensed insect exterminator sprayed homes in the Chicago metropolitan area with methyl-parathion, an insecticide illegal for indoor use. Methyl-parathion can worsen respiratory symptoms such as asthma in children. It is unknown how many unrecognized exposures are occurring in civilian populations. Hundreds or thousands of patients could be, for years, appearing at various clinics with unusual symptoms from such exposures.

Human malevolence can also create threats to public health. In 1982, seven people in the Lake County community of Illinois died from mysterious causes. Their deaths were ultimately traced to cyanide-laced Tylenol tablets. Shortly after this event, Goody's headache powder was poisoned followed in 1986 by Lipton's cup of soup, Excedrin, and Tylenol (again); in 1991, Sudafed. The FBI has noted that over 53 poisonings have occurred in the Cook and Lake County regions of Illinois. Similar poisonings have occurred across the country. Given current world events and the global threat of terrorism, the risk of malevolent acts is even greater. Although the anthrax attacks of 1991 were not widespread, models of effectively orchestrated bioattacks suggest deaths could number in the thousands.

Few communities have automated "watchdog" surveillance systems to detect new biothreats, despite the significant risks. The frequency of these events and potentially preventable morbidity and mortality strongly suggest the need for systems and approaches to detect, alert, track, manage, and mitigate biothreats.

A DEFINITION OF BIOSURVEILLANCE AND BIOTHREATS

Biosurveillance has generally been defined as the effort to identify new or emerging threats to public health. As research on biosurveillance continues, it is increasingly being recognized that this definition should extend beyond simple detection. Biosurveillance may or may not be effective in initial detection in some situations, but the more important benefit may be an ability to provide ongoing assessment and management of biothreats once they have emerged. The aim of biosurveillance is therefore to promote early detection, maintain situational awareness, and facilitate rapid interventional responses aimed to improve public health outcomes. Biosurveillance efforts often focus on detecting events, which when analyzed across a cohort of practicing clinicians are detectible, but might not typically be noticed as abnormal by a single practicing clinician. Ongoing biosurveillance efforts provide the ability to measure whether a perceived threat is widespread and whether interventions are creating the desired effect.

Biothreats are defined as any event or process that can lead to morbidity and mortality in the human population. Biothreats can come in multiple forms including: biological agents (emerging disease like SARS, avian flu, West Nile virus, and anthrax); chemical agents (e.g., toxic spills and environmental contamination); and nuclear agents (e.g., dirty bomb attack, nuclear reactor meltdown).

THE NEED FOR EARLY INTERVENTION

Biothreats can have extremely early and narrow windows of opportunity for intervention. Models of diseases such as anthrax and smallpox suggest potential devastating impact on civilian populations without early interventions. Estimates from a model of 100,000 people exposed to a large-scale release of aerosolized anthrax spores indicated that a delay in detection of just *one hour could incur a cumulative cost of $200 million per hour during the peak days of exposure.* A delay of even one day with certain diseases such as smallpox can mean the "*difference between the loss and salvage of as much as 90% of an exposed population.*" The goal of biosurveillance is to detect a public health threat as early in the epidemiologic trajectory as possible in order to facilitate interventions to mitigate mortality and morbidity.

Biosurveillance efforts are likely to be more successful if they can facilitate early detection and intervention, enhancing the traditional reporting done by astute clinicians.

THE NEED FOR LOCAL, REGIONAL, AND NATIONAL COOPERATION FOR BIOSURVEILLANCE

Biosurveillance is most effective when data are shared across a region. Biothreats can present in manners that can only be detected when analyzed across a cohort of different physicians' patients and are not detectable statistically by the single practicing clinician. The death of a young patient noticed by a practicing clinician might not trigger concerns of a public health threat in even an "astute" clinician, especially if the cause is believed known. A cluster of five deaths across five different hospitals in young adults may, however, be an indication for something more ominous like a meningitis outbreak, contaminated drugs of abuse, or youth targeting influenza (similar to the Spanish flu).

Biosurveillance effectiveness is enhanced when participation is comprehensive, includes rural and urban centers, and inpatient and outpatient facilities. When the first SARS case presented in Hong Kong, a single admitted patient infected over 50 health-care workers in less than 1 week. No known, prevalent disease today matches such a level of virulence. With a mortality rate of up to 10%, undetected SARS in communities could be devastating. Because small regions can become seeding areas to global pandemics, *the need for biosurveillance systems in rural communities is just as high as in urban centers.*

Biosurveillance is more effective when retrospective data are available. The anomaly detection capability of surveillance systems is greatly affected by the amount of baseline data that are available. Short-term biosurveillance efforts using "drop-in" systems have found the lack of baseline patterns as a detrimental factor to their ability to detect anomalies by confounding detection thresholds. "Back-loading" biosurveillance systems with retrospective data should be a significant part of any effort.

Biosurveillance is a national public health priority that is most effective when it is comprehensive geographically, demographically, and historically. The United States may gain insight by study of comprehensive systems overseas. The Danish National Patient Registry contains information on all patient contacts with clinical hospital departments in Denmark, spanning emergency department visits, outpatient visits, admissions, and discharges, since 1977. The original purpose of the registry was to support health planning but the efforts have since expanded to include biosurveillance, research, and quality assurance. Increased funding in the United States to grow national repositories for biosurveillance could have dramatic benefits.

THE NEED FOR HETEROGENEOUS DATA INTEGRATION FOR BIOSURVEILLANCE

Heterogeneous data, beyond standard clinical data, are needed for biosurveillance efforts to be most effective. Potential high-yield sources of nonclinical data include: environmental data, zoonotic data, preclinical data, and surrogate markers of disease such as social upheavals and unrest.

Environmental Data in Biosurveillance

Combining environmental data with clinical data has the potential to avert public health disasters. In 1993, more than 400,000 cases of disease (including 54 deaths) occurred in a cryptosporidium outbreak that resulted from the contamination of the Milwaukee, WI, water supply. A contributing factor in the contamination was heavy rainfall and runoff that resulted in a decline in the quality of raw surface water arriving at the Milwaukee drinking water plant. Retrospective review has shown that biosurveillance systems could have potentially caught the outbreak much earlier. For more than a year before the outbreak, increasing water turbidity was associated with increasing rates of gastroenteritis. This finding suggests that waterborne cryptosporidiosis was occurring in Milwaukee for over a year before the large-scale outbreak. Another study shows that tracking the incidence of gastroenteritis cases alone through biosurveillance could have prevented 85% of the cases through earlier detection.

The "Coal Mine Canary" Approach to Biosurveillance

Zoonotic diseases are another potential source for data useful in biosurveillance. Up to 70% of newly emerging diseases are of zoonotic origin. The difference in presentation of disease between animals and humans can potentially be used to predict the arrival of a disease or biothreat to an area. For example, West Nile virus is more often fatal to horses and birds than human populations. Urban zoos noticed an increased frequency of dead birds on pavement paths in zoos before West Nile was recognized in human populations. Disease in animals can be a harbinger of biothreats to human. From 1911 to 1986, coal miners in order to detect dangerous gasses underground used canaries in cages. Mice were also used, but canaries were found preferable due to the detectable effect of even small amounts of carbon monoxide. Today, veterinary populations, livestock, zoological parks, insect vector surveillance, and other zoonotic disease sources can serve as the modern equivalent of the "Coal Miner's Canary"—an early warning system of an exigent biothreat.

Preclinical Data Sources

Public behavior can be an early indicator of emerging biothreats. Such behaviors include calls to regional poison control centers, nurse help lines, and water utility complaint lines; sales of over-the-counter (OTC) remedies; and school and work absenteeism. Of 31,000 calls to a poison center in the year 2000, 2.5% of calls (783) involved suspected foodborne illness or illness related to food ingestion. Calls to nurse help lines increased more than 17-fold during the 1993 Milwaukee cryptosporidiosis outbreak. Evidence suggests that surveillance of calls to water utility complaint lines could be useful. One study found up to 10% of the annual cases of gastrointestinal illness in France are related to consumption of tap water. OTC remedies have also been identified as potentially useful. There is a close correlation between physician-coded diagnoses of "influenza" and OTC sales of "flu" remedies. Sales of electrolyte products preceded hospital diagnoses of respiratory and diarrheal illness by an average of 1.7 weeks. Surveillance of pharmaceutical sales of antidiarrheal medication was used to draw the conclusion that an outbreak in Florida of 865 patient with gastrointestinal disease was

confined to the Greenville area. *Campylobacter jejuni* was isolated from 11 clinically ill patients. The researchers noted that "the city water plant, a deep well system, had numerous deficiencies including an unlicensed operator, a failure of chlorination, and open-top treatment towers. Birds were observed perching on the open-top treatment tower" with 37% found to harbor *C. jejuni*. The outbreak suggested that water systems that are unprotected from contact with birds may become sources for contamination with *Campylobacter*. Sales of other OTC remedies and prescription drugs have also been correlated to emerging disease. School and work absenteeism also correlate to disease in the community. Preclinical data sources can be a valuable adjunct to clinical data sources in biosurveillance.

Digital Media, Internet and Telecommunications Data Sources

Many diseases emerge in human populations within foreign countries. Millions of passengers travel from overseas into the United States each year. Project Argus is one example of an automated system to detect emerging disease in foreign countries. Using natural language processing software, the system scans thousands of overseas newspapers for warning signs of societal disruption. Such warning events include school closings, surges in refugees, increases in homelessness, riots for food, creation of quarantine zones, reports of disease, factory closings, and others. The identification of foreign countries in the midst of a biothreat event can serve as a trigger for biosurveillance in neighboring countries or for screening of passengers from those countries of origin.

The Need for "Actionable Knowledge"

The challenge of heterogeneous data is related to specificity. Using data that are chronologically earlier than specific diagnostic information often comes at the expense of specificity. A surge in OTC medication sales for Tylenol being used for headaches is likely not specific enough to identify an underlying viral meningitis epidemic in a community. In the absence of specificity, public health decisions are more challenging. "Unless it produces action, knowledge is overhead. Timeliness of data must be balanced with the requirement for 'actionable knowledge'."

Apart from heterogeneous data, flexible algorithmic methods of disease detection are needed. To accomplish this task, digital approaches are necessary.

BIOSURVEILLANCE AND MEDICAL INFORMATICS

To accomplish comprehensive surveillance efforts that integrate heterogeneous data that is demographically diverse, geographically disperse, and algorithmically flexible, digital systems for biosurveillance are necessary.

Use of Automated and Manual Data Collection Systems

Automated systems have several advantages over manual methods of data collection including timeliness and compliance. Automated systems can provide a substantial alerting timeliness advantage over traditional public health monitoring approaches. Automated methods can exceed the speed of human effort for compiling and analyzing data. Where available, reuse of existing data that can be scavenged from other systems can avoid failure modes in manual data collection. Manual data collection methods can be hampered by noncompliance, particularly if data collection changes workflows for caregivers and there is inadequate coaching and training surrounding the process change. During the SARS outbreak, some communities were able to collect data by implementing new processes. However, a study at Northwestern University on volunteer SARS screening during the epidemic by triage nurses found compliance to be less than 0.1% in the computer system despite the system being designed to require only a single mouse click by the users within the existing triage data entry page.

When using automated systems, systems with flexible data structures are highly desirable. Surveillance systems that could be easily linked with laboratory data and are flexible in adding new variables have been found most useful. Though manual methods of data collection have been shown to lose momentum and can fail to capture data adequately, they can be particularly effective for "drop in" surveillance for short-term sporting events or public gatherings.

The "Doctrine of Daily Routine"

When implementing manual methods for data collection, it is prudent to adhere to the "*doctrine of daily routine.*" This doctrine states that in the face of confusion, people generally do what they know and what they do regularly. New workflow patterns required only during disasters or biothreats (such as special steps to be taken or data to be collected) will often be forgotten, or ignored. Data that can be collected as the natural product of routine workflow or routine patient care is most likely to be effective. Adhering to the *doctrine of daily routine* can improve the likelihood of successful data capture in systems requiring manual data capture.

"GOLD STANDARD" VERSUS "SYNDROMIC" SURVEILLANCE

Biosurveillance aims to identify both known and unknown types of biothreats. To this end, two categories of surveillance are possible. In traditional disease surveillance, or "gold standard surveillance," a gold standard model of disease detection is applied to determine the frequency and distribution of a known disease. Such approaches are useful in detecting and tracking outbreaks of *Neisseria meningitis* through cerebrospinal fluid cultures, or West Nile virus through serologic testing. In contrast, "syndromic surveillance" aims to identify diseases for which presentation patterns and clinical appearance might not be known. Syndromic surveillance categorizes patient's symptoms into syndromes meant to represent a particular physiologic manifestation of a set of diseases. There is no universally agreed standard syndromic set for biosurveillance, but often these syndromes include such categories as "gastrointestinal symptoms" or "rash with fever," and so on. The effective balance between these approaches for optimal biosurveillance remains a matter of research and debate.

CURRENT EFFORTS IN BIOSURVEILLANCE

The following are an overview of current national efforts in biosurveillance. This alphabetic list is not meant to be fully inclusive, but rather broadly representative of the types of activities that are occurring.

BioSense is a project sponsored by the Centers for Disease Control aimed to aggregate data of potential public health significance to support early detection, quantification, and localization of biothreats events. The intent is to collect structured, standardized data from hospitals and health-care systems in major metropolitan cities across the nation, connecting existing health information to public health in a way not previously possible. The goal is to provide the immediate, constant, and comparable information needed to inform local, state, and national public health and to support national preparedness.

EMSystem is a regional emergency medicine Internet (REMI) application used for communication and incident management during disasters and biothreats. Hospitals, health departments, and emergency medicine providers use the system to manage incidents affecting over 34% of the population of the United States (over 100 million patient lives.) The system supports bidirectional communication between frontline clinical providers and health departments for rapid event notification and data collection during disaster and biothreat incidents using unstructured flexible web-based forms. REMIs of this type can permit rapid deployment of new syndromic surveillance approaches across widely disparate jurisdictions.

Early notification of community-based epidemics (ESSENCE) uses syndromic and nontraditional health information to facilitate detection of biothreats in the National Capital Area (NCA). Clinical data sets include emergency room syndromes, private practice ICD-9 codes grouped into syndromes, and veterinary syndromes. Nonclinical data include school absenteeism, calls to nursing hotlines, frequency of prescribed medications, and veterinary syndromes. Temporal and spatial analysis tools are provided through secure Internet Web sites.

The Frontlines of Medicine is a consensus-based data exchange standard developed by emergency physicians for exchange of surveillance-related data generated during emergency triage. The standard is XML-based, open-standards compliant, and nonproprietary.

The National Emergency Encounter Registry (NEER) is an effort through the American College of Emergency Physicians to create a national registry of emergency department visits for cross-institutional quality metric comparisons and biosurveillance. The National Biosurveillance Testbed (NBT) is a sister effort to create a widely heterogeneous, research quality repository for use by scientists to discover new methods for biosurveillance.

The National Retail Data Monitor (NRDM) collects sales data from over 15,000 retail stores and makes them available to public health officials. The project aims to serve as a national data utility for public health surveillance.

The Real-time Outbreak and Disease Surveillance (RODS) system is an open-source biosurveillance system utilizing ED chief complaint data across over 200 EDs to categorize patients into seven syndromic categories. The system integrates time-series detection algorithms to trigger electronic alarms to researchers and public health physicians.

Multiple other efforts to develop biosurveillance systems are underway across the country. In 2005, the International Society for Disease Surveillance was launched, with a mission to improve population health by advancing the field of disease surveillance. The society provides an education and scientific forum where stakeholders can collaborate to advance the field. Healthy People 2010 is also one of many national calls for improved surveillance systems as a key objective in the nation's pursuit of improved health status for its citizens.

FUTURE OF BIOSURVEILLANCE

The most significant improvements in biosurveillance in the next decade will emerge from improved use of information technologies. Areas with the great potential for impact will likely include improved local, regional, and national data sharing to create automated "weather maps" of disease; and the development of evidence-based public health responses to outbreaks.

Today, rainfall predictions and pollen counts are easily available from the broadcast news, newspapers, or the Internet. Health-care practitioners practice with relatively static mental models of the world. These models are encapsulated with such clinical phrases as "this is the flu season" or "this is the croup season." Local and regional "weather maps of disease" could create an environment where health-care decision-making is placed into a more dynamic context.

Automated regional "weather maps of disease" could substantially impact the quality of delivered care. Knowing when regional hospitals have found more frequent cases of bacterial meningitis could decrease local provider's threshold of performing lumbar punctures on children with fevers and a headache, or change the frequency of ordered tests.

Preemptive public health interventions to impact a region become possible with widespread data sharing. In 1992, McDonald et al. demonstrated that computer-generated reminders to administer influenza vaccine were able to blunt the regional peak incidence of influenza. As regional and national data sharing grows, the possibilities of early intervention into growing epidemics could dramatically shift the epidemiologic trajectory of disease and improve public health outcomes.

Biosurveillance efforts aim to prevent everything from the spread of disease in a local neighborhood to preventing the next great pandemic. Ironically, the greatest evidence of biosurveillance success in the future will be events that never happen.

Suggested Reading

Andersen TF, Mellemkjoer L, Olsen JH. The Danish National Hospital Register: a valuable source of data for modern health sciences. *Dan Med Bull.* 1999 Jun;46(3):263–8.

Barthell EN, Aronsky D, Cochrane DG, et al., Frontlines Work Group. The Frontlines of Medicine Project progress report: standardized communication of emergency department triage data for syndromic surveillance. *Ann Emerg Med.* 2004 Sep;44(3):247–52.

Barthell EN, Cordell WH, Moorhead JC, et al. The Frontlines of Medicine Project: a proposal for the standardized communication of emergency department data for public health uses including syndromic surveillance for biological and chemical terrorism. *Ann Emerg Med.* 2002 Apr;39(4):422–9.

Beaudeau P, Payment P, Bourderont D, et al. A time series study of anti-diarrheal drug sales and tap water quality. *Int J Environ Health Res.* 1999;9:293–311.

Berger M, Shiau R, Weintraub JM. Review of syndromic surveillance: implications for waterborne disease detection. *J Epidemiol Community Health.* 2006 Jun;60(6):543–50.

Bradley CA, Rolka H, Walker D, Loonsk J. BioSense: implementation of a National Early Event Detection and Situational Awareness System. *MMWR.* 2005 Aug 26;54 Suppl:11–9.

British Broadcasting Company. 1986: Coal Mine Canaries made Redundant. *http://news.bbc.co.uk/onthisday/hi/dates/stories/december/30/newsid_2547000/2547587.stm* Accessed: July 2, 2006.

Burkom HS, Elbert Y, Feldman A, et al., Centers for Disease Control and Prevention (CDC). Role of data aggregation in biosurveillance detection strategies with applications from ESSENCE. *MMWR.* 2004 Sep 24;53 Suppl:67–73.

California Department of Food & Agriculture. *http://www.cdfa.ca.gov/ahfss/ah/wnv_info.htm* Accessed: July 2, 2006.

Centers for Disease Control and Prevention (CDC). Strength training among adults aged >/=65 years—United States, 2001. *MMWR.* 2004 Jan 23;53(2):25–8.

Cho J, Kim J, Yoo I, et al. Syndromic surveillance based on the emergency department in Korea. *J Urban Health*. 2003;80: i124.

Collmann J. Project Argus. Georgetown U niversity ISIS Center. *http://www.advamed.org/policy/hit/collmann30905.pdf* Access date: July 2, 2006.

Davies GR, Finch RG. Sales of over-the-counter remedies as an early warning system for winter bed crises. *Clin Microbiol Infect*. 2003 Aug;9(8):858–63.

Department of Health, Hong Kong Special Administrative Region, People's Republic of China. Outbreak of severe acute respiratory syndrome (SARS) at Amoy Gardens, Kowloon Bay, Hong Kong—main findings of the investigation. Hong Kong: Department of Health, Hong Kong SAR, 2003. (*http://www. info.gov.hk/info/ap/pdf/amoy_e.pdf*). Access date: October 25, 2003.

Derby MP, McNally J, Ranger-Moore J, et al. Poison control center-based syndromic surveillance for foodborne illness. *MMWR*. 2005 Aug 26;54 Suppl:35–40.

Eisenberg JN, Lei X, Hubbard AH, et al. The role of disease transmission and conferred immunity in outbreaks: analysis of the 1993 Cryptosporidium outbreak in Milwaukee, Wisconsin. *Am J Epidemiol*. 2005 Jan 1;161(1):62–72.

Eisenberg JN, Seto EY, Colford JM, et al. An analysis of the Milwaukee cryptosporidiosis outbreak based on a dynamic model of the infection process. *Epidemiology*. 1998 May; 9(3):255–63.

Foldy S, Biedrzycki PA, Barthell EN, et al. Syndromic surveillance using regional emergency medicine internet. *Ann Emerg Med*. 2004 Sep;44(3):242–6.

Foldy SL, Barthell E, Silva J, et al. SARS Surveillance Project: Internet-enabled multiregional surveillance for rapidly emerging disease. *MMWR*. 2004;53(Suppl):215–20.

Foldy SL, Barthell EN, Silva JC, et al. SARS surveillance project: Internet-enabled multi-region syndromic surveillance for rapidly emerging disease. *MMWR*. September 9, 2004;53 (Suppl RR).

Gillam, Feied, Handler. The National Emergency Encounter Registry (NEER). SAEM Academic Informatics Section Presentation, New York City, NY. May, 2005

Graham J, Buckeridge D, Choy M, et al. Conceptual heterogeneity complicates automated syndromic surveillance for bioterrorism. *Proc AMIA Annu Fall Symp*. 2002:1030.

Handler J, Feied C, Gillam M. The National Biosurveillance Testbed. Emergency Department Information System 9th Annual Symposium Pennsylvania ACEP. 2004.

Henig, Robin Marantz. *Flu Pandemic: Once and Future Menace*. New York Times Magazine, November 19, 1992.

Ho AS, Sung JJ, Chan-Yeung M. An outbreak of severe acute respiratory syndrome among hospital workers in a community hospital in Hong Kong. *Ann Intern Med*. 2003 Oct 7; 139(7):564–7.

Hogan WR, Tsui FC, Ivanov O, et al, Indiana-Pennsylvania-Utah Collaboration. Detection of pediatric respiratory and diarrheal outbreaks from sales of over-the-counter electrolyte products. *J Am Med Inform Assoc*. 2003 Nov–Dec;10(6): 555–62.

Hryhorczuk D, Persky V, Piorkowski J, et al. Residential mercury spills from gas regulators. *Environ Health Perspect*. 2006 Jun;114(6):848–52.

Lapinsky SE, Granton JT. Critical care lessons from severe acute respiratory syndrome. *Curr Opin Crit Care*. 2004 Feb;10(1): 53–8.

Lombardo J, Burkom H, Elbert E, et al. A systems overview of the Electronic Surveillance System for the Early Notification of Community-Based Epidemics (ESSENCE II). *J Urban Health*. 2003 Jun;80(2 Suppl 1):i32–42.

MacKenzie WR, Schell WL, Blair KA, et al. Massive outbreak of waterborne cryptosporidium infection in Milwaukee, Wisconsin: recurrence of illness and risk of secondary transmission. *Clin Infect Dis*. 1995 Jul;21(1):57–62.

Magruder SF, Lewis SH, Najmi A, et al, Centers for Disease Control and Prevention (CDC). Progress in understanding and using over-the-counter pharmaceuticals for syndromic surveillance. *MMWR*. 2004 Sep 24;53 Suppl:117–22.

McDonald CJ, Hui SL, Tierney WM. Effects of computer reminders for influenza vaccination on morbidity during influenza epidemics. *MD Comput*. 1992 Sep–Oct;9(5):304–12.

Okumura T, Suzuki K, Fukuda A, et al. The Tokyo subway sarin attack: disaster management, Part 2: hospital response. *Acad Emerg Med*. 1998;5:618–24.

Osaka K, Takahashi H, Ohyama T. Testing a symptom-based surveillance system at high-profile gatherings as a preparatory measure for bioterrorism. *Epidemiol Infect*. 2002 Dec;129 (3): 429–34.

Personal correspondence. Illinois Poison Center. 2003.

Personal Correspondence. Lincoln Park Zoologic Conservatory. 2004

Petzinger, Thomas Jr. Wall Street Journal. *http://picardmarketing. com/survey/* Accessed: March 15, 2005.

Population and Public Health Branch (PPHB), Health Canada. Summary of severe acute respiratory (SARS) cases: Canada and International. *http:// www.hc-sc.gc.ca/pphb-dgspsp/sars-sras/eu-ae/sars20030501_e.html* Accessed: May 1, 2003.

Proctor ME, Blair KA, Davis JP. Surveillance data for waterborne illness detection: an assessment following a massive waterborne outbreak of cryptosporidium infection. *Epidemiol Infect*. 1998;120:43–54.

Rodman JS, Frost F, Jakubowski W. Using nurse hot line calls for disease surveillance. *Emerg Infect Dis*. 1998 Apr–Jun;4(2): 329–32.

Rydman RJ, Rumoro DP, Silva JC, et al. The rate and risk of heat related illness in hospital emergency departments during the 1995 Chicago heat disaster. *J Med Systems*. 1999;23:41–56.

Sacks JJ, Lieb S, Baldy LM, et al. Epidemic campylobacteriosis associated with a community water supply. *Am J Public Health*. 1986 Apr;76(4):424–8.

Scott Evans, Ken Kleinman, Marcello Pagano. Statistics in Defense and National Security: Bioterrorism and Biosurveillance. Harvard University. *http://www.amstat.org/sections/ sdns/amstat4.pdf* Accessed: July 1, 2006.

Taylor LH, Latham SM, Woolhouse MEJ. Risk factors for human disease emergence. Philosophical Transactions—Royal Society of London Series B Biological Sciences. 2001;356 (1411):983–990.

Testimony of Peter H. Morris to US Senate Committee on Appropriations. February 2, 2002 *http://appropriations. senate.gov/releases/record.cfm?id=180450* Accession Date: July 3, 2006.

Tsui FC, Wagner MM, Dato V, et al. Value of ICD-9 coded chief complaints for detection of epidemics. *Proc AMIA Symp.* 2001:711–5.

Tsui FC, Espino JU, Dato VM, et al. Technical description of RODS: a real-time public health surveillance system. *J Am Med Inform Assoc.* 2003 Sep–Oct;10(5):399–08.

Wagner MM, Tsui FC, Espino JU, et al. The emerging science of very early detection of disease outbreaks. *J Public Health Manag Pract.* 2001;7:51–9.

Wagner MM, Tsui FC, Espino J, et al, Centers for Disease Control and Prevention (CDC). National Retail Data Monitor for public health surveillance. *MMWR.* 2004 Sep 24;53 Suppl:40–2.

Wong TW. An outbreak of SARS among healthcare workers. *Occup Environ Med.* 2003 Jul;60(7):528.

Wong W, Moore AW, Cooper G, et al. Rule-based anomaly pattern detection for detecting disease outbreaks. Presented at the 18th National Conference on Artificial Intelligence (AAAI-02), 2002.

Zelicoff A, Brillman J, Forslund DW, et al. The Rapid Syndrome Validation Project (RSVP). *Proc AMIA Symp.* 2001:771–5.

56

VACCINES

Susan Shoshana Weisberg

VACCINES

- Neither smallpox, anthrax, nor botulinum vaccines are currently commercially available for general use in the United States.
- Smallpox vaccine has a poorer safety profile than any vaccine currently in routine use in the United States.
- Smallpox vaccination is helpful both pre- and postexposure.
- Smallpox vaccine has many contraindications for routine use, but the disease has such a high mortality rate that in the event of widespread exposures and outbreaks, there may be no absolute contraindications.
- Research has shown the effectiveness of diluted, smaller smallpox vaccine doses that would greatly stretch available vaccine supplies.
- Previous experience has shown the effectiveness of isolation and ring immunization in stopping smallpox outbreaks.
- The anthrax vaccine has a favorable safety profile.
- Anthrax vaccination is useful for both pre- and postexposure prophylaxis.
- Both active and passive forms of botulism protection exist. The role of antitoxin administration for postexposure prophylaxis in asymptomatic people has yet to be defined, but antitoxin has proven beneficial when given quickly to patients with early signs of botulism.

SMALLPOX VACCINATION

The History of Smallpox Vaccination and Vaccine Development

No one knows exactly when or where attempts to immunize people against smallpox began. Legend has it that centuries ago the Chinese Prime Minister Wang Tan consulted a

Tibetan Buddhist nun as to how to protect his precious last son after losing all his other children to smallpox. The nun told him to blow smallpox scabs up the boy's nostrils. It worked, and when the nun returned to the mountains, she was worshipped by other women as the "Goddess of Smallpox." Aged or powdered smallpox scabs were delivered into susceptible people's nostrils in China through tubes. Donors were smallpox survivors whose infections had been relatively benign. In India, fluid from smallpox pustules or scabs was also scratched into susceptible people's skin. This process of inducing smallpox immunity via deliberate but hopefully mild infection was called "variolation." It was described as early as 590 BC in the Sung Dynasty, and is also recorded in early Sanskrit texts. It was performed by a variety of different healers in Africa and Eurasia centuries before Edward Jenner's famed 1796 smallpox work. In the early 1700s, variolation was introduced to western nations when Lady Mary Montegu, wife of the British Ambassador to Constantinople, heard about its use in the Ottoman Court. Lady Montegu was particularly interested in smallpox prevention after losing her brother to the disease. She herself survived infection but was left disfigured by severe facial scarring and the loss of her eyelashes. Lady Mary Montague had her children inoculated (the first without her husband's knowledge), and the news spread. In researching variolation, the British royal family gave leniency to prisoners in exchange for participation in their "Royal Experiment." Up to 3% of people died of smallpox after being variolated, but as of 1717 in Boston, the death rate among people who had undergone variolation was only one-sixth the rate of those who were left susceptible. Edward Jenner himself was variolated as a child. In 1775, General George Washington agonized over whether or not to immunize his Revolutionary War troops with an imperfect smallpox vaccine. After smallpox in his troops contributed to military defeat in his Canadian campaign, General Washington ordered vaccination of susceptible soldiers at Valley Forge.

The connection between cowpox and smallpox was evidenced by the first known oral vaccine. Around 1700, in China, a pill of fleas from cows was used to prevent smallpox. In agricultural, rural European and Mexican communities, it was common knowledge for centuries that previous cowpox infection protected milkmaids from smallpox. The next link came when Englishman Dr Fewster reported to the Medical Society of London that people with a history of cowpox failed to react to variolation. Later in the eighteenth century, at least two individuals, a British farmer and a schoolmaster, preceded Edward Jenner in using cowpox to vaccinate against smallpox. Unfortunately, in each instance, severe inflammation ensued. The farmer's wife almost lost her arm, and the daughter of the schoolmaster's employer suffered extreme swelling of her hand. The novice researchers were frightened away from further trials. Dr Edward Jenner, an English country doctor, had better success inoculating with animal pox to prevent smallpox. In 1790, he tried it out on his own son and a few others, later challenging them with variolation. He then began inoculating extracts from human cowpox lesions directly from person to person. In 1796, Jenner inoculated an 8-year-old with cowpox. Variolation 6 weeks later produced no response, demonstrating immunity to smallpox. The term "vaccination" is derived from the Latin word for cow, honoring the bovine origin of the smallpox vaccine.

The History of Smallpox Vaccine Use

Within a decade, Jenner's vaccine was used throughout the world. By 1801, over 100,000 Englishmen had been vaccinated with Jenner's vaccine. Within 15 years, 1.7 million Frenchmen and 2 million Russians were also vaccinated. In the United States, the first American vaccinated was the 5-year-old son of Dr Benjamin Waterhouse, in 1800. Dr Waterhouse appealed to the then president Thomas Jefferson for approval for promoting smallpox vaccination. Jefferson studied the issue, became a vaccine expert, and supported vaccination efforts from the White House. The older variolation was outlawed in Britain in 1840 by an act of Parliament. In 1853, another such act required smallpox vaccination of the entire British population. The "vaccinia" virus that replaced the original cowpox used in smallpox vaccination is of uncertain origin. Vaccinia is a laboratory virus with no known natural host. It is an orthopox virus, but with a genome different from either smallpox or modern cowpox. It may be a derivative of horsepox, which disappeared in the late 1800s. Multiple strains of vaccinia virus exist.

In the 1940s, researcher Leslie Collier of the Lister Institute took Jenner's work a step forward in developing techniques for producing heat-stable, freeze-dried vaccines that withstood storage for years. Another advance came when Dr Benjamin Rubin, experimenting with sewing needles in the early 1960s, invented the bifurcated smallpox needle. Dr Rubin's needle allowed the efficient delivery of tiny amounts of smallpox vaccine. By 1980, when the world was declared smallpox free, about 2.4 billion doses of smallpox vaccine had been used worldwide in global elimination programs. As the risk of indigenous smallpox fell, recommendations for routine smallpox vaccination for the general population were withdrawn by the United States Public Health Service in 1971. After 1976, American health-care workers were no longer vaccinated, and after 1982, recommendations for international travelers were likewise changed. Military use of the vaccine ceased in 1990. Between then and 2001, only laboratory workers in contact with related orthopox viruses were immunized. After terrorist attacks in 2001, the United States reinstituted smallpox vaccination in selected military personnel and civilian workers most likely to be exposed to the virus if it were used as a bioterror weapon.

In the absence of actual, confirmed smallpox cases or exposures, immunization is a military and not a medical decision. The risk of indigenous smallpox in the United States is essentially zero. In the United States, our last smallpox case was in 1949. Worldwide, the last case of community-acquired smallpox was in Somalia in 1977. If smallpox reappears now, it will be most likely as a deliberate act of war. And given the risks of smallpox vaccination, if Americans are offered the immunization it will most likely be as part of a public health program instead of as an elective vaccine given by private physicians.

Over 200 years since Edward Jenner's experiments using live cowpox germs to purposefully infect people and induce an immunity that crossed over to provide them with smallpox protection, not much has really changed. Our "modern" smallpox vaccine is basically more of the same—a live "vaccinia" virus vaccine. The smallpox vaccine licensed in the United States is manufactured by Wyeth Laboratories, and is a lyophilized preparation made from calf lymph with seed vaccinia virus from the New York City Board of Health strain of vaccinia virus. It has a minimum of 100 million pock-forming units per milliliter. Research on macaques and monkeypox seem to indicate that protection from the vaccine is B cell mediated. After vaccination, over 95% of people being smallpox immunized for the first time develop neutralizing or hemagglutination inhibition antibody titers $\geq 1:10$. The antibody response to smallpox vaccination is genus-specific and cross-protective for other orthopox viruses such as monkeypox and cowpox. Protection from the smallpox vaccine begins soon after vaccination. If given within the first few days after an actual exposure to smallpox germs, it will prevent or lessen smallpox disease. As late as 5 days into smallpox's 12–14-day incubation period, vaccination offers some protective benefit.

Smallpox Vaccine Administration

The vaccinia virus vaccine is administered intradermally by puncturing it into the skin over the arm. A double-pointed, "bifurcated" needle that holds a droplet of the vaccine is perpendicularly jabbed into but not through the skin 15 times, within a 5-mm diameter area, evoking a trace of blood after 15–30 seconds. The skin at the immunization site should not be cleansed first as doing so will lessen the effectiveness of the vaccine. After vaccination, the Centers for Disease Control and Prevention (CDC) now recommends that the site be kept covered until a scab is formed. It is further recommended that before discarding them, shed scabs and used bandages should be placed in plastic zip bags. Newly vaccinated people should also be instructed not to touch, rub, or scratch their vaccination site, and to separately launder their clothing and bedding. A successful result from injection with the live vaccinia virus immunization is a localized infection from it. The desired response to smallpox vaccination, that is, to the injection of vaccinia virus, is a pimple at the site that progresses to a blister and then a pustule in 8–10 days. By 2–3 weeks, a scab should have formed and shed, leaving a scar. If there is no local reaction or infection, the vaccine is considered a failure in that recipient, and they should be given another dose.

Side Effects of Smallpox Vaccination

Besides the scar, which anyone who has been successfully immunized against smallpox should be left with, there are many other side effects of smallpox vaccination (see Table 56-1).

There are also rare allergic reactions to the smallpox vaccine, either immediately or up to 10 days later. Treatment for other complications of smallpox vaccination is with vaccinia immunoglobulin, fractionated from the plasma of people previously smallpox vaccinated.

In America, during the 2003 smallpox immunization campaign for military workers and civilian first responders, there were 16 cases of heart attacks, 3 fatal, within weeks after vaccination. The CDC reported that its analysis showed a "growing body of evidence suggesting that" those heart attacks "might have been unrelated to vaccine." An analysis of civilian vaccinees concluded that the rate of ischemic cardiac events, including sudden death, "does not appear to be greater than expected in a comparable, nonvaccinated population." On a larger scale, the same smallpox shots were given to 6 million New Yorkers in 1947. That mass immunization campaign was followed by no increase in cardiac deaths.

Regarding neurological adverse events following smallpox vaccination, analysis of data from the 2003 American smallpox immunization program showed no increased rates of any serious events, including Guillain-Barre syndrome, Bell's palsy, or encephalitis, in excess of baseline expected estimates.

Because the vaccinia immunization is a live virus vaccine that works by causing an active infection, it can also cause infection, and therefore side effects, in people who are not actual vaccine recipients but simply contacts of others who were recently immunized. People with immune system impairment or underlying health problems such as human immunodeficiency virus (HIV) are at greatest risk

TABLE 56-1

OVERALL ADVERSE EVENT RATES AFTER SMALLPOX VACCINATION

Adverse Event Following Smallpox Vaccination	Incidence per Number of Vacinees
Fever >100°F for 1 or more days, starting Up to 4–14 days after vaccination	7:10 children
Fever higher than 102°F	up to 1:5 children
Autoinnoculation of vaccinia virus infection to other sites, including the eye	1:1900
"Generalized vaccinia," most often concentrated on the trunk that can cause scarring. It is usually self-limited, but sometimes recurs in 4–6 week cycles for up to a year	1:2500 in infants <1 year old 1:5000 for older recipients
"Eczema vaccinatum," a severe skin infection by the vaccine virus that affects people with eczema, active or healed, that can be fatal, or result in severe scarring	1:26,000
"Progressive vaccinia," a severe reaction that starts as sloughing of the skin at the vaccination site and spreads to other areas and can be fatal	1:313,000 in infants <1 year old 1:667,000 overall
Vaccinia encephalitis	1:23,000 in infants <1 year old 1:81,000 overall
Death from vaccination	1:1,000,000

for "contact" vaccinia, as are children less than 5 years of age. Up to one-third of eczema vaccinatum cases occur as a result of contact spread. Overall, for every million smallpox vaccines given, there are at least 27 contact infections.

Almost three decades after immunization of American health-care workers was stopped, the CDC resumed vaccinating civilians against smallpox in January 2002 in response to concerns about use of the germ as a terrorist weapon. A half-million military personnel were immunized, and it was planned to vaccinate as many civilian health-care workers, followed by another 10 million other public safety responders. Within 6 months, state health department directors were asking to slow things down after the first 37,000 civilian vaccinations. Work proceeded, however, on planning for mass population immunization programs if the need should arise. By March 2004, smallpox shots had been given to approximately 665,000 military and civilian workers, 435,000 of whom were first-time vacinnees. The programs were monitored, and adverse events were investigated. See Table 56-2 for combined published adverse event data from the 2003 campaigns.

No deaths have been reported from smallpox immunization in the military since 1943. Spread of the smallpox vaccine germ to contacts of recipients occurred 30 times from the 578,000 doses given in the military between 2002 and 2004. In two of the cases, the transfer was via an unvaccinated "secondary" contact to a third party. As a special precautionary measure, the Food and Drug Administration (FDA) now calls for a 3-week waiting period after vaccination before recipients can donate blood.

T A B L E   5 6 - 2

COMBINED PUBLISHED RATES OF TEMPORALLY ASSOCIATED ADVERSE EVENTS FOLLOWING SMALLPOX VACCINATION DURING THE 2003 AMERICAN VACCINATION CAMPAIGN

Adverse Event Following Smallpox Vaccination	Incidence per Number of Vaccinees
Generalized vaccinia	1:12,550
Inadvertent autoinoculation of vaccinia from the vaccination site to other body locations	1:8440 to 1:5555
Ocular vaccinia	1:12,000 to 1:37,660
Myocarditis and/or pericarditis	1:7777 to 1:8440
Encephalitis or encephalomyelitis	1:221,666 to 1:489,500
Fever	up to 1:20
Headache, muscle aches	up to 1:5
Body rash	up to 1:12
Local rash, itching	up to 2:3
Superinfection of the vaccination site or regional lymph notes	1:19,000

There have been about 50 cases where women who were smallpox vaccinated while pregnant, or within a month of conception, gave birth to infants with evidence of harm from the vaccinia virus. Three of those cases occurred in the United States, in 1924, 1959, and 1968. The results in these cases of "fetal vaccinia" have included skin scars, internal organ damage, and "often" death. For the strain of vaccinia used to make the smallpox vaccine now in use in America, the risk of fetal vaccinia has been calculated to be one case per 90,000–280,000 pregnant women immunized. Between 2001 and 2003, there were 103 American women smallpox vaccinated who were either pregnant at the time, or who conceived within 4 weeks. No harm has been documented in those cases, but monitoring is ongoing. Elective smallpox immunization during pregnancy is still not recommended, and vaccinated women are advised to avoid conceiving within the next month.

In the United States, there are about 120 million people born after smallpox vaccination was stopped. The other 155 million residents were vaccinated before 1971. Small studies found good results when previously immunized adults were revaccinated with smallpox shots diluted to less than a tenth the normal dose. Also using diluted, partial vaccine doses, another small study found good results immunizing never vaccinated people, which would stretch vaccine supplies in the event of sudden outbreaks. There is also ongoing research working toward the development of safer smallpox vaccines. One in particular, from Germany, is named "MVA," for Modified Vaccinia Ankara. In the 1970s, MVA was used to vaccinate about 150,000 Germans who were at high risk for complications from the older smallpox immunization. Another vaccine, from Japan, was tried on 10,000 people in 1974 with relatively few side effects. Highly attenuated strains of fowlpox and canarypox viruses have also been researched for recombinant vaccine development.

Factors that Influence Who Should Be Smallpox Vaccinated

The side effects of the vaccinia vaccine against smallpox make it much more dangerous than any other immunization currently in use. As late as 1968, there were nine smallpox vaccine associated deaths in the United States. Exactly who should be smallpox vaccinated changes depending upon the risk of exposure to the disease, or whether an exposure has already occurred. Here are the main issues:

1. People with eczema or a history of eczema should generally not be smallpox immunized because of their increased risk of eczema vaccinatum. This may also include people with impetigo, burns, shingles, Darier's disease, and other dermatological issues. Household contacts of such people should likewise not be immunized due to the risk of household spread of the vaccine virus. If exposure to actual smallpox virus has already occurred, these precautions may no longer apply.

2. Pregnancy is a reason to withhold smallpox immunization, because the live vaccinia virus can infect fetuses, usually resulting in stillbirth or death soon after birth. If a pregnant woman has already been smallpox exposed, however, it might be the lesser of two risks to immunize her at that point. It is currently recommended that breastfeeding women likewise not be immunized. It is unknown whether vaccinia virus or antibodies may be transmitted via breast milk.

3. Children and infants are at increased risk of side effects from smallpox immunization. Most strategies to control actual or threatened smallpox virus release will probably involve immunizing adults first.

4. People allergic to certain substances are at risk of allergic reactions to smallpox immunization. The vaccine may contain polymixin B, streptomycin, a chlortetracycline, neomycin, and latex.

5. Immunosuppressed people are at increased risk for complications from smallpox immunization, but following a definite exposure it might be safer to vaccinate them, anyway. Such people include anyone with HIV or cancer, anyone who is on chemotherapy or high-dose steroid drugs, anyone who has had a recent bone marrow or organ transplant, or anyone with any other form of immunosuppression.

6. People with known cardiac disease are also listed by the CDC as being among those who should avoid smallpox vaccination in the absence of known exposure or disease outbreak. Included in this group are patients with cardiomyopathy, stroke or transient ischemic attacks (TIAs), or known coronary artery disease.

Smallpox is so dangerous that after an actual exposure there are almost no absolute contraindications to immunization. The disease is assumed to be worse than vaccination even for people at particularly high risk for side effects from the shot. However, in less clear cut situations, it is especially dangerous to immunize people with HIV. In America, it is believed that there are 300,000 HIV-positive people who are unaware of it. Patients with any risk factors for HIV infection should be aware that there might not be much time for testing once mass immunization programs are begun.

In June 2002, the United States' Advisory Committee on Immunization Practices resisted public pressure for mass immunization and reaffirmed a policy of surveillance and containment. They made smallpox vaccine available to response and health-care teams only, allowing for states to expand immunization to "additional groups, up to and including their entire population" depending on special circumstances. The same year the American Academy of Pediatrics issued a policy statement that "at present, the AAP supports the ring vaccination approach to contain smallpox cases that might develop as a result of bioterrorism." During one of our planet's last smallpox outbreaks in Nigeria, a delay in supply delivery stalled a mass vaccination program. Medical missionary Dr William Foege developed an interim, alternative strategy with intense but limited vaccination surrounding known cases. When the awaited additional vaccine arrived, there was no smallpox left in eastern Nigeria.

ANTHRAX VACCINATION

The History of Anthrax Vaccine Development

The first anthrax vaccinations were given to 24 sheep on April 28, 1881. The original vaccines were developed and administered not by a physician, but by a trained chemist. The researcher's interests extended from studying tartrate chemicals to learning about fermentation and wine and beer production, drawing him next into investigating microorganisms. The researcher's name was Louis Pasteur. To honor Dr Edward Jenner and his smallpox work, Pasteur coined the term "vaccine" from the Latin word for cow in reference to the bovine role in Jenner's research. Pasteur's sheep were revaccinated 3 weeks later, and then both they and an unvaccinated control group of sheep were challenged with implanted anthrax bacilli. All vaccinated sheep survived. All unvaccinated ones died.

Epidemic in humans in the eighteenth and nineteenth centuries in France and England as an industrial disease striking factory workers processing horsehair and sheep's wool, anthrax was initially addressed via public health measures. The British Factory and Workshops Act of 1895 made anthrax a notifiable disease, and the later Anthrax Prevention Act of 1919 stopped the importation of manufacturing materials most likely to be contaminated. The advent of antibiotics subsequently also lowered the human death toll from anthrax.

The History of Anthrax Vaccine Use

For animals, anthrax control initially focused on vaccination. Pasteur's original anthrax vaccine was a preparation of live, attenuated anthrax strains. By the 1940s, veterinary researchers had developed a better vaccine using a live, unencapsulated avirulent variant of the *Bacillus anthracis*. The vaccine is still widely used for livestock. Human vaccination took a different turn after 1904, when it was demonstrated that sterilized edema fluid from anthrax lesions provided protection in laboratory animals without the risks of live cell inoculation. Trials of filtrates of cultivated anthrax bacilli led, in 1954, to the first "acellular" anthrax vaccine that was effective in monkeys and humans with fewer side effects than previous live vaccines. The vaccine was refined and improved through the development of a better adjuvant and protein-free media, and through the use of better anthrax strains capable of producing more protective antigens.

The final version, "AVA" or "Anthrax Vaccine Adsorbed" was patented in the United States in 1965, and FDA approved for use in adults only in 1970. It is a sterile filtrate of a toxigenic, nonencapsulated V770-NP1-R strain of *B. anthracis* adsorbed to aluminum hydroxide as an adjuvant. It contains all three toxins that allow anthrax to overcome the immune system—(1) "lethal factor," a mitogen-activated protein kinase-kinase inhibiting protease, (2) "edema factor," a cytoplasmic cyclic adenosine monophosphate generating adenylate cyclase, and (3) "protective antigen" that binds and translocates both of these into host cells. The vaccine also contains benzethonium chloride as a preservative, and formaldehyde as a stabilizer. It is administered subcutaneously in a recommended schedule of 0, 2, and 4 weeks for primary vaccination, followed by booster doses at 6, 12, and 18 months and then annually thereafter. Vaccine contraindications include a history of anaphylactic reaction to any vaccine component or previous anthrax vaccination, or a past history of anthrax infection.

Anthrax vaccine efficacy has been demonstrated in macaque monkeys subjected to later aerosol challenge in five studies published between 1954 and 1995. Vaccination routes and dosage schedules, challenge strains, and intervals between vaccination and challenge varied between researchers. After the longest interval studied, 100 weeks, there was 88% protection. Combining data, 52 of 55 monkeys given two doses of anthrax vaccine survived later aerosol anthrax challenge. Other animal studies have involved guinea pigs and rabbits. The single controlled anthrax vaccine trial in humans was published in 1962 and it utilized the vaccine developed prior to the one currently used in the United States, an alum precipitate. It involved mill workers at risk for industrial exposure to anthrax, 379 of whom were given actual vaccine, 414 of whom were given placebo, and 340 of whom received neither. During an outbreak of inhalation anthrax, which concurrently hit the mill, all five workers afflicted were unvaccinated. No vaccinated employees were infected. Calculations based on person time of occupational exposure declared a vaccine efficacy of 92.5% against cutaneous and inhalation anthrax. After three primary doses of anthrax vaccine, 95% of people seroconvert, demonstrating a fourfold rise in antiprotective antibody IgG titers.

Research on Newer Anthrax Vaccines

There are newer anthrax vaccines in a variety of different stages of research and development, and there are also ongoing studies regarding simpler schedules and different routes of administration of the existing AVA vaccine. Some of the vaccines being studied are purified from recombinant sources, and others are derived from antigen subunits using different adjuvants. Still others are live vaccines using anthrax strains with auxotrophic mutations. The first contract awarded through the American Project BioShield law signed by President Bush in 2004 was for $878,000,000 for new, recombinant anthrax vaccine.

TABLE 56-3

COMBINED DATA ON THE RATES OF ADVERSE SYMPTOMS FOLLOWING ANTHRAX VACCINATION

Symptom	Incidence per Number of Vaccinees
Mild local reactions, with 1–3 cm erythema, and mild local tenderness and arm pain	1:33 to 1:3
Moderate local reactions, with 3–12 cm local inflammation	1:200 to 1:25
Severe local reactions, with >12 cm inflammation	<1:100 to 1:25
Mild systemic reactions including malaise, fever, chills, headache, muscle or joint aches, heartburn, or nausea	1:500 to 1:6

Side Effects of Anthrax Vaccination

In December 1997, the United States Department of Defense announced its decision to immunize all military personnel. Between 1998 and 2001, there were 1,985,654 anthrax vaccinations administered in the United States. For combined data from active monitoring in prelicensure studies, manufacturer surveillance reports, and Canadian and American armed forces postvaccination questionnaires regarding the risks of anthrax vaccination, see Table 56-3.

For the risks of anthrax vaccination listed for vaccine recipients in the vaccine information statement provided by the CDC, see Table 56-4.

Women report more side effects than men after anthrax vaccination. A cohort study published by military researchers in 2002 looked at pregnancy and birth outcomes among

TABLE 56-4

SYMPTOMS FOLLOWING ANTHRAX VACCINE LISTED BY THE CDC IN THE VACCINE INFORMATION STATEMENT PROVIDED TO VACCINEES

Symptom	Incidence per Number of Vaccinees
Vaccine site "soreness, redness, or itching"	1:10 men and 1:6 women
Lump at the shot site	1:2
"Large areas of redness" at the shot site	1:20
Muscle or joint aches	1:5
Headaches	1:5
Fatigue	1:15 men and 1:6 women
Chills, fever, or nausea	1:20
"Serious allergic reaction"	once in 100,000 doses

American army women. There was no evidence that prepregnancy anthrax vaccination had any effect on pregnancy or birth rates or birth outcomes. Between January 1990 and August 2000, there were 1,859,000 anthrax vaccine doses distributed in the United States and 1544 reports filed in the vaccine adverse event reporting system (VAERS). Aside from local reactions and mild systemic symptoms, there were two reports of anaphylaxis. The one report of a death following anthrax vaccination was attributed to coronary arteritis at autopsy. A second fatality following anthrax vaccination occurring subsequent to 2000 was due to aplastic anemia. In neither case was a causal association with vaccination established. Although they likewise show no pattern clearly consistent with vaccine causality, other events reported to VAERS in temporal association with anthrax vaccination have included cellulitis, pneumonia, Guillain-Barre syndrome, seizures, cardiomyopathy, systemic lupus erythematosus, multiple sclerosis, collagen vascular disease, sepsis, angioedema, and transverse myelitis. Each of these associations occurred less than 10 times during the 1990 and 2000 reporting period. In Canadian Armed Forces data, there is also a single report of an individual with a persistent nodule at the injection site and multiple other nodules that developed at several distant sites following vaccination.

An Institute of Medicine report released in 2002 concluded the anthrax vaccine to be acceptably safe. A civilian anthrax vaccine expert committee, assembled by the U.S. Department of Health and Human Services at the request of the Department of Defense, also reviews VAERS reports. In Congressional testimony in 1999, the committee declared that data thus far did "not signal concerns about the safety of the vaccine." Monitoring by that committee is ongoing.

Current Recommendations Regarding the Use of Anthrax Vaccine

Anthrax vaccine is recommended not only for disease prevention, but also as part of postexposure prophylaxis. The Working Group on Civilian Biodefense is a 23-member organization of medical academicians and researchers, and government, military, public health, and emergency medical specialists. In 2002, they published recommendations for managing anthrax exposures. They concluded that "optimal protection" following anthrax exposure consists of vaccination in conjunction with 60 days of antibiotic administration. The same year, the Institute of Medicine offered similar advice for simultaneous vaccination along with antibiotic therapy after anthrax exposure. In 2004, the CDC's report on responding to the detection of aerosolized anthrax in workplaces also advocated combined postexposure vaccination and antibiotic use. In a 2002 statement by the Advisory Committee on Immunization Practices, it was noted that postexposure prophylaxis "could have additional benefits" in supplementing antimicrobial therapy. With antibiotic

compliance in the 60-day regimen as low as 42% after the 2001 American anthrax attacks, any additional benefit could be of great significance. Because anthrax vaccine is licensed only for pre-exposure prophylaxis in adults, postexposure use can only be accomplished as an emergency intervention under investigational drug protocols. In their 2002 statement on the use of anthrax vaccine in bioterrorism response, the Advisory Committee on Immunization Practices specifically recommended studies on the safety and effectiveness of the vaccine in children and pregnant women. They have not yet been done. Published guidelines for postexposure use of anthrax vaccine in adults recommend that it be given as a 3-dose regimen starting as soon as possible, then 2 and 4 weeks later.

BOTULINUM ANTITOXIN AND TOXOID

The History of Preparation for the Use of Botulinum Toxin as a Bioterrorism Agent

The CDC began addressing the threat of biological warfare as early as 1949. Late that year, the National Security Resources Board ordered planning for all types of enemy attack including bacteriological or chemical assaults. News of the potential threat did not become common knowledge in the scientific community, however, until then President Harry S. Truman's Executive Office issued a manual in December 1950 warning of the possibility of pathogenic aerosol clouds and food supply contamination. The general public, in turn, was first informed about the risk in a pamphlet from the Federal Civil Defense Administration, which specifically listed botulinus toxin as a likely agent. Americans were aware of the dangers of mass disease spread after the amebiasis epidemic that spread from the 1933 Chicago World's Fair.

Botulinum neurotoxin may be the most poisonous substance known to man. It is 275 times more potent than cyanide. Yet over half a century after acknowledging botulism's potential as a bioweapon, we lack a widely available, well-tested vaccine against it. Most research on the toxin has focused, instead, on putting it to good use. Botulinum toxin is the first toxin to be licensed for therapeutic purposes. As of 2005, it was FDA approved for the treatment of adult cervical dystonia, severe primary axillary hyperhidrosis, and dystonia-associated strabismus and blepharospasm. Though not officially FDA sanctioned for such, it is also widely used for multiple additional conditions from migraine headaches to cerebral palsy. And widespread cosmetic use has made botulinum toxin a household word.

The History of Passive and Active Immunization against Botulism

There is progress in both passive and active botulism immunization. For passive immunization in the treatment of diagnosed botulism, there are two licensed and one investigational botulism antitoxin preparations in existence in the United States. Whichever is used, early administration maximizes effectiveness, because antitoxin can only neutralize circulating toxin. By the time weakness is clinically apparent, about 75% of neuromuscular junction receptors are already occupied by a blocker. When diaphragmatic function is impaired, over 90% of receptors are already affected. Pregnancy is not considered a contraindication to the administration of botulinum antitoxin. While recommended dosages of the antitoxins provide more than enough antibody to neutralize toxin concentrations seen with foodborne disease acquisition, botulism acquired via bioterrorism may involve greater exposures. Treatment dosages may need to be titrated by repeated monitoring of serum for the presence of toxin. Given the risks of equine botulinum antitoxin administration and the limits of its supply, the role of antitoxin as a postexposure measure in asymptomatic people has yet to be defined. In foodborne outbreaks, public health recommendations have generally been to carefully observe but withhold treatment of exposed people until the development of symptoms. A small primate study looked at monkeys exposed to aerosolized botulinum toxin. Of the monkeys antitoxin treated while asymptomatic, but postexposure, all seven lived. Of four other monkeys not treated until the signs of illness, half died. U.S. Army researchers found that antitoxin given to rhesus monkeys up to 24 hours after an aerosol challenge was highly protective. All monkeys left untreated until symptomatic, 29–46 hours postexposure, died unless mechanically ventilated.

Botulinum Antitoxin Preparations

The oldest of the botulinum antitoxin preparations is a trivalent antitoxin against types A, B, and E, the most likely causes of foodborne outbreaks. It is an equine product manufactured by immunizing horses and then collecting serum from them after they mount an immune response. The process is complicated and takes about 2 years to complete, but the end product can be freeze-dried and stored indefinitely. Only a few sources exist, primarily Connaught Laboratories, a few smaller European companies, and another facility that supplies only to Japan. Because equine products are so allergenic, it has been recommended that antitoxin use be preceded by skin testing with an intradermal 0.1 mL injection of a 1:10 dilution of the antitoxin. Desensitization can be attempted over 3–4 hours for reactors to skin testing. Even for nonreactors, infusion should be slow, with anaphylaxis treatment supplies at hand. Limited data have shown that up to 2% of the recipients of the trivalent antitoxin suffer anaphylaxis within 10 minutes. Overall, up to 9% show urticaria, serum sickness, or other hypersensitivity symptoms.

A broader spectrum botulinum antitoxin preparation, with neutralizing antibodies against all seven serotypes,

has been developed by the U.S. Army. Although also of equine origin, the product is "despeciated" by the cleavage of the Fc fragments from the horse IgG proteins. Only 4% of the horse antigens are left in the final product. When used in a 1991 Egyptian foodborne outbreak, there were no anaphylactic reactions but 10 out of 50 recipients suffered milder side effects, including one case of serum sickness. The heptavalent antitoxin is an investigational product.

In late 2003, the FDA licensed a human botulism immune globulin product. It is made from pooled plasma of adults immunized with pentavalent botulinum toxoid vaccine, and contains neutralizing antibodies against types A and B toxins. It was developed for use in infant botulism, and was approved following a 5-year placebo-controlled randomized clinical trial in infants.

Botulinum Toxoid Preparations

Passive immunization against botulism is nothing new. During World War II, over a million doses of a botulinum toxoid vaccine were made for Allied troops in anticipation of D-day. There were fears that Germany had and would use botulism as a bioweapon. In 1997, Philadelphia researchers reported having developed a modified recombinant neurotoxin vaccine against serotype C that was effective in mice when given either subcutaneously or orally.

In the 1970s, public health and military researchers devised the only botulism vaccine now in use in humans. It is a pentavalent toxoid against strains A, B, C, D, and E. It is difficult to mass produce and is most safely manufactured in a dedicated facility. For obvious reasons, efficacy testing in humans is hardly possible, though serum antitoxin levels stimulated by it seem to match protective levels in experimental animals. It is therefore not FDA approved, and is available only as an investigational agent through the CDC. The pentavalent toxoid contains alum, formaldehyde, and thimerosal, and it is contraindicated in anyone with allergies to any of these substances or a history of sensitivity reactions to previous doses of the vaccine. The primary series consists of doses at 0, 2, and 12 weeks. Over 90% of recipients seroconvert, but antibody levels fall by a year. Annual boosters are therefore recommended. Up to 4% of those vaccinated complain of local site reactions after their first dose. Subsequent injections elicit more frequent local reactions, with up to a 10% incidence after second and third doses, and up to 20% after boosters. Up to 3% of recipients report fever, malaise, headache, and myalgia. It has been used to vaccinate over 3000 laboratory workers internationally, and has also been used by the military. Because immunity develops after several months, this agent would be of little use in a postexposure situation. For pre-exposure prophylaxis, mass vaccination might also interfere with the efficacy of botulinum toxin for therapeutic uses. A separate monovalent serotype F vaccine is also available as an investigational agent.

Research on New Botulinum Antitoxins and Toxoids

Several attempts are underway to develop newer and better botulism vaccines. One group is working toward identifying a synthetic peptide harboring a neutralizing epitope. Another approach involves the use of a Venezuelan equine encephalitis virus replicon vector to make in vivo botulism neurotoxin protective antigens. U.S. Army researchers at Fort Detrick have been working on a botulinum vaccine since the late 1980s. Their laboratory uses recombinant technology to genetically engineer yeast to produce dismantled botulinum toxins. Vaccine-induced protective immunity to neurotoxin challenges has been demonstrated in both mice and nonhuman primates.

Suggested Reading

ACIP weighs public demand but comes out against mass smallpox vaccination. *Infect Dis in Children.* 2002 August:36.

FDA approves rapid HIV test. *Infect Dis in Children.* 2002 December;12:51.

Medicine's People: Needle in Time. *Am Med News.* 1992 March 9.

Abbey DM. Letter to the editor. *J Am Med Assn.* 2002 October 9; 288(14):1717.

Advisory Committee on Immunization Practices. Vaccinia (smallpox) vaccine. *MMWR.* June 22, 2001;50(RR-10):1–25.

Allergan, Inc., Irvine, California. Package Insert, Botox (Botulinim Toxin Type A, Purified Neurotoxin Complex), revised July, 2004.

Altemeier WA III. Smallpox vaccine. Letters to the editor. *Pediatr Ann.* 2000 May;29(5):263.

Anderson DC, Stiehm ER. Immunization. *JAMA.* 1992 November 25;268(20):2959–63.

Arnon SS, Schechter R, Inglesby TV, et al. Botulism toxin as a biological weapon; medical and public health management. *JAMA.* 2001 February 28;285(8):1059–70.

Baker JP, Pearson HA. Dedicated to the health of all children: 75 years of caring 1930-2005. *Am Acad Pediatr.* 2005:12.

Bechtel Bryan. ACIP suggests making vaccinia immune globulin available for prophylaxis. *Infect Dis in Children.* 2003 April; 16(4).

Bechtel Bryan. FDA restricts blood donation by smallpox vaccine recipients. *Infect Dis in Children.* 2003 February;16(2):3–15.

Bechtel Bryan. Saint Louis University to study new smallpox vaccines. *Infect Dis in Children.* 2004 April.

Bechtel Bryan. States want pause in smallpox vaccination efforts. *Infect Dis in Children.* 2003 July:17–8.

Berman JG, Henderson DA. Diagnosis and management of smallpox. *N Engl J Med.* 2002 Apr 25;346(17):1300–8.

Black RE, Gunn RA. Hypersensitivity reactions associated with botulinal antitoxin. *Am J Med.* 1980;69:567–70.

Bollet, Alfred J. Smallpox—the biography of a disease: part I. *Resident Staff Physician.* 1983 May:29–31.

Brachman PS, Gold G, Plotkin SA, et al. Field evaluation of a human anthrax vaccine. *Am J Public Health.* 1962;52:632–45.

Bray RS. *Armies of Pestilence: The Impact of Disease on History.* New York, NY: Barnes & Noble Books; 1996: 121.

Byrne MP, Smith LA. Development of vaccines for prevention of botulism. *Biochimie.* 2000 September–October;82(9–10): 955–66.

Casey CG, Iskander JK, Roper MH, et al. Adverse events associated with smallpox vaccination in the United States, January–October 2003. *JAMA.* 2005 December 7;294(21): 2734–43.

CDC: Notice to Readers: 25th Anniversary of the Last casr of Naturally Acquired Smallpox. *MMWR;* October 25, 2002; 51 (42): 952.

Center for Disease Control. *www.bt.cdc.gov/training/smallpox-vaccine/reactions*

Centers for Disease Control and Prevention, U.S. Department of Health and Human Services. Use of anthrax vaccine in the United States. *MMWR.* 2000 December 15;49(RR–15):5.

Centers for Disease Control and Prevention. Cardiac adverse events following smallpox vaccination—United States, 2003. *MMWR.* 2003;52:248–50.

Centers for Disease Control and Prevention. Cardiac deaths after a mass smallpox vaccination campaign—New York City, 1947. *MMWR.* 2003 October 3;52(39):933–6.

Centers for Disease Control and Prevention. Responding to detection of aerosolized *Bacillus anthracis* by autonomous detection systems in the workplace. *MMWR.* 2004 June 4;53 (RR-7): 8–9.

Centers for Disease Control and Prevention. Secondary and tertiary transfer of vaccinia virus among U.S. military personnel—United States and worldwide, 2002–2004. *MMWR.* 2004 February 13;53(5):103–5.

Centers for Disease Control and Prevention. Smallpox pre-vaccination information packet: contents and instructions. Smallpox Vaccine Information Statement, November 15, 2003:1–6.

Centers for Disease Control and Prevention. Smallpox vaccination and adverse reactions. *MMWR.* 2003 February 21;52(RR-4).

Centers for Disease Control and Prevention. Surveillance for adverse events associated with anthrax vaccination—U.S. Department of Defense, 1998-2000. *MMWR.* 2000 April 28;49(16):341–5.

Centers for Disease Control and Prevention. Surveillance for safety after immunization: vaccine adverse event reporting system (VAERS)—United States, 1991–2001. *MMWR.* 2003 January 24;52(SS-1):11.

Centers for Disease Control and Prevention. Update: adverse events following civilian smallpox vaccination—United States, 2003. *MMWR.* 2004 February 13;53(5):106–7.

Centers for Disease Control and Prevention. Update: cardiac and other adverse events following civilian smallpox vaccination—United States, 2003; *MMWR.* 2003 July 11;52(27): 639–42.

Centers for Disease Control and Prevention. Use of anthrax vaccine in the United States. *MMWR.* 2000 December 15; 49 (RR-15):9.

Centers for Disease Control and Prevention. Use of anthrax vaccine in response to terrorism: supplemental recommendations of the Advisory Committee on Immunization Practices. *MMWR.* 2002 November 15;51(45):1024–6.

Centers for Disease Control and Prevention. Use of anthrax vaccine in response to terrorism: supplemental recommendations of the Advisory Committee on Immunization Practices. *MMWR.* 2002 November 15;51(45):1024–6.

Centers for Disease Control and Prevention. Vaccine Information Statement, *Anthrax*. April 24, 2003.

Centers for Disease Control and Prevention. Vaccinia(Smallpox) Vaccine. *MMWR*. 2001 June 22;50(RR-10):1–25.

Centers for Disease Control and Prevention. Women with smallpox vaccine exposure during pregnancy reported to the National Smallpox Vaccine in Pregnancy Registry—United States, 2003. *MMWR*. 2003 May 2;52(17):386–8.

Centers for Disease Control and Prevention. Wound botulism—California, 1995. *MMWR*. 1995 December 8;44(48):889–91.

Chase, Marilyn. German, U.S. researchers aim at safer vaccines for smallpox. *Wall St J*. 2002 December 24; D2.

Cohen Jon. Smallpox vaccinations: how much protection remains? *Science*. 2001 November;294:985.

Cohen, Jon, Marshall E. Vaccines for biodefense: a system in distress. *Science*. 2001 October 19;294:498–501.

Committee on Infectious Diseases, American Academy of Pediatrics. Policy statement: smallpox vaccine. *Pediatrics*. 2002 October;110(4):841–6.

Committee to Assess the Safety and Efficacy of the Anthrax Vaccine; Medical Follow-Up Agency. *The Anthrax Vaccine: Is It Safe? Does is Work?* Washington, DC: Institute of Medicine, National Academy Press. 2002 March.

Couch D. *The U.S. Armed Forces Nuclear, Biological, and Chemical survival manual*. New York, NY; Basic Books, 2003:192.

Crookshank EM. *History and pathology of vaccination. Volume I: a critical inquiry*. London: H.K. Lewis, 1889.

Dixon TC, Meselson M, Guillemin J, et al. Anthrax. *N Engl J Med*. 1999 September 9;341(11):815–26.

Edwards EG. *A Concise History of Smallpox and Vaccination in Europe*. London: H. K. Lewis; 1902.

Etheridge, Elizabeth W. Sentinel for Health; A History of the Centers for Disease Control. Berkeley and Los Angeles, CA; the University of California Press, 1992:38–9.

Fauci AS, et al, eds. *Harrison's Principles of Internal Medicine*. 14th ed. New York, NY: McGraw-Hill; 1998:1095–6.

Fenn, Elizabeth A. *Pox Americana: The Great Smallpox Epidemic of 1775–1782*. New York, NY; Hill & Wang, 2001.

Fox CK, Keet CA, Strober JB. Recent advances in infant botulism. *Pediatr Neurol*. 2005;32:149–54.

Frey SE, Newman FK, Yan L, et al. Response to smallpox vaccine in persons immunized in the distant past. *J Am Med Assn*. 2003 June 25;289(24):3295–9.

Friedlander AM, Pittman PR, Parker GW. Anthrax vaccine: evidence for safety and efficacy against inhalational anthrax. *JAMA*. 1999;282:2104–6.

Grabenstein JD, Winkenwerder W. US military smallpox vaccination program experience. *J Am Med Assn*. 2003 June 25; 289(24):3278–82.

Halsell JS, Riddle JR, Atwood JE, et al. Myopericarditis following smallpox vaccination among vaccinia-naïve US military personnel. *J Am Med Assn*. 2003 June 25;289(24): 3283–9.

Hampton T. New smallpox vaccine shows promise. *J Am Med Assn*. 2004 April 21;291(15):1825.

Hibbs RG, Weber JT, Corwin A, et al. Experience with the use of an investigational F(ab')2 heptavalent botulism immune globulin of equine origin during an outbreak of type E botulism in Egypt. *Clin Infect Dis*. 1996;567–70.

Inglesby TV, O'Toole T, Henderson DA, et al. Anthrax as a biological weapon, 2002; updated recommendations for management. *JAMA*. 2002 May 1;287(17):2236–52.

Ivins BE, Fellows PF, Pitt MLM, et al. Efficacy of a standard human anthrax vaccine against *Bacillus anthracis* aerosol spore challenge in rheses monkeys. *Salisbury Medical Bulletin*. 1995 September 19–21;87(suppl.):125–6.

Kiple, Kenneth F, ed. *The Cambridge World History of Human Disease*. New York, NY: Cambridge University Press; 1993: 1008–9.

Kipple, Kenneth F, ed. *The Cambridge World History of Human Disease*. Cambridge, Great Britain: Cambridge University Press, 1993: 582–4.

Kiyatkin, Nikita M, Andrew B, et al. Induction of an immune response by oral administration of recombinant botulinum toxin. *Infection and Immunity*. 1997 November;65(11): 4586–91.

Monzo Jill. HHS makes plans to develop safer smallpox vaccine. *Infect Dis in Children*. 2003 March.

Nature Med doi:10.1038/nm1261(2005).

Paton WDM, Waud DR. The margin of safety of neuromuscular transmission. *J Physiol*. 1967;37(suppl), 417–428.

Patt HA, Feigin RD. Diagnosis and management of suspected cases of bioterrorism: a pediatric perspective. *Pediatrics*. 2002 April;109(4):685–92.

Pitt MLM, Ivins BE, Estep JE, et al. Comparison of the efficacy of purified protective antigen and MDPH (AVA) to protect non-human primates from inhalation anthrax. *Salisbury Medical Bulletin*. 1995 September 19–21;87(suppl):130.

Pittman P, Gibbs P, Cannon T, et al. Anthrax vaccine. *Vaccine*. 2001;20:972–8.

Plotkin SA, Mortimer EA Jr, eds. *Vaccines*. 2nd ed. Philadelphia, PA: Saunders; 1994: 1–11.

Porter Roy, ed. *The Cambridge Illustrated History of Medicine*. Cambridge, Great Britain: Cambridge University Press, 1996: 184.

Puziss M, Wright GG. Studies on immunity in anthrax. *J Bacteriol*. 1963;85:230–6.

Radetskky M. Smallpox: a history of its rise and fall. *Pediatr Infect Dis J*. 1999;18(2):85–93.

Redfield RR, Wright DC, James WD, et al. Disseminated vaccinia in a military recruit with human immunodeficiency virus (HIV) disease. *N Engl J Med*. 1987 March 12;316(11):673–6.

Robin L, Herman D, Redett R. Botulism in a pregnant woman. Letter to the editor. *N Engl J Med*. 1996 September 12; 335(11):823–4.

Sejvar JJ, Labutta RJ, Chapman LE, et al. Neurological adverse events associated with smallpox vaccination in the United States, 2002–2004. *JAMA*. 2005 December 7;294(21): 2744–50.

Sejvar JJ, Labutta RJ, Chapman LE, et al. Neurological adverse events associated with smallpox vaccination in the United States, 2002–2004. *JAMA*. 2005 December 7;294(21): 2744–50.

Shapiro RL, Hatheway CH, Becher J, et al. Botulism surveillance and emergency response; a public health strategy for a global challenge. *JAMA*. 1997 August 6;278(5):433–5.

Shapiro RL, Hatheway CH, Swerdlow DL. Botulism in the United States: a clinical and epidemiologic review. *Ann Intern Med*. 1998;129:221–8.

Shepard CW, Soriano-Gabarro M, Zell ER, et al. Antimicrobial postexposure prophylaxis for anthrax: adverse events and adherence. *Emerg Infect Dis.* 2002;8:1124–32.

Shulman ST. Important history. *Pediatr Ann.* 2003 March; 32(3):135.

Smallpox Vaccine. The Medical Letter 2003 Jan 6;45(1147):1–3.

Stephenson J. Smallpox vaccine program launched amid concerns raised by expert panel, unions. *J Am Med Assn.* 2003 February 12;289(6):685–6.

Stockman JA III. Clinical facts and curios. *Curr Prob Pediatr.* 1998;27:200–202.

Talbot TR, Stapleton JT, Brady RC, et al. Vaccination success rate and reaction profile with diluted and undiluted smallpox vaccine. *J Am Med Assn.* 2004 September 8;292(10):1205–12.

The Medical Letter. Post-exposure anthrax prophylaxis. *The Medical Letter.* 2001 October 29;43(Issue 1116-1117):91–2.

Turnbull PC. Anthrax vaccines: past, present, and future. *Vaccine.* 1991;9:533–9.

Turnbull PCB, Broster MG, Carman JA, et al. Development of antibodies to protective antigen and lethal factor components of anthrax toxin in humans and guinea pigs and their relevance to protective antibody. *Infect Immun.* 1986;52:356–63.

Vaccinia (smallpox) vaccine: recommendations of the Advisory Committee on Immunization Practices (ACIP), 2001. *MMWR.* 2001;50(RR-10):1–25.

Vastag B. Experts weigh prevention, therapy for ocular vaccinia in smallpox vaccines. *J Am Med Assn.* 2003 May 7;289(17): 2198–9.

Weisen AR, Littell CT. Relationship between prepregnancy anthrax vaccination and pregnancy and birth outcomes among US army women. *JAMA.* 2002 March 27;287(12):1556–60.

Wright GG, Green TW, Kanode RG Jr. Studies on immunity in anthrax. *J Immunol.* 1954;73:387–91.

Wysocki Bernard Jr. U.S. struggles for drugs to counter biological threats. *Wall Street Journal.* 2005 July 11;1:A10.

A

CDC CHEMICAL EMERGENCIES: Overview

The CDC has a key role in protecting the public's health in an emergency involving the release of a chemical that could harm people's health. This document provides information to help people be prepared to protect themselves during and after such an event.

What chemical emergencies are

A chemical emergency occurs when a hazardous chemical has been released and the release has the potential for harming people's health. Chemical releases can be unintentional, as in the case of an industrial accident, or intentional, as in the case of a terrorist attack.

Where hazardous chemicals come from

Some chemicals that are hazardous have been developed by military organizations for use in warfare. Examples are nerve agents such as sarin and VX, mustards such as sulfur mustards and nitrogen mustards, and choking agents such as phosgene. It might be possible for terrorists to get these chemical warfare agents and use them to harm people.

Many hazardous chemicals are used in industry (for example, chlorine, ammonia, and benzene). Others are found in nature (for example, poisonous plants). Some could be made from everyday items such as household cleaners. These types of hazardous chemicals also could be obtained and used to harm people, or they could be accidentally released.

Types and categories of hazardous chemicals

Scientists often categorize hazardous chemicals by the type of chemical or by the effects a chemical would have on people exposed to it. The categories/types used by the Centers for Disease Control and Prevention are as follows:

- **Biotoxins**—poisons that come from plants or animals (see *www.bt.cdc.gov/agent/agentlistchem-category.asp#biotoxins*)
- **Blister agents/vesicants**—chemicals that severely blister the eyes, respiratory tract, and skin on contact (see *www.bt.cdc.gov/agent/vesicants*)
- **Blood agents**—poisons that affect the body by being absorbed into the blood (see *www.bt.cdc.gov/agent/agentlistchem-category.asp#blood*)
- **Caustics (acids)**—chemicals that burn or corrode people's skin, eyes, and mucus membranes (lining of the nose, mouth, throat, and lungs) on contact (see *www.bt.cdc.gov/agent/agentlistchem-category. asp#acids*)
- **Choking/lung/pulmonary agents**—chemicals that cause severe irritation or swelling of the respiratory tract (lining of the nose and throat, lungs) (see *www. bt.cdc.gov/agent/agentlistchem-category.asp#choking*)
- **Incapacitating agents**—drugs that make people unable to think clearly or that cause an altered state of consciousness (possibly unconsciousness) (see *www. bt.cdc.gov/agent/agentlistchem-category. asp#incapacitating*)
- **Long-acting anticoagulants**—poisons that prevent blood from clotting properly, which can lead to uncontrolled bleeding (see *www.bt.cdc.gov/agent/ agentlistchem-category.asp#anticoagulant*)
- **Metals**—agents that consist of metallic poisons (see *www.bt.cdc.gov/agent/agentlistchem-category. asp#metals*)
- **Nerve agents**—highly poisonous chemicals that work by preventing the nervous system from working properly (see *www.bt.cdc.gov/agent/agentlistchem-category. asp#nerve*)
- **Organic solvents**—agents that damage the tissues of living things by dissolving fats and oils (see *www.bt. cdc.gov/agent/agentlistchem-category. asp#organicsolvents*)

Information for the appendix provided by the Centers for Disease Control (CDC) at www.bt.cdc.gov.

- **Riot control agents/tear gas**—highly irritating agents normally used by law enforcement for crowd control or by individuals for protection (for example, mace) (see *www.bt.cdc.gov/agent/agentlistchem-category.asp#riotcontrol*)
- **Toxic alcohols**—poisonous alcohols that can damage the heart, kidneys, and nervous system (see *www.bt.cdc.gov/agent/agentlistchem-category.asp#toxicalcohols*)
- **Vomiting agents**—chemicals that cause nausea and vomiting (see *www.bt.cdc.gov/agent/agentlistchem-category.asp#vomiting*)

Hazardous chemicals by name (A-Z list)

If you know the name of a chemical but aren't sure what category it would be in, you can look for the chemical by name on the "A–Z List of Chemical Agents" (*www.bt.cdc.gov/agent/agentlistchem.asp*) on the CDC Emergency Preparedness and Response website.

Protecting yourself if you don't know what the chemical is

You could protect yourself during a chemical emergency, even if you didn't know yet what chemical had been released. For general information on protecting yourself, read the fact sheets on evacuation (*www.bt.cdc.gov/planning/evacuationfacts.asp*), sheltering in place (*www.bt.cdc.gov/planning/shelteringfacts.asp*), and personal cleaning and disposal of contaminated clothing (*www.bt.cdc.gov/planning/personalcleaningfacts.asp*).

Basic information on chemical emergencies

Basic chemical emergency information designed for the public can be found in the general fact sheets (*www.bt.cdc.gov/chemical/genfactsheets.asp*) and chemical-specific fact sheets (*www.bt.cdc.gov/chemical/factsheets.asp*) and in the toxicology FAQs (*www.bt.cdc.gov/chemical/toxfaqs.asp*) on the CDC Emergency Preparedness and Response website.

In-depth information on chemical emergencies

Chemical emergency information designed for groups such as first responders, clinicians, laboratorians, and public health practitioners can be found in the case definitions (*www.bt.cdc.gov/chemical/casedef.asp*), toxic syndrome descriptions (*www.bt.cdc.gov/chemical/tsd.asp*), toxicological profiles (*www.bt.cdc.gov/chemical/toxprofiles.asp*), medical management guidelines (*www.bt.cdc.gov/chemical/mmg.asp*), emergency response cards (*www.bt.cdc.gov/chemical/erc.asp*), First Responders page (*www.bt.cdc.gov/chemical/responders.asp*), and Laboratory Information page (*www.bt.cdc.gov/chemical/lab.asp*).

For more information...

For more information about chemical emergencies, you can visit the following websites:

- **Centers for Disease Control and Prevention (CDC)**
  - National Center for Environmental Health (NCEH)
    - Chemicals: Health Studies Program Activities (*www.cdc.gov/nceh/hsb/chemicals*)
    - Chemical Weapons Elimination (*www.cdc.gov/nceh/demil*)
    - Childhood Lead Poisoning Prevention Program (*www.cdc.gov/nceh/lead/lead.htm*)
    - National Report on Human Exposure to Environmental Chemicals (*www.cdc.gov/exposurereport*)
  - National Institute for Occupational Safety and Health (NIOSH)
    - Chemical Agent Information (*www.cdc.gov/niosh/topics/emres/chemagent.html*)
    - Chemical Safety Cards (*www.cdc.gov/niosh/ipcs/icstart.html*)
    - NIOSH Pocket Guide to Chemical Hazards (*www.cdc.gov/niosh/npg/npg.html*)
- **Agency for Toxic Substances and Disease Registry (ATSDR)**
  - Fact Sheet: Hazardous Substances Emergency Events Surveillance System (*www.bt.cdc.gov/surveillance/hsees.asp*)
  - Hazardous Substances in the Environment (*www.atsdr.cdc.gov/2p-hazardous-substances.html*)
  - Medical Management Guidelines for Acute Chemical Exposures (*www.atsdr.cdc.gov/mmg.html*)
  - ToxFAQs (*www.atsdr.cdc.gov/toxfaq.html*)
- **American Association of Poison Control Centers** (*www.aapcc.org*)
  - 2003 Annual Report of the American Association of Poison Control Centers (*www.aapcc.org/Annual%20Reports/03report/Annual%20Report%202003.pdf*)
- **Environmental Protection Agency (EPA)**
  - Pollutants/Toxics (*www.epa.gov/ebtpages/pollutants. html*)
- **Material Safety Data Sheets** (*www.eh.doe.gov/chem_safety/Msds.html*) (from the Department of Energy website)
- **National Library of Medicine**
  - Chemical Information (*http://sis.nlm.nih.gov/Chem/ChemMain.html*)
  - Household Products Database (*http://householdproducts.nlm.nih.gov*)
  - Tox Town (*http://toxtown.nlm.nih.gov*)
- **Regional poison control center** (1-800-222-1222)
- **State and local health departments** (*www.cdc.gov/other.htm#states*)

B

CDC LABORATORY PREPAREDNESS FOR EMERGENCIES: Response to Suspicious Substances

In October 2001, a series of letters containing spores of *Bacillus anthracis* was sent to Florida, New York City, and Washington, D.C. through the U.S. Postal Service. Since then there have been several incidents where threatening letters containing suspicious substances have been discovered. Determining whether suspicious letters pose a real danger to postal workers and the public requires a detailed threat assessment and accurate laboratory testing. This fact sheet explains how federal, state, and local agencies respond to threatening letters and how laboratories play a role in detection and response.

Notifying agencies and determining response

Biological and chemical terrorism come in two forms—announced (overt) and unannounced (covert). An overt incident involves the announced release of an agent, often with some type of threat made. For example, a letter containing a powder and a note saying the recipient has been exposed to anthrax is considered overt.

Response to these types of threats normally begins with law enforcement, followed by notification of the Federal Bureau of Investigation (FBI), state emergency management, and state or local public health officials. The FBI and public health authorities contact the Centers for Disease Control and Prevention (CDC). Together, federal, state and local authorities determine whether the threat is real. If the threat is real, the FBI arranges for samples of

Information for the appendix provided by the Centers for Disease Control (CDC) at www.bt.cdc.gov.

the suspicious substance to be sent to a special laboratory that can perform the necessary testing. The lab is likely to be a state or local public health lab that is part of the Laboratory Response Network (LRN), a national network of labs coordinated by CDC.

Notification of federal, state and local authorities, assessment of the situation, and transfer to a laboratory for testing can take about 4 hours.

Lab testing

Lab workers can do a number of tests to identify an unknown substance. One of those tests is called PCR (polymerase chain reaction). PCR tests for the presence of DNA unique to each disease agent. Test results usually take between 3 to 5 hours. PCR can confirm whether earlier tests, such as those used by postal facilities to screen letters, were accurate.

Some postal facilities have or will have on-site air collectors that use PCR to test samples. These tests are considered screens and detect a limited number of agents.

PCR tests performed by LRN labs are considered more accurate and reliable because lab workers have been trained to use CDC-developed tests, which are performed in controlled laboratory conditions.

A positive result from a screening test is considered presumptive, meaning additional tests must be performed to confirm the original test result. An LRN laboratory performs confirmatory tests. A positive result from a confirmatory test sets off a chain of actions. These include a criminal investigation to uncover the person or persons who mailed the letter and a public health investigation to determine how many people were exposed and the best course of treatment.

Response plans

Depending on the agent that was detected, a response plan is set into motion. The immediate concern is the health of those who may have been exposed. One of the actions that may be taken is to give medicine to those who may have been exposed to the threat agent to prevent them from getting sick or to reduce the effects of their illness. Whether people are given medicine, such as antibiotics, depends upon the agent and their risk for getting sick. Anthrax, for example, calls for antibiotics like ciprofloxacin. Other threat agents, such as ricin toxin, have no drug treatment and call for supportive care if a person develops symptoms. For treatment information on specific terrorism-related diseases, visit CDC's Emergency Preparedness and Response Website at *http://www.bt.cdc.gov*.

LRN Laboratories

Because of threats of terrorism using disease and chemical agents, the CDC created the LRN in 1999. The LRN played a critical role in the anthrax investigation in 2001, as well as other incidents where suspicious substances were found. (For more information, see "Facts About the Laboratory Response Network" at *www.bt.cdc.gov/lrn/ factsheet.asp*.)

Labs that are part of the LRN are labeled as either National, Reference, or Sentinel.

Labs at CDC and the U.S. Army Medical Research Institute for Infectious Diseases (USAMRIID) in Ft. Detrick, MD, are the national labs. These labs perform confirmatory testing for disease agents that other labs are not capable of testing. They can also detect specific strains of disease agents and perform other specialized tests. Clinical specimens involving known or unknown chemical agents are also sent directly to CDC.

Reference labs include state and local public health, federal, military, veterinary, food, water and environmental testing labs. Reference labs perform confirmatory tests for biological agents. This allows local authorities to respond quicker to "positive" results rather than having to wait for CDC confirmation.

Sentinel labs are the thousands of private, commercial, and hospital-based labs that test patient specimens as part of their daily routine. These labs are in a unique position to spot unusual results, alert public health and law enforcement authorities, and refer suspicious specimens to LRN reference laboratories for confirmatory testing.

CDC is working with state and local health authorities to prepare for biological and chemical terrorism. Specifically, it continues to expand its network of laboratories and provide support to these labs so that they can detect threat agents. Also, CDC and other federal partners are working on procedures to ensure that proper authorities are notified quickly so that response is efficient and that the public is protected.

C

CDC LABORATORY PREPAREDNESS FOR EMERGENCIES: Facts About the Laboratory Response Network

In 1999, the Centers for Disease Control and Prevention (CDC) established the Laboratory Response Network (LRN). The LRN's purpose is to run a network of labs that can respond to biological and chemical terrorism. The LRN has grown since it was set up. It now includes state and local public health, veterinary, military, and international labs. This fact sheet provides a brief description of the LRN, and how it works.

The LRN Mission

The LRN and its partners will maintain an integrated national and international network of laboratories that are fully equipped to respond quickly to acts of chemical or biological terrorism, emerging infectious diseases, and other public health threats and emergencies.

What Is the LRN?

The LRN is a national network of about 140 labs. The network includes the following types of labs:

- **Federal**—These include labs at CDC, the U.S. Department of Agriculture, the Food and Drug Administration (FDA), and other facilities run by federal agencies.
- **State and local public health**—These are labs run by state and local departments of health. In addition to being able to test for Category A biological agents, a few LRN public health labs are able to measure

human exposure to toxic chemicals through tests on clinical specimens.

- **Military**—Labs operated by the Department of Defense, including the Naval Medical Research Center in Bethesda, MD.
- **Food testing**—The LRN includes FDA and USDA labs, and others that are responsible for ensuring the safety of the food supply.
- **Environmental**—Includes labs that are capable of testing water and other environmental samples.
- **Veterinary**—Some LRN labs, such as those run by USDA, are responsible for animal testing. Some diseases can be shared by humans and animals, and animals often provide the first sign of disease outbreak.
- **International**—The LRN has labs located in Canada, the United Kingdom, and Australia.

The LRN in Action

Anthrax Attacks of 2001

The LRN has been put to the test on several occasions. In 2001, a Florida LRN reference laboratory discovered the presence of *Bacillus anthracis* in a clinical specimen. *B. anthracis* causes anthrax. LRN labs tested 125,000 samples by the time the investigation was completed. This amounted to more than 1 million separate tests.

BioWatch

BioWatch is a program using air samplers to test for threat agents. The samplers are located in undisclosed cities and

---

Information for the appendix provided by the Centers for Disease Control (CDC) at www.bt.cdc.gov.

monitor the air 24 hours a day, 7 days a week. LRN BioWatch labs test filters from these samplers. Tests include polymerase chain reaction (PCR). PCR can quickly detect the presence of an agent's unique DNA.

Severe Acute Respiratory Syndrome

CDC labs identified the unique DNA sequence of the virus that causes severe acute respiratory syndrome (SARS). The LRN developed tests and materials needed to support these tests. LRN gave member labs access to the tests and materials.

The LRN Structure for Bioterrorism

LRN labs are designated as either national, reference, or sentinel. Designation depends on the types of tests a laboratory can perform and how it handles infectious agents to protect workers and the public.

> **National labs** have unique resources to handle highly infectious agents and the ability to identify specific agent strains.
>
> **Reference labs,** sometimes referred to as "confirmatory reference," can perform tests to detect and confirm the presence of a threat agent. These labs ensure a timely

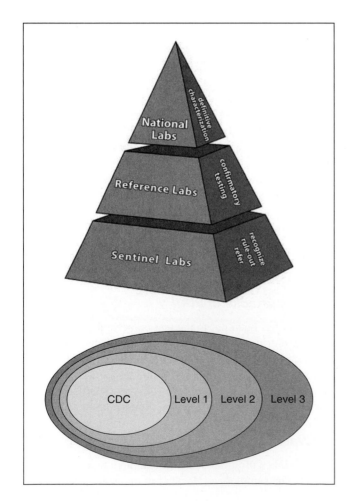

local response in the event of a terrorist incident. Rather than having to rely on confirmation from labs at CDC, reference labs are capable of producing conclusive results. This allows local authorities to respond quickly to emergencies.

> **Sentinel labs** represent the thousands of hospital-based labs that are on the front lines. Sentinel labs have direct contact with patients. In an unannounced or covert terrorist attack, patients provide specimens during routine patient care. Sentinel labs could be the first facility to spot a suspicious specimen. A sentinel laboratory's responsibility is to refer a suspicious sample to the right reference lab.

LRN structure for Chemical Terrorism

Currently, 62 state, territorial and metropolitan public health laboratories are members of the chemical component of the network. A designation of Level 1, 2, or 3 defines network participation, and each level builds upon the preceding level. (Please note that the level designations were changed in early 2005 so that laboratories previously designated "Level 1" are now "Level 3," and laboratories previously designated "Level 3" are now "Level 1.")

Level 3 Laboratories

Each chemical network member participates in Level 3 activities. Level 3 laboratories are responsible for:

- Working with hospitals in their jurisdiction;
- Knowing how to properly collect and ship clinical specimen;
- Ensuring that specimens, which can be used as evidence in a criminal investigation, are handled properly and chain-of-custody procedures are followed;
- Being familiar with chemical agents and their health effects;
- Training on anticipated clinical sample flow and shipping regulations; and
- Working to develop a coordinated response plan for their respective state and jurisdiction.

Level 2 Laboratories

Thirty-seven labs also participate in Level 2 activities. At this level, laboratory personnel are trained to detect exposure to a limited number of toxic chemical agents in human blood or urine. Analysis of cyanide and toxic metals in human samples are examples of Level 2 laboratory activities.

Level 1 Laboratories

Ten laboratories participate in Level 1 activities. At this level, personnel are trained to detect exposure to an expanded number of chemicals in human blood or urine, including all Level 2 laboratory analyses, plus analyses for mustard agents, nerve agents, and other toxic chemicals.

How Do Public Health Labs Become LRN Members?

State lab directors determine whether public health labs in their states should be included in the network. Membership is not automatic. Prospective reference labs must have the equipment, trained personnel, properly designed facilities, and must demonstrate testing accuracy. State lab directors determine the criteria for inviting sentinel labs to join the LRN.

Partnerships

The LRN is also a partnership between government and private organizations that have a stake in bioterrorism and chemical preparedness. CDC runs the program with direction and recommendations provided by the following agencies and organizations:

- The Association of Public Health Laboratories;
- The Federal Bureau of Investigation (Department of Justice);
- The American Association of Veterinary Laboratory Diagnosticians;
- The American Society for Microbiology;
- The Environmental Protection Agency;
- The US Department of Agriculture;
- The Department of Defense;
- The US Food and Drug Administration;
- The Department of Homeland Security.

D

CDC LABORATORY PREPAREDNESS FOR EMERGENCIES: Laboratory Network for Biological Terrorism

National Laboratories

National laboratories, including those operated by CDC, U.S. Army Medical Research Institute for Infectious Diseases (USAMRIID), and the Naval Medical Research Center (NMRC), are responsible for specialized strain characterizations, bioforensics, select agent activity, and handling highly infectious biological agents.

Reference Laboratories

Reference laboratories are responsible for investigation and/or referral of specimens. They are made up of more than 100 state and local public health, military, international, veterinary, agriculture, food, and water testing laboratories. In addition to laboratories located in the United States, facilities located in Australia, Canada, and the United Kingdom serve as reference laboratories abroad.

Sentinel Laboratories

The LRN is currently working with the American Society for Microbiology and state public health laboratory directors to ensure that private and commercial laboratories are part of the LRN. There is an estimated 25,000 private and commercial laboratories in the United States. The majority of these laboratories are hospital-based, clinical institutions, and commercial diagnostic laboratories.

Sentinel laboratories play a key role in the early detection of biological agents. Sentinel laboratories provide routine diagnostic services, rule-out, and referral steps in the identification process. While these laboratories may not be equipped to perform the same tests as LRN reference laboratories, they can test samples.

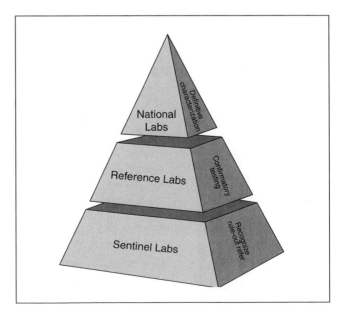

Information for the appendix provided by the Centers for Disease Control (CDC) at www.bt.cdc.gov.

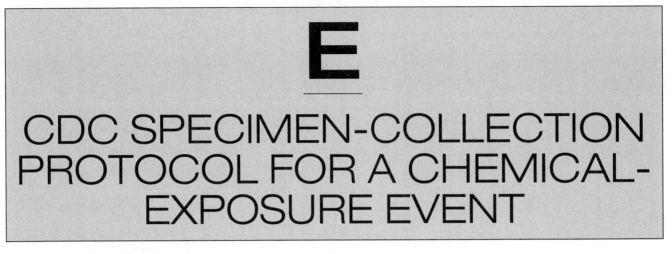

E

CDC SPECIMEN-COLLECTION PROTOCOL FOR A CHEMICAL-EXPOSURE EVENT

Information for the appendix provided by the Centers for Disease
Control (CDC) at www.bt.cdc.gov.

Collect blood and urine samples for each person involved in the chemical-exposure event.

Note: For children, collect only urine samples unless otherwise directed by CDC.

For detailed instructions see CDC's Shipping Instructions for Specimens Collected from People Who May Have Been Exposed to Chemical-Terrorism Agents.

Blood-Sample Collection

For each person, collect blood in glass tubes in the following order: **1st**: collect three (3) purple-top (EDTA) glass tubes; **2nd**: collect one (1) gray- or green-top glass tube. Collect the specimens by following the steps below.

① Collect three (3) purple-top glass tubes of blood.
Do not use gel separators or plastic tubes.

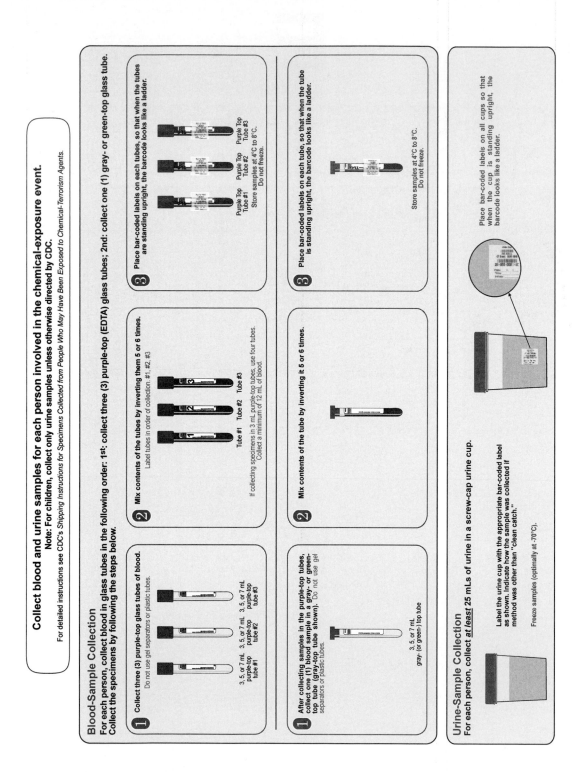

3, 5, or 7 mL purple-top tube #1
3, 5, or 7 mL purple-top tube #2
3, 5, or 7 mL purple-top tube #3

② Mix contents of the tubes by inverting them 5 or 6 times.
Label tubes in order of collection: #1, #2, #3

Tube #1   Tube #2   Tube #3

If collecting specimens in 3 mL purple-top tubes, use four tubes. Collect a minimum of 12 mL of blood.

③ Place bar-coded labels on each tubes, so that when the tubes are standing upright, the barcode looks like a ladder.

Purple Top Tube #1   Purple Top Tube #2   Purple Top Tube #3

Store samples at 4°C to 8°C. Do not freeze.

① After collecting samples in the purple-top tubes, collect one (1) blood sample in a gray- or green-top tube (gray-top tube shown). Do not use gel separators or plastic tubes.

3, 5, or 7 mL gray- (or green-) top tube

② Mix contents of the tube by inverting it 5 or 6 times.

③ Place bar-coded labels on each tube, so that when the tube is standing upright, the barcode looks like a ladder.

Store samples at 4°C to 8°C. Do not freeze.

Urine-Sample Collection

For each person, collect **at least 25 mLs** of urine in a screw-cap urine cup.

Label the urine cup with the appropriate bar-coded label as shown. Indicate how the sample was collected if method was other than "clean catch."

Freeze samples (optimally at -70°C).

Place bar-coded labels on all cups so that when the cup is standing upright, the barcode looks like a ladder.

F

CENTERS FOR DISEASE CONTROL AND PREVENTION SHIPPING INSTRUCTIONS FOR SPECIMENS COLLECTED FROM PEOPLE WHO MAY HAVE BEEN EXPOSED TO CHEMICAL-TERRORISM AGENTS

COLLECTING SPECIMENS

Required Specimens

Unless otherwise directed, collect the following specimens from each person who may have been exposed:

Urine

- Collect at least 25 mL. Use a screw-capped plastic container; do not overfill.
- Freeze specimen as soon as possible (−70°C or dry ice preferred).
- Ship the specimen on dry ice. Do not use large chunks or flakes of dry ice.
- For children, collect only urine unless directed otherwise by CDC.

Information for the appendix provided by the Centers for Disease Control (CDC) at www.bt.cdc.gov.

Whole Blood

- Collect a minimum of 12 mL of blood.
- Use three vacuum-fill (unopened) 5, or 7 mL or four vacuum–fill (unopened) 3 mL purple-top (EDTA) tubes to collect specimen. Collect in non-gel tubes.
- Using indelible ink, mark each purple-top tube of blood *in the order collected* (e.g., # 1, # 2, # 3, # 4 [if using 3 mL tubes]).
- In addition, use one 3-mL or larger gray-top or one 3-mL or larger green-top tube, vacuum-fill only (unopened) to collect the specimen.

Blanks

For each lot number of tubes and urine cups used for collection, provide the following to be used as blanks for measuring background contamination:

- Two (2) empty, unopened purple-top tubes.
- Two (2) empty, unopened green- or gray-top tubes.
- Two (2) empty, unopened urine cups.

LABELING SPECIMENS

- Label specimens with labels generated by your facility. These labels may include the following information: medical records number, specimen identification number, collector's initials, and date and time of collection.
- If you use bar-coded labels, place the labels on blood tubes and urine cups so that when these containers are upright, the bar code looks like a ladder.
- Follow your facility's procedures for proper specimen labeling. The collector's initials and date and time of collection will allow law enforcement officials to trace the specimen to the collector should investigations lead to legal action and the collector has to testify that he or she collected the specimen.
- Information provided on labels may prove helpful in correlating the results obtained from CDC's Rapid Toxic Screen and subsequent analysis with the people from whom the specimens were collected.
- Maintain a list of names with corresponding specimen identification numbers at the collection site so that results can be reported to patients.

PACKAGING SPECIMENS

Packaging consists of the following components: primary receptacles (blood tubes or urine cups), secondary packaging (materials used to protect primary receptacles), and outer packaging (polystyrene insulated corrugated fiberboard shippers).

Secondary Packaging for Blood Tubes

- Separate each tube of blood collected from other tubes, or wrap tubes to prevent glass-to-glass contact between tubes. Examples of some ways to do this are to—
  - Use a gridded box wrapped with absorbent material and sealed inside a clear waterproof plastic bag.
  - Use a sealable polystyrene container or blood tube shipment sleeve and transport tube, with individually wrapped tubes sealed inside a clear waterproof plastic bag.
- To facilitate processing, package blood tubes so that similar tubes are packaged together (e.g., package all purple-top tubes together).
- Place absorbent material between the primary receptacle and the secondary packaging. Use enough absorbent material to absorb the entire contents of primary receptacles.
- Wrap the package containing specimens (e.g., the closed gridded box or transport tube) with absorbent

material. Use evidence tape to seal, writing initials half on the evidence tape and half on the absorbent material.
- Place one wrapped box in a clear, waterproof plastic bag and seal. Place this bag inside a white Tyvek Saf-T-Pak ® (or equivalent) and seal the opening of this bag with a continuous strip of tamper-evident forensic evidence tape initialed half on the packaging and half on the evidence tape by the individual making the seal.
- According to 49 CFR 173.199(b), if specimens are to be transported by air, either the primary receptacle or the secondary packaging used must be capable of withstanding, without leaking, an internal pressure producing a pressure differential of not less than 95 kPa (0.95 bar, 14 psi). Verify in advance that the manufacturer of either the blood tube or secondary packaging used in your facility is in compliance with the pressure differential requirement.

Secondary Packaging for Urine Cups

- Separate each urine cup from other urine cups, or wrap urine cups to prevent contact between urine cups. For example you could use—
  - A gridded box lined and wrapped with absorbent material and sealed inside a clear, waterproof plastic bag.
  - Individually wrapped urine cups sealed inside a clear, waterproof plastic bag.
- Secure absorbent material using a single strip of tamper-evident forensic evidence tape initialed half on the packaging and half on the evidence tape by the individual making the seal.
- Place urine cups (boxed or individually wrapped and secured properly with evidence tape) in secondary packaging.
- Secondary packaging must have its closure secured with a single strip of tamper-evident forensic evidence tape initialed half on the packaging and half on the evidence tape by the individual making the seal.
- Verify that the urine cup or secondary packaging complies with the requirement stated in 49 CFR173.199 (b).

Outer Packaging

Use polystyrene insulated corrugated fiberboard shippers (may be available from your transfusion service or send-outs department). Do not ship blood tubes and urine cups together in the same package.

Blood Tubes

- Ship at 4°C to 8°C.
- For cushioning, place additional absorbent material in the bottom of the shipper.

- Add a single layer of refrigerator packs on top of absorbent material.
- Place the packaged boxes of specimens on top of the refrigerator packs.
- Use additional cushioning material to minimize shifting while the shipper is in transit.
- Place additional refrigerator packs on top of the secondary packaging.
- Place blood shipping manifest in a sealable plastic bag and put on top of packs inside the shipper.
- Keep chain-of-custody documents for your files.
- Place lid on shipper and secure with filamentous shipping tape.
- Place your shipping address in the upper left-hand corner of the shipper top and put CDC's receiving address in center.
- Affix labels and markings adjacent to the shipper's/consignee's address that appears on the shipper.
- Place the UN 3373 label and the words "Biological Substance, Category B" adjacent to the label on the front of the shipper.

Urine Cups

- Ensure that specimens will remain frozen or will freeze during transport.
- For cushioning, place additional absorbent material in the bottom of the shipper.
- Place a layer of dry ice on top of the absorbent material. Do not use large chunks or flakes of dry ice for shipment because large chunks have the potential for shattering urine cups during transport.
- Place packaged urine cups in the shipper.
- Use additional absorbent or cushioning material between wrapped urine cups to minimize shifting while shipper is in transit.
- Place an additional layer of dry ice on top of samples.
- Place the urine shipping manifest in a sealable plastic bag and put on top of dry ice inside the shipper.
- Keep chain-of-custody documents for your files.
- Place lid on shipper and secure with filamentous shipping tape.
- Place your shipping address in the upper left-hand corner of the shipper top and put CDC's receiving address in center.
- Place the UN 3373 label and the words "Biological Substance, Category B" adjacent to the label on the front of the shipper.
- Place a Class 9/UN1845 hazard label on the same side of the shipper as the UN 3373 marking.
- If the proper shipping name, (either dry ice or carbon dioxide, solid) and 9/UN 1845 is not preprinted on the hazard label, add it in an area adjacent to the label.
- Note the weight of dry ice (in kg) on the preprinted area of the hazard label, or place that information adjacent to the class 9/UN 1845 hazard label.
- Orientation arrows are not required on a shipper containing "Biological substance, category B." If you use arrows, be sure to orient the inner packaging so that closures are aligned with the arrows.
- If the shipper will be transported by a commercial air carrier, complete an airway bill. On the airway bill, note the proper shipping name and UN number for each hazardous material and identify a person responsible for the shipper per IATA packing instruction 650.

PREPARING DOCUMENTATION

- Since blood tubes and urine cups cannot be shipped together in the same package, prepare a separate shipping manifest for each.
- Place each shipping manifest (with specimen identification numbers) in a plastic zippered bag on top of the specimens before closing the lid of the polystyrene insulated corrugated fiberboard shipper.
- Do not transport chain-of-custody forms with specimens. Each entity or organization handling the specimens is responsible for the specimens only during the time that it has control of the specimens.
- Each entity or organization receiving the specimens must sign-off on the chain-of-custody form of the entity or organization relinquishing the specimens to close that chain. Electronic procedures such as electronic chain-of-custody and barcode readers will expedite this process.
- When receiving specimens, each new entity or organization must begin its own chain of custody. The entity or organization relinquishing the specimens must sign its chain of custody to start the chain and indicate that they have transferred the specimens.

Note: When the individual relinquishing the specimens (relinquisher) and the individual receiving the specimens (receiver) are not together at the time of specimen transfer, the relinquisher must document on its chain-of-custody form that the receiver is FedEx (and must document the FedEx Tracking Number) or have the individual transporting the specimens sign the chain-of-custody to indicate that he or she has taken control of the specimens. Likewise, when the receiver receives the specimens, he or she will document on his or her chain-of-custody form that the relinquisher is FedEx (and provide the Tracking Number) or have the individual transporting the specimens sign the chain-of-custody form.

Shipping Specimens
- Follow the guidance provided in your state's chemical-terrorism comprehensive response plan.

- If you are directed to ship the specimens to CDC, please ship the specimens to the following address:

Centers for Disease Control and Prevention
Attn: Charles Dodson
4770 Buford Hwy.
Building 110 Loading Dock
Atlanta, GA 30341
(770) 488-4305

QUESTIONS

If you have any questions or problems with specimen packaging or shipment, please send an e-mail to or call one of the following contacts:

- Jacob Wamsley, DLS Incident Response Laboratory Coordinator, at *jwamsley@cdc.gov*, 770-294-2491, or Jessica Mitchell, Battelle Contractor, at *JCMitchell@cdc.gov*, 770-488-4166.
- Dr. Jerry Thomas, Medical Officer, Emergency Response and Air Toxicants Branch, Division of Laboratory Sciences, 770-488-7279
- DLS administrative office, 770-488-7950

G

CONTINUATION GUIDANCE–BUDGET YEAR FOUR, Focus Area D: Laboratory Capacity–Chemical Agents

BACKGROUND

The purpose of this focus area is to develop nationwide laboratory capacity that provides rapid and effective analysis of clinical specimens (e.g., blood and urine) for chemical agents likely to be used in terrorism. These laboratory measurements will help guide emergency medical care, public health management of a chemical terrorism incident, and follow up of a chemical terrorism incident event by identifying the chemical agent(s) used, determining who has been exposed and how much exposure each person has had.

This focus area also addresses laboratory analyses of food specimens for chemical agents likely to be used in terrorism. The intent is to enable awardees to gain access to capabilities needed in their jurisdictions. This may be done by contracting for services with laboratories that possess the requisite capabilities, by sponsoring such capability development within collaborating organizations (e.g., food regulatory laboratories), and/or by developing the requisite capabilities directly within public health department laboratories. Technical assistance with respect to selection of analytic methods will be provided by FDA in consultation with CDC (see Appendix 1 for FDA contact information).

With respect to analysis of clinical specimens, the envisioned nationwide capability has three levels of laboratory capacity.

Information for the appendix provided by the Centers for Disease Control (CDC) at www.bt.cdc.gov.

Level-One Laboratories

Awardees are eligible to receive funding to support a chemical terrorism laboratory coordinator and technical assistance/training to assist in management of laboratory assets and to properly collect and ship human blood and urine specimens in response to a chemical terrorism incident. Chemists and/or medical technologists will staff this function. Awards for Level-One laboratories will be limited to $400,000 per awardee.

Level-Two Laboratories

Awardees that already have established or are in the process of establishing the capabilities of Level-One laboratories are eligible to receive financial support, technical assistance, equipment and training for analysis of human samples for Level-Two industrial chemicals, selected chemical threat agents (such as heavy metals, lewisite, and cyanide), or their metabolites. Development of Level-One and Level-Two capabilities may be concurrent activities. Level-Two laboratories will be equipped with state-of-the–art instrumentation including automated sample preparation equipment. These laboratories should be staffed with one Ph.D. chemist, or an individual with equivalent experience, and multiple laboratory support personnel.

To be eligible for Level-Two funding, the recipient must document a basic level of staff competency in analytical/clinical chemistry and laboratory quality control in measurements of low concentrations of chemicals or metabolites in clinical samples. Evidence of such competency would include a laboratory program in existence for at least one year involving the quantitative measurement of low levels of a toxic chemical, chemical metabolite, or biochemical indicator of health status or disease risk in blood, urine, or other human specimens, or in environmental specimens (e.g., blood lead analysis program, EPA certification for chemical contaminant analyses of drinking water, or Clinical Laboratory Improvement Amendments (CLIA) certification for clinical chemistry measurements).

Level Three Laboratories

Laboratories will be funded to maintain capabilities of Level-Two laboratories, plus they will receive financial support, technical assistance, equipment and training for analysis of human samples for chemical threat agents that require a higher level of analytical expertise (e.g. tandem mass spectrometry). Such laboratories will be equipped with state-of-the-art instrumentation similar to the Level-Two laboratories but also will have more extensive automated sample preparation equipment and tandem mass spectrometers as necessary. These laboratories will be staffed with multiple Ph.D. chemists, or individuals with equivalent experience (M.S. with 5 years experience), and multiple support personnel. This will bring the total number of states funded at Level-Three to approximately 10. Acceptance into Level-Three will be contingent upon demonstrated analytical competency at Level-Two, including success in an accepted proficiency testing program for all Level-Two chemical agents. Level-Three laboratories will be chosen on the basis of the technical review, information provided in the application, program needs, national goals, and geographic location.

CRITICAL CAPACITY #10 (LEVEL-ONE LABORATORIES)

To develop and implement a jurisdiction-wide program that provides rapid and effective laboratory response for chemical terrorism by establishing competency in collection and transport of clinical specimens to laboratories capable of measuring chemical threat agents.

Recipient Activities

1. **CRITICAL BENCHMARK #15—APPLICABLE TO LEVEL-ONE LABORATORIES:** Hire and train a chemical terrorism laboratory coordinator (chemist or medical technologist) and assistant coordinator to advise the laboratory director, the State Terrorism Coordinator and other public health and environmental health officials about chemical terrorism incidents and preparedness. These individuals are responsible for ensuring the proper collection, labeling, and shipment

of blood, urine, and other clinical specimens required in response to known or suspected chemical terrorism incidents and for ensuring associated data and communication requirements are met.

2. Develop a component, incorporated within the comprehensive response plan, that directs how public health, food testing, environmental testing, and other laboratories within your jurisdiction will respond to a chemical terrorism incident. The plan must include (a) roles and responsibilities, (b) inter- and intra-jurisdictional surge capacity, (c) a description of how the plan integrates with other department-wide emergency response efforts, (d) protocols for the safe transport of specimens by air and ground, and (e) a mechanism for reporting laboratory data to public health officials, law enforcement agencies, and other chemical terrorism LRN laboratories. (**LINK WITH ALL OTHER FOCUS AREAS**)

3. Establish and document in the comprehensive response plan, relationships with local members of HazMat teams, first responders, local, state, and federal law enforcement, and the Army National Guard (WMD-CST) to coordinate laboratory support for response to chemical terrorism with their response activities.

4. Join the chemical terrorism component of the Laboratory Response Network (LRN) and ensure that capacity exists (within the state, through partnerships with Level-Two and/or Level-Three laboratories in other states, or CDC) for validated testing of chemical agents in clinical specimens.

5. Enhance relationships with other chemical terrorism-related resources such as poison control centers, emergency medical personnel, medical toxicologists, food regulatory laboratories, schools of public health, and other partners with a view to ensuring that medical and public health officials have the benefit of at least preliminary chemical laboratory analyses in time to facilitate both the care of victims and the management of the incident. To this end, sponsor outreach efforts, professional conferences, and meetings.

ENHANCED CAPACITY #7 (LEVEL-TWO LABORATORIES)

In addition to establishing Level-One capacity, Level-Two Laboratories are to establish adequate and secure laboratory facilities, reagents, and equipment (e.g., ICP-MS, GC-MSD) to rapidly detect and measure in clinical specimens Level-Two chemical agents (such as cyanide-based compounds, heavy metals, and lewisites). Currently, CDC methods for Level-Two chemical agents use analytical techniques of inductively coupled plasma mass spectrometry and gas chromatography mass spectrometry. The list of Level-Two chemical agents may expand as better methods are developed. Tandem mass spectrometry methods are not required for Level-Two chemical agents. *Prerequisite: To be eligible for Level-Two funding, the recipient must document a basic level competency in analytical chemistry and laboratory quality control in measurements of low concentrations of chemicals in clinical samples. Evidence of such competency would include a laboratory program in existence for at least one year that includes the quantitative measurement of low levels of a chemical in blood, urine, or environmental specimens (e.g., blood lead analysis program, EPA certification for chemical contaminant analyses of drinking water, or CLIA certification for clinical chemistry measurements).*

Recipient Activities

1. Develop or enhance plans and protocols that address: (a) clinical specimen transport and handling, (b) worker safety, (c) appropriate Bio-Safety Level (BSL) conditions for working with clinical specimens, (d) staffing and training of personnel, (e) quality control and assurance, (f) internal and external proficiency testing, (g) triage procedures for prioritizing intake and testing of specimens or samples before analysis, (h) secure storage of critical agents and samples of forensic value, and (i) appropriate levels of supplies and equipment needed to respond to chemical terrorism events. This should be documented in your comprehensive response plans.
2. Level-Two laboratories must, in collaboration with CDC, purchase equipment, hire and train staff, implement analytical methods, participate in proficiency testing programs, and demonstrate competency in the analysis of Level-Two chemical agents or their metabolites in human specimens. Level-Two laboratories must achieve CLIA certification within 18 months of funding.
3. **CRITICAL BENCHMARK #16—APPLICABLE TO LEVEL-TWO LABORATORIES ONLY:** Participate in at least one exercise per year that specifically tests chemical terrorism laboratory readiness and capability to detect and identify at least one chemical-threat agent.
4. Use BSL-2 practices, as outlined in the CDC-NIH publication "Bio-safety in Microbiological and Biomedical Laboratories, 4th Edition" (BMBL), to process clinical specimens (e.g., blood and urine)—see *www.cdc.gov/od/ohs*. CDC also recognizes the need that state laboratories have to safely handle unknown environmental samples. Laboratories are encouraged to participate with federal partners, the LRN, HAZMAT, first responders, and other state public health laboratories to develop and disseminate standardized methods, procedures, and protocols to safely triage, aliquot, transfer, ship, and store unknown clinical or environmental specimens potentially containing chemical, biological, radiological, or explosive agents. **(LINK WITH FOCUS AREA C)**
5. At a minimum, ensure that laboratory security is consistent with standards set forth in the Select Agent Rule or subsequent updates. Note that pursuant to 18 USC section 175b, as amended by section 817 of the USA PATRIOT Act of 2001, P.L. 107-56, aliens (other than aliens lawfully admitted to the United States for permanent residence) are prohibited from possessing select agents if they are nationals of countries about which the Secretary of State (pursuant to provisions of the Export Administration Act of 1979, the Foreign Assistance Act of 1981, or the Arms Export Control Act) has made an unrevoked determination that such countries have repeatedly provided support for acts of international terrorism.
6. Enhance and document Internet connectivity to enable rapid communication via the Internet for information and data transfer with chemical laboratories in the LRN. **(LINK WITH FOCUS AREA C & E)**

ENHANCED CAPACITY #8 (LEVEL-THREE LABORATORIES)

In addition to maintaining Level-One and Level-Two capacity, Level-Three laboratories are to establish adequate and secure laboratory facilities, reagents, and equipment (e.g., tandem mass spectrometer) to rapidly detect and measure in clinical specimens Level-Three chemical agents (such as nerve agents, mustards, mycotoxins, and selected toxic industrial chemicals). Level-Three laboratories will also provide surge capacity to CDC and serve as referral laboratories for Level-One and Level-Two laboratories. The five laboratories currently funded under Focus Area D (California, Michigan, New Mexico, New York and Virginia) are considered Level-Three laboratories. It is CDC's intent in the future to add up to five additional laboratories at Level-Three. *Prerequisite: To be considered for acceptance into Level-Three, a laboratory must demonstrate analytical competency at Level-Two, including success in an accepted proficiency testing program for all Level-Two chemical agents (e.g., heavy metals, lewisites, cyanide).*

Recipient Activities

1. Level-Three laboratories must, in collaboration with CDC, purchase equipment, hire and train staff, implement analytical methods, participate in proficiency testing programs, and demonstrate competency in the analysis of Level-Three chemical agents or their metabolites in blood and urine.
2. **CRITICAL BENCHMARK #17—APPLICABLE TO LEVEL-THREE LABORATORIES ONLY:**

Participate in at least one exercise per year that specifically tests chemical terrorism laboratory readiness and capability to detect and identify at least two chemical-threat agents.

3. In collaboration with CDC and other Level-Three laboratories, participate in method development and validation studies.

4. Provide surge capacity to CDC and serve as a referral laboratory for Level-One and Level-Two laboratories.

5. Develop and implement a plan for 24/7 staff coverage in the event of a chemical terrorism emergency. Documentation of this plan should be provided to CDC to coordinate efforts.

H

INSTRUCTIONS FOR SHIPPING BLOOD SAMPLES TO CDC AFTER A CHEMICAL-EXPOSURE EVENT

Information for the appendix provided by the Centers for Disease Control (CDC) at www.bt.cdc.gov.

Guidance in Accordance with Packaging Instructions International Air Transport Authority (IATA) 650 Biological Substance Category B

For detailed instructions see CDC's *Shipping Instructions for Specimens Collected from People Who May Have Been Exposed to Chemical-Terrorism Agents.*

1
Place purple- and gray- or green- top tubes by patient number into gridded- type box with absorbent pad.

Prevent glass-to-glass contact.

2
Wrap box with absorbent material. Use evidence tape to seal. Write initials half on the evidence tape and half on the absorbent material.

3
Place one wrapped box in clear waterproof bag (or equivalent) and seal. Note: If primary receptacles have not been shown to meet the internal pressure differential of 95 kPa, use compliant secondary packaging materials.

4
Place this bag inside a white Tyvek Saf-T-Pak® bag (or equivalent).

5
Seal the opening of this bag with a continuous piece of evidence tape. Write initials half on the evidence tape and half on the bag.

6
Use a polystyrene insulated corrugated, fiberboard shipper to ship boxes to CDC.

7
Place absorbent material in the bottom of the shipper.

8
Place refrigerator packs in a single layer on top of the absorbent material.

9
Place the packaged boxes in the shipper. Use cushioning material to minimize shifting while box is in transit. Place additional refrigerator packs on top of samples.

10
Place the blood shipping manifest in a sealable plastic bag and put on top of the sample boxes inside the shipper. Keep your chain-of-custody documents for your files. Place lid on the shipper.

11
Secure the shipper lid with filamentous shipping tape. Place your shipping address in the upper left-hand corner of the shipper top and put the CDC Laboratory receiving address in the center.

12
UN 3373

BIOLOGICAL SUBSTANCE
CATEGORY B

Add the UN3373 label and the words "Biological Substance Category B" on the front of the shipper. UN3373 is the code identifying the shipper's contents as "Biological Substance, Category B."

13
Send shipment via FedEx to:

Centers for Disease Control and Prevention
Attn: Charles Dodson
4770 Buford Hwy.
Building 110 Loading Dock
Atlanta, GA 30341
(770) 488-4305

I

INSTRUCTIONS FOR SHIPPING URINE SAMPLES TO CDC AFTER A CHEMICAL-EXPOSURE EVENT

Information for the appendix provided by the Centers for Disease Control (CDC) at www.bt.cdc.gov.

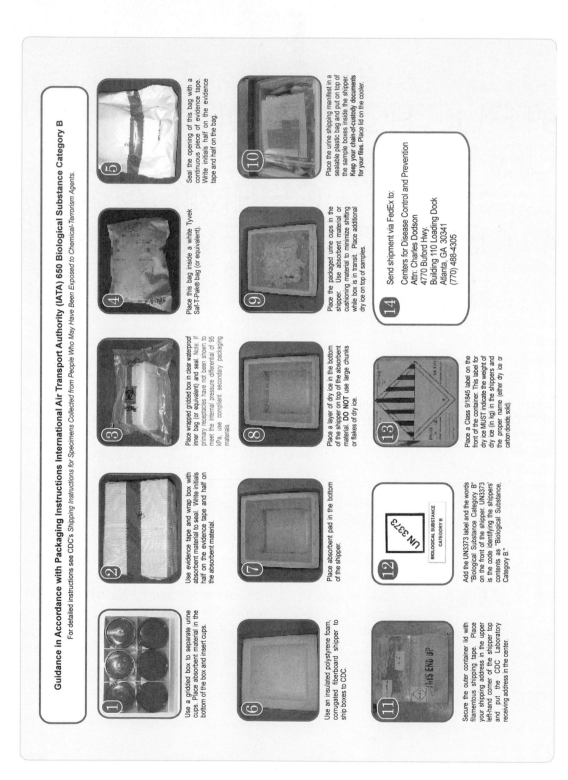

Guidance in Accordance with Packaging Instructions International Air Transport Authority (IATA) 650 Biological Substance Category B

For detailed instructions see CDC's Shipping Instructions for Specimens Collected from People Who May Have Been Exposed to Chemical-Terrorism Agents.

1 Use a gridded box to separate urine cups. Place absorbent material in the bottom of the box and insert cups.

2 Use evidence tape and wrap box with absorbent material to seal. Write initials half on the evidence tape and half on the absorbent material.

3 Place wrapped gridded box in clear waterproof inner bag (or equivalent) and seal. Note: If primary receptacles have not been shown to meet the internal pressure differential of 95 kPa, use compliant secondary packaging materials.

4 Place this bag inside a white Tyvek Saf-T-Pak® bag (or equivalent).

5 Seal the opening of this bag with a continuous piece of evidence tape. Write initials half on the evidence tape and half on the bag.

6 Use an insulated polystyrene foam, corrugated fiberboard shipper to ship boxes to CDC.

7 Place absorbent pad in the bottom of the shipper.

8 Place a layer of dry ice in the bottom of the shipper on top of the absorbent material. **DO NOT** use large chunks or flakes of dry ice.

9 Place the packaged urine cups in the shipper. Use absorbent material or cushioning material to minimize shifting while box is in transit. Place additional dry ice on top of samples.

10 Place the urine shipping manifest in a sealable plastic bag and put on top of the sample boxes inside the shipper. **Keep your chain-of-custody documents for your files.** Place lid on the cooler.

11 Secure the outer container lid with filamentous shipping tape. Place your shipping address in the upper left-hand corner of the shipper top and put the CDC Laboratory receiving address in the center.

12 Add the UN3373 label and the words "Biological Substance Category B" on the front of the shipper. UN3373 is the code identifying the shippers' contents as "Biological Substance, Category B."

UN 3373
BIOLOGICAL SUBSTANCE
CATEGORY B

13 Place a Class 9/1845 label on the front of the container. This label for dry ice MUST indicate the weight of dry ice (in kg) in the shippers and the proper name (either dry ice or carbon dioxide, solid).

14 Send shipment via FedEx to:
Centers for Disease Control and Prevention
Attn: Charles Dodson
4770 Buford Hwy.
Building 110 Loading Dock
Atlanta, GA 30341
(770) 488-4305

J

SENTINEL LABORATORY GUIDELINES FOR SUSPECTED AGENTS OF BIOTERRORISM: Clinical Laboratory Bioterrorism Readiness Plan

Retrieved from: *http://www.asm.org/ASM/files/LeftMargin HeaderList/DOWNLOADFILENAME/000000001206/ BTtemplateRevised8-10-6.doc* November 11, 2006.

Revised—10 August 06

NOTE: Amended to include link to State Public Health Laboratory Emergency Contacts and Table J7, Bioterrorism (BT) Readiness Checklist for Sentinel Laboratories.

Credits: Clinical Laboratory Bioterrorism Readiness Plan

Subject Matter Experts, ASM:

Daniel S. Shapiro, M.D.
Lahey Clinic
Burlington, MA

Susan E. Sharp, Ph.D.
Kaiser Permanente
Portland, OR

ASM Laboratory Protocol Working Group

Vickie Baselski, Ph.D.
University of Tennessee at Memphis
Memphis, TN

Roberta B. Carey, Ph.D.

Peter H. Gilligan, Ph.D.
University of North Carolina
Hospitals/Clinical Microbiology and Immunology Labs
Chapel Hill, NC

Larry Gray, Ph.D.
TriHealth Laboratories and
University of Cincinnati College of Medicine
Cincinnati, OH

Rosemary Humes, MS, MT (ASCP) SM
Association of Public Health Laboratories
Silver Spring, MD

Karen Krisher, Ph.D.
Clinical Microbiology Institute
Wilsonville, OR

Judith Lovchik, Ph.D.
Public Health Laboratories, NYCDOH
New York, NY

Chris N. Mangal, MPH
Association of Public Health Laboratories
Silver Spring, MD

Alice Weissfeld, Ph.D.
Microbiology Specialists, Inc.
Houston, TX

David Welch, Ph.D.
Medical Microbiology Consulting
Dallas, TX

Mary K. York, Ph.D.
MKY Microbiology Consultants
Walnut Creek, CA

Coordinating Editor:

James W. Snyder, Ph.D.
University of Louisville
Louisville, KY

The purpose of this template is to provide a model for laboratories to use for developing a bioterrorism (BT) preparedness plan. The components of this template can be used to develop a readiness plan to meet the needs of the institution. It is not meant to be all-inclusive. Rather, it is to serve as an aid in the process of developing a specific plan for each institution.

The laboratory BT preparedness plan should be integrated into the institutional BT preparedness plan.

Some of the specific laboratory protocols for the BT agents included in this template contain flowcharts. Ideally, these flowcharts should be integrated into laboratory procedures so that technologists have ready access to this information.

NOTE: It is quite possible that the laboratory will not be contacted in advance and informed that one of the potential agents of bioterrorism is suspected. As a result, it is essential that appropriate safeguards be taken, including subculture of all blood cultures in a biosafety cabinet or behind a safety shield, following the flowcharts for suspicious agents, and always considering the possibility of bioterrorist agents.

I. LABORATORY BT CONTACT PROTOCOL: WHEN TO IMPLEMENT

A. If a possible BT agent is grown in the laboratory or detected by other laboratory means (as outlined in the laboratory protocols included in this document), place phone calls to the responsible physician and the following individuals noted below immediately. Contacting these individuals and the procedures required in the laboratory are NOT one-person tasks. Additional assistance from other technologists and laboratory support personnel is essential.

or

B. If a specimen is submitted for detection of a BT agent as the result of a possible BT event, place phone calls to the individuals noted below immediately.

NOTE: Certain geographic areas are known to have natural human cases of infection due to BT agents (e.g., tularemia in Nantucket and Martha's Vineyard, Massachusetts, as well as Missouri, Oklahoma, and neighboring areas; and plague in much of the southwestern United States, especially New Mexico).

- Microbiology Laboratory Supervisor: (xxx) xxx-xxxx
- Microbiology Manager: (xxx) xxx-xxxx
- Microbiology Laboratory Director: (xxx) xxx-xxxx
- Infection Control Officer: (xxx) xxx-xxxx
- Infectious Disease Physician: (xxx) xxx-xxxx
- Local Health Department: (xxx) xxx-xxxx
- State Health Department: (xxx) xxx-xxxx
- Laboratory Director on Call (beeper no.): (xxx) xxx-xxxx
- Clinical Pathologist on Call (beeper no.): (xxx) xxx-xxxx
- Chief of Infectious Diseases: (xxx) xxx-xxxx
- Chief of Pathology: (xxx) xxx-xxxx
- Other: (xxx) xxx-xxxx

(Include contacts pertinent to your institution in a predetermined order, and delete those who are not to be contacted in your institution.)

II. THE LRN: LABORATORY RESPONSE NETWORK FOR BIOTERRORISM

The Laboratory Response Network (LRN) is a consortium and partnership of laboratories that provide immediate and sustained laboratory testing and communication in support of public health emergencies, particularly in response to acts of bioterrorism. The LRN is currently comprised of local, state, and federal public health laboratories in addition to private and commercial clinical laboratories, and selected food, water, agricultural, military, and veterinary testing laboratories. Other key federal partners include the Federal Bureau of Investigation (FBI), the Department of Defense (DOD), the Environmental Protection Agency (EPA), the Department of Agriculture (USDA), the Department of Justice (DOJ), the Department of Energy (DOE), the Food and Drug Administration (FDA), the Association of Public Health Laboratories (APHL), the National Institutes of Health (NIH), the American Association of Veterinary Laboratory Diagnosticians (AAVLD), and the American Society for Microbiology (ASM). All laboratories are regarded as partners and in some cases, registered members of the LRN. Preliminary testing and screening are performed primarily in a distributed rather than a centralized fashion to ensure a prompt and rapid initial response; a system of triage and referral of specimens ensures transfer of appropriate materials to specialty laboratories where sophisticated equipment, technologies, and expertise are applied to specimen analysis.

The goals of the LRN are to:

1. Ensure that the nation's public health, clinical, and other select laboratories are prepared to detect and respond to a bioterrorism or chemical terrorism event in an appropriate and integrated manner.
2. Ensure that all member reference laboratories collectively maintain state-of-the-art biodetection and diagnostic capabilities and surge capacity as well as secure electronic communication of test results for the biological and chemical agents likely to be used in the commission of a biocrime or bioterrorism event.
3. Work with other departments and agencies to ensure a successful federal response to an act of bioterrorism and to facilitate and optimize the ability of states to competently respond independently to biocrimes or public health emergencies in the state.
4. Promote the CDC's and HHS' bioterrorism research agenda and CDC's internal response needs.
5. Enlist an optimal number of registered participating LRN laboratories throughout the United States as determined by the LRN working group.

The LRN maintains the following:

1. A registry and linkage of clinical and private laboratories in the U.S. that would include Sentinel and Reference laboratories.
2. Complete, accurate, and standardized protocols for all levels of testing for agents deemed critical and likely to be used in the commission of biocrimes or acts of bioterrorism.
3. Secure but accessible supply of standardized reagents and diagnostic technologies produced and maintained by the CDC.
4. Secure electronic laboratory reporting that integrates with key epidemiologic, surveillance, and emergency response components
5. Training and proficiency testing essential to the diagnostic process

Clinical laboratories play a critical role in the LRN. Their heightened awareness to the possibility of recovering the agents of bioterrorism from patient specimens and referral of suspect isolates to the appropriate public health reference laboratory is crucial (see *ASM's Laboratory Guideline on Packing and Shipping Diagnostic and Clinical Specimens, Infectious Substances, and Biological Agents, which can be downloaded from ASM's Web site at http://www.asm.org/Policy/index.asp?bid=6342*

Bioterrorism is defined as the "intentional use of microorganisms, or toxins, derived from living organisms, to produce disease and death in humans, animals, or plants." A bioterrorism event may be either overt or covert.

An **overt** attack would be accompanied by an announcement that a specific agent was released. These attacks elicit an immediate response by law enforcement and HAZMAT personnel. Public health officials will also be involved to assist in evaluating the risk and control of the disease. Samples (environmental, food, water, animals) for testing would be submitted directly to a public health reference laboratory, usually a state health laboratory.

A **covert** attack involves the release of an organism or toxin without an announcement. Days or weeks may pass before the release is noticed. The event would probably be signaled by a cluster of disease appearing after the incubation period. Emergency departments may be the first to observe unusual patterns of illness, while clinical laboratories would almost certainly detect the first cases of disease and raise suspicion of a possible event. Organisms isolated by the clinical laboratory must be forwarded to the appropriate LRN reference laboratory, and public health officials are to be notified of the suspicious event that may be indicative of a bioterrorism incident. Public health officials in concert with law enforcement officials would determine if an attack has occurred, in addition to confirming the identification of the agent, and institute protective and preventive measures designed to minimize the spread of disease.

THE LRN STRUCTURE FOR BIOTERRORISM: LRN LABORATORIES ARE DESIGNATED AS SENTINEL, REFERENCE, AND NATIONAL LABORATORIES (SEE APPENDICES C AND D)

Sentinel Laboratories

Depending on the level of diagnostic testing, there are two kinds of sentinel clinical laboratories. **Advanced sentinel clinical laboratories** function at the local front line and have the most capability. Laboratories with less analytical capability that are also in a position to handle specimens that might contain agents of bio-terrorism or emerging infectious disease are referred to as **basic sentinel clinical laboratories**. These latter facilities need at a minimum a communication link to each jurisdiction's LRN reference laboratory for completion of the network. Characteristics of these two kinds of laboratory are as follows:

Advanced Sentinel Clinical Laboratory:

1. The laboratory is certified under the Clinical Laboratory Improvement Amendments of 1988 (CLIA) by the Centers for Medicare & Medicaid Services (CMS) for the applicable subspecialty within

the specialty of microbiology, and meets the requirements to perform high complexity testing.

2. The laboratory is inspected successfully by CMS, a CMS agent, a CMS-approved accreditation organization, or, for a CLIA-exempt laboratory, by that laboratory's State.

3. The laboratory has policies and procedures for direct referral of **suspicious** specimens or isolates to the nearest LRN reference laboratory in its jurisdiction.

In addition to the above criteria, Advanced Sentinel Laboratories shall meet the following:

4. Have a Class II or higher Certified Biological Safety Cabinet.

5. Comply with Biosafety Level II (BSL-2) practices[1] AND

6. Have policies and procedures in place for use of additional respiratory protection, including a definition of when such use is necessary, as well as documentation of safe use (e.g., N95 fit-testing).

7. Have policies and procedures that include the LRN Sentinel Level Clinical Microbiology Laboratory Guidelines that are available and can be downloaded from the ASM Web site: (*http://www.asm.org/ Policy/ index.asp?bid=6342*).

8. All personnel have been trained, with demonstrated competency, and are fully aware of the details contained within each LRN Sentinel Level Clinical Microbiology Laboratory Guideline.

9. Personnel have been trained and certified in Packing and Shipping of Infectious Substances Guidelines.[2]

10. Have procedures to track and account for decontamination of laboratory biological waste (specimens, cultures). At a minimum, ensure that any contract or procedure for waste/disposal is available for inspection in the laboratory safety or waste disposal manual.

It is further highly recommended that Advanced Sentinel Laboratories comply with the following:

11. The microbiology laboratory operates under negative pressure as recommended by the American Institute of Architecture (AIA) Guidelines for Construction of Healthcare Facilities.[3] If a microbiology laboratory is planning to remodel or construct a new facility, it should be designed to operate under negative air pressure as recommended by the AIA. This only applies to new construction or remodeling.

[1]Biosafety in Microbiological and Biomedical Laboratories 4th ed, U. S. Department of Health and Human Services.

[2]Federal Register, Part IV, Department of Transportation, 49 CFR Part 172, Hazardous Materials: Security Requirements for Offerors and Transporters of Hazardous Materials; Final Rule.

[3]American Institute of Architecture, Guidelines for Construction of Healthcare Facilities, 2001 Edition.

12. There is on-site terminal decontamination capability, e.g., autoclaving, for disposal of wastes categorized as BSL-3 or Select Agent.

Basic Sentinel Clinical Laboratory

1. The laboratory is certified under the Clinical Laboratory Improvement Amendments of 1988 (CLIA) by the Centers for Medicare & Medicaid Services (CMS) for the applicable subspecialty within the specialty of microbiology.

2. The laboratory is inspected successfully by CMS, a CMS agent, a CMS-approved accreditation organization, or, for a CLIA-exempt laboratory, by that laboratory's State.

3. The laboratory has policies and procedures for referral of diagnostic specimens to an Advanced Sentinel Laboratory.

4. The laboratory has policies and procedures for direct referral of **suspicious** specimens or isolates to the nearest LRN reference laboratory in its jurisdiction.

LRN Reference Laboratories

LRN reference laboratories are local and state public health laboratories, selected academic- or university-based laboratories, designated specialty laboratories (veterinary, water, food, chemical, military, agricultural) that possess the reagents and technology for definitive confirmation of organisms including toxin testing, referred by Sentinel laboratories. LRN Reference laboratories follow BSL-3 containment and practice guidelines. Contact your designated state public health laboratory for more information about the LRN reference laboratory located closest to you. A list of state public health laboratories can be downloaded at: *http://www.asm.org/ASM/files/LeftMarginHeaderList/DO-WNLOADFILENAME/000000000527/emcontactlist8-6.pdf*

LRN National Laboratories

LRN National Laboratories are Federal laboratories that have BSL-4 containment facilities and practice guidelines. The primary laboratory at this level is located at the CDC and specializes in the isolation and identification of BSL-4 agents such as Ebola, Marburg, and Smallpox virus. This laboratory also possesses the capability of advanced genetic characterization and archiving of all bioterrorism agents. (See Appendices C and D.)

III. THE CLINICAL LABORATORY'S RESPONSIBILITY

As members of the LRN, Sentinel laboratories have access to the network and serve as "sentinels" for the early detection of and raising suspicion regarding a suspicious agent that cannot be ruled out as a possible bioterrorism-associated organism. Sentinel laboratories do not have access to the CDC secure website for Reference Laboratory Testing Protocols or reagents. Instead, Sentinel laboratories must utilize standardized testing protocols (ASM Sentinel Clinical Microbiology Laboratory Guidelines) that have been designed to utilize conventional tests to facilitate the "rule-out" or "referral" of a suspicious isolate to an LRN Reference laboratory.

The Sentinel laboratory is NOT responsible for and SHOULD NOT make the decision that a bioterrorism event has occurred; that responsibility rests with local, state, and federal health and law enforcement officials. A designated individual within your facility (preferably the Infection Control Officer) should be notified of a suspicious agent, who in turns notifies the local public health officials. Under no circumstances should the laboratory contact law enforcement or public health officials. The exception is the need to contact the LRN Reference Laboratory for guidance in the disposition of the suspicious agent prior to referral for confirmatory testing.

NOTE: In no case should the Sentinel laboratory accept environmental (powders, letters, packages), animal, food, or water specimens for examination, culture, or transport for bioterrorism-associated agents. Such specimens should be submitted directly to the nearest LRN Reference laboratory.

IV. SHIPPING AND HANDLING OF INFECTIOUS MATERIALS GUIDELINES

United States, international, and commercial regulations mandate the proper packing, documentation, and safe shipment of dangerous goods in order to protect the public, airline workers, couriers, and other persons who work for commercial shippers and who handle the dangerous goods during the many segments of the shipping process. In addition, proper packing and shipping of dangerous goods will reduce the exposure of the shipper to the risks of criminal and civil liabilities associated with shipping dangerous goods, particularly infectious substances.

The process of properly packing and shipping an infectious substance, a diagnostic specimen, or a biological agent is composed of the following sequential steps:

A. Training of all persons involved in the shipping process
B. Determination of the applicability of the regulations
C. Determination of any applicable shipping limitations
D. Classification of the substance to be shipped
E. Identification of the substance to be shipped
F. Selection of the appropriate packing instructions to use
G. Selection of appropriate packaging

H. Marking and labeling the package
I. Documentation of the shipment

Failure to follow governmental and commercial regulations for the packing and shipping of infectious substances and other dangerous goods can result in criminal prosecution and substantial financial penalties.

NOTICE: Many important packing and shipping regulations have changed, been added, and been deleted in 2005. ASM's Laboratory Guideline on Packing and Shipping Diagnostic and Clinical Specimens, Infectious Substances, and Biological Agents has been revised and is available at *http://www.asm.org/Policy/index.asp?bid =6342*

V. INFORMATION CHECKLIST

This checklist (**Figure K1**) may help in the gathering of information in a suspected bioterrorism event. The checklist is to be filled out by the shift operations manager, shift supervisor, or other designated personnel.

VI. HANDLING OF POSSIBLE BT AGENT

NOTE: Under no circumstances are viral cultures to be set up if smallpox, Ebola virus, or another of the viral agents of bioterrorism is suspected.

A. A lead BT technologist should be appointed and be notified immediately that a suspected BT specimen or agent is in the laboratory. Laboratory workers are to be informed promptly of the name and medical record number of the person(s) with the suspected infection and, if appropriate, to treat other specimens from the patient(s) appropriately. This must be done in a manner that is in compliance with the Health Insurance Portability and Accountability Act (HIPAA).

B. All suspected BT specimens are to be processed in the biological safety cabinet located in **{fill in institution-specific information; whenever possible, this should be in a biological safety cabinet in a room that is under negative pressure}** while wearing appropriate personal protective equipment, such as gown, gloves, and mask.

C. Each of the plates, tubes, and blood culture bottles for which this applies must be labeled prominently: **"Possible highly infectious agent: [fill in name of agent]"**

D. All plates that have been streaked for culture or subculture will be sealed with shrink seal or the equivalent and labeled as in step C above.

E. Any growth from specimens is to be manipulated in the biological safety cabinet **{fill in institution-specific information}** while wearing appropriate personal protective equipment, such as gown, gloves, and mask.

F. As the culture is being worked up, the technologist(s) working on the culture(s) must be in close touch with the microbiology supervisor and medical director.

G. An identification of the organism is **NOT** the role of the Sentinel microbiology laboratory. An organism that is consistent with, for example, *Yersinia pestis*, will be forwarded to a LRN Reference or higher laboratory for definitive identification. **Do not perform any more manipulation of the cultures than is absolutely essential.**

VII. TABLES

TABLE J-1

CDC BIOSAFETY LEVEL (BSL) DESIGNATIONS FOR LABORATORIES

BSL	Agents	Practices	Safety Equipment	Facility
1	Not known to cause disease in healthy adults	Standard microbiological procedures	None required	Open bench top sink required
2	Associated with human disease. Hazard = autoinoculation, ingestion, or mucous membrane exposure	BSL-1 practice plus limited access, biohazard warning signs, Sharps precautions, and a biosafety manual defining waste decontamination or medical surveillance policies	Class I or II biosafety cabinet (BSC), splash guards and other devices to prevent splashes or aerosols. PPE = Lab coats, gloves, and face protection as needed	BSL-1 plus autoclave available
3	Indigenous or exotic agents with potential aerosol transmission. Disease may have serious or lethal consequences	BSL-2 practice plus controlled access, decontamination of all waste, decontamination of clothing before laundering, baseline serum	BSL-2 safety equipment plus respiratory protection as needed	BSL-2 plus physical separation from access corridors, self-closing double-door access, exhausted air not recirculated, negative airflow into the lab
4	Dangerous and exotic agents that pose high risk of life-threatening disease; aerosol transmitted	BSL-3 practices plus clothing change before entering, shower on exit, all materials decontaminated on exit from facility	All procedures conducted in Class III BSC or Class I or II BSC in combination with full-body, air-supplied, positive-pressure personnel suit	BSL-3 plus separate building or isolated zone, dedicated supply/exhaust, vacuum and decon system

RECOMMENDED BSL FOR BT AGENTS

Agent	BSL Specimen Handling	BSL Culture Handling	Specimen Exposure Risk	Recommended Laboratories Precautions
Alphaviruses	2	3	Blood, CSF. Tissue culture and animal inoculation studies should be performed at BSL-3 and are **NOT** Sentinel **(Level A) laboratory procedures.**	BSL-2: Activities involving clinical material collection and transport BSL-3: Activities with high potential for aerosol or droplet production
Bacillus anthracis	2	3	Blood, skin lesion exudates, CSF, pleural fluid, sputum, and rarely urine and feces	BSL-2: Activities involving clinical material collection and diagnostic quantities of infectious cultures BSL-3: All activities involving manipulations of cultures
Brucella spp.[a]	2	3	Blood, bone marrow, CSF, tissue, semen, and occasionally urine	BSL-2: Activities limited to collection,transport, and plating of clinical material BSL-3: All activities involving manipulations of cultures
Burkholderia pseudomallei	2	3	Blood, sputum, CSF, tissue, abscesses, and urine	BSL-2: Activities limited to collection, transport, and plating of clinical material
Burkholderia mallei	2	3	Blood, sputum, CSF, tissue, abscesses, and urine	BSL-2: Activities limited to collection, transport, and plating of clinical material BSL-3: All activities involving manipulations of cultures
Coxiella burnetii[b]	2	3	Blood, tissue, body fluids, feces. Manipulation of tissues from infected animals and tissue culture should be performed at BSL-3 and are **NOT Sentinel laboratory procedures**	BSL-2: Activities limited to collection and transport of clinical material, including serological examinations
Clostridium botulinum[c]	2	3	Toxin may be present in food specimens, clinical material (serum, gastric, and feces). **TOXIN IS EXTREMELY POISONOUS!**	BSL-2: Activities with materials known to be or potentially containing toxin must be handled in a BSC (class II) with a lab coat, disposable surgical gloves, and a face shield (as needed). BLS-3: Activities with high potential for aerosol or droplet production
Francisella tularensis[d]	2	3	Skin lesion exudates, respiratory secretions, CSF, blood, urine, tissues from infected animals, and fluids from infected arthropods	BLS-2: Activities limited to collection, transport, and plating of clinical material BLS-3: All activities involving manipulations of cultures

(Continued)

T A B L E   J - 2
RECOMMENDED BSL FOR BT AGENTS (CONTINUED)

Agent	BSL		Specimen Exposure Risk	Recommended Laboratories Precautions
	Specimen Handling	Culture Handling		
Yersinia pestis[e]	2	3	Bubo fluid, blood, sputum, CSF, feces, and urine	BSL-2: Activities involving clinical material collection and diagnostic quantities of infectious cultures BSL-3: Activities with high potential for aerosol or droplet production
Smallpox[f]	4	4	Lesion fluid or crusts, respiratory secretions, or tissue	BSL-2: Packing and shipping. Do **NOT** put in cell culture.
Staphylococcal enterotoxin B	2	2	Toxin may be present in food specimens, clinical material (serum, gastric, urine, respiratory secretions, and feces), and isolates of S. aureus.	BSL-2: Activities involving clinical material collection and diagnostic quantities of infectious cultures
VHF[g]	4	4	Blood, urine, respiratory, and throat secretions, semen, and tissue	BSL-2: Packing and shipping. Do **NOT** put in cell culture.

[a]Laboratory-acquired brucellosis has occurred by "sniffing" cultures; aerosols generated by centrifugation; mouth pipetting; accidental parenteral inoculations; and sprays into eyes, nose, and mouth; by direct contact with clinical specimens; and when no breach in technique could be identified.

[b]Laboratory-acquired infections have been acquired from virulent phase I organisms due to infectious aerosols from cell culture and the use of embryonated eggs to propagate C. burnetii.

[c]Exposure to toxin is the primary laboratory hazard, since absorption can occur with direct contact with skin, eyes, or mucous membranes, including the respiratory tract. The toxin can be neutralized by 0.1 M sodium hydroxide. C. botulinum is inactivated by a 1:10 dilution of household bleach. Contact time is 20 min. If material contains both toxin and organisms, the spill must be sequentially treated with bleach and sodium hydroxide for a total contact time of 40 min.

[d]Laboratory-acquired tularemia infection has been more commonly associated with cultures than with clinical materials or animals. Direct skin/mucous membrane contact with cultures, parenteral inoculation, ingestion, and aerosol exposure have resulted in infection.

[e]Special care should be taken to avoid the generation of aerosols.

[f]Ingestion, parenteral inoculation, and droplet or aerosol exposure of mucous membranes or broken skin with infectious fluids or tissues are the primary hazards to laboratory workers.

[g]Respiratory exposure to infectious aerosols, mucous membrane exposure to infectious droplets, and accidental parenteral inoculation are the primary hazards to laboratory workers.

SPECIMEN SELECTION: BIOTERRORISM AGENTS[a]

Disease/Agent	Specimen Selection	Transport & Storage	Specimen Plating and Processing					
			SBA	CA	MAC	Stain	Other	
Anthrax (Bacillus anthracis)	Possible Bacillus anthracis exposure in an asymptomatic patient	Swab of anterior nares: Only to be collected if so advised by local public health authorities	≤24 h, RT	No	No	No	None	Follow public health instructions on anterior nares swab ONLY if advised to collect these.
	Cutaneous	Vesicular stage: Collect fluid from intact vesicles on sterile swab(s). The organism is best demonstrated in this stage.	≤24 h, RT	X	X	X	Gram stain	
		Eschar stage: Without removing eschar, insert swab moistened in sterile saline beneath the edge of eschar, rotate, and collect lesion material.	≤24 h, RT	X	X	X	Gram stain	
		Vesicular stage and eschar stage: collect 2 punch biopsies Place one biopsy in 10% formalin to be sent to CDC for histopathology, immunohistochemical staining, and PCR.	One punch biopsy in 10% formalin. Once in formalin, can be stored until transported to CDC	No	No	No	Performed at CDC	Arrange for transport to CDC.
		Submit second biopsy in an anaerobic transport vial for culture	Second punch biopsy in anaerobic transport vial ≤24 h, RT	X	X	X	Gram stain	
		Blood cultures: Collect 2 sets (1 set is 2 bottles) per institutional procedure for routine blood cultures.	Transport at RT. Incubate at 35–37°C per blood culture protocol	Blood culture bottles				Positive in some cases during late stages of disease

(Continued)

T A B L E J - 3

SPECIMEN SELECTION: BIOTERRORISM AGENTS[a] (CONTINUED)

Disease/Agent	Specimen Selection	Transport & Storage	Specimen Plating and Processing				
			SBA	CA	MAC	Stain	Other
Anthrax (Bacillus anthracis) (Continued)	Cutaneous (Continued)	Purple-top tube (EDTA): for inpatients only, collect for direct Gram stain	No	No	No	Gram stain	
		Red-top or blue-top tubes for serology; White Tube for PCR	No	No	No	No	Arrange for transport to CDC.
	Gastro-intestinal	Stool: Collect 5–10 g in a clean, sterile, leakproof container.	Inoculate routine stool plating media plus CNA or PEA.				Minimal recovery
		Blood cultures: Collect 2 sets (1 set is 2 bottles) per institutional procedure for routine blood cultures.	Blood culture bottles				Positive in late stages of disease
		Purple-top tube (EDTA): for inpatients only, collect for direct Gram stain	No	No	No	Gram stain	
		Red-top or blue-top tubes for serology; White Tube for PCR	No	No	No		
	Inhalation	Sputum: Collect expectorated specimen into a sterile, leakproof container.	X	X	X	Gram stain	Minimal recovery
		Pleural fluid: Collect specimen into sterile, leakproof container.	X	X	X	Gram stain	Save excess (if any) for PCR.
		Blood cultures: Collect 2 sets (1 set is 2 bottles) procedure per institutional for routine blood cultures.	Blood culture bottles				Positive in late stages of disease

Transport & Storage notes:
- Purple-top rows: ≤2 h, RT
- Red-top / blue-top rows: ≤24 h, 4°C
- Stool: ≤24 h, 4°C
- Blood cultures: Transport at RT. Incubate at 35–37°C per blood culture protocol.
- Sputum: ≤24 h, 4°C
- Pleural fluid: ≤24 h, 4°C

Disease	Specimen	Transport/Storage					Comments
	Purple-top tube (EDTA): for inpatients only, collect for direct Gram stain.	≤2 h, RT	No	No	No	No	Gram stain
	Red-top or blue-top tubes for serology; White Tube for PCR	≤24 h, 4°C	No	No	No	No	
Meningitis	Cerebrospinal fluid culture: Aseptically collect CSF per institutional procedure.	≤24 h, RT	X	X		Gram stain	May be seen in late stages of disease; consider adding broth medium such as brain heart infusion.
	Blood cultures: Collect 2 sets (1 set is 2 bottles) per institutional procedure for routine blood cultures.	Transport at RT. Incubate at 35–37°C per blood culture		Blood culture bottles		Positive in late stages of disease	
Brucellosis (Brucella melitensis, B. abortus, B. suis, B. canis)	Serum: Collect 10–12 cc (ml) of acute-phase specimen as soon as possible after disease onset. Follow with a convalescent-phase specimen obtained 21 days later.	≤ ransport in ≤ 2 h, at RT. Store at –20°C.	Specimen should be stored and shipped frozen at –20°C to State Laboratory or other LRN Reference (Level B/C) laboratory.			Serologic diagnosis: 1. Single titer: ≤ 1:160 2. 4-fold rise 3. IgM NOTE: B. canis does not cross-react with standard serologic reagents.	
	Blood: Collect 2 sets (1 set is 2 bottles) per institutional procedure for routine blood cultures.	Transport at RT. Incubate at 35–37°C	Blood culture bottles: Subculture at 5 days and hold 21 days.			Blood culture isolation rates vary from 15–70% depending on methods and length of incubation. Cultures should be manipulated in a biological safety cabinet. Personal protective equipment includes gloves, gown, mask, and protective faceshield. All cultures should be taped shut during incubation.	

(Continued)

547

TABLE J-3

SPECIMEN SELECTION: BIOTERRORISM AGENTS[a] (CONTINUED)

Disease/Agent	Specimen Selection	Transport & Storage	Specimen Plating and Processing				
			SBA	CA	MAC	Stain	Other
	Bone marrow, spleen, or liver: Collect per institution's surgical/pathology procedure.	£ 24 h, RT	X	X	Hold cultures for at least 7 days.	Gram stain	Cultures should be manipulated in a biological safety cabinet. Personal protective equipment includes gloves, gown, mask, and protective faceshield. All cultures should be taped shut during incubation.
Meningitis	Cerebrospinal fluid culture: Aseptically collect CSF per institutional procedure.	£ 24 h, RT	X	X	Hold cultures for at least 7 days.	Gram stain	Cultures should be manipulated in a biological safety cabinet. Personal protective equipment includes gloves, gown, mask, and protective faceshield. All cultures should be taped shut during incubation. Consider adding broth medium such as brain heart infusion.
	Cerebrospinal fluid for antibody testing	–20°C			Specimen should be stored and shipped frozen at –20°C or lower temperature to State Laboratory or other LRN Reference laboratory.	None	

Disease/Agent	Specimen Selection						Transport & Storage	Specimen Handling
	Specimen type	Clinical syndrome						Specimen(s) of choice for confirming botulism:
		Foodborne	Infant	Wound	Intentional release (airborne)			1. Serum
								2. Wound/tissue
								3. Stool
								4. Incriminated food
Botulism (botulinum toxin)	Enema fluid—20 ml	X	X		X		4°C	Purge with a minimal amount of sterile nonbacteriostatic water to minimize dilution of toxin.
	Food sample—10–50g	X	X		X		4°C	Foods that support C. botulinum growth will have a pH of 3.5–7.0; most common pH is 5.5–6.5. Submit food in original container, placing individually in leakproof sealed transport devices.
	Gastric fluid—20 ml	X,A					4°C	Collect up to 20 ml.
	Intestinal fluid—20 ml	A	A				4°C	Autopsy: Intestinal contents from various areas of the small and large intestines should be provided.
	Nasal swab (anaerobic swab)				X		RT	For aerosolized botulinum toxin exposure, obtain nasal cultures for C. botulinum and serum for mouse toxicity testing.
	Serum—15–20 ml	X,A		X	X		4°C	Serum should be obtained as soon as possible after the onset of symptoms and before antitoxin is given. Whole blood (30 ml [3 red-top or gold-top tubes]) is required for mouse toxicity testing. In infants, serum is generally not useful, since the toxin is quickly absorbed before serum can be obtained.
	Stool >25 g	X	X	X	X		4°C	Botulism has been confirmed in infants with only "pea-size" stools. Please note: Anticholinesterase given orally, as in patients with myasthenia gravis, has been shown to interfere with toxin testing.
	Vomitus—20 ml	X					4°C	Collect up to 20 ml.
	Wound, tissue—anaerobic swab or transport system						Anaerobic swab or transport system Transport at RT	Exudate, tissue, or swabs must be collected and transported in an anaerobic transport system. Samples from an enema or feces should also be submitted, since the wound may not be the source of botulinum toxin.

(Continued)

SPECIMEN SELECTION: BIOTERRORISM AGENTS[a] (CONTINUED)

	Specimen Selection				
Disease/Agent	Specimen type	Foodborne	Airborne (intentional release)	Transport and Storage	Specimen Handling
Staphylococcal enterotoxin B (From Staphylococcus aureus)	Serum—10 ml	X	X	2–8°C	1. Obtain as soon as possible after the onset of symptoms to detect the toxin. 2. Also collect 7–14 days after onset of illness to compare acute and convalescent antibody titers. 3. Do not send whole blood, since hemolysis during transit will compromise the quality of the specimen.
	Nasal swab—dacron or rayon swab		X	2–8°C	Collect a nasal swab within 24 h of exposure by rubbing a dry, sterile swab (Dacron or rayon) on the mucosa of the anterior nares. Place in protective transport tube.
	Induced respiratory secretions		X	2–8°C	Collect sputum induced by instilling 10–25 ml of sterile saline into nasal passages into a sterile screw-top container.
	Urine—20–30 ml	X	X	2–8°C	Collect into a sterile, leakproof container with screw-top lid.
	Stool or gastric aspirate—10–50 g	X	X	2–8°C	Collect into a sterile, leakproof container with screw-top lid.
	Postmortem 10 g	X	X	2–8°C	Obtain specimens of the intestinal contents from different levels of the small and large bowel. Place 10 g of specimen into a sterile, leakproof container with screw-top lid. Obtain serum as previously described.
	Culture isolate	X	X	2–8°C	Send S. aureus isolate for toxin testing on appropriate agar slant.
	Food specimen	X	X	2–8°C	Food should be left in its original container if possible or placed in sterile unbreakable containers and labeled carefully. Place containers individually in leakproof containers (i.e., sealed plastic bags) to prevent cross-contamination during shipment. Empty containers with remnants of suspected contaminated foods can be examined.

Disease/Agent	Specimen Selection	Transport & Storage	Specimen Plating and Processing				
			SBA	CA	MAC	Stain	Other
Plague (Yersinia pestis)	Possible Y. pestis exposure in asymptomatic patient	No cultures or serology indicated					Follow public health instructions if advised to collect specimens.
	Bubonic	Blood cultures: Collect 2 sets (1 set is 2 bottles) per institutional procedure for routine blood cultures.	Transport at RT. Incubate at 35–37°C per blood culture protocol.	Blood culture bottles			Gram stain of positive cultures	If suspicion of plague is high, obtain an additional set for incubation at RT (22–28°C) without shaking
		Tiger-top, red-top, or gold-top tube: For serology (acute and, if needed for diagnosis, convalescent serum in 14 days) Green-top (heparin) tube: For PCR	£ 20h, 4°C		No		No	Patients with negative cultures having a single titer, £ 1:10, specific to F1 antigen by agglutination would meet presumptive criteria.
		Lymph node (bubo) aspirate: Flushing with 1.0 ml of sterile saline may be needed to obtain material.	Transport at RT or 4°C if transport is delayed. Store at £ 24 h, 4°C.	X	X	X	Gram stain, Giemsa, Wright's stain	Contact LRN Reference lab or above laboratory to prepare smears for DFA.
		Tissue: Collect in sterile container with 1 to 2 drops of sterile, nonbacteriostatic saline.	Transport at RT or 4°C if transport is delayed. Store at £ 24 h, 4°C.	X	X	X	Gram stain, Giemsa, Wright's stain	Contact LRN Reference lab or above laboratory to prepare smears for DFA.

(Continued)

SPECIMEN SELECTION: BIOTERRORISM AGENTS^a *(CONTINUED)*

Disease/Agent	Specimen Selection	Transport & Storage	Specimen Plating and Processing				
			SBA	CA	MAC	Stain	Other
Plague (*Yersinia pestis*) (*Continued*)	Bubonic (*Continued*)	Throat: Collect routine throat culture using a swab collected into a sterile, leakproof container.	X	X	X	Gram stain	Contact LRN Reference lab or above laboratory to prepare smears for DFA.
	Pneumonic	Sputum/throat: Collect routine throat culture using a swab or expectorated sputum collected into a sterile, leakproof container.	X	X	X	Gram stain	Contact LRN Reference lab or above laboratory to prepare smears for DFA.
		Bronchial/tracheal wash: Collect per institution's procedure in an area dedicated to collecting respiratory specimens under isolation/containment circumstances, i.e., isolation chamber/"bubble."	X	X	X	Gram stain	Contact LRN Reference lab or above laboratory to prepare smears for DFA.
		Blood cultures: Collect 2 sets (1 set is 2 bottles) per institutional procedure for routine blood cultures.	Blood culture bottles			Gram stain of positive cultures	If suspicion of plague is high, obtain an additional set for incubation at RT (22–28°C) without shaking.
		Tiger-top, red-top, or gold-top tube: For serology (acute and, if needed for diagnosis, convalescent serum in 14 days) Green-top (heparin) tube: For PCR	No	No			Patients with negative cultures having a single titer, ≤ 1:10, specific to F1 antigen would meet presumptive criteria.

Transport & Storage:
- Throat (Bubonic): ≤ 24 h, 4°C
- Sputum/throat (Pneumonic): ≤ 24 h, 4°C
- Bronchial/tracheal wash: ≤ 24 h, 4°C
- Blood cultures: Transport at RT. Incubate at 35–37°C per blood culture protocol.
- Tiger-top, red-top, or gold-top tube: ≤ 24 h, 4°C

			Blood culture bottles			
Meningitis	Blood cultures: Collect 2 sets (1 set is 2 bottles) per institutional procedure for routine blood cultures.	Transport at RT Incubate at 35–37°C per blood culture protocol.			Gram stain of positive cultures	If suspicion of plague is high, obtain an additional set for incubation at RT (22–28°C) without shaking.
	Tiger-top, red-top, or gold-top tube: For serology (acute and, if needed for diagnosis, convalescent serum in 14 days) Green-top (heparin) tube: For PCR	≤ 24 h, 4°C	No	No		Patients with negative cultures having a single titer, ≤ 1:10, specific to F1 antigen by agglutination would meet presumptive criteria.
	Cerebrospinal fluid	Transport at RT. Store incubated at 35–37°C.	X	X	Gram stain	Can add broth culture at RT (22–28°C) without shaking
Tularemia (Francisella tularensis)	Possible Francisella tularensis exposure in asymptomatic patient No cultures or serology indicated					Follow public health instructions if advised to collect specimens.
	Oculo-glandular Conjunctival scraping	≤ 24 h, 4 ≤ C	X	X	Gram stain; prepare smears for DFA referral.	Add a BCYE plate and a plate selective for Neisseria gonorrhoeae such as modified Thayer-Martin. Manipulate cultures in a biological safety cabinet. Personal protective equipment includes gloves, gown, mask, and protective faceshield. All cultures should be taped shut during incubation.

(Continued)

SPECIMEN SELECTION: BIOTERRORISM AGENTS[a] (CONTINUED)

Disease/Agent		Specimen Selection	Transport & Storage	Specimen Plating and Processing				
				SBA	CA	MAC	Stain	Other
Tularemia (Francisella tularensis) (Continued)	Oculo–glandular (Continued)	Lymph node aspirate: Flushing with 1.0 ml of sterile saline may be needed to obtain material.	Transport at RT, 4°C if transport is delayed. Store at £ 24 h, 4°C.	X	X	X	Gram stain; prepare smears for DFA referral.	Add a BCYE plate and a plate selective for Neisseria gonorrhoeae such as modified Thayer-Martin. Manipulate cultures in a biological safety cabinet. Personal protective equipment includes gloves, gown, mask, and protective faceshield. All cultures should be taped shut during incubation.
		Blood cultures: Collect 2 sets (1 set is 2 bottles) per institutional procedure for routine blood cultures. Growth is more likely from aerobic bottle.	Transport at RT. Incubate at 35–37°C per blood culture protocol.	Blood culture bottles; subculture the broth to BCYE plate and incubate aerobically.				Cultures should be manipulated in a biological safety cabinet. Personal protective equipment includes gloves, gown, mask, and protective faceshield. All cultures should be taped shut during incubation.

	Specimen and collection	Transport/storage			Comments
Ulcero-glandular	Blood cultures: Collect 2 sets (1 set is 2 bottles) per institutional procedure for routine blood cultures. Growth is more likely from aerobic bottle.	Transport at RT. Incubate at 35–37°C per blood culture protocol.	Blood culture bottles; subculture the broth to BCYE plate and incubate aerobically		Cultures should be manipulated in a biological safety cabinet. Personal protective equipment includes gloves, gown, mask, and protective faceshield. All cultures should be taped shut during incubation.
	Ulcer or tissue: Collect biopsy (best specimen), scraping, or swab. Lymph node aspirate: Flushing with 1.0 ml of sterile saline may be needed to obtain material.	≤ 24 h, 4°C Transport at RT. 4°C if transport is delayed. Store at ≤ 24 h, 4°C.	X X	Gram stain Gram stain; prepare smears for DFA referral.	Add a BCYE plate and a plate selective for *Neisseria gonorrhoeae* such as modified Thayer-Martin. Prepare smears for DFA referral. Manipulate cultures in a biological safety cabinet. Personal
Pneumonic	Sputum/throat: Collect routine throat culture using a swab or expectorated sputum collected into a sterile, leakproof container.	≤ 24 h, 4°C.	X	Gram stain	protective equipment includes gloves, gown, mask, and protective fasecshield. All cultures should be taped shut during incubation.
	Bronchial/tracheal wash: Collect per institution's procedure in an area dedicated to collecting respiratory specimens under isolation/containment circumstances, i.e., isolation chamber/"bubble."	≤ 24 h, 4°C.	X	Gram stain	

(Continued)

SPECIMEN SELECTION: BIOTERRORISM AGENTS[a] (CONTINUED)

Disease/Agent	Specimen Selection	Transport & Storage	Specimen Plating and Processing				
			SBA	CA	MAC	Stain	Other
Tularemia (Francisella tularensis) (Continued)	Pneumonic (Continued) Blood cultures: Collect 2 sets (1 set is 2 bottles) per institutional procedure for routine blood cultures. Growth is more likely from aerobic bottle.	Transport at RT. Incubate at 35–37°C per blood culture protocol.	Blood culture bottles; subculture the broth to BCYE plate and incubate aerobically				Cultures should be manipulated in a biological safety cabinet. Personal protective equipment includes gloves, gown, mask, and protective faceshield. All cultures should be taped shut during incubation.
	2 Red-top or gold-top tubes: For PCR and serology (acute and, if needed for diagnosis, convalescent serum in 14 days)	£ 2 h RT, £ 24 h, 4°C	No				Positive serology test would meet presumptive criteria. Confirmation requires culture identification or a 4-fold rise in titer.

Disease/Agent	Specimen Selection and Transport	Specimen Handling

Smallpox (Variola virus)	See CDC document "Specimen Collection and Transport Guidelines" for detailed instructions http://www.bt.cdc.gov/agent/smallpox/response-plan/index.asp#guidec (Click on Guide D)
	
	NOTE: Only recently, successfully *vaccinated* personnel (within 3 years) wearing appropriate barrier protection (gloves, gown, and shoe covers) should be involved in specimen collection for suspected cases of smallpox. Respiratory protection is not needed for personnel with recent, successful vaccination. Masks and eyewear or faceshields should be used if splashing is anticipated.
	
	If unvaccinated personnel must be utilized to collect specimens, only those without contraindications to vaccination should be utilized, as they would require immediate vaccination if the diagnosis of smallpox is confirmed. Fit-tested N95 masks should be worn by unvaccinated individuals caring for suspected patients.
		1. **A suspected case of smallpox should be reported <u>immediately to</u> the respective Local and State Health Departments for review.**
		2. And if, after review, smallpox is still suspected, one of the following should be contacted immediately:
		  A. CDC Emergency Response Hotline (24 hours): 770-488-7100
		  B. Poxvirus Section, Division of Viral and Rickettsial Diseases, NCID, CDC, Atlanta, Georgia 30333. Laboratory: 404-639-4931
		  C. Bioterrorism Preparedness and Response Program, NCID, CDC: 404-639-0385 or 404-639-2468. (8 am to 5 pm weekdays)
		NOTE: Approval must be obtained prior to the shipment of potential smallpox patient clinical specimens to CDC
		3. At this time, review the packaging/shipping requirements with CDC and request assistance in coordinating a carrier for transport/shipment.
		4. **Hand carry all specimens and do not send specimens via pneumatic tube system.**
		5. Do not attempt viral cultures: this is a Biosafety Level 4 agent, and this could result in a very unsafe situation in which there is a significant amount of infectious virus.

	Rash	Biopsy specimens	See CDC document "Specimen
		Scabs	Collection and Transport Guidelines"
		Vesicular fluid	for detailed instructions (Guide D).
	Posterior tonsillar tissue swab	Swab	
	Blood	Use plastic tubes	
	Autopsy	Portions of skin containing lesions, liver, spleen, lung, lymph nodes, and/or kidney	

(Continued)

SPECIMEN SELECTION: BIOTERRORISM AGENTS[a] (CONTINUED)

Disease/Agent	Specimen Selection	Transport & Storage	Specimen Handling
VHF (Various viruses including Ebola, Marburg, Lassa, Machupo, Junin, Guanarito, Sabia, Crimeancongo hemorrhagic fever Rift Valley fever, Omsk hemorrhagic fever, Kyasanur Forest disease virus, and others)	Serum for antibody testing: Collect blood in red-top or gold-top or gold-top tubes. Obtain convalescent serum at least 14 days acute specimen is obtained. Use a Vacutainer or other sealed sterile dry tube for blood collection. Viral culture, blood: Collect serum, heparinized plasma (green-top tube), or whole blood during acute febrile illness. Throat wash specimens: Mix with equal volume of viral transport medium Urine: Mix with equal volume of viral transport medium.	Transport within ~2 h, at RT. Store at −20°C to −70°C. Transport at RT. Store 4°C or frozen on dry ice and liquid nitrogen. Transport on wet ice. Store at −40°C or colder. Transport on wet ice. Store at −40°C or colder.	Specific handling conditions are currently under development. Contact CDC to discuss proper collection and handling. 1. Double-bag each specimen. 2. Swab the exterior of the outside bag with disinfectant *before* removal from the patient's room 3. Do not use glass tubes. 4. Hand carry all specimens and do not send specimens via pneumatic tube system. **NOTE:** Disposable equipment and sharps go into rigid containers containing disinfectant that are then autoclaved or incinerated. Double-bag refuse. The exterior of the outside bag is to be treated with disinfectant and then autoclaved or incinerated. **Do not attempt tissue culture isolation.** This is only to be done in a Biosafety Level 4 facility.
	CSF, tissue, other specimens	As per discussion with CDC	In laboratory: 1. Strict barrier precautions are to be used. Personal protective equipment includes gloves, gown, mask, shoe covers, and protective faceshield. 2. Handle specimens in biological safety cabinet if possible. 3. Consider respiratory mask with HEPA filter. 4. Specimens should be centrifuged at low speed.
	Blood cultures: If clinical and travel history warrants, collect 2 sets (1 set is 2 bottles) of blood cultures per institutional procedure for routine blood cultures. Malaria smear of peripheral blood: If clinical and travel history warrants	Transport at RT. Incubate at 35–37°C per blood culture protocol. Lavender-top tube at RT	Bacteremia with disseminated intravascular coagulation and malaria due to *Plasmodium falciparum* are two life-threatening and treatable clinical entities that can present with prominent clinical findings of hemorrhage and fever in a patient with a travel history to areas with VHF. Handle with precautions noted above. Continue to use the same precautions as above.

Agent	Specimen	Transport/Storage	Comments
Q. fever (*Coxiella burnetii*)	Serum: Collect 10 ml of serum (red-top, tiger-top, or gold-top tube) as soon as possible after onset of symptoms (acute) and with a follow-up specimen (convalescent) at ≥14 days for serological testing.	Transport within ~6 h, at 4°C. Store at −20° to −70°C	**Do not attempt tissue culture isolation,** as that could result in a very unsafe situation in which there is a significant amount of infectious organism.
	Blood: Collect blood in EDTA (lavender) or sodium citrate (blue) and maintain at 4°C for storage and shipping for PCR or special cultures. If possible, collect specimens prior to antimicrobial therapy.	Transport within ~6 h, at 4°C. Store at 4°C.	Sentinel laboratories should consult with State Public Health Laboratory Director (or designate) prior to or concurrent with testing if *C. burnetii* is suspected by the attending physician.
	Tissue, body fluids, others, including cell cultures and cell supernatants: Specimens can be kept at 2–8°C if transported within 24 h. Store frozen at −70°C or on dry ice.	Transport within <24 h, at 2–8°C. Store at −70°C or on dry ice.	Serology is available through commercial reference as well as public health laboratories.
Alphaviruses (Includes Eastern equine, Western equine, Venezuelan equine encephalitis viruses and others)	Serum: Collect 10 ml of serum (red-top, tiger-top, or gold-top tube) as soon as possible after onset of symptoms (acute) and with a follow-up specimen (convalescent) at ≥14 days for serological testing.	Transport within ~6 h, at 4°C. Store at −20°C to 70°C	**Do not attempt tissue culture isolation,** as that could result in a very unsafe situation in which there is a significant amount of infectious organism.
	Blood: Collect blood in EDTA (lavender) or sodium citrate (blue) and maintain at 4°C for storage and shipping for PCR or special studies.	Transport within ~6 h, at 4°C. Store at 4°C.	
	Cerebrospinal fluid: Specimens (greater than 1 ml) can be kept at 2–8°C if transported within 24 h. If frozen, store at −70°C and transport on dry ice.	Transport on wet ice. If already frozen, store at −70°C and transport on dry ice.	
	Tissue, body fluids, others, including cell cultures and cell supernatants: Specimens can be kept at 2–8°C if transported within 24 h. If frozen, store at −70°C and transport on dry ice.	Transport on wet ice. If already frozen, store at 70°C and transport on dry ice.	

(Continued)

SPECIMEN SELECTION: BIOTERRORISM AGENTS[a] (CONTINUED)

Disease/Agent	Specimen Selection	Transport & Storage	Specimen Plating and Processing					
			SBA	CA	MAC	PC	Stain	Other
Melioidosis and glanders (Burkholderia pseudomallei and Burkholderia mallei)	Possible Burkholderia pseudomallei or Burkholderia mallei exposure in asymptomatic patient	No cultures or serology indicated						Follow public health instructions if advised to collect specimens.
	Clinical illness	Bone marrow		X				B. pseudomallei is a small gram-negative bacillus that may demonstrate bipolar morphology on stain.
		Transport within £ 2 h, at RT. Store £ 24 h, at 4°C					Gram stain	B. mallei is a small gram-negative coccobacillus. Incubation should be at 35 to 37°C, ambient atmosphere; CO_2 incubation is acceptable.
	Blood cultures: Collect 2 sets (1 set is 2 bottles) per institutional procedure for routine blood cultures OR collect lysis-centrifugation (e.g., Isolator) blood cultures.	Transport at RT. Incubate at 35–37°C per blood culture protocol				Blood culture bottles OR Collect lysis-centrifugation (e.g., Isolator) blood cultures and plate to:		Cultures should be manipulated in a biological safety cabinet. Personal protective equipment includes gloves gown, mask, and protective faceshield. All cultures should be taped shut during incubation. Incubation should be at 35 to 37°C, ambient atmosphere; CO_2 incubation is acceptable.
				X				

Specimen	Transport/Storage					Comments
Respiratory specimens, abscess material, wound specimens, urine	Transport within ≤ 2 h, at RT. Store ≤ 24 h, at 4°C.	X	X	X	X	If the laboratory has *B cepacia* selective agar medium, it has been shown useful in isolation of *B. pseudomallei* for specimens in which indigenous microflora is likely to be encountered. Ashdown medium is a selective medium specifically designed for recovery of *B. pseudo mallei*. This medium is not likely to be available in most Sentinel laboratories. Incubation should be at 35 to 37°C; ambient atmosphere; CO_2 incubation is acceptable. Obtain if serologic diagnosis of *B. pseudomallei* infection is being considered.
Serum: Red-top or gold-top tube for both acute and convalescent (obtained 14 days after the acute specimen)	Transport within ~6 h, at 4°C. Store at −20°C to 70°C.					

Gram stain

*a*Abbreviations: A, autopsy; BCYE, buffered charcoal-yeast extract agar; C, centigrade; CA, chocolate agar; CNA, colistin–nalidixic acid agar; DFA, direct fluorescent antibody; MAC, MacConkey agar; PEA, phenylethyl alcohol blood agar; RT, room temperature; VHF, viral hemorrhagic fever; PC, selective medium for *Burkholderia cepacia*.

AGENT CHARACTERISTICS SUMMARY: MICROORGANISMS

Characteristic	B. anthracis	Y. pestis	Burkholderia Pseudomallei and B. mallei	F. tularensis	Brucella spp.	Variola Virus (smallpox)
Gram stain morphology	• Large gram-positive rod • Nonmotile • From blood agar: no capsule, central to subterminal spores that do not enlarge the cell • From blood: capsule, no spores	• Plump gram-negative rod • Gram stain: ± bipolar or "safety pin" appearance • Wright-Giemsa: bipolar or "safety pin" appearance	• B. pseudomallei: small gram-negative rod • B. mallei: small gram-negative coccobacillus • Gram stain: ± bipolar or "safety pin" appearance (B. pseudomallei) • Wright-Giemsa: bipolar or "safety pin" appearance (B. pseudomallei)	• Minute GNCB • Poorly staining • Smaller than Haemophilus influenzae • Pleomorphic	• Tiny GNCB • Faintly staining	
Growth	• Standard conditions • Extremely rapid	• 28°C optimal, without agitation • 35–37°C more slowly	• 35–37°C • Ambient atmosphere, though CO_2 is acceptable	• Aerobic conditions • Growth is best on media containing cysteine, such as BCYE, but will often grow initially on chocolate or BA	• Grows in blood culture media • Can require blind subculturing	• Grows in most cell lines • Unusual or unrecognizable CPE
Colonial morphology (BA)	• Nonhemolytic • Ground glass • Irregular/wavy edges • Tenacious • "Beaten egg whites" when touched with loop	• Pinpoint at 24–48 h • "Fried egg" or "hammered copper" or shiny at 48–72 h • Nonhemolytic	B. pseudomallei: • SBA: small, smooth creamy colonies in first 1 to 2 days, gradually changing after a few days to dry, wrinkled colonies similar to Pseudomonas stutzeri B. mallei: • SBA: smooth, gray, translucent colonies without pigment	• Does not pass well on BA	• Small colonies • Punctate after 48 h • Nonhemolytic	
Tests	• Cat (+)	• Cat (+) • Ox (−) • Urease (−) • MAC: Lac (−) • Indole (−)	• Cat (+) • Colistin (10 µg) and polymyxin B (300 U) (R) • Motility (+) B. pseudomallei • Motility (−) B. mallei • Indole (−) • Oxidase (+) B. pseudomallei • Oxidase (+/−) B. mallei • MAC: Lac (−) (B. pseudomallei) • MAC: Lac (−) or NG (B. mallei)	• Cat wk (+) • Ox (−) • Urease (−) • β-Lac (−) • Satellite (−) • MAC: NG	• Ox (+) • Urease (+), though some are negative • Satellite (−) • MAC: Poor to NG	• CPE can be passed

BIOTERRORISM AGENT CLINICAL SUMMARY

Disease	Virulence Factor(s)	Infective Dose (ID)	Incubation Period	Duration of Illness	Person-to-Person Transmission[e]	Isolation Precautions for Hospitalized[f]	Persistence of Organism
Inhalation anthrax	Exotoxin[a] capsule	Lower limit unknown, ID2 estimated at 9 spores[b]	1–6 days	3–5 days	No	Standard	>40 yr
Brucellosis	LPS;[c] PMN survival	10–100 organisms	5–60 days (usually 1–2 mo)	Weeks to months	Via breast milk[g] and sexually[h] (rare)	Standard	Water/soil, ~10 wk
Botulism	Neurotoxin	0.001 μg/kg is LD_{50} for type A	6 h to 10 days (usually 1–5 days)	Death in 24–72 h; lasts months if not lethal	No	Standard	Food/water, ~weeks
Glanders	Little studied, possible antiphagocytic capsule	Low	10–14 days via aerosol	Death in 7–10 days in septicemic form	YES (low)	Standard	Very stable
Melioidosis	Possibly LPS, exotoxin, intracellular survival, antiphagocytic capsule	Low	2 days to 26 yr	Days to months	YES (rare)[i]	Standard	Very stable in water/soil
Pneumonic plague	V and W antigens LPS (endotoxin) F1 antigen[d]	<100 organisms	2–3 days	1–6 days	YES (high)	Droplet[f]	Soil, up to 1 yr
Q fever	Intracellular survival LPS (endotoxin)	1–10 organisms	10–40 days	~2 wk (acute), months to years (chronic)	Rare[j]	Standard	Very stable
Smallpox		10–100 particles	7–17 days	~4 wk	YES (high)	Airborne[f]	Very Stable

(Continued)

BIOTERRORISM AGENT CLINICAL SUMMARY (CONTINUED)

Disease	Virulence Factor(s)	Infective Dose (ID)	Incubation Period	Duration of Illness	Person-to-Person Transmission[e]	Isolation Precautions for Hospitalized[f]	Persistence of Organism
Staphylococcal enterotoxin B	Superantigen	0.0004 µg/kg incapacitation; LD_{50} is 0.02 µg/kg	3–12 h after inhalation	Hours	No	Standard	Resistant to freezing
Tularemia	Intracellular survival	10–50 organisms	2–10 days	≥2 wk	Single case report during autopsy	Standard	Moist soil, ~ months
VHF	Varies with virus	1–10 particles	4–21 days	7–16 days	YES (moderate)	Airborne and contact[f]	Unstable

[a]*B. anthracis* exotoxin or exotoxins consist of three components: the **edema factor** and **lethal factor** exert their effect within cells by interacting with a common transport protein designated **"protective antigen"** (so named because, when modified, it contributes to vaccine efficacy). Expression of toxic factors is mediated by one plasmid, and that of the capsule (D-glutamic acid polypeptide) is mediated by a second plasmid. Strains repeatedly subcultured at 42°C become avirulent as a result of losing virulence-determining plasmids, which is thought to be the basis for Pasteur's attenuated anthrax vaccine used at Pouilly-le-Fort in 1881.

[b]The estimate that nine inhaled spores would infect 2% of the exposed human population is based on data from Science **266**:1202–1208, 1994. The dose needed to infect 50% of the exposed human population may be 8,000 or higher.

[c]The major virulence factor for brucellosis appears to be an endotoxic lipopolysaccharide (LPS) among smooth strains. Pathogenicity is related to an LPS containing poly N-formyl perosamine O chain, Cu-Zn superoxide dismutase, erythrulose phosphate dehydrogenase, intracellular stress-induced proteins, and adenine and guanine monophosphate inhibitors of phagocyte functions.

[d]The V and W antigens and the F1 capsular antigens are only expressed at 7°C and not at the lower temperature of the flea (20 to 25°C).

[e]Periods of communicability are as follows: for **inhalation anthrax and botulism, none;** no evidence of person-to-person transmission; **pneumonic plague,** 72 h following initiation of appropriate antimicrobial therapy or until sputum culture is negative; **smallpox, approximately 3 weeks;** usually corresponds with the initial appearance of skin lesions to their final disappearance and is most infectious during the first week of rash via inhalation of virus released from oropharyngeal lesion secretions of the index case; **VHF, varies with virus, but at minimum, all for the duration of illness,** and for Ebola/Marburg transmission through semen may occur up to 7 weeks after clinical recovery.

[f]Guidelines for isolation precautions in hospitals can be found in Infect. Control Hosp. Epidemiol. **17:**53–80, 1996, in addition to the standard precautions that apply to all patients.

[g]Published reports of possible transmission of brucellosis via human breast milk may be found in Int. J. Infect. Dis. **4:**55–56, 2000; Ann. Trop. Paediatr. **10:**305–307, 1990; J. Infect. **26:**346–348, 1993; and Trop. Geogr. Med. **40:**151–152, 1988.

[h]Published reports of possible sexual transmission of brucellosis can be found in Lancet **i:**773, 1983; Aten Primaria **8:**165–166, 1991; Lancet **337:**848–849, 1991; Lancet **337:**14–15, 1991; Infection **11:**313–314, 1983; and Lancet **348:**615, 1996.

[i]See Lancet **337:**1290–1291, 1991.

[j]Published reports of possible sexual transmission of Q fever can be found in Clin. Infect. Dis. **22:**1087–1088, 1996; and Clin. Infect. Dis. **33:**399–402, 2001.)

TABLE J-6

ALTERNATIVE NAMES FOR BIOTERRORISM AGENTS FOR USE AT SPECIMEN RECEIVING AREA

Agent(s)	Other Information that May Appear on Requisition
Bacillus anthracis	Anthrax, cutaneous anthrax, gastrointestinal anthrax, inhalation anthrax, anthrax meningitis, patient with hemorrhagic mediastinitis
Brucella melitensis, B. suis, B. abortus, B. canis	Brucellosis; history of ingestion of goat's milk; history of consumption of Mexican cheese; slaughterhouse worker; history of consumption of unpasteurized milk or cheese; contact with goats, sheep, cattle, or camels; laboratory worker with accident
Burkholderia mallei	*Pseudomonas mallei*, glanders, laboratory worker with accident
Burkholderia pseudomallei	*Pseudomonas pseudomallei*, melioidosis
Clostridium botulinum toxin	Botulism, botulinum toxin, botulism toxin, infant botulism, wound botulism, food from patient with botulism
Coxiella burnetii	Q fever, pneumonia and sheep exposure, pneumonia and goat exposure, culture-negative endocarditis
Crimean-Congo hemorrhagic fever virus	Congo-Crimean hemorrhagic fever virus, CCHF, viral hemorrhagic fever, VHF, hemorrhagic fever
Ebola virus	Ebola, viral hemorrhagic fever, VHF, hemorrhagic fever
Francisella tularensis	Tularemia, *Pasteurella tularensis*, rabbit fever, deerfly fever, history of skinning animals, history of rabbit contact, tularemic pneumonia, typhoidal tularemia, oculoglandular tularemia, ulceroglandular tularemia, glandular tularemia, pharyngeal tularemia
Guanarito virus	Venezuelan hemorrhagic fever virus, viral hemorrhagic fever, VHF, hemorrhagic fever
Hantaviruses (one causes a VHF)	Korean hemorrhagic fever, Sin Nombre virus, hantavirus pulmonary syndrome, viral hemorrhagic fever, VHF, hemorrhagic fever
Junin virus (a VHF)	Argentinian hemorrhagic fever virus, viral hemorrhagic fever, VHF, hemorrhagic fever
Lassa fever virus	Viral hemorrhagic fever, VHF, hemorrhagic fever
Machupo virus	Bolivian hemorrhagic fever virus, viral hemorrhagic fever, VHF, hemorrhagic fever
Marburg virus	Marburg, viral hemorrhagic fever, VHF, hemorrhagic fever
Nipah virus	Hendra-like virus, pig contact with encephalitis
Smallpox virus	Variola, smallpox
Staphylococcal enterotoxin B	*Staphylococcus aureus* enterotoxin B, *Staphylococcus aureus* enterotoxin, staphylococcal enterotoxin, food from patient with food poisoning
Viral hemorrhagic fever	Hemorrhagic fever, VHF
Yersinia pestis	Plague, bubonic plague, pneumonic plague, septicemic plague, bubo, *Pasteurella pestis*, plague meningitis

TABLE J-7

BIOTERRORISM (BT) READINESS CHECKLIST FOR SENTINEL LABORATORIES

Does the laboratory have a biological safety cabinet?	YES ___ NO ___
Is the biological safety cabinet certified at least annually?	YES ___ NO ___
Does the laboratory have an autoclave?	YES ___ NO ___
Does the laboratory perform BSL2 or BSL3 practices?	YES ___ NO ___
Has someone in the laboratory attended state- or city-sponsored BT agent training?	YES ___ NO ___
Is someone in the laboratory certified in packaging and shipping of infectious substances?	YES ___ NO ___
Does the laboratory participate in the BT readiness proficiency testing program offered by CAP or the CDC?	YES ___ NO ___
Can the laboratory provide standard microbiological methods to investigate potential BT incidents?	YES ___ NO ___
Does the laboratory have guidelines or protocols in place to handle clinical specimens suspected of containing a BT agent?	YES ___ NO ___
Do they include:	
Safe collection, processing and labeling of specimens?	YES ___ NO ___
Chain of custody?	YES ___ NO ___
Safe disposal/decontamination protocols?	YES ___ NO ___
Coordination with the institution's internal emergency management system?	YES ___ NO ___
Are there protocols to presumptively identify/rule out the following:	
Bacillus anthracis?	YES ___ NO ___
Brucella species?	YES ___ NO ___
Francisella tularensis?	YES ___ NO ___
Yersinia pestis?	YES ___ NO ___
Does the laboratory have a copy of the most recent ASM sentinel laboratory BT guidelines?	YES ___ NO ___
Does the laboratory staff know how and whom to contact at the state laboratory regarding suspect BT agents?	YES ___ NO ___

ACKNOWLEDGMENT

ASM would like to thank the Oregon State Public Health Laboratory (*http://www.ohd.hr.state.or.us/phl/index.cfm*) for information from its web site that was useful in the drafting of this document.

VIII. REFERENCES

1. **Department of Health and Human Services.** 1999. Biosafety in microbiological and biomedical laboratories, 4th ed. U.S. Government Printing Office, Washington, D.C.

2. **Department of Health and Human Services.** 1999. Public Health Service, Centers for Disease Control and Prevention, and National Institutes of Health.

3. **Department of Health, Education, and Welfare.** 1974. Biohazards safety guide. Department of Health, Education, and Welfare, Bethesda, Md.

4. **Pike, R. M.** 1976. Laboratory-associated infections. Summary and analysis of 3921 cases. Health Lab. Sci. **13:**105–114.

Step	Task/data		Date/time completed	Signature
1. Name of patient(s), medical record number(s), patient location (s) and other pertinent information.				
A.				
B.				
C.				
D.				
E.				
F.				
G.				
H.				
2.	Who contacted lab about possibility of bioterrorism?			
3.	Person's (in step 4) phone number			
4.	Suspected bioterrorism agent(s) (e.g., anthrax, plague, etc., or unknown)	1. 2. 3. 4. 5.		

FIGURE J-1

INFORMATION CHECKLIST

Step	Task/data		Date/time completed	Signature
5.	Contacted microbiology personnel	❏ Yes ❏ No Who		
6.	Contacted clinical pathologist on call	❏ Yes ❏ No		
7.	Contacted ID physician **(if instructed) and/or** IC practitioner **(if instructed)**	❏ Yes ❏ No		
8.	If instructed to contact others *within* facility, write who and whether the person was available	Who: Contacted: ❏ Yes ❏ No Who: Contacted: ❏ Yes ❏ No		
9.	If instructed to contact others *outside* facility, write who and whether the person was available.	Who: Contacted: ❏ Yes ❏ No Who: Contacted: ❏ Yes ❏ No		
10.	Specimens for suspected bioterrorism agents placed in the biological safety cabinet in the _____ part of the laboratory.	❏ Yes ❏ No		

FIGURE J-1

(*CONTINUED*)

A P P E N D I X

K

RIOT CONTROL AGENTS

Katherine A. Martens, Christina Hantsch Bardsley, and Brian L. Bardsley

BACKGROUND

Civil disturbances and other uncontrolled demonstrations have been a part of history for years. When intervening in such situations, law enforcement and military personnel have employed various techniques including aggressive use of force at times. For example, in the New York Draft Riots of 1863, an angry mob numbering 50,000 was responsible for 1.5 million dollars in damage and as many as 100 injuries and deaths over the course of 3 days. President Lincoln ordered Federal Army combat troops to the scene to assist with restoration of order. Techniques utilized by the troops included the exchange of gunfire with the mob; multiple injuries and fatalities on both sides resulted.

Modern approaches to control of civil disturbances are more humanitarian. Rather than seriously injure or kill the victims, methods utilized are intended to deter or render temporary inability to fight or resist due to pain or discomfort. Nonchemical methods, such as water cannons, plastic or rubber bullets, and low friction polymers may be used. Chemical methods, however, are more commonly used. This discussion will focus on chemical riot control agents (RCAs.)

Modern use of chemical RCAs dates back to 1910–1914, just before World War I, when French police reportedly used ethylbromoacetate to dispel rioters. Subsequent battlefield use of RCAs continued during World War I including experimentation with likely 30 different compounds. Ongoing military experience with RCAs, including extensive use during the Vietnam War, has led to their emergence in law enforcement operations and an emphasis on safer and more effective agents with ease of dissemination. In addition, RCAs are now commonly used even by lay public individuals as a means of personal protection.

Examples of RCAs are chlorobenzylidene malonitrile (CS) and chloroacetophenone (CN.) CN is commercially available as Mace,™ a personal protection agent. CN use by the military has been replaced by use of the less toxic agent, CS. Oleoresin capsicum (OC, pepper spray) is another RCA. It is a naturally occurring substance found in peppers but it can also be produced synthetically.

RCAs are not recognized by the United States as official chemical warfare agents. Other agents excluded from official classification as chemical warfare agents include chemical herbicides and smoke and flame materials. Herbicides and smoke and flame materials are discussed in other sections of this book.

CHARACTERISTICS

RCAS, like incapacitating agents, are designed as non-lethal, less-than-lethal or, perhaps more accurately, less-lethal weapons. Rather than seriously injure or kill the victims, RCAs are intended to deter or impair performance due to discomfort. RCAs have a high safety ratio. Their specific mechanisms of action on the sensory nervous system include depletion of substance P and interference with sensory C fiber function. They produce irritation and pain of exposed mucous membranes and skin within seconds of contact. These peripheral effects of chemical RCAs are in contrast to the systemic effects of incapacitating agents. In addition, RCA effects are of shorter duration than incapacitating agent effects with symptoms often ending shortly after cessation of RCA exposure.

Under typical conditions, RCAs are liquids or solids. Fine particles or solutions of RCAs can be disseminated via dispersing devices such as spray cans or spray tanks or other munitions such as grenades or mortar shells. There are no field mechanisms for detection of RCAs in the environment.

CLINICAL MANIFESTATIONS

The clinical effects produced by RCA exposure depend on several factors including the specific agent as well as the concentration of the agent, duration of exposure, and route of exposure. With mild exposure, the effects are short and self-limited.

Irritation of the eyes, nose, mouth and skin are typical. The eyes are particularly sensitive to RCAs. Excessive lacrimation, blepharospasm and a sensation of conjunctival and corneal burning are common. If exposed individuals are able to keep their eyes open, conjunctival injection but baseline visual acuity are found on examination.

Erythema and a burning sensation occur with skin exposure. Dermal effects may be more severe in high temperature and/or high humidity conditions. A burning sensation, rhinorrhea and increased salivation are caused by nasal and oral contact.

Inhalational RCA exposure produces airway irritation and burning accompanied by bronchorrhea, cough, and a sensation of chest tightness. Individuals with asthma or allergies are more likely to have symptoms and more likely to have severe symptoms compared to those without asthma or allergies. Bronchospasm may occur. Individuals who are unable to leave the area of exposure quickly are also more likely to have pulmonary effects.

Nausea, vomiting and other nonspecific gastrointestinal symptoms may occur with inhalational RCA exposure. CS, CN or excessive OC ingestion are uncommon but are associated with diarrhea as well as gastrointestinal membrane irritation.

DIFFERENTIAL DIAGNOSIS

Exposure to blister agents including Lewisite and phosgene oxime (but not sulfur mustard) produces rapid onset of burning pain and irritation similar to RCAs. However, the effects of blister agents are more significant and do not subside with elimination of ongoing exposure. These factors, in addition to circumstances of the exposure event help differentiate blister agent exposure from RCA exposure.

TREATMENT

Effects of RCAs typically end shortly after cessation of exposure. The primary goals of treatment therefore are removal from the area of exposure, decontamination, and supportive measures. There are no specific laboratory tests to support or confirm the diagnosis of RCA exposure. There are no specific antidote therapies for RCAs.

Decontamination

Individuals exposed to RCAs should be moved to a well-ventilated, fresh air environment as soon as possible. Contaminated clothing should be removed and secured to avoid ongoing exposure to the victims as well as secondary exposure to health-care workers due to off-gassing. Those involved in decontamination should wear protective gear including impermeable gloves, gown, and mask. A full-face respirator with an organic vapor cartridge and high efficiency particulate filter may be needed in poorly ventilated areas.

Skin decontamination should be completed with soap and water. Cool water may help reduce irritation. Decontamination using any bleach solution should be avoided as the bleach reacts with some RCAs to produce a more toxic chemical. A slightly alkaline solution however, such as that made with sodium bicarbonate, will enhance RCA skin decontamination.

Ocular decontamination after RCA eye exposure should include irrigation with copious amounts of water or saline. Contact lenses and cosmetics should be removed. Topical ocular anesthetics may facilitate decontamination. Alkaline solution should not be used for ocular decontamination. Since many RCAs are solids dispersed as aerosols, it is possible for particles to be caught under the eyelid or otherwise trapped in the eyes. Ocular decontamination and evaluation should address this possibility.

Supportive Measures

Rather than seriously injure or kill the victims, RCAs are intended to deter or impair performance due to discomfort. Symptoms often end shortly after cessation of RCA exposure. However, conditions of some RCA exposures (e.g., high RCA concentration, prolonged exposure, individuals with certain underlying medical conditions) can lead to more prolonged or severe effects.

Administration of supplemental oxygen and airway support may be required for treatment of respiratory symptoms. Beta agonists, systemic steroids, and other bronchodilators are effective for RCA-related bronchospasm.

Ophthalmologic evaluation should be obtained for eye symptoms that persist more than 30–60 minutes after decontamination as corneal epithelial damage may be present. Skin erythema alone does not usually require treatment beyond decontamination. However, more extensive rashes, vesicles or bullae development should be treated with standard chemical burn management.

Suggested Reading

Hankin SM, Ramsay CN. Investigation of accidental secondary exposure to CS agent. *Clinical Toxicology* 2007. 45:409.

Olajos EJ, Stopford W, eds. *Riot Control Agents–Issues in Toxicology, Safety, and Health*, CRC Press, Boca Raton 2004.

United States Army FM 3-11/MCRP 3-3.7.2 *Flame, Riot Control Agents, and Herbicide Operations*. Washington DC 1996.

L

CHLORINE USE AS A WEAPON

Robin B. McFee

In early April, 2007 several chlorine gas suicide attacks occurred in Iraq, including a truck bomb explosion in Ramadi, releasing chlorine and killing at least 20 people. These attacks have resulted in numerous injuries and deaths, and raise the specter of greater use of chemical weapons by terrorist groups world wide. The first large scale use of chlorine occurred during World War I by German and British forces. The imagery captured in photographs often referred to as "the march of the blind" as hundreds of soldiers are lead hand to shoulder after being exposed to chlorine gas in trench warfare serves as a haunting reminder of the power chlorine poses as a weapon. In 1997 a serial bomber in Australia detonated several chlorine chemical bombs in Sydney. Not long after, chlorine was found in Japanese subway stations apparently to commemorate the Tokyo Sarin events. The use of combination weapons that include chemicals is not new. In the 1980's Saddam Hussein attacked Kurdish areas with chemical weapons during the Iran-Iraq war. More recently it has been reported that Hamas used pesticides, rat poison, cyanide and even infectious agents as part of their improvised explosive devices.

Increasingly appearing in the headlines are articles covering federal and state agencies attempting to enhance security and protective legislation for hazardous materials manufacturing, transportation and storage facilities. Of concern, security issues often get entangled in political and turf battles as Federal Authorities and State Regulators clash—often leaving local preparedness concerns dangling unsolved in the interim. Never the less, there remains a persistent threat of highly toxic industrial chemicals which can be adapted to become 'weapons of convenience"—such as chlorine. According to the General Accounting Office (GAO), Department of Transportation (DOT), and other federal agencies, among chemical accidents in the United States occurring between 1994–1998, chlorine was the number 2 leading toxicant associated with 518 incidents. Argonne National Labs listed chemicals it determined as posing the greatest risk: chlorine was number two on their list. From 1998–2001 the average annual rail car loads of chlorine was 32, 150. Most chemicals on a Ton-Mile basis are transported by truck (43%), railroad (29%) and pipeline (28%). Six toxic by inhalation (TIH) chemicals posed 90% greatest risk according to hazardous materials in transport safety (HMIS) data—of which chlorine represented over 57.5% of that risk! This became painfully evident in South Carolina, January 2005 when a railcar crash involving chlorine caused 9 deaths, 69 hospitalizations, 529 treat and release and the evacuation of 5453 people living within a 1 mile radius of the event. This was an accident; imagine the impact if such events were planned given the ubiquitous nature of chlorine in virtually every community, highway, and railway nationwide.

Combining suicide bombing with weapons of mass destruction including weapons of convenience such as hazardous materials, or even medical toxicants like blood thinners poses increasing difficulty for responders, ranging from greater on scene risk for providers and potentially delayed diagnosis or worsening clinical outcomes for patients due to added pathology resulting from the toxicant.

Chlorine is the prototypical moderately water soluble irritant gas—see chapter 34. Patients with irritant gas exposure are likely to require medical attention. However, it is likely that the majority of patients seeking care may be the worried well. Any patient exhibiting signs of airway compromise after irritant gas exposure should be considered in the immediate triage category. Likewise patients having severe shortness of breath should also be considered immediate. Patients exhibiting mild shortness of breath and no airway compromise should be considered delayed and those complaining only of mild mucous membrane symptoms should be considered minimal. Patients who are in respiratory arrest should be considered expectant unless an airway can be obtained immediately and the patient ventilated.

Saving lives and minimizing detrimental health risks are the most important challenges facing emergency medical providers and emergency medical services (EMS) arriving on scene of a mass-casualty event. Considering the possibility of chemical terrorism allows the early recognition of a toxicant being involved. Suspicion of a toxic exposure risk followed by reporting to emergency authorities should start implementation of predesigned and well practiced contingency plans. The two main dilemmas throughout the process are: (1) Is there a chemical toxicant involved in the scene?; and (2) Which clinical syndrome (toxidrome) is involved, i.e. which toxicant (s) ? Bear in mind that multiple toxicants can be used simultaneously, which can confound the diagnosis.

As recent events in Iraq underscore the risk of chlorine as a weapon, the preparedness community must recognize there has been an escalation in the use of improvised weapons that goes beyond simple explosives to include toxic gases. The reader is encouraged to obtain from the DOT the most up to date version of the Emergency Response Guide (ERG) "a guidebook for emergency responders during the initial phase of a hazardous materials incident." It is available from the US Government at http://hazmat.dot.gov/pubs/erg/gydebook.htm. The sections in *Emergency Toxicoterrorism* covering hazardous materials, chemical weapons and explosives provide an in depth discussion how to prepare for and respond to chlorine and other improvised mass casualty incidents.

M

INTENTIONAL USE OF RADIATION AS A POISON

Robin B. McFee and Jerrold B. Leikin

Of all the Weapons of Mass Destruction (WMD) agent categories—chemical, biological, radiologic, nuclear and explosive that exist as terrorist threats—radiological and nuclear agents represent the ultimate lethal mass casualty as well as psychological threat, yet remain the most under-emphasized and least prepared for among these weapons. Almost half of hospitals lack a plan for nuclear terrorism. Even when they exist, few have been practiced. This is not just a domestic problem. According to the British Medical Journal, while the United Kingdom has one of the longest established systems of public protection after radiation incidents, such plans are not well known by health professionals, making them thus less than ideally placed to advise or protect their patients. The daily use of radioactive materials within our communities is a persistent threat as is the risk associated with transporting radioactive waste across the country. The case report that follows contains critical information in this respect.

CASE REPORT—THE INTENTIONAL USE OF RADIATION AS A POISON—WHEN THE POSSIBILITY BECAME REALITY. LONDON, NOVEMBER 2006.

"The chilling reality is that nuclear materials and technologies are more accessible now than at any other time in history." Former Director—Central Intelligence, John Deutch.

This reality became all too evident in November 2006 when former KGB agent Alexander Litvinenko was murdered by poisoning with radioactive polonium—210 in the United Kingdom. He was not the only person exposed in this saga of espionage, murder and intrigue. At least 12 people tested positive for contamination as of January 2007.

Moreover, fears of polonium-210 contamination have led literally thousands of people to contact the National Health Services (NHS) Direct helpline, which was established in the aftermath of the assassination. The British initiated an investigation, which uncovered traces of ^{210}Po at a restaurant and bar, both in Mayfair—a posh section of London. Some traces had been found on British Airways (BA) aircraft; fortunately none of the 1700 passengers on BA flights or 250 patrons of the restaurants and bar have become sick or were contaminated. A former KGB agent and former Russian army officer both tested positive for ^{210}Po in Moscow; both have received medical treatment.

The lack of emphasis on radiation preparedness became evident when Mr. Litvinenko presented to a British hospital in early November. Clinicians initially believed his symptoms were due to radiation exposure but the detectors they used failed to support their concern. What the clinicians did not understand was that their equipment could not detect alpha emissions. As a result, physicians looked to other etiologies—taking valuable time in useless pursuit of exotic illnesses all the while the radiation continued to poison Mr. Litvinenko. Prior to his death, samples were sent for advanced testing which eventually determined the toxicant was an alpha emitter Polonium 210 [^{210}Po]. By then the likelihood of treatment success was nil; he died shortly thereafter.

Polonium was discovered and chemically separated by Marie and Pierre Curie; Madame Curie named it after her native Poland. There are over 20 isotopes of Po; ^{210}Po is the most stable form. ^{210}Po was an important component during the early development of nuclear weapons; it has a 138 day half life ($t^{1}/_{2}$) and is an alpha emitter. Po can be used in radioisotope thermoelectron generators (RTGs), producing electricity to operate satellites. However owing to the short t$^{1}/_{2}$ of Po, it is being replaced by plutonium, as a longer lived alpha emitter. In recent years obtaining quantities of polonium requires neutron bombardment of bismuth. As a poison, it is highly toxic; ^{210}Po is several orders of magnitude more toxic, on a milligram per milligram basis than hydrogen cyanide. It is estimated that one gram of ^{210}Po could kill 50 million and sicken another 50 million.

While alpha particles cannot travel great distances in air, personal protective equipment, intact skin and clothes are effective barriers; unlike other radioactive elements; ^{210}Po is relatively safe to transport. However, if inhaled, ingested or inserted into abraded skins or wounds, they can damage tissue. Within minutes the cells lining the gastrointestinal tract of Mr. Litvinenko would begin to die and slough off, causing nausea, pain and severe internal bleeding. ^{210}Po would also damage other systems. Unless early decorporative (chelation) treatment is initiated to lower the body burden, significant morbidity and ultimately death can be anticipated.

There are several treatment options available to treat the radiation poisoned patient, from colony stimulating factors to increase blood cell counts and decorporative antidotes (chelators), these must be initiated early. Currently available chelators—domestic and foreign include Dimercaptosuccinic acid (DMSA) [an oral agent], mono-N—(1-butyl)-meso-2,3-dimercapto succinamide (Mi-BDMA), N,N'-di (2-hydroxyethyl_ethylenediamine-N, N'-biscarbodithioate (HOEtTTC), N-(2,3-dimercaptopropyl) phthalamidic acid (DMPA) as well as British Anti-Lewisite (BAL)—oxytiol or oxathiol (Russian); each demonstrating varying degrees of capabilities in reducing body burden and toxicity. From a rapid deployment perspective, oral agents are ideal, especially if the toxicant is ingested. Under laboratory conditions HOEtTTC appears to be superior to other options. A Russian radiation expert asserted that oxytiol and other countermeasure based upon electrochemical characteristics of cyclic acetals and other similarly acting thiols, dithiols and azathiols could have conferred a survival benefit to Mr. Litvinenko. Not all chelators are available worldwide; guidance from on site radiation expertise, and REAC-TS are essential; rapid treatment is critical to survival.

Whether thought of as first responders or last preemptors, emergency medical professionals need to be able to identify rapidly a possible radiologic event, control potential public anxiety or outright panic and protect themselves with appropriate personal protective equipment. It is critical to understand the performance capabilities of equipment and detectors, realize that the initial diagnosis of radiation, like most WMD is clinical (Litvinenko clinicians' initial instincts were correct—it was radiation) and to obtain expertise immediately. Reach out to experts very early on– either poison control centers, REAC TS for radiation, CDC or WHO for biologicals—not hours or days later, as occurred in the Litvinenko case. Responding to a radiation incident requires advanced planning, training, and information sharing with agencies tasked with public protection.

Suggested Reading

Bogdan GM, Aposhian HV. N-(2,3-dimercaptopropyl)phthalamidic acid (DMPA) increases polonium—210 excretion. *Biol Met.* 1990;3(3-4):232–6.

Day M. Former spy's death causes public health alert. *BMJ.* 2006;333:1117.

Dirty bomb threat puts spotlight on unprepared Eds: do you have a plan? *ED Manag.* 2002;14:97–100.

Dyer O. More cases of polonium-210 contamination are uncovered in London. *BMJ.* 2007;334:65.

Gower-Thomas K, Lewis M, Shiralkar S, et al. Doctors knowledge of radiation exposure is deficient. *BMJ.* 2002;324:919.

International Atomic Energy Agency and World Health Organization. Follow up of delayed health consequences of acute accidental radiation exposure; lessons to be learned from their medical management. Viena IAEA 2002;129 (IAEA Tec Doc 1300).

Kaplan K, Maugh TH. Polonium-210's Quiet Trail of Death. Jan. 1, 2007. http://ww.mjwcorp.com/rad_dose_assessments_poloniumarticle.php. Last accessed 1/27/07.

Komarov S. Litvinenko Could Have Been Saved. *Moscow News.* http://english.mn.ru/english/issue.php?2006-48-11. Last accessed 1/27/07.

Leikin JB, McFee RB, Walter F, et al. A primer for nuclear terrorism. *Dis Mon.* 2003;49:485–516.

McFee RB, Leikin JB, Kiernan K. Preparing for an era of weapons of mass destruction (WMD)—Are we there yet? Why we should all be concerned, Part II. *Vet Human Tox.* 2004;46(6):347–51.

McFee RB, Leikin JB. Radiation terrorism: the unthinkable possibility, the ignored reality. *JEMS.* 2005 April:78–92.

Meineke V, van Beuningen D. Sohns TG, Fleidner TM. Medical management principles for radiation accidents. *Mil Med.* 2003;168:219–22.

Rencova J, Volf V, Jones MM, Singh PK. Mobilization and detoxification of polonium—210 in rats by 2,3 dimercaptosuccinic acid and its derivatives. *Int J Radiat Biol.* 2000 Oct;76(10):1409–15.

Rencova J, Volf V, Jones MM, et al. Bis-dithiocarbamates: effective chelating agents for mobilization of polonium-210 from rat. *Int J Radiat Biol.* 1995 Feb;67(2):229–34.

Roy RK, Bagaria P, Naik S, Kavala V, Patel BK. Chemoselectivities in acetalization, thioacetalization, oxathioacetalization and azathioacetalization. *J Phys Chem A Mol Spectrosc Kinet Environ Gen Theory.* 2006 Feb 16;110(6):2181–7.

Skomorkhova TN, Borisov VP. Eliminatory effect of oxathiol upon exposure to fumes of metallic mercury 203 Hg. *Gig Tr Prof Zabol.* 1982 Mar;(3):46–7.

Timins JK, Lipoti JA. Radiological terrorism. *NJ Med.* 2003;100:14–21.

Turai I, Veress K, Gunalp B, Souchkevitch G. Medical response to radiation incidents and radionuclear threats. *BMJ.* 2004;328:568–72.

INDEX

Note: Figures are indicated by *f* and tables by *t* following the page reference.